The M.D. Anderson Surgical Oncology Handbook

Third Edition

M.D. Anderson Cancer Center
Department of Surgical Oncology
Houston, Texas

Editors

Barry W. Feig, M.D.
David H. Berger, M.D.
George M. Fuhrman, M.D.

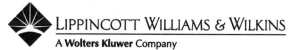

LIPPINCOTT WILLIAMS & WILKINS
A **Wolters Kluwer** Company

Philadelphia • Baltimore • New York • London
Buenos Aires • Hong Kong • Sydney • Tokyo

Acquisitions Editor: Brian Brown
Developmental Editor: Lloyd Unverferth
Production Editor: Emily Lerman
Manufacturing Manager: Ben Rivera
Cover Illustrator: Patricia Gast
Compositor: TechBooks
Printer: RR Donnelley—Crawfordsville

© 2003 by M.D. Anderson Cancer Center
Department of Surgical Oncology

Published by Lippincott Williams & Wilkins
530 Walnut Street
Philadelphia, PA 19106 USA
LWW.com

Printed in the USA

Library of Congress Cataloging-in-Publication Data

The M.D. Anderson surgical oncology handbook / M.D. Anderson Cancer Center, Department of Surgical Oncology, Houston, Texas; editors, Barry W. Feig, David H. Berger, George M. Fuhrman.— 3rd ed.
    p. ; cm.
  Includes bibliographical references and index.
  ISBN 0-7817-3307-3 (alk. paper)
  1. Cancer—Surgery—Handbooks, manuals, etc. I. Title: Surgical oncology handbook. II. Feig, Barry W., 1959– III. Berger, David H., 1959– IV. Fuhrman, George M. V. University of Texas M.D. Anderson Cancer Center. Dept. of Surgical Oncology.
  [DNLM: 1. Neoplasms—surgery—Handbooks. QZ 39 M111 2003]
RD651 .M17 2003
616.99′4059—dc21

                              2002030102

10 9 8 7 6 5 4 3 2 1

*To our wives (Barbara, Adrianne, and Laura)
and families, for their support, enthusiasm,
and patience through our many years of training
and continued long hours spent in the care
of patients with cancer.*

Contents

Contributing Authors

Eddie K. Abdalla, M.D., *Hepatobiliary Fellow, Service de Chirugie Digestive, Hôpital Beaujohn, Paris, France*

Paul M. Ahearne, M.D., *Surgical Oncologist, Asheville VA Medical Center, Asheville, North Carolina*

Syed A. Ahmad, M.D., *Assistant Professor, Department of Surgery, University of Cincinnati Medical Center, Cincinnati, Ohio*

Daniel Albo, M.D., Ph.D., *Assistant Professor, Department of Surgery, Division of Surgical Oncology, The Medical College of Georgia, Augusta, Georgia*

Carlton C. Barnett, Jr., M.D., *Assistant Professor, Department of Surgery, Medical University of South Carolina, Charleston, South Carolina*

David H. Berger, M.D., *Associate Professor, Department of Surgery, Baylor College of Medicine, Vice Chairman, Department of Surgery, Veterans Administration Hospital, Houston, Texas*

Diane C. Bodurka Bevers, M.D., *Assistant Professor, Department of Gynecologic Oncology, The University of Texas M.D. Anderson Cancer Center, Houston, Texas*

Michael W. Bevers, M.D., *Associate Professor, Department of Gynecologic Oncology, The University of Texas M.D. Anderson Cancer Center, Houston, Texas*

Richard J. Bold, M.D., *Assistant Professor, Department of Surgery, University of California, Davis, Davis, California; Assistant Professor, Department of Surgery, University of California Davis Cancer Center, Sacramento, California*

Michael Bouvet, M.D., *Associate Professor of Surgery, University of California San Diego, San Diego, California*

Judy L. Chase, Pharm.D., F.A.S.H.P., *Clinical Pharmacy Coordinator, Division of Pharmacy, The University of Texas M.D. Anderson Cancer Center, Houston, Texas*

Janice N. Cormier, M.D., *Assistant Professor, Department of Surgical Oncology, The University of Texas M.D. Anderson Cancer Center, Houston, Texas*

James C. Cusack, M.D., *Assistant Professor, Department of Surgery, Harvard Medical School; Assistant in Surgery, Division of Surgical Oncology, Massachusetts General Hospital, Boston, Massachusetts*

Colin P.N. Dinney, M.D., *Associate Professor, Department of Urology, The University of Texas M.D. Anderson Cancer Center, Houston, Texas*

Nestor F. Esnaola, M.D., M.P.H., *Clinical Fellow, Department of Surgical Oncology, The University of Texas M.D. Anderson Cancer Center, Houston, Texas*

Barry W. Feig, M.D., *Associate Professor, Department of Surgical Oncology, The University of Texas M.D. Anderson Cancer Center, Houston, Texas*

Wayne A.I. Frederick, M.D., *Surgical Oncology Fellow, Department of Surgical Oncology, The University of Texas M.D. Anderson Cancer Center, Houston, Texas*

George M. Fuhrman, M.D., *Department of Surgery, Ochsner Clinic, New Orleans, Louisiana*

Jeffrey E. Gershenwald, M.D., *Assistant Professor, Department of Surgical Oncology, The University of Texas M.D. Anderson Cancer Center, Houston, Texas*

Ana M. Grau, M.D., *Assistant Professor, Department of Surgery, Meharry Medical College / Vanderbilt University, Nashville, Tennessee*

Keith M. Heaton, M.D., *Clinical Instructor, Department of Surgery, University of Minnesota, Minneapolis, Minnesota; Department of Surgery, Park Nicolett Health Systems, St. Louis Park, Minnesota*

Samuel F. Huang, M.D., *Clinical Specialist, Department of Urology, The University of Texas M.D. Anderson Cancer Center, Houston, Texas*

Kelly K. Hunt, M.D., *Associate Professor, Department of Surgical Oncology and Chief, Surgical Breast Section, The University of Texas M.D. Anderson Cancer Center, Houston, Texas*

Rosa F. Hwang, M.D., *Surgical Oncology Fellow, Department of Surgical Oncology, The University of Texas M.D. Anderson Cancer Center, Houston, Texas*

Marina E. Jean, *Resident, Cincinnati University Hospital, Cincinnati, Ohio*

Steven D. Leach, M.D., *Associate Professor and Chief, Department of Surgical Oncology, The Johns Hopkins Hospital, Baltimore, Maryland*

Jeffrey E. Lee, M.D., *Associate Professor, Department of Surgical Oncology, The University of Texas M.D. Anderson Cancer Center, Houston, Texas*

Jeffrey T. Lenert, CDR, MC, USNR, *Assistant Professor, Department of Surgery, Uniform Services University of Health Sciences; Surgical Oncologist, Department of Surgery, National Naval Medical Center, Bethesda, Maryland*

Phillip B. Ley, M.D., *Clinical Assistant Professor, Department of Surgery, University of Mississippi Medical Center; Attending Surgical Oncologist, Mississippi Baptist Medical Center, Jackson, Mississippi*

Funda Meric, M.D., *Assistant Professor, Department of Surgical Oncology, The University of Texas M.D. Anderson Cancer Center, Houston, Texas*

Sarkis H. Meterissian, M.D.C.M., M.Sc., *Associate Professor of Surgery and Oncology, McGill University Health Center, Montreal, Quebec, Canada*

Gregory P. Midis, M.D., *Surgical Oncologist, Premier Surgical, Knoxville, Tennessee*

Kresimira M. Milas, M.D., *Assistant Professor, Department of General Surgery, Ohio State University; Staff, Department of General Surgery, The Cleveland Clinic Foundation, Cleveland, Ohio*

Alexander A. Parikh, M.D., *Surgical Oncology Fellow, Department of Surgical Oncology, The University of Texas M.D. Anderson Cancer Center, Houston, Texas*

David B. Pearlstone, M.D., *Palmetto State Surgical Associates; Department of Surgery, Greenville Hospital System, Greenville, South Carolina*

A. Scott Pearson, M.D., *Department of Surgery, Vanderbilt Medical Center North, Nashville, Tennessee*

James A. Reilly, Jr., M.D., *Clinical Associate Professor, Department of Surgery, University of Nebraska Medical Physicians' Clinic Surgery West, Omaha, Nebraska*

Emily K. Robinson, M.D., *Assistant Professor, Department of Surgery, The University of Texas—Houston; Assistant Professor, Department of Surgery, Lyndon B. Johnson Hospital, Houston, Texas*

Jorge A. Romaguera, M.D., *Associate Professor, Department of Lymphoma/Myeloma, The University of Texas M.D. Anderson Cancer Center, Houston, Texas*

Barry J. Roseman, M.D., *Chief, Department of Surgery, Blount Memorial Hospital, Maryville, Tennessee*

Dennis L. Rousseau, Jr., M.D., *Surgical Oncology Fellow, Department of Surgical Oncology, The University of Texas M.D. Anderson Cancer Center, Houston, Texas*

Carmen C. Solorzano, M.D.,   *Assistant Professor,
Department of Surgery, Division of Surgical Oncology,
University of Miami, Miami, Florida*

Francis R. Spitz, M.D.,   *Assistant Professor, Division of
Surgical Oncology, University of Pennsylvania Medical Center,
Philadelphia, Pennsylvania*

Charles A. Staley, M.D.,   *Holland W. Ware Professor,
Department of Surgery, Emory University School of Medicine,
Atlanta, Georgia*

Jeffrey J. Sussman, M.D.,   *Assistant Professor, Department
of Surgery, Division of Surgical Oncology, University of
Cincinnati Medical Center, Cincinnati, Ohio*

Stephen G. Swisher, M.D.,   *Associate Professor, Department
of Thoracic and Cardiovascular Surgery, The University of
Texas M.D. Anderson Cancer Center, Houston, Texas*

Hiroomi Tada, M.D., Ph.D.,   *Assistant Professor, Department
of Surgery, University of Massachusetts Medical School;
Department of Surgery, UMass Memorial Health Center,
Worcester, Massachusetts*

Kenneth K. Tanabe, M.D.,   *Associate Professor, Department
of Surgery, Harvard Medical School; Chief, Division of
Surgical Oncology, Massachusetts General Hospital, Boston,
Massachusetts*

Paula M. Termuhlen, M.D.,   *Assistant Professor and
Associate Program Director, Department of Surgery, Wright
State University, Kettering, Ohio*

Douglas S. Tyler, M.D.,   *Associate Professor of Surgery and
Chief of Surgical Oncology, Department of Surgery, Duke
University Medical Center, Durham, North Carolina*

Ara A. Vaporciyan, M.D.,   *Assistant Professor, Department
of Thoracic and Cardiovascular Surgery, The University of
Texas M.D. Anderson Cancer Center, Houston, Texas*

Thomas N. Wang, M.D., Ph.D.,   *Assistant Professor,
Department of Surgery, Medical College of Georgia,
Augusta, Georgia*

Jeffrey D. Wayne, M.D.,   *Assistant Professor, Northwestern
Medical Faculty Foundation, Chicago, Illinois*

Judith K. Wolf, M.D.,   *Associate Professor, Department of
Gynecologic Oncology, The University of Texas M.D. Anderson
Cancer Center, Houston, Texas*

Alan M. Yahanda, M.D.,   *Indiana Surgical Specialists, L.L.C.,
Fort Wayne, Indiana*

Foreword

What are the components of contemporary surgical care for the patient burdened by cancer? The answer to this question is to be found in the discipline of surgical oncology, which is arguably more of a cognitive than a technical surgical specialty. Other than several surgical procedures that are only infrequently performed outside of cancer centers (such as trisegmentectomy, hemipelvectomy, and regional pancreatectomy), the specialty of surgical oncology focuses on integrating surgery with other modalities of cancer treatment such as radiation oncology and systemic chemotherapy approaches. This integration is achieved via the crucible of prospective clinical trials that have emerged as the hallmark of clinical scientific research in oncology. To be effective, the surgical oncologist must understand the natural biology of solid tumors including their inception, proliferation, and dissemination. Such an understanding also implies a more than passing awareness of the underlying basic and translational science that is currently pushing the frontiers of our understanding in oncology further and further.

In addition to knowledge about the natural biology of tumors, the surgical oncologist must be intimately aware of the diagnostic options in the initial evaluation of the tumor and the staging systems by which a given tumor can be described, prognosis ascertained, and therapeutic algorithms accessed. The applicable treatments and their indications, risks, and benefits are critically important as part of this cognitive armamentarium. Moreover, in this era of managed care and cost containment, outcomes and research-defined surveillance strategies are also a part of the knowledge base of the practicing surgical oncologist.

The targeted audience of *The M.D. Anderson Surgical Oncology Handbook,* now in its third edition, includes surgeons-in-training as well as surgeons of all specialties who are in practice. Other healthcare professionals will no doubt find this concise manual to be of use as a ready reference as well, in much the same manner as the first and second editions of this book has been utilized by the oncology community at large. The credit for this current handbook belongs to the present and former surgical oncology fellows at The University of Texas M.D. Anderson Cancer Center. These efforts, coupled with your own interest, will help ensure that the solid tumor oncology patient receives the best possible multimodality care available. We hope that you find this handbook useful in this critical effort.

Raphael E. Pollock, M.D., Ph.D.
Head, Division of Surgery
Professor and Chairman
Department of Surgical Oncology
M.D. Anderson Cancer Center
Houston, Texas

Preface

The *M.D. Anderson Surgical Oncology Handbook* was written in an attempt to document the philosophies and practices of the Department of Surgical Oncology at the M.D. Anderson Cancer Center. The purpose of the book is to outline basic management approaches based on our experience with surgical oncology problems at M.D. Anderson. The book is intended to serve as a practical guide to the established surgical oncology principles for treating cancer as it involves each organ system in the body. This third edition has included new chapters on basic science and the treatment of tumors of unknown primary origin. In addition, updated information has been added on new treatments and procedures including lymphatic mapping for breast cancer and melanoma, hyperthermic isolated limb perfusion for extremity melanoma and sarcoma, cryosurgery for liver tumors, as well as many other new advances in treatment.

This book is written by current and former surgical oncology fellows at M.D. Anderson. Although the target audience for the first edition was the surgical house staff and surgical oncology trainees, we found that there was a significantly wider appeal for the book across multiple disciplines and at various levels of training and experience. We have, therefore, widened the scope of the third edition to reach this broader group. The authors represent various training programs, and they have spent at least two years at the M.D. Anderson Cancer Center studying only surgical oncology. The diversity of authors allows us to present the current opinions and practices of the M.D. Anderson Department of Surgical Oncology, along with other opinions and treatment options practiced in our far-ranging surgical training. Although there is no "senior" well-known name associated with the book, the authors represent 160 years of surgical training; we have not, however, become dogmatic and unyielding in our medical practices.

This handbook is not meant to encompass all aspects of oncology in minute detail. Rather, it is an attempt to address commonly encountered as well as controversial issues in surgical oncology. While other authors present their opinions and approaches as firmly established, we have tried to point out controversies and show alternative approaches to these problems besides our own.

We would like to thank the surgical staff at the M.D. Anderson Cancer Center for their assistance with the content of this book and for their devoted teaching in the hospital clinics, wards, and operating rooms. In addition, we would particularly like to thank the patients seen and treated at M.D. Anderson for their warmth and appreciation of our care, as well as for their patience and understanding of the learning process.

B.W.F.
D.H.B.
G.M.F.

NOTICE

Care has been taken to confirm the accuracy of the information presented and to describe generally accepted practices. However, the authors, editors, and publisher are not responsible for errors or omissions or for any consequences from application of the information in this book and make no warranty, expressed or implied, with respect to the contents of the publication.

The indications and dosages of all drugs in this book have been recommended in the medical literature and conform to the practices of the general medical community. The medications prescribed do not necessarily have specific approval by the Food and Drug Administration for use in the diseases and dosages for which they are recommended. The package insert for each drug should be consulted for use and dosage as approved by the FDA. Because standards for usage change, it is advisable to keep abreast of revised recommendations, particularly those concerning new drugs.

Noninvasive Breast Cancer

Funda Meric, Emily K. Robinson,
and Kelly K. Hunt

Noninvasive breast cancer comprises two separate entities: ductal carcinoma in situ (DCIS) and lobular carcinoma in situ (LCIS). DCIS is defined as a proliferation of epithelial cells confined to the mammary ducts. LCIS is defined as a proliferation of epithelial cells confined to the lobules, without demonstrable evidence of invasion through the basement membrane. Because they are noninvasive, DCIS and LCIS do not pose a risk of metastasis. The term "minimal breast cancer," once used to describe in situ lesions and invasive cancers less than 5 mm in diameter, has been abandoned because the prognoses and treatment strategies for these in situ lesions differ from those for invasive cancer.

DUCTAL CARCINOMA IN SITU

Epidemiology

Since the introduction of routine screening with mammography, the reported incidence of DCIS has increased threefold from that observed in older series, when DCIS remained undetected until it became palpable. In the United States, the incidence is now 10 to 20 per 100,000 woman-years. The reported prevalence of DCIS has increased as the quality and sensitivity of mammography have improved, and DCIS currently accounts for 20% to 44% of all new screen-detected breast neoplasms.

The median age reported for patients with DCIS ranges from 47 to 63 years, which is similar to that reported for patients with invasive carcinoma. Some studies have noted a trend toward a lower median age of patients whose DCIS was detected during screening examinations. The frequency of a family history of breast cancer among first-degree relatives of patients with DCIS (i.e., 10%–35%) is the same as that reported for women with invasive breast malignancies.

Pathology

DCIS is thought to arise from ductal epithelium in the region of the terminal lobular-ductal unit and probably represents one stage in the continuum from atypical ductal hyperplasia to invasive carcinoma. DCIS comprises a heterogeneous group of lesions with variable histologic architecture, cellular characteristics, and clinical behavior. Malignant cells proliferate to obliterate the ductal lumen, and there may be an associated inflammatory reaction, stromal response, or lymphoid infiltration surrounding the duct.

DCIS is generally classified as one of five subtypes—comedo, solid, cribriform, micropapillary, and papillary—based on differences in the architectural pattern of the cancer cells and nuclear features. Cribriform, comedo, and micropapillary are the most common subtypes, although two or more patterns coexist in up to 50% of cases.

The identification of factors indicative of aggressive biology has led to a fundamental change in the way noninvasive breast cancer is classified. The old classification system, a strictly descriptive histologic nomenclature, has been abandoned in favor of a system that incorporates these prognostic factors and stratifies lesions based on their likelihood of recurrence. Lagios et al. (1989) identified high nuclear grade and comedo necrosis as factors predictive of local recurrence. At 8 years, patients with high nuclear grade and comedo necrosis had a 20% local recurrence rate after breast conservation surgery and irradiation, compared with 5% for patients without necrosis and with a lower nuclear grade. Subsequently, Silverstein et al. (1995) developed the Van Nuys classification in which three groups were distinguished based on the presence or absence of high nuclear grade and comedo-type necrosis (1) non-high-grade DCIS without comedo-type necrosis, (2) non–high-grade DCIS with comedo-type necrosis, and (3) high-grade DCIS with or without comedo-type necrosis. Silverstein et al. found 31 cases of local recurrence among 238 patients treated with breast-conserving surgery; the local recurrence rate was 3.8% in group 1, 11.1% in group 2, and 26.5% in group 3. The 8-year actuarial disease-free survival rates were 93% for group 1, 84% for group 2, and 61% for group 3.

Multifocality

Multifocal DCIS is generally defined as DCIS having two or more foci separated by 5 mm in the same breast quadrant. However, some investigators believe that multifocal disease may in fact represent intraductal spread from a single focus of DCIS. By careful serial subsectioning, Holland et al. (1990) demonstrated that multifocal lesions that appeared to be separate using traditional pathologic techniques actually originated from the same focus in 81 of 82 mastectomy specimens.

Multicentricity

Multicentric DCIS is defined as DCIS having a separate focus outside the index quadrant. The reported incidence of multicentricity may depend on the extent of the pathologic review and therefore varies from 18% to 60% but is more likely around 30% to 40%. Because mammary lobules are not constrained by the artificially imposed quadrant segregations, cursory pathologic examination may incorrectly interpret contiguous intraductal spread as multicentricity. Approximately 96% of all local recurrences after treatment for DCIS occur in the same quadrant as the index lesion, implicating residual untreated disease rather than multicentricity, and raising questions about the importance of multicentricity. The incidence of detection of DCIS is higher in autopsy studies than in the general population, suggesting that not all DCIS lesions become clinically significant.

Microinvasion

The American Joint Commission on Cancer (AJCC) staging system (1997) defines microinvasion as invasion by breast cancer through the basement membrane at one or more foci, none of which exceeds a depth of 1 mm. A breast cancer with microinvasion is classified as a "T1mic" tumor, whereas DCIS is classified as "T0". Microinvasion upstages the cancer from stage 0 to stage 1 in the AJCC staging system.

The incidence of microinvasion in DCIS varies according to the size and extent of the index lesion. Lagios et al. (1989) reported a 2% incidence of microinvasion in patients with DCIS measuring less than 25 mm in diameter, compared with a 29% incidence of microinvasion in index lesions larger than 26 mm. Some investigators have questioned whether it is useful to distinguish pure DCIS from DCIS with microinvasion. In a series by Wong et al. (1990), 41 patients presenting with DCIS and microinvasion had axillary nodal dissection as part of their treatment. There were no cases of nodal metastases, and none of the patients had recurrence of their disease, with a median follow-up of 37 months. When patients with DCIS were retrospectively compared with patients with DCIS with microinvasion, Silverstein et al. (1993) found no difference in axillary node positivity, disease-free survival, or overall survival and concluded that therapy for both forms of DCIS should be based on tumor size, margin status, ability to observe the patient with mammography, and the patient's desires and needs. Mirza et al. (2000) recently reported the long-term results of breast-conserving therapy in DCIS and early stage (T1) breast cancer: 20-year disease-specific survival rates were better among patients with DCIS than among patients with DCIS with microinvasion or T1 invasive tumors. Patients with microinvasion and those with T1 tumors had similar survival rates. This study suggests that lesions with microinvasion require a therapeutic approach similar to that for invasive cancer. However, the management of microinvasion remains controversial and further study is needed to investigate the biology of microinvasion.

Diagnosis

Clinical Presentation

Before the advent of routine mammography, most patients with DCIS presented with a palpable mass, nipple discharge, or Paget's disease of the nipple. Occasionally, DCIS was an incidental finding in an otherwise benign biopsy specimen. The palpable lesions were large, and up to 25% demonstrated associated foci of invasive disease. Now that screening mammography is more prevalent, most cases of DCIS are diagnosed with the use of mammography alone.

Mammographic Features

Microcalcifications are the most common manifestation of DCIS found on mammography. DCIS accounts for 80% of all breast carcinomas presenting with calcifications. Any interval change from a previous mammogram is associated with malignancy in 15% to 20% of cases and most often indicates in situ disease. Holland et al. (1990) described two different classes of microcalcifications: (1) linear-branching type microcalcifications which are associated with high–nuclear-grade, comedo-type lesions; and

(2) fine, granular calcifications, which are associated with micropapillary or cribriform lesions of lower nuclear grade that do not show necrosis. These investigators demonstrated that the mammographic findings significantly underestimated the pathologic extent of disease, particularly among cases of micropapillary tumors. Lesions were more than 2 cm larger by histologic examination than by mammographic estimate in 44% of cases of micropapillary lesions, compared with only 12% of cases of the pure comedo subtype. However, when magnification views were used in the mammographic examination, the extent of disease was underestimated in only 14% of cases of micropapillary tumors.

Diagnostic Biopsy

Stereotactic core-needle or vacuum-assisted biopsy is the preferred method for diagnosing DCIS. Calcifications that appear faintly on mammograms or that are deep in the breast and close to the chest wall may be difficult to target with stereotactic biopsy. In addition, it may be impossible to use stereotactic biopsy in patients above the weight limit of the stereotactic system (about 135 kg [297 lb]), and in patients with small breasts. Patients who cannot remain prone or who cannot cooperate for the duration of the procedure are also not candidates for stereotactic biopsy. Bleeding disorders and the concomitant use of anticoagulants are relative contraindications. Biopsy specimens should be radiographed to document the sampling of suspicious microcalcifications. Care should be taken not to completely excise all microcalcifications without placing a metallic marker to guide future surgical excision.

Because stereotactic core-needle and vacuum-assisted biopsy specimens represent only a sample of an abnormality observed on mammography, the results are subject to sampling error. Invasive carcinoma is found on excisional biopsy in 20% of patients in whom DCIS was diagnosed using a stereotactic core-needle biopsy. If the core-needle biopsy results disagree with the findings of imaging studies, an excisional biopsy should be performed to confirm the diagnosis. After diagnosis using stereotactic core-needle biopsy, 50% of patients with atypical ductal hyperplasia and 20% of patients with radial scar are found to have a coexistent carcinoma near the site of the biopsy. Therefore, when the final pathologic studies from core-needle biopsy indicate either of these diagnoses, this should be followed by surgical excisional biopsy.

Patients who are not candidates for stereotactic biopsy or who have stereotactic biopsy results that are inconclusive or that disagree with the mammographic findings should undergo excisional biopsy. This technique is performed with the assistance of preoperative needle localization of the mammographic abnormality. The excisional biopsy should aim to perform a margin-negative resection that can serve as a definitive surgery. The margins should be at least 1 cm. This recommendation is based on the data provided by Holland et al. (1990), which demonstrated that up to 44% of lesions were found to extend more than 2 cm further on histologic examination than was estimated by mammography.

Specimen radiography is essential to confirm the removal of all microcalcifications. After whole-specimen radiography, the specimen should be inked and then serially sectioned for repeat radiographic examination and pathologic examination to evaluate margin status and extent of disease. If the microcalcifications extend to the cut edge of the specimen, further excision is performed at the same setting. The boundary of the lumpectomy cavity is marked with radio-opaque clips to aid in the planning of postoperative radiotherapy and in mammographic follow-up. If the margins are deemed inadequate on pathologic analysis, reexcision is indicated.

Treatment

The diagnosis of DCIS is followed by a mastectomy or breast-conserving surgery (also referred to as segmental mastectomy, lumpectomy, or wide local excision) with needle localization. Most patients receive postoperative radiation therapy to improve local control. Postoperative hormonal therapy with tamoxifen can also be considered.

Mastectomy Versus Breast-Conserving Therapy

Traditionally, mastectomy has been the preferred treatment of DCIS. However, as breast-conserving techniques for invasive disease have been shown to be effective local therapy, the practice of treating a noninvasive condition with a surgery more radical than that used to treat its invasive counterpart has been questioned. The rationale for performing total mastectomy in patients with DCIS is based on the high incidences of multifocality and multicentricity as well as the risk of occult invasion associated with the disease. Thus, mastectomy remains the standard with which other proposed therapeutic modalities should be compared. A retrospective review by Balch et al. (1993) documented a local relapse rate of 3.1% and a mortality rate of 2.3% after mastectomy for DCIS. The cancer-related mortality following mastectomy for DCIS was 1.7% in a series reported by Fowble (1989) and ranged from 0% to 8% in a review by Vezeridis and Bland (1994).

In one of the largest studies comparing breast-conserving therapy with mastectomy, Silverstein and colleagues (1992) examined 227 cases of DCIS without microinvasion. In this nonrandomized study, patients with tumors smaller than 4 cm with microscopically clear margins were treated with breast-conserving surgery and radiation therapy, whereas patients with tumors larger than 4 cm or with positive margins were treated with mastectomy. The rate of disease-free survival at 7 years was 98% in the mastectomy group compared with 84% in the breast-conserving surgery group ($p = 0.038$), with no difference in overall survival rates. The recent National Surgical Adjuvant Breast and Bowel Project (NSABP) B-17 trial update demonstrated that patients with localized DCIS were successfully treated with breast conservation surgery and postoperative radiation therapy. The rate of ipsilateral breast tumors was 1.9 per 100 patients per year; 30 of the 47 ipsilateral breast tumors were noninvasive breast cancer, and the other 17 were invasive.

At The University of Texas M.D. Anderson Cancer Center, the choice of surgical therapy is based on several factors, including tumor size and grade, margin width, mammographic appearance, and patient preference. Most patients with DCIS are candidates for breast-conserving therapy. Mastectomy is indicated in patients with diffuse, malignant-appearing calcifications in the breast and persistent positive margins after attempts at surgical excision. Although tumor size is not an absolute indication for mastectomy, mastectomy is often preferred for patients with large (>3 cm in diameter), high-grade DCIS. There are few data on the efficacy of breast-conserving surgery for DCIS with index lesions greater than 4 cm in diameter.

The benefits and risks of breast-conserving surgery and mastectomy should be discussed in detail with each patient. Breast-conserving therapy is associated with a higher local recurrence rate, including a risk of invasive breast cancer. However, for most patients, the choice of local treatment does not influence overall survival. Mastectomy may be a better choice when a patient's anxiety over the possibility of recurrence outweighs the impact a mastectomy would have on her quality of life. Immediate breast reconstruction should be considered for all patients who require or elect mastectomy.

Axillary Node Staging

Because DCIS is a noninvasive disease, lymph node involvement is not expected; thus, theoretically the role for axillary lymph node dissection is limited. In cases of larger tumors or extensive microcalcifications, a focus of invasion can be missed due to pathologic sampling error. Patients who are treated with mastectomy for large high-grade DCIS are often staged with a dissection of low-level axillary nodes. Patients with large high-grade tumors who are undergoing breast-conserving surgery are potential candidates for intraoperative lymphatic mapping and sentinel lymph node biopsy (discussed in detail in Chapter 2). Diagnosis of DCIS using stereotactic core-needle biopsy is associated with a 20% rate of concomitant invasive cancer, further enhancing the importance of sentinel lymph node biopsy at the time of mastectomy for large, high-grade lesions. In a study by Cox et al. (1998), the combination of hematoxylin-eosin staining and immunohistochemistry showed that 6% of patients with newly diagnosed DCIS had metastatic disease in the sentinel nodes. Kauber-DeMore et al. (2000) found that sentinel lymph nodes were positive for cancer among 12% of patients with DCIS considered to be at high risk for invasion and among 10% of patients who had DCIS with microinvasion.

Radiation Therapy

Most patients with DCIS who undergo breast-conserving surgery receive postoperative radiation therapy. The efficacy of radiation therapy for local control of DCIS treated with breast conservation surgery was demonstrated with the NSABP B-17 trial. Women with localized DCIS were randomized to breast conservation surgery or breast conservation surgery plus radiation therapy after margin-negative resections. At a follow-up time of

8 years, radiation therapy was associated with a reduction in the incidence of noninvasive ipsilateral breast tumors from 13.4% to 8.2% and with a reduction in the incidence of ipsilateral invasive breast tumors from 13.4% to 3.9%.

The overall benefit of radiation therapy for patients with DCIS was also confirmed with the European Organization for Research and Treatment of Cancer (EORTC) Trial (Julien et al., 2001). Women with DCIS were randomized to breast conservation surgery or breast conservation surgery plus radiation therapy. At a follow-up time of 4.25 years, radiation therapy was associated with a reduction in the incidence of noninvasive ipsilateral breast tumors from 8% to 5% and with a reduction in the incidence of ipsilateral invasive breast tumors from 8% to 4%.

It has recently been suggested that breast-conserving surgery alone (i.e., without radiation therapy) may be sufficient in a select subgroup of patients with DCIS. Initial data that supported the use of breast-conserving surgery alone in the treatment of DCIS came from a study by Lagios et al. (1989) in which 79 patients with mammographically detected DCIS were treated with margin-negative excision alone. After a follow-up of 124 months, local recurrence was 16% overall—33% for the subgroup of patients with high-grade lesions and comedo necrosis versus only 2% for the patients with low- or intermediate-grade lesions.

Subsequently, Silverstein et al. (1996) developed the Van Nuys Prognostic Index (VNPI) by combining three statistically significant predictors of local recurrence: tumor size, margin width, and pathologic classification. Numerical values ranging from 1 (best prognosis) to 3 (worst prognosis) are assigned for each of the three predictors. A size score of 1 is given to small tumors ($\leq$15 mm), 2 to intermediate tumors (16–40 mm), and 3 to large tumors ($\geq$41 mm). Margin width is assigned a score of 1 if 10 mm or greater, 2 if 1 to 9 mm, and 3 if less than 1 mm. The pathologic classification is 1 for non-high-grade DCIS without necrosis, 2 for non-high-grade DCIS with necrosis, and 3 for high-grade DCIS with or without necrosis. The sum of these results is the VNPI score, with 3 being the lowest possible score and 9 the highest possible score. The VNPI scores of 333 patients with DCIS treated with breast-conserving therapy were retrospectively determined and the outcomes were compared using local recurrence as the end point. Among patients with VNPI scores of 3 or 4, the addition of radiation therapy did not appear to confer an advantage over excision alone for local recurrence-free survival. In contrast, for patients with VNPI scores of 5, 6, or 7, the local recurrence-free survival rate was 17% higher among those treated with radiation therapy and excision than among those who received excision alone (85% vs. 68%, $p = 0.017$). Although patients with VNPI scores of 8 or 9 showed the greatest benefit with the addition of radiation therapy, local recurrence rates still exceeded 60% in 8 years, regardless of irradiation. Silverstein et al. (1995) proposed a treatment schema based on the VNPI score: wide local excision alone was recommended for patients with VPNI scores of 3 or 4; excision plus radiotherapy for scores of 5, 6, or 7; and mastectomy for those with scores of 8 or 9. The VNPI may become a useful adjunct in therapeutic decision making; however, its validity has yet to be tested prospectively.

The role of postoperative radiation therapy for patients with margin-negative resections was recently investigated by Silverstein et al. (1999). This retrospective study evaluated the outcomes of 469 patients with DCIS treated with breast-conserving surgery with or without radiation therapy. Postoperative radiation therapy was not found to lower the local recurrence rate among patients with margins of excision that were at least 10 mm. In contrast, even on reanalysis of the NSABP B-17 data, all patient cohorts benefited from radiation therapy, regardless of clinical or mammographic tumor characteristics.

At M.D. Anderson Cancer Center, breast-conserving surgery alone (without radiation therapy) is usually considered for selected patients with small (<1 cm in diameter), low-grade lesions that have been excised with margins of at least 5 mm and who can be observed diligently for recurrence.

Hormonal Therapy

Tamoxifen may be beneficial as adjuvant therapy for DCIS. In the NSABP B-24 trial, 20 mg/day tamoxifen was given for 5 years following breast-conserving therapy in 1,804 women with DCIS, including those in whom resected sample margins were positive for cancer. Women who received tamoxifen had fewer breast-cancer events at 5 years follow-up than did the placebo group (8.2% vs. 13.4%). Among those treated with tamoxifen, the rate of ipsilateral invasive breast cancer was 2.1% at 5 years compared with 4.2% in the control group. Tamoxifen also decreased the incidence of contralateral breast neoplasms (invasive and noninvasive) to 0.4% per year compared with 0.8% per year among the control group. The benefit of tamoxifen therapy also extended to patients with positive margins or margins of unknown status.

The decision of whether to use adjuvant tamoxifen for DCIS should be made on an individual basis. The use of tamoxifen has been associated with vasomotor symptoms, deep venous thrombosis, pulmonary emboli, and cataracts. The risk of endometrial cancer among patients treated with the drug is two to seven times the norm. Tamoxifen may be associated with increased rates of stroke and benign ovarian cysts. Therefore, the effects of tamoxifen to reduce ipsilateral breast tumors and to prevent contralateral breast disease should be weighed against the risk of tamoxifen use in each patient.

Predictors of Local Relapse

There are several features of DCIS that are associated with a less favorable clinical course. Traditional pathologic variables, such as large tumor size (>3 cm), high nuclear grade, comedo-type necrosis, and involved margins of excision, are associated with a greater risk of local recurrence, as has been previously discussed. Involved margins of resection constitute the most important independent prognostic variable for predicting local relapse. As previously described, the VNPI combines three significant predictors of local recurrence: tumor size, margin width, and pathologic classification. Other clinical parameters associated with a higher risk of local recurrence are young age (less than 50 years) and a positive family history of breast cancer; however, these factors are not considered contraindications for breast-conserving therapy. Molecular markers, such as overexpression of HER-2/*neu*, nm23, heat shock protein, and metallothionein; low expression of p21Waf1 and Bcl2; and DNA aneuploidy have been associated with high-grade comedo lesions, but their importance as independent prognostic variables in DCIS has not been clarified.

Treatment and Outcome of Local Relapse

In cases of local recurrence in a patient who underwent breast-conserving surgery without radiation therapy, reexcision with negative margins and postoperative radiation therapy constitute a treatment option. For patients who have recurrent breast cancer after receiving breast-conserving surgery and radiation therapy, a mastectomy is usually the preferred treatment. If the recurrent tumor is invasive, staging of axillary nodes is performed with lymphatic mapping and sentinel lymph node biopsy or with axillary lymph node dissection.

In general, the overall survival rate of patients with DCIS is excellent. In a recent series, Weng et al. (2000) reported an overall survival rate of 97% at 8 years. The local recurrence rates in this series were 25% for patients with DCIS treated with breast-conserving surgery only, 13% for those treated with breast-conserving surgery and radiation therapy, and 4% for those treated with mastectomy. About 50% of patients with recurrences after DCIS have invasive tumors. Silverstein et al. (1998) found that among patients with invasive recurrent disease, the 8-year disease-specific mortality rate is 14.4% and the distant-disease probability 27.1%. Although most patients with recurrent disease after DCIS do survive, an invasive recurrence is a serious event. Patients with DCIS should receive long-term follow-up both for recurrent disease and for the development of a new ipsilateral or contralateral primary tumors.

Surveillance

Following breast-conserving surgery, a postsurgical mammogram should be obtained to screen for residual microcalcifications. In addition, a mammogram should be obtained 4 to 6 months after the completion of radiation therapy to establish a new baseline. Follow-up of patients after breast-conserving surgery with or without radiation therapy should include a twice-yearly physical examination and annual mammography for the first 5 years, with an annual physical examination and mammogram thereafter. Both patients treated with breast-conserving therapy and patients treated with mastectomy should be monitored closely for new primary cancers in the contralateral breast. The risk that a new primary cancer will develop in the contralateral breast after treatment for DCIS is two to five times the risk of the development of a first primary breast cancer and is approximately the same as the risk of the development of a contralateral new primary cancer after invasive cancer.

LOBULAR CARCINOMA IN SITU

LCIS was first described as a distinct pathologic entity in 1941. During the era that followed, the treatment for LCIS was the same as that for invasive carcinoma—radical mastectomy. Haagensen is credited with altering the treatment philosophy for LCIS. In his review of 211 cases, Haagensen et al. (1978) noted a 17% incidence of subsequent invasive carcinomas among women in whom disease was diagnosed as LCIS and who were treated by observation alone (without surgery). The risk of developing a subsequent carcinoma was equal for both breasts, and only six patients died of breast cancer. Haagensen concluded that close observation for LCIS allowed for early detection of subsequent malignancy, with associated high cure rates. Haagensen's rationale for observation as a treatment philosophy for LCIS was based on his view that patients with LCIS were at increased risk for invasive breast cancer but that LCIS itself did not progress into a malignancy.

Epidemiology

The incidence of LCIS is difficult to estimate because the diagnosis is most often made following a purely incidental finding. LCIS is not detectable by palpation, gross pathologic examination, or mammography. The incidence of LCIS has increased dramatically in recent years as a result of the increased use of screening mammography and therefore increased numbers of biopsies performed for mammographically detected breast abnormalities. In a review of breast biopsies for mammographic abnormalities, LCIS was found in 1.3% of biopsy specimens.

LCIS occurs most commonly in premenopausal women. In Haagensen's series (1978), 90% of the patients were premenopausal, and most studies have reported mean ages between 45 and 50 years. Estrogens are hypothesized to play an important role in the pathogenesis of LCIS. Postmenopausal regression of LCIS has been noted and may explain the decreased incidence in the elderly. The theory that LCIS represents a marker of increased risk for invasive breast carcinoma is supported by the fact that the mean age at diagnosis is 10 to 15 years less than that for invasive cancer.

When the diagnosis of LCIS is established, there is a 0% to 6% chance that the patient has a synchronous invasive breast lesion. It is estimated that the risk of developing a subsequent invasive lesion is 0.5% per year of follow-up. The invasive malignancies in women with LCIS are ductal carcinomas in 60% to 70% of cases. This finding supports the theory that LCIS does not differentiate into invasive carcinoma; if this were the case, invasive lobular carcinoma should develop in a larger percentage of patients. Thus, LCIS is not considered a premalignant lesion but rather a marker that identifies women at high risk for subsequent development of breast cancer. More recently it has been suggested that LCIS may be morphologically and biologically more heterogenous. It has been proposed that although classic LCIS is not associated with invasive lobular carcinoma, cases of larger, more pleomorphic LCIS lesions may represent a clonal proliferation of cells that may progress to invasive lobular carcinoma. Further study of the biology of LCIS is needed.

Pathology

LCIS is characterized by an intraepithelial proliferation of the terminal lobular-ductal unit. The cells are slightly larger and paler than those that line the normal acini, but the lobular architecture remains intact. The cells have a homogeneous morphology and do not display prominent chromatin. The cytoplasm-to-nucleus ratio is normal, with infrequent mitoses and no necrosis. The proliferating cells do not penetrate the basement membrane.

The diagnosis of LCIS involves the differentiation of LCIS from other forms of benign disease and from invasive lesions. In the absence of complete replacement of the lobular unit, "atypical lobular hyperplasia" is the designated pathologic term. Papillomatosis in the terminal ducts may resemble LCIS but lacks the characteristic involvement of the acini. DCIS may extend retrograde into the acini but has a more characteristic anaplastic cell morphology. LCIS is contained within the basement membrane and is thus distinguished from invasive lobular carcinoma.

Numerous studies have documented that LCIS is multifocal and multicentric. If diligently sought, foci can be found elsewhere in the breast in almost all cases. In addition, LCIS is identified in the contralateral breast in 50% to 90% of cases. Thus, the presence of LCIS reflects a phenotypic manifestation of a generalized abnormality present throughout both breasts. As a result, the treatment of LCIS should be directed not only at the index lesion but at both breasts.

Diagnosis

Clinical Presentation

Because LCIS is not detectable by physical examination or mammography, this disease is most commonly diagnosed as an incidental finding in a breast biopsy specimen. Therefore, the clinical presentation of patients with LCIS is similar to that of patients requiring breast biopsy for fibroadenoma, benign ductal disease, DCIS, and invasive breast cancer.

Treatment

Most patients with LCIS can be treated with close clinical observation alone, as recommended by Haagensen et al. (1978). There are no data suggesting a need for reexcision to achieve negative margins for LCIS. Further study of the various LCIS subtypes is needed to determine if patients with some subtypes would indeed benefit from reexcision. Contralateral mirror-image breast biopsy, a procedure advocated for LCIS in the past, has fallen out of favor because a negative mirror-image biopsy does not eliminate the need for close observation of the remaining breast tissue in the contralateral breast.

The second treatment option for patients with LCIS is chemoprevention with tamoxifen. In the NSABP breast cancer prevention trial P-1, the incidence of breast cancer in the subset of women with LCIS who received tamoxifen was 56% lower than that in patients with LCIS who received observation alone. The annual hazard rate for invasive cancer was 5.69 per 1,000 women who received tamoxifen compared with 12.99 per 1,000 women who did not. Postmenopausal women with LCIS may be eligible to be randomized between tamoxifen and raloxifene in the ongoing NSABP P-2 trial (STAR).

A third therapeutic option to treat patients with LCIS is bilateral prophylactic mastectomy. This approach is usually reserved for patients who have other additional risk factors or who experience extreme anxiety over the observation or chemoprevention options. Because LCIS poses no risk of regional metastasis, axillary node dissection is not required. Immediate breast reconstruction should be offered for patients undergoing prophylactic mastectomy for LCIS.

RECOMMENDED READING

Balch CM, Singletary SE, Bland KI. Clinical decision-making in early breast cancer. *Ann Surg* 1993;217:207.

Cox CE, Pendas S, Cox JM, et al. Guidelines for sentinel node biopsy and lymphatic mapping of patients with breast cancer. *Ann Surg* 1998;227:645.

Fleming ID, Cooper JS, Henson DE. *AJCC Cancer Staging. American Joint Commission on Cancer.* Philadelphia: Lippincott-Raven, 1997.

Fisher B, Costantino J, Redmond C, et al. Lumpectomy compared with lumpectomy and radiation therapy for the treatment of intraductal breast carcinoma. *N Engl J Med* 1993;328:1581.

Fisher ER, Costantino J, Fisher B, et al. Pathological findings from the National Surgical Adjuvant Breast Project (NSABP) Protocol B-17. *Cancer* 1995;75:1310.

Fisher B, Dignam J, Wolmark N, et al. Tamoxifen in treatment of intraductal breast cancer: National Surgical Adjuvant Breast and Bowel Project B-24 randomised controlled trial. *Lancet* 1999; 353:1993.

Fowble B. Intraductal noninvasive breast cancer: a comparison of three local treatments. *Oncology* 1989;3:51.

Frykberg ER, Bland KI. Overview of the biology and management of ductal carcinoma in situ of the breast. *Cancer* 1994;74:350.

Goedde TA, Frykberg ER, Crump JM, et al. The impact of mammography on breast biopsy *Am Surg* 1992;58:661.

Haagensen CA, Lome N, Lattes R, et al. Lobular neoplasia (so-called lobular carcinoma in situ) of the breast. *Cancer* 1978;42:757.

Holland R, Hendricks JH, Verbeek AL, et al. Extent, distribution, and mammographic/histological correlations of breast ductal carcinoma in situ. *Lancet* 1990;335:519.

Julian J-P, Bijker N, Fentiman IS, et al. Radiotherapy in breast-conserving treatment for ductal carcinoma in situ: first results of the EORTC randomised phase III trial 10853. *Lancet* 2001;355:528.

Klauber-DeMore N, Tan LK, Liberman L, et al. Sentinel lymph node biopsy: is it indicated in patients with high-risk ductal carcinoma-in-situ and ductal carcinoma-in-situ with microinvasion? *Ann Surg Oncol* 2000;2:636.

Lagios MD, Margolin FR, Westdahl PR, et al. Mammographically detected duct carcinoma in situ. *Cancer* 1989;63:618.

Mirza NQ, Vlastos G, Meric F, et al. Ductal carcinoma-in-situ: long-term results of breast-conserving therapy. *Ann Surg Oncol* 2000;7:656.

Nielson M, Thomsen JL, Primdahl U, et al. Breast cancer and atypia among young and middle-aged women: a study of 110 medicolegal autopsies. *Br J Cancer* 1987;56:814.

Page DL, Dupont WD, Rogers LW, et al. Continued local recurrence of carcinoma 15–25 years after a diagnosis of low grade ductal carcinoma in situ of the breast treated only by biopsy. *Cancer* 1995;76:1197.

Schwartz GF, Finkel GC, Garcia JC, et al. Subclinical ductal carcinoma in situ of the breast. *Cancer* 1992;70:2468.

Silverstein MJ, Waisman JR, Gierson ED, et al. Intraductal breast carcinoma (DCIS) with and without microinvasion: is there a difference in outcome? [abstract 24]. *Proc Am Soc Clin Oncol* 1993:53.

Silverstein MJ, Cohlan BF, Gierson ED, et al. Ductal carcinoma in situ: 227 cases without microinvasion. *Eur J Cancer* 1992;28:630.

Silverstein ML, Lagios MD, Craig PH, et al. A prognostic index for ductal carcinoma in situ of the breast. *Cancer* 1996;77:2267.

Silverstein MJ, Lagios MD, Groshen S, et al. The influence of margin width on local control of ductal carcinoma in situ of the breast. *N Engl J Med* 1999;340:1455.

Silverstein MJ, Lagios MD, Martino S, et al. Outcome after invasive local recurrence in patients with ductal carcinoma in situ of the breast. *J Clin Oncol* 1998;16:1367.

Silverstein MJ, Poller DN, Waisman JR, et al. Prognostic classification of breast ductal carcinoma in situ. *Lancet* 1995;345:1154.

Solin LJ, Yeh IT, Kurtz J, et al. Ductal carcinoma in situ (intraductal carcinoma) of the breast treated with breast-conserving surgery and definitive irradiation. *Cancer* 1993;71:2532.

Vezeridis MP, Bland KI. Management of ductal carcinoma in situ. *Surg Oncol* 1994;3:309.

Weng EY, Juillard GJF, Parker RG, et al. Outcomes and factors impacting local recurrence of ductal carcinoma in situ. *Cancer* 2000;88:1643.

Wong JH, Kopald KH, Morton DL. The impact of microinvasion on axillary node metastases and survival in patients with intraductal breast cancer. *Arch Surg* 1990;125:1298.

Invasive Breast Cancer

Carmen C. Solorzano, Paul M. Ahearne,
Steven D. Leach, and Barry W. Feig

EPIDEMIOLOGY

Breast cancer has become a leading health concern in the United States, accounting for approximately 30% of all cancers among women. Each year 44,000 women die of breast cancer, making it the second leading cause of deaths among American women, after lung cancer, and the leading cause of death among women aged 40 to 50 years. For an American woman the lifetime risk of being diagnosed with breast cancer is 1 in 8, or 12.5%, and the lifetime risk of dying from breast cancer is approximately 3.4%.

The incidence of breast cancer increases rapidly during the fourth decade of life and becomes substantial before age 50 years. After menopause, the incidence continues to increase but at a much slower rate. Breast cancer incidence rates have been increasing steadily since the start of data collection in the 1930s. In Connecticut, which has one of the oldest cancer registries in the country, the incidence of breast cancer rose by 1.2% per year from 1940 to 1982. According to the National Cancer Institute Surveillance, Epidemiology, and End Results Program (SEER), the incidence of breast cancer increased by 33% from 1973 to 1988. Because the breast cancer incidence rate increased by only 3% from 1973 to 1980, the majority of the increase occurred during the 1980s, indicating that this dramatic increase may be related to the increased use of mammographic screening during that time. If screening, and therefore increased detection, is responsible for the dramatic increase in incidence, a plateau should occur over the next few years. In fact, the incidence rates for localized disease have stabilized or increased more slowly since 1987. The incidence rates for regional disease decreased after 1987, and distant disease incidence rates have remained level over the past 20 years. Survival rates increased steadily and significantly for women with localized and regional disease in all age groups from 1980 through 1989, and the age-adjusted breast cancer mortality rate for white women in the United States dropped 6.8% from 1989 through 1993.

The decrease in the diagnosis of regional disease in the late 1980s in women older than 40 years likely reflects the increased use of mammography earlier in the 1980s, whereas the increase in survival rates, particularly for women with regional disease, likely reflects improvements in systemic adjuvant therapy. However, the recent decrease in the breast cancer mortality rate is too rapid to be explained solely by the increased use of mammography and the increase in survival rates is not dramatic enough to be explained by improved therapy alone. Thus, both screening mammography and improved therapy are likely to be involved in the recent decline in breast cancer mortality rates in the United States.

RISK FACTORS

The most important risk factor for the development of breast cancer is gender. The female-to-male ratio for breast cancer is 100:1. We will therefore focus on risk factors related to the development of breast cancer in women.

Age is an important risk factor for the development of breast cancer. The risk that breast cancer will develop in a white American woman in a single year increases from 1:5,900 at age 30 years to 1:290 at age 80.

Any family history of breast cancer increases a woman's risk of breast cancer.

A more important increase in risk is associated with the presence of breast cancer in a first-degree relative. The overall risk depends on the number of relatives with cancer, their ages at diagnosis, and whether the disease was unilateral or bilateral. For a 30-year-old woman whose sister had bilateral breast cancer before age 50, the cumulative probability of breast cancer by age 70 is 55%. This cumulative probability decreases to 8% for a woman whose sister developed unilateral breast cancer after age 50.

Genetic alterations predisposing individuals to breast cancer have received much attention recently. Although these gene mutations are inherited, only 5% to 10% of all breast cancers are believed to result from inheritance of a mutated gene. Autosomal dominant conditions associated with an increased risk of breast cancer include Li-Fraumeni syndrome, BRCA-1 and BRCA-2 mutations, Muir-Torre syndrome, Cowden disease, and Peutz-Jeghers syndrome. Although autosomal dominant, these conditions do not always exhibit 100% penetrance. Other inherited conditions include the autosomal recessive disorder ataxia-telangiectasia.

The most extensively publicized disorders associated with an increased risk of breast cancer have been the hereditary mutations in the BRCA-1 and BRCA-2 genes. The BRCA-1 gene is found on the long arm of chromosome 17q. Risks of developing breast or ovarian cancer differ with the site of the mutation but are in the range of 37% to 87% by age 70 for breast cancer and 11% to 42% by age 60 for ovarian cancer. The BRCA-2 gene is found on chromosome 13. In contrast to BRCA-1 mutation, BRCA-2 mutations are believed to be associated with breast cancer but not with ovarian cancer.

Prior breast cancer is a significant risk factor for the development of cancer in the contralateral breast, with an incidence of 0.5% to1.0% per year of follow-up.

Nonproliferative breast diseases such as adenosis, fibroadenomas, apocrine changes, duct ectasia, and mild hyperplasia carry no increased risk of breast cancer. However, proliferative breast diseases can be divided according to their association with a slightly increased, moderately increased, or high risk of breast cancer. Moderate or florid hyperplasia without atypia, papillomas, and sclerosing adenosis carry a slightly increased risk of breast cancer (one and a half to two times that of the general population). Atypical ductal or lobular hyperplasia is associated with a moderately increased risk of developing breast cancer (four to five times). Lobular carcinoma in situ is associated with a high risk of breast cancer (eight to ten times). These risks apply equally to both breasts, even if the breast disease was unilateral.

A number of endogenous endocrine factors have also been implicated as risk factors in breast cancer, including age at menarche, age at menopause, parity, and age at first full-term pregnancy. The risk of breast cancer for women who experience menopause after age 55 is twice that of women who experience menopause before age 44. Although age at menarche is important, age at onset of regular menses may be even more critical. Women who have regular ovulatory cycles before age 13 have a fourfold greater risk than those whose menarche occurred after age 13 and who had a 5-year delay to the development of regular cycles. The cumulative duration of menstruation also may be important. Women who menstruate for more than 30 years are at greater risk than those who menstruate for fewer than 30 years. Age at first birth has a greater impact on risk than the number of pregnancies, with a woman who had her first child before age 19 having half the risk of a nulliparous woman. Interestingly, women who have their first child between 30 and 34 years of age have the same risk as nulliparous women, and women who have their first child after age 35 have a greater risk than nulliparous women. These observations indicate that the hormonal milieu at different times in a woman's life may affect her risk of breast cancer.

The potential of exogenous hormones to increase a woman's risk of breast cancer remains controversial. Recent evidence suggests that the benefits of hormone replacement therapy in postmenopausal women outweigh the risks. The benefits include decreased risk of coronary artery disease and stroke, as well as increased bone density. The longevity benefits extend especially to women in high-risk groups for coronary artery disease. However, after long-term use of hormone replacement therapy, the risk of breast cancer increases to a point at which continued use becomes of questionable benefit. Other studies suggest that prolonged use of oral contraceptives (greater than 10 years) may be associated with an increased risk of breast cancer.

Exposure to ionizing radiation for the treatment of Hodgkin's disease has been associated with an increased risk of breast cancer if the exposure was before age 30. The risk for the first 15 years after treatment is less than the risk after 15 years.

Both obesity and alcohol consumption have been proposed as potential risk factors for breast cancer. In general, however, obesity has not been identified as an important risk factor for breast cancer. Among premenopausal women, obesity is associated with a decreased incidence of breast cancer. In postmenopausal women, there is a clinically unimportant association of obesity with breast cancer. Furthermore, despite the fact that a high-fat diet promotes mammary tumors in animals, only weak or nonexistent associations have been observed in human studies. Similarly, no conclusive evidence has been published to link alcohol consumption with an increased risk of breast cancer.

PATHOLOGY

Invasive carcinomas of the breast tend to be histologically heterogeneous tumors. Overwhelmingly, these tumors are adenocarcinomas that arise from the terminal ducts. There are five common
histologic variants of mammary adenocarcinoma.

1. *Infiltrating ductal carcinoma* accounts for 75% of all breast
   cancers. This lesion is characterized by the absence of special histologic features. It is hard when palpated and gritty
   when transected. It is associated with various degrees of fibrotic response. Often there is associated ductal carcinoma
   in situ (DCIS) within the specimen. Infiltrating ductal carcinomas commonly metastasize to axillary lymph nodes. The
   prognosis for patients with these tumors is poorer than that
   for patients with some of the other histologic subtypes. Distant metastases are found most often in the bones, lungs,
   liver, and brain.
2. *Infiltrating lobular carcinoma* is seen in 5% to 10% of breast
   cancer cases. Clinically, this lesion often presents as an area
   of ill-defined thickening within the breast. Microscopically,
   small cells in a single-file arrangement are seen. Infiltrating lobular cancers have a tendency to grow around ducts
   and lobules. Multicentricity is observed more frequently in
   infiltrating lobular carcinoma than in infiltrating ductal carcinoma. The prognosis for lobular carcinoma is similar to that
   for infiltrating ductal carcinoma. In addition to metastasizing to axillary lymph nodes, lobular carcinoma is known to
   metastasize to unusual sites, such as meninges and serosal
   surfaces, more often than do other forms of breast cancer.
3. *Tubular carcinoma* accounts for only 2% of breast carcinomas. The diagnosis of tubular carcinoma is made only when
   more than 75% of the tumor demonstrates tubule formation.
   Axillary nodal metastases are uncommon with this type of
   tumor. The prognosis for patients with tubular carcinoma is
   considerably better than that for patients with other types of
   breast cancer.
4. *Medullary carcinoma* accounts for 5% to 7% of breast cancers. Histologically, the lesion is characterized by poorly
   differentiated nuclei, a syncytial growth pattern, a well-
   circumscribed border, intense infiltration with small lymphocytes and plasma cells, and little or no DCIS. The prognosis
   for patients with medullary carcinoma is favorable only if all
   these characteristics are present.
5. *Mucinous or colloid carcinoma* constitutes approximately 3%
   of breast cancers. It is characterized by an abundant accumulation of extracellular mucin surrounding clusters of tumor cells. Colloid carcinoma is slow-growing and tends to be
   bulky. If a breast carcinoma is predominantly mucinous, the
   prognosis is favorable.

Rarer histologic types of breast malignancy include papillary,
apocrine, secretory, squamous cell, and spindle cell carcinomas,
cystosarcoma phyllodes, and carcinosarcoma. Infiltrating ductal carcinomas occasionally have small areas containing one or
more of these special histologic types. Tumors with these mixed

histologic appearances behave similarly to pure infiltrating ductal carcinomas.

STAGING

Typically, breast cancer is staged using the American Joint Committee on Cancer (AJCC) guidelines. The TNM classifications and stage groupings for breast cancer are summarized in Table 2-1. Please refer to www.cancerstaging.org for a summary of changes in the upcoming sixth edition of the *AJCC Staging Manual*.

DIAGNOSIS

History and Physical Examination

The diagnosis of breast cancer has undergone a dramatic evolution since the mid-1980s. Previously, 50% to 75% of all breast cancers were detected by self-examination. Subsequent to the widespread availability of mammographic screening programs, there has been a shift toward the diagnosis of clinically occult, nonpalpable lesions. Despite this trend, evaluation of the woman with potential breast cancer continues to be based on a careful history and physical examination.

The history is directed at assessing cancer risk as well as establishing the presence or absence of symptoms potentially related to breast disease. It should include the age at menarche, menopausal status, previous pregnancy, and use of oral contraceptives or postmenopausal replacement estrogens. A personal history of breast cancer is of obvious importance. In addition, a family history of breast cancer in first-degree relatives (i.e., mother or sister) should be sought.

After determination of cancer risk, the history should establish the presence or absence of specific symptoms potentially referable to breast cancer. It is worthwhile to inquire about breast pain and nipple discharge, although these symptoms are more commonly associated with benign processes, including fibrocystic disease and intraductal papilloma. Malaise, bony pain, and weight loss are rare but may indicate metastatic disease.

Physical examination of patients with potential breast cancer must constantly take into consideration the comfort and emotional well-being of the patient. Examination is initiated by careful visual inspection with the patient sitting upright. Nipple changes, gross asymmetry, and obvious masses are all noted. The skin must be carefully inspected for subtle changes; these can range from slight dimpling to the more dramatic *peau d'orange* appearance associated with locally advanced or inflammatory breast cancer.

Following careful inspection and with the patient remaining in the sitting position, the periclavicular regions are examined for potential nodal disease. Both axillae are then carefully palpated. If palpable, nodes should be characterized as to their number, size, and whether they are mobile or fixed. Examination of the axilla always includes palpation of the axillary tail of the breast; assessment of this area is often overlooked once the patient is placed in a supine position.

Palpation of the breast parenchyma itself is accomplished with the patient in a supine position and the ipsilateral arm placed

Table 2-1. Current AJCC TNM classification and stage grouping for breast carcinoma

TNM Classification		Stage Grouping			
Primary tumor (T)					
TX	Primary tumor cannot be assessed	Stage 0	Tis	N0	M0
T0	No evidence of primary tumor	Stage I	T1	N0	M0
Tis	Carcinoma *in situ*	Stage IIa	T0	N1	M0
T1	Tumor ≤ 2 cm in		T1	N1	M0
	greatest dimension		T2	N0	M0
T2	Tumor > 2 cm but ≤ 5 cm	Stage IIb	T2	N1	M0
T3	Tumor > 5 cm		T3	N0	M0
T4	Tumor of any size with	Stage IIIa	T0	N0	M0
	direct extension to		T1	N2	M0
	chest wall or skin;		T2	N2	M0
	includes inflammatory		T3	N1,2	M0
	carcinoma				
Regional lymph nodes (N)					
NX	Regional lymph nodes cannot be assessed	Stage IIIb	T4	Any N	M0
N0	No regional lymph node metastases		Any T	N3	M0
N1	Metastasis to movable ipsilateral axillary lymph node(s)	Stage IV	Any T	Any N	M1
N2	Metastases to ipsilateral axillary lymph nodes fixed to one another or to other structures				
N3	Metastasis to ipsilateral internal mammary lymph nodes				
Distant metastasis (M)					
MX	Presence of distant metastasis cannot be assessed				
M0	No distant metastasis				
M1	Distant metastasis (includes ipsilateral supraclavicular node[s])				

AJCC, American Joint Committee on Cancer.

over the head. The subareolar tissues and each quadrant of both breasts are systematically palpated. Masses are noted with respect to their size, shape, location, consistency, and mobility.

When subjected to critical analysis, physical examination often proves to be inadequate in differentiating benign from malignant breast masses. Various series have identified a 20% to 40% error rate, even among experienced examiners. Given this rate of inaccuracy, any persistent breast mass occurring in a patient older than age 30 years requires additional evaluation.

Evaluation of Palpable Lesions

The choice of initial evaluation following the detection of a breast mass should be individualized for each patient according to age, perceived cancer risk, and characteristics of the lesion in question. For most patients, mammographic evaluation is an important initial step. Mammography in this setting serves two purposes: (a) the risk of malignancy for the palpable lesion is further assessed, and (b) both breasts are screened for nonpalpable lesions. Bilateral synchronous cancers occur in approximately 3% of all cases; at least half of these lesions are nonpalpable.

For a palpable lesion, mammography may demonstrate the stellate or spiculated appearance typical of malignancy. Calcifications, nipple changes, and axillary adenopathy may also be visualized. Together, the presence or absence of these mammographic findings can predict malignancy with an overall accuracy of 70% to 80%. Mammography is least accurate in younger patients with dense breasts; it is rarely applied in patients under the age of 30 years.

Following mammographic evaluation, palpable masses suspected to be malignant should undergo fine-needle aspiration biopsy or core-needle biopsy. Some clinicians advocate needle biopsy at the time of initial evaluation, before mammography. For most patients, we defer biopsy until after mammographic examination is completed, because a needle-puncture hematoma will occasionally confuse future radiographic evaluation. For young patients with dense breasts in whom mammography is not contemplated, needle biopsy with or without the aid of ultrasonography remains an ideal primary mode of evaluation.

Fine-needle aspiration with a 22-gauge needle allows for accurate differentiation between cystic and solid masses and provides material for cytologic examination. Cystic lesions are not well visualized by mammography but are very well characterized by ultrasonography. Benign breast cysts typically yield nonbloody fluid and become nonpalpable after aspiration. Bloody fluid should be submitted for cytologic analysis. The incidence of malignancy among breast cysts is typically 1%; this is limited almost exclusively to those cysts that yield bloody fluid or have a residual mass following aspiration. Aspiration is often curative; only one in five breast cysts will recur following aspiration, and most of these are obliterated with a second drainage.

For solid lesions, several passes through the lesion with the syringe under constant negative pressure will typically yield ample material for cytologic evaluation. The material is evacuated onto a microscopic slide and immediately fixed in 95% ethanol. Multiple reports have demonstrated fine needle aspiration to be simple, safe, and accurate in evaluating benign and malignant breast masses. For lesions interpreted as malignant, cytologic evaluation is unable to differentiate between in situ and invasive carcinoma. Core-needle biopsy allows the pathologist to distinguish invasive from in situ carcinoma by providing a core of tissue for histopathologic evaluation.

Although physical examination, mammography, and needle biopsy all carry error rates when used as single modalities, the combination of these three investigations has proven extremely accurate in predicting whether a palpable lesion is benign or malignant. For lesions with equivocal or contradictory results, open biopsy remains the definitive test.

Evaluation of Nonpalpable Lesions

Because of the increasing availability of mammographic screening programs, there has been a rapid increase in the diagnosis of nonpalpable breast cancer in the United States. Since 1997, the American Cancer Society, National Cancer Institute, and American College of Radiologists have released updated guidelines for breast cancer screening, in large part based on new data published in 1997. Each organization recommends that women begin regular screening mammography in their 40s.

Mammographic signs of malignancy can be divided into two main categories: microcalcifications and density changes. Microcalcifications can be either clustered or scattered. Density changes include discrete masses, architectural distortions, and asymmetries. Mammographic findings most predictive of malignancy include spiculated masses with associated architectural distortion, clustered microcalcifications in a linear or branching array, or microcalcifications with a mass. The American College of Radiology has suggested the following categories for reporting mammographic results: I = negative (no findings), II = benign appearance, III = probably benign appearance, IV = findings suspicious for breast cancer, and V = findings highly suspicious for breast cancer.

Once screening mammography demonstrates a suspicious lesion, further evaluation is necessary. For lesions interpreted as "probably benign" (well-defined, solitary masses), careful counseling and repeat mammography in 6 months may be undertaken in patients at low risk for breast cancer. For appropriate lesions, ultrasonography may identify a subset of cystic lesions that will not require biopsy. Ultrasonography may also be used to guide fine-needle or core-needle biopsy. For suspicious lesions, some form of biopsy is required. Ultrasound-guided biopsy is not useful in the evaluation of microcalcifications; these are typically not sonographically visible. Mammography-guided stereotactic breast biopsy has emerged as a useful technique for nonpalpable lesions and microcalcifications.

Breast Biopsy Technique

For either palpable or nonpalpable lesions, planning an optimal open biopsy mandates careful consideration of at least three issues. First, the biopsy site may require future reexcision, even under a strategy of breast conservation. Second, the biopsy site must be able to be incorporated into a future mastectomy incision should this form of treatment be chosen. Third, the biopsy must be constructed in a cosmetically optimal manner. All breast biopsies should be performed with the assumption that the target lesion is malignant.

Biopsies are typically performed in an outpatient setting using local anesthesia. In general, incisions must be planned carefully so that they can be incorporated into a mastectomy if that becomes necessary. Curvilinear incisions are often used to take advantage of decreased lines of tension along Langer's lines. Radial scars are generally avoided, except in the extreme medial aspect of the breast, where mastectomy incisions become radially oriented; lesions in the inner-lower quadrant are often best approached through a radial incision. Circumareolar incisions have obvious cosmetic advantage but carry the potential disadvantage of leading to sacrifice of areolar tissue should reexcision be required. Although a modest amount of peripheral tunneling is acceptable to maintain an incision within a potential mastectomy scar, extreme tunneling to the periphery of the breast from a central periareolar incision not only makes it virtually impossible to identify the tumor bed if reexcision is required, but also exposes an inordinate amount of breast tissue to potential contamination by tumor cells. In patients in whom breast conservation with axillary dissection is contemplated, the biopsy site should not be contiguous with the axillary incision. Separating these incisions provides a better cosmetic outcome (as the axillary drain will cause the biopsy cavity to become distorted if they are not separated) and may prevent tumor seeding of a previously negative axilla, thus avoiding the need to irradiate a dissected axilla.

The excisional breast biopsy has the potential to serve both diagnostic and local treatment purposes. It is reserved as a diagnostic tool when needle biopsy is impossible or inappropriate. The entire mass and a surrounding 1-cm rim of normal tissue should be excised. An excisional biopsy such as this will fulfill the requirements for lumpectomy and avoid subsequent reexcision.

For nonpalpable lesions, preoperative needle localization with a self-retaining hookwire is required. This procedure requires careful communication between radiologist and surgeon. For most lesions, the localizing needle is placed under mammographic guidance into the breast via the shortest direct path to the lesion. The self-retaining wire is placed through the needle, and the needle is removed. Postlocalization mammograms are then reviewed. Biopsy is done by excising a core of breast tissue surrounding the wire tip. For superficial lesions, an ellipse of skin at the point of wire insertion may be removed en bloc with the underlying breast tissue. Postexcision specimen radiographs are essential to confirm successful biopsy.

Once the biopsy specimen has been excised, careful handling is critical. The surgeon should meticulously note the orientation of the excised breast tissue and hand-deliver the specimen to the pathology department. The lateral, medial, superior, inferior, superficial, and deep margins should be inked in a color-coded manner. Material should be processed for receptor analysis and flow cytometry.

Closure of the biopsy incision requires meticulous hemostasis. Deep parenchymal sutures often cause cosmetically unpleasing distortion of the residual breast and should be avoided. Drains are not used in the breast. The skin is closed with a subcuticular suture, and a light dressing is placed.

PRETREATMENT EVALUATION

Once the diagnosis of breast cancer has been made, appropriate treatment planning involves the possibility of metastatic disease. For patients with stage I or stage II breast cancer, this is typically limited to a complete history and physical examination, a chest radiograph, and evaluation of serum liver chemistries. The routine use of bone scans in asymptomatic patients with apparent early stage breast cancer carries an extremely low yield; several series have demonstrated only a 2% incidence of positive scan results in this setting. In contrast, up to 25% of asymptomatic patients with apparent stage III cancer have positive bone scan results; routine scanning in this population appears worthwhile. In the absence of increased serum liver chemistries or palpable hepatomegaly, liver imaging is not used routinely in the preoperative evaluation of patients with early stage disease. Supraclavicular ultrasonography may be useful to rule out metastatic disease in patients with clinical nodal disease.

TREATMENT

Many of the current recommendations regarding therapy for invasive breast cancer have been influenced by the results of randomized, prospective clinical trials performed by the National Surgical Adjuvant Breast and Bowel Project (NSABP). A summary of selected trials is presented in Table 2-2.

Early Stage Breast Cancer (T1, T2, N0, N1)

Approximately 75% of patients with breast cancer present with tumors less than 5 cm in diameter and no evidence of fixed or matted nodes. These patients with early stage breast cancer are generally treated by one of three surgical options: (a) breast conservation surgery with irradiation, (b) modified radical mastectomy, or (c) modified radical mastectomy with either immediate or delayed reconstruction. With careful patient selection, the goal of maintaining either a conserved or reconstructed breast can be achieved in most cases.

Breast Conservation Versus Mastectomy

It is now clear that many patients with breast cancer can be effectively treated with breast conservation. Since 1970, seven different prospective randomized trials comparing breast conservation strategies with radical or modified radical mastectomy have failed to demonstrate any survival benefit to the more aggressive approach. Among these trials, the two most widely known were conducted by Harris et al. (1992) at the National Cancer Institute in Milan, Italy, and by Fisher et al. (1995) in conjunction with the NSABP in the United States. The Milan trial was limited to patients with stage I breast cancer (tumor <2 cm, negative axillary nodes) and compared radical mastectomy with a

**Table 2-2.   Summary of selected NSABP
therapeutic trials for invasive breast cancer**

Trial	Treatments	Outcome
NSABP B-04	Total mastectomy vs. total mastectomy with XRT vs. radical mastectomy	No difference in disease-free or overall survival
NSABP B-06	Total mastectomy vs. lumpectomy vs. lumpectomy with XRT	No difference in disease-free or overall survival; addition if XRT to lumpectomy reduced local recurrence rate from 39% to 10%
NSABP B-13	Surgery alone vs. surgery plus adjuvant chemotherapy in node-negative patients with ER-negative tumors	Improved disease-free survival for adjuvant chemotherapy group
NSABP B-14	Surgery alone vs. surgery plus adjuvant tamoxifen in node-negative patients with ER-positive tumors	Improved disease-free survival for adjuvant tamoxifen group
NSABP B-21	Lumpectomy plus tamoxifen vs. lumpectomy plus tamoxifen plus XRT vs. lumpectomy plus XRT for node-negative tumors < 1 cm	Combination of XRT and tamoxifen was more effective than either adjuvant treatment alone in reducing IBTR

ER, estrogen receptor; IBRT, ipsilateral breast tumor recurrence; NSABP, National Surgical Adjuvant Breast and Bowel Project; XRT, radiation therapy.

breast conservation strategy involving quadrantectomy, axillary dissection, and radiation therapy. No differences in local control, disease-free survival, or overall survival have been noted.

NSABP trial B-06 examined an expanded patient population that included women with primary tumors up to 4 cm in diameter and either N0 or N1 nodal status. Patients were randomized to one of three treatment strategies: modified radical mastectomy, lumpectomy with axillary dissection and radiation therapy, or lumpectomy and axillary dissection alone. Histologically negative margins were required in the breast conservation groups. There were no differences in disease-free survival or overall survival among the three groups. The local recurrence rate, however, was markedly reduced by the addition of radiation therapy to lumpectomy and axillary dissection (12% with radiation therapy vs. 53% without radiation therapy, at 10 years). These results upheld breast conservation as an appropriate treatment for patients with stage I or stage II breast cancer and made it clear that radiation therapy is required as an integral part of any breast conservation strategy. At The University of Texas M.D. Anderson Cancer Center, we typically initiate radiation therapy 2 to 3 weeks following surgery or at the completion of postoperative adjuvant chemotherapy. A dose of 50 Gy is given to the whole breast followed by a 10 Gy boost to the operative site using tangential ports and computerized dosimetry.

Although it is clear that breast conservation is equal to mastectomy for patients with stage I or II disease, the decision to embark on a treatment strategy involving breast conservation must be individualized for each patient. Numerous factors contribute to this decision. The patient's motivation and commitment to breast conservation must be strong, because daily outpatient radiation treatments over 5 to 6 weeks are required. The patient also must be willing to accept the 10% to 12% risk of a local recurrence within the conserved breast.

Other factors contributing to the choice between mastectomy and breast conservation surgery include the size of the breast, tumor size, tumor histologic characteristics, tumor multicentricity, and patient age. For extremely small breasts, the cosmetic result may be unacceptable following local excision, especially for larger lesions. For large, pendulous breasts, lack of uniformity in radiation dosing may result in unattractive fibrosis and retraction. Patients with either extreme may benefit from a strategy of mastectomy and reconstruction, occasionally coupled with surgical augmentation or reduction of the contralateral breast. Patients with larger tumors also might be best served by mastectomy. At this point, there are no data to suggest that T3 lesions (i.e., >5 cm) can be adequately treated by breast conservation. From a purely practical point of view, local excision of such lesions rarely results in a cosmetically acceptable result. However, preoperative (neoadjuvant) chemotherapy may be able to downstage T3 tumors to the point where breast conservation may become an option.

The use of neoadjuvant chemotherapy has its origins in the management of inoperable locally advanced breast cancer. Several important trials including NSABP B-18 have demonstrated that neoadjuvant chemotherapy can increase the resectability rate of locally advanced primary breast cancer, can allow more patients to successfully undergo breast conservation surgery, and does not confer a survival disadvantage compared to standard adjuvant postoperative chemotherapy. Based on these findings, neoadjuvant chemotherapy is the preferred initial treatment for patients with locally advanced or inflammatory breast carcinoma (covered later in the chapter). However, if a patient is predicted to derive little advantage from chemotherapy in the adjuvant setting, it is equally unlikely that she will benefit from neoadjuvant chemotherapy. But if a woman desires breast conservation surgery and her primary tumor size precludes this approach, neoadjuvant chemotherapy should be offered regardless of clinical disease stage. The potential for a higher risk of recurrence in the breast (as compared to mastectomy) in this setting should be discussed with the patient. The clinical and pathologic responses of the primary breast tumor to neoadjuvant chemotherapy appear to be a surrogate marker for the response of occult micrometastases and patient outcomes.

The role of neoadjuvant chemotherapy in operable breast cancer remains undefined. There appears to be no rationale, outside of a clinical trial, for its use in patients with early stage breast cancer who are suitable candidates for breast conservation or who choose mastectomy.

A number of attempts have been made to identify patients with a high rate of local recurrence following breast conservation based on the histology of the primary tumor. To date, there have been no documented differences in local recurrence among the various histologic subtypes. The risk of local recurrence has been shown to be higher for women younger than 35 years and for women whose tumors are greater than 2 cm in diameter regardless of lymph node status. For patients with positive lymph nodes, nuclear grade is also significantly correlated with recurrence.

Axillary Dissection

A substantial portion of patients with apparent early stage breast cancer present with axillary nodal metastases. In one series, 17% of patients with clinically T1N0 disease had histologically positive nodes; this figure rose to 27% for patients with clinically T2N0 disease. Other series have reported that 10% of patients with tumors smaller than 0.5 cm have positive axillary lymph nodes. Tumors 0.5 to1.0 cm are associated with positive axillary lymph nodes in 13 to 22% of patients. Tumors 1.1 to 2.0 cm in size are associated with lymph node metastases in up to 30% of patients. Although axillary dissection contributes little to overall survival, it is important for staging and local control in women undergoing breast conservation surgery or modified radical mastectomy. Axillary dissection is also a source of significant potential morbidity.

The contribution of axillary dissection to local control is small but measurable. In the NSABP B-04 trial comparing radical mastectomy with simple mastectomy (without axillary dissection) with and without irradiation, 40% of patients with clinically negative axillae were found to have positive nodes at the time of radical mastectomy, and 1% of these patients eventually recurred in the axilla. In patients with unoperated axillae, 18% (65 of 365) eventually developed clinical adenopathy requiring delayed axillary dissection. Four of these patients eventually experienced recurrence in the axilla despite delayed dissection. No survival disadvantage was seen for patients undergoing delayed versus immediate axillary dissection. Radiation was less effective than axillary dissection in preventing eventual recurrence in the axilla; this was especially true for patients with clinically positive nodes.

In addition to contributing to local control, axillary dissection provides important staging and prognostic information. As noted earlier, clinical staging of the axilla remains relatively inaccurate. However, nodal status remains a major predictor of outcome. For all patients with node-negative cancer, at least a 70% 10-year survival rate may be anticipated. This drops to 40% for patients with one to three positive nodes and to less than 20% for patients with four to ten positive nodes. Micrometastatic nodal disease (<2 mm in diameter) carries a better prognosis than macrometastatic disease. As discussed later, the contribution of axillary dissection to local control and treatment planning is currently in flux.

The current standard of care is an anatomic level I and II axillary lymph node dissection for all patients with stage I and II breast cancer. For patients with invasive breast cancer undergoing breast conservation therapy, axillary dissection should be performed via a separate axillary incision that does not extend anterior to the pectoralis fold. Axillary dissection should consist of en bloc removal of level I and level II nodal tissue. The addition of level III nodes to the dissection often requires division or resection of the pectoralis minor muscle and is of little benefit with respect to staging; only 1% to 3% of stage I/II patients show level III involvement in the absence of level I or II disease. On the other hand, level III dissections carry a substantially higher risk of subsequent lymphedema, especially if radiation therapy is also used. The level I and II axillary dissection should preserve the long thoracic and thoraco-dorsal nerves and avoid stripping of the axillary vein. A closed-suction drain is placed and removed later after the drainage has sufficiently decreased.

Whether a full axillary node dissection is necessary for all patients with invasive carcinoma remains controversial. Patients with early stage disease with a low risk of axillary node involvement may not require axillary dissection (patients with T1a and T1b tumors that are not high grade). However, before such a treatment regimen can be recommended there must be (a) identification of the subgroup of patients who is truly at low risk (see "Sentinel Lymph Node Biopsy"), and (b) randomized prospective trial to evaluate the issue. Another group of patients who may not benefit from axillary dissection consists of those who are receiving chemotherapy and radiotherapy regardless of the nodal findings (i.e., premenopausal women with tumors >1 cm). Certainly the best approach for patients with T1c tumors might be the use of sentinel lymph node (SLN) biopsy to detect lymph node metastases, this would provide prognostic information with presumably less morbidity and help formulate a treatment strategy. Radiation portals can then be adjusted to minimize the risk of axillary regional failure, or axillary dissection.

Sentinel Lymph Node Biopsy

There has been increasing difficulty in recent years in justifying the practice of routine axillary dissection. Furthermore, the breast cancer size on presentation has been progressively smaller because of widespread use of screening mammography; thus, the probability of nodal involvement is smaller. The challenge is to employ axillary dissection only in patients with nodal metastases. A newer approach that enables selective lymphadenectomy is lymphatic mapping and SLN biopsy. The SLN is the first lymph node to receive lymphatic drainage from a primary breast cancer and therefore the node most likely to contain metastatic tumor cells. When the SLN biopsy is performed by an experienced team consisting of the surgeon, the nuclear medicine physician, the pathologist, and the operating room nurses and technicians, the finding of a tumor-free SLN almost invariably indicates that the patient has node-negative breast cancer and need not undergo further axillary dissection. However, SLN biopsy should not be undertaken without completion axillary dissection until the SLN biopsy team has documented consistently a high rate of SLN identification and low rate of falsely negative SLN. SLN biopsy can be performed using radiolabeled colloid, vital blue dye or both. Preoperative lymphoscintigraphy is used to identify the SLN and document patterns of lymphatic drainage. Intraoperatively a handheld gamma counter, the aid of visible blue dye, or both can be used to locate the SLN.

In patients with certain clinical presentations, SLN biopsy is more likely to be unsuccessful or uninformative:

Palpable axillary adenopathy

Medial hemisphere location of the primary tumor where preoperative lymphoscintigraphy did not identify an axillary SLN

Large primary tumors (>5 cm)—the lymphatic drainage may be to multiple nodes

Previous axillary surgery—the lymphatic drainage from the primary may be distorted

Large biopsy cavity (>6 cm)—the lymphatic drainage from the surrounding breast tissue may not be the same as that of the primary tumor

Tumors treated with neoadjuvant chemotherapy in patients with nodal disease at presentation—metastases may be eradicated in the SLN while still being present in other regional lymph nodes.

Before SLN biopsy, patients should be informed of the experimental nature of this technique and the necessity of performing an axillary node dissection in the event the SLN is not identified. The ultimate objective of SLN biopsy is to identify node-negative patients who would not benefit from axillary dissection. Therefore, the false-negative rate of this new technique needs to be low. The most recent large SLN mapping studies for breast cancer reported rates of successful SLN detection of 79% to 98%, accuracy rates of 97% to 100%, and false-negative rates of 0% to 29%. A recent validation study of SLN biopsy involving 11 centers reported similar findings.

The most important question resulting from the emergence of SLN biopsy technology is whether SLN biopsy can replace routine axillary dissection. At M.D. Anderson we believe that the answer is yes, if the procedure is performed at an experienced center in patients with small primary breast tumors and clinically negative axilla. Another important question posed by this new technique is the significance of SLN positivity by immunohistochemistry but not by routine hematoxylin and eosin staining. Knowing whether subsequent full axillary dissection, axillary radiation therapy, or adjuvant chemotherapy is needed in patients with micrometastasis in the SLN necessitates a better understanding of the natural history of the disease. Several regional and national studies (American College of Surgeons Oncology Group Z0010/Z0011 and

NSABP B-32) are being conducted to address the multiple issues associated with this new technique.

BREAST RECONSTRUCTION

For patients not undergoing breast conservation, breast reconstruction should be considered a standard component of cancer therapy. Reconstruction may involve autologous tissue, synthetic implants, or a combination. Although satisfactory results can be obtained with either immediate or delayed reconstruction, we favor immediate reconstruction for most patients. Immediate reconstruction carries a substantial psychologic benefit for many women and often allows a better cosmetic result. The initiation of adjuvant chemotherapy is not significantly delayed, and concerns that local recurrence may go undetected in a reconstructed breast are not well founded, especially for T1 and T2 lesions.

In our institution, 50% of all patients with breast cancer treated with mastectomy undergo immediate reconstruction. Although the method of reconstruction is individualized for each patient, either pedicled or free transverse rectus abdominis myocutaneous (TRAM) flaps are most commonly used. Contralateral augmentation or reduction may be performed to maximize symmetry. For premenopausal women with a perceived high risk for a contralateral second primary lesion, simultaneous contralateral mastectomy with bilateral free TRAM flap reconstruction is available.

We typically perform a skin-sparing mastectomy in patients undergoing immediate breast reconstruction; the preservation of breast skin allows for a more natural contour to the reconstructed breast. To date, no increased risk of local recurrence has been observed for patients treated with skin-sparing techniques.

Although breast mound reconstruction may be undertaken immediately following mastectomy, nipple reconstruction is typically delayed 6 to 12 weeks to allow time for the reconstructed breast to remodel and attain its final shape and position. Only then can appropriate nipple position be determined. The nipple is formed by raising local skin flaps using local anesthesia; pigment is provided using tattooing techniques.

CURRENT TREATMENT STANDARDS FOR SYSTEMIC ADJUVANT THERAPY

For node-positive and node-negative patients, decisions regarding adjuvant chemotherapy must be individualized. Current standards are based largely on the histologic status of the axilla, age of the patient, level of estrogen receptors expressed by the tumor, and size of the primary tumor. Other factors are also considered, including overall health status, ploidy, S-phase fraction, c-erbB-2 oncogene amplification, and cathepsin D expression. General guidelines regarding the use of adjuvant chemotherapy are presented in Table 2-3. Current standards favor the use of multidrug combination chemotherapy in all patients except those with the most favorable presentation (node-negative, primary tumor <1 cm). Results from the Early Breast Cancer Trialists' Collaborative Group indicated that multidrug chemotherapy significantly reduces recurrence and death in both lymph node–positive and lymph node–negative patients. The most widely used

Table 2-3. Adjuvant chemotherapy recommendations for patients with invasive breast carcinoma based on axillary nodal status, menopausal status, estrogen receptor expression, and tumor size

Nodal Status	Menopausal Status	ER Status	Tumor Size	Therapy	Comments
Positive	Premenopausal	Negative	Any	Multidrug combination chemotherapy (CMF,CAF, or AC;[a] AC + T)	4 to 8 cycles is standard duration of treatment. Addition of 4 cycles of paclitaxel to 4 cycles of AC improves overall survival in high-risk patients.
		Positive		Multidrug combination chemotherapy (CMF,CAF, or AC; AC + T) + tamoxifen	Addition of tamoxifen to chemotherapy results in additional survival benefit.
	Postmenopausal	Negative		Multidrug combination chemotherapy (CMF,CAF, or AC; AC + T)	20% reduction in recurrence and 11% reduction in mortality in patients aged 50 to 69. Minimal data for patients aged ≥ 70.
		Positive		Tamoxifen 10 mg bid +/– multidrug combination chemotherapy (CMF,CAF, or AC; AC + T)	Combination chemotherapy and tamoxifen results in better survival than tamoxifen alone.

Negative	Pre- or postmenopausal	Postive or negative	<1 cm	None; consider tamoxifen for contralateral risk reduction	Survival after local treatment alone is >90%. Low toxicity and beneficial effects of tamoxifen may justify its use.
		Negative	≥1 cm <2	Consider multidrug combination chemotherapy (CMF,CAF, or AC)	Prognostic factors, such as grade and S-phase, may be useful in selecting patients for chemotherapy.
		Negative	≥2 cm	Multidrug combination chemotherapy (CMF,CAF or AC)	Reduction in risk of recurrence is equal to that observed in node-positive disease.
		Positive	≥1 cm	Tamoxifen 10 mg bid ± multidrug combination chemotherapy (CMF,CAF, or AC)	Chemotherapy is recommended for women with high-grade tumors or T2 lesions. Tamoxifen therapy is recommended for tumors 1 to 2 cm. Decisions about the addition of cytotoxic therapy for pre- or postmenopausal women should be made on the basis of ER levels, performance status, and tumor factors.

A, doxorubicin (Adriamycin); C, cyclophosphamide; ER, estrogen receptor; F, 5-flourouracil; M, methotrexate; T, taxane.
[a]Addition of the taxane paclitaxel to 4 cycles of AC as treatment alternative.
Adapted from Singletary SE. *J Am Coll Surg* 2001;192;220.

regimen is cyclophosphamide, methotrexate, and 5-flourouracil, although anthracycline-based chemotherapy is gaining popularity, especially for high-risk node-positive patients. The usual duration of treatment for chemotherapy is four to eight cycles. Data from clinical trials have indicated that fewer than three cycles is not advantageous, and no additional benefit is likely after 12 cycles.

Tamoxifen, originally recommended for the treatment of postmenopausal women with estrogen receptor–positive breast cancer, is now indicated for a much broader range of patients. Regardless of patient age or menopausal status, when used for 5 years, tamoxifen is associated with a 47% reduction in the risk of breast cancer recurrence and a 26% reduction in the risk of death. Tamoxifen therapy is generally well tolerated; treatment-limiting adverse effects develop in less than 5% of patients. Beneficial effects on bone density and serum cholesterol, as well as an overall reduction in the mortality rate due to cardiovascular diseases, may offset concerns regarding an increased incidence of endometrial cancer and thromboembolic events in women taking tamoxifen. For these reasons, many practitioners recommend the use of tamoxifen for low-risk breast cancer patients who would not otherwise receive systemic therapy. Standard treatment with tamoxifen is 5 years. A metaanalysis of five randomized clinical trials showed that patients who had 3 to 5 years of tamoxifen treatment had a greater reduction in recurrence than did patients who had 1 to 2 years of treatment (22% ± 8% vs. 7% ± 11%, respectively). Data from the NSABP B-14 study indicated that 10 years of tamoxifen use offers no survival advantage over 5 years. For postmenopausal women with either node-positive or node-negative breast cancer, chemotherapy used in combination with Tamoxifen increases disease-free survival compared with tamoxifen alone.

EVOLVING MODALITIES IN ADJUVANT CHEMOTHERAPY

Taxanes

The taxane family of drugs work by stabilizing microtubule polymerization, leading to arrest in the G2/M phase of the cell cycle. The mechanism of action of taxanes results in lack of cross-resistance with other active agents. Because of this, the taxanes, which include paclitaxel and docetaxel, have a growing role in crossover protocols in patients with anthracycline-resistant tumors. A recent analysis of a Cancer and Leukemia Group B trial found that the addition of sequential paclitaxel to doxorubicin and cyclophosphamide further reduced the annual odds of recurrence and death in node-positive breast cancer patients (22% and 26%, respectively). Clinical trials are now looking at the efficacy of combinations of taxanes with doxorubicin and the integration of taxanes into other combination regimens.

Herceptin

Trastuzumab (Herceptin) is a monoclonal antibody that targets the *HER-2/neu* gene, which codes for a growth factor that is overexpressed in 25% of breast cancers. The antibody works by binding to the HER-2 growth factor receptors present on the surface of the cancer cells. The effects of trastuzumab seem to be restricted to patients with *HER-2/neu*-overexpressing tumors. Preliminary phase II trials indicate that trastuzumab may increase the effectiveness of various chemotherapeutic agents without adding significant toxicity. The NSABP B-31 trial is currently looking at the effectiveness of a regimen containing doxorubicin and cyclophosphamide, followed by paclitaxel with or without trastuzumab.

High-Dose Chemotherapy

Researchers have attempted to treat metastatic and high-risk primary breast cancers with increasingly higher doses of chemotherapeutic agents. Initial work using high-dose chemotherapy with stem cell rescue showed promising results. However, these initial encouraging results have not been supported by recently reported, more mature studies. At this time, there is no good evidence that high-dose chemotherapy with stem cell rescue is preferable to standard treatment for high-risk breast cancer patients. Therefore, the use of this treatment regimen cannot be recommended outside of a well-designed clinical trial.

One potentially promising approach is dose-dense treatment regimens. This approach is based on the idea that more frequent exposure to chemotherapeutic agents reduces the possibility that growth-resistant clones will emerge and grow during the inter-treatment intervals. Patients receive active drugs at reduced doses separated by shorter inter-treatment intervals than standard chemotherapy regimens. The efficacy of this approach remains undetermined.

LOCALLY ADVANCED BREAST CANCER

Locally advanced breast cancer encompasses tumors with a broad range of biologic behaviors. This category is generally believed to include tumors that are large and/or have extensive regional lymph node involvement without evidence of distant metastatic disease at initial presentation. These tumors are classified as stage III disease according to the AJCC system. Approximately 10% to 20% of all patients with breast cancer have stage III disease, which includes T3 tumors with N1, N2, or N3 disease; T4 tumors with any N classification; or any T classification with N2 or N3 regional lymph node involvement. Stage III disease is further subdivided into stage IIIa and stage IIIb (Table 2-1). Approximately 25% to 30% of stage III breast cancers are inoperable at the time of diagnosis.

Because of the advanced stage of disease at diagnosis, many locally advanced breast cancers are discovered by the patient or her spouse. The rest are discovered during routine physical examination. On occasion, a discrete mass may not be present; rather, there is a diffuse infiltration of the breast tissue. These patients present with a breast that is asymmetric, immobile, and different in consistency from the contralateral breast. Seventy-five percent of patients with stage III disease will have clinically palpable axillary or supraclavicular lymph nodes at the time of diagnosis. This clinical finding is confirmed on pathologic examination in 66% to 90% of patients. Of the patients with positive nodes, 50% will have more than four nodes involved by tumor. When appropriate staging is performed, 20% of patients with stage III disease will have distant metastases at presentation. Distant metastases are also the most frequent form of treatment failure, usually appearing within 2 years of the initial diagnosis.

Both fine-needle aspiration and core-needle biopsy can be used to confirm the suspicion of breast cancer in these patients. These procedures usually are easily performed because of the large tumor size at presentation.

The Halsted radical mastectomy was initially believed to be the treatment of choice for locally advanced breast cancer; however, it proved to be inadequate in terms of both local control and long-term survival. In 1942, Haagensen reported a 53% local recurrence rate and 0% 5-year survival rate in a group of 1,135 patients with stage III breast cancer who had Halsted radical mastectomies.

The failure of surgery alone to control stage III breast cancer led to the use of radiation therapy as a single-agent treatment modality in this group of patients. However, the results with radiation therapy were in some cases inferior to those seen with surgery alone. The 5-year survival and local recurrence rates seen with radiation therapy alone were 10% to 30% and 25% to 70%, respectively.

The subsequent combination of surgery and radiation therapy for locally advanced breast cancer also resulted in poor overall results. The lack of efficacy with the combination of two local treatment modalities confirmed the fact that stage III breast cancer is a systemic disease. Although there was a slight improvement in local control with surgery plus radiation therapy, the 5-year survival rate was unchanged, because patients continued to die of distant metastases.

In the early 1970s, systemic combination chemotherapy was added to the local treatments for locally advanced breast cancer. Initial protocols were designed to administer the chemotherapy following local treatment. However, this sequence of treatment does not allow for any assessment of the efficacy of the chemotherapy, as all measurable disease is removed before administration of the drugs. This led to the current practice of administering induction chemotherapy prior to any local treatment. This sequencing affords several advantages, including reduction of the initial tumor burden before surgery, ability to treat the potential systemic disease without delay, and ability to assess the response of the tumor to the treatment being rendered.

Several centers have reported experiences with combined-modality therapy for locally advanced disease. Although the protocols differ among institutions with respect to the specific chemotherapy regimens and the type of local treatment, all the studies have used induction chemotherapy followed by local treatment (surgery and/or radiation therapy) and subsequent adjuvant chemotherapy. Based on these reports, it has now become the standard of care to treat patients with locally advanced breast cancer using this chemotherapy sandwich approach. Chemotherapy should consist of a doxorubicin-based regimen for four to six cycles, followed by surgery. After surgery, adjuvant chemotherapy should precede radiation therapy to avoid interrupting the treatment of systemic disease, because distant metastases are the most frequent form of treatment failure. The role of adjuvant hormonal therapy in this group of patients is still under investigation.

INFLAMMATORY BREAST CANCER

Inflammatory breast cancer is a rare, virulent form of locally advanced breast cancer. It represents 1% to 6% of all breast cancers and presents as erythema, warmth, and edema of the breast. Rapid onset of symptoms (within 3 months) is necessary to make the diagnosis of inflammatory carcinoma. The time course distinguishes it from locally advanced breast cancer with secondary lymphatic invasion, which usually progresses slowly over more than 3 months. Pain is also present in approximately one half of patients with inflammatory breast cancer. The physical findings are often confused with an infectious process, resulting in frequent delays in diagnosis and treatment. Tumor emboli are seen in the subdermal lymphatics on microscopic examination. Biopsy for diagnosis should include a segment of involved skin because there is usually no dominant mass palpable on physical examination.

Inflammatory carcinoma, like other forms of locally advanced breast cancer, is a systemic disease. This was manifest in the poor outcome seen when local therapy was used as the only treatment modality. Median survival was less than 2 years, with 5-year survival rates around 5%.

The use of multimodality therapy in these patients has improved local control and survival compared with local therapy alone. Current therapy for inflammatory breast carcinoma at M.D. Anderson begins with chemotherapy. Patients with a complete or partial response proceed to surgery, which is followed by adjuvant chemotherapy and radiation therapy. Patients with progression of disease during chemotherapy proceed to preoperative radiation therapy. Patients with less than partial response to chemotherapy but no progression receive a second chemotherapeutic regimen, followed by surgery for a partial or complete response or radiation therapy for disease progression.

FOLLOW-UP AFTER PRIMARY TREATMENT OF INVASIVE BREAST CANCER

Following primary therapy for invasive breast cancer, patients must be made aware of the long-term risk for recurrent or metastatic disease. Although most series report most recurrences within the first 5 years after primary therapy, recurrences more than 20 years after primary therapy have been reported.

For each patient with breast cancer, the follow-up evaluation should be individualized based on the treatments applied, perceived risk of disease recurrence, and specific patient needs. Despite the availability of multiple biochemical and radiographic tests, periodic history taking and physical examination remain the most effective modalities for detecting recurrent disease. Numerous studies have demonstrated that 65% to 85% of all breast cancer recurrences may be detected by a history and physical examination alone.

For patients who have undergone breast conservation therapy, follow-up examination should be undertaken every 4 months for the first 2 years, every 6 months for the third through fifth years, and yearly thereafter. Monthly self-examination of the breasts is also required. Mammography is done 6 months following the completion of breast conservation therapy to allow surgical and radiation changes to stabilize, and then yearly. For patients who have undergone mastectomy, a contralateral mammogram is obtained yearly. For both groups, further evaluation should be limited to a yearly serum biochemical evaluation in patients who receive chemotherapy and a yearly chest radiograph. The routine use of bone scans, skeletal surveys, and computed tomography scans of the abdomen and brain yields an extremely low rate of occult metastases in otherwise asymptomatic patients and is not cost-effective for patients with early stage breast cancer.

LOCALLY RECURRENT BREAST CANCER

The time course, significance, and prognosis of locally recurrent breast cancer vary dramatically for patients undergoing breast conservation versus those undergoing mastectomy. Local recurrence rates of 5% to 10% at 8 to 10 years are reported in the conserved breast. This typically occurs over a protracted time and is associated with systemic metastases in less than 10% of the patients. Local recurrence following lumpectomy remains curable in most cases; 50% to 63% of patients with local recurrence will remain disease-free 5 years after salvage mastectomy.

In contrast, local chest wall recurrence following mastectomy typically occurs within the first 2 to 3 years after surgery. It is associated with distant metastases in as many as two thirds of the patients and predicts eventual death from breast cancer for many of the patients. One third of patients with chest wall recurrence will have distant metastatic disease concurrent with their local recurrence; within 1 year, half will demonstrate distant disease. The median survival in this setting is 2 to 3 years.

Patients with an apparently isolated local recurrence can often be treated without systemic cytotoxic chemotherapy. These patients should undergo complete restaging following detection of the recurrence; for patients with a purely local recurrence, surgical excision combined with radiation therapy provides better local control than does either modality used alone.

METASTATIC BREAST CANCER

Metastatic breast cancer generally cannot be cured; the median survival following the detection of distant metastases is 2 years. Treatment in this setting is purely palliative, although significant prolongation of survival can be obtained with appropriate therapy. The most common site of distant metastatic spread is the osseous skeleton, followed by the soft tissues, distant lymph nodes, lungs, pleura, liver, and other tissues. Certain subtypes of breast cancer present different patterns of metastases. For example, patients with rapidly growing, hormone receptor-negative, and poorly differentiated tumors are more likely to have metastases to visceral organs, such as the liver, the lungs, and the brain.

On the other hand, tumors that are well-differentiated, express hormone receptors, and have a slower growth rate are more likely to develop metastases to bone and soft tissues, and are less likely to produce life-threatening manifestations.

For patients with overt metastases, the decision to treat with either systemic chemotherapy or hormonal therapy rests on several issues: site and extent of disease, hormone receptor status, disease-free interval, age, and menopausal status. In general terms, patients with slow-growing, limited, and non-life-threatening metastatic disease, who have hormone receptor–positive or known hormone-responsive tumors should be offered hormonal therapy as the first therapeutic modality. Because all hormonal manipulations used today have a better therapeutic ratio than do cytotoxic therapies, the practical result of sequential hormonal therapies is adding many months, sometimes several years, of high-quality life to the survival of patients with hormone-responsive metastatic breast cancer. For patients with more extensive (symptomatic) or life-threatening disease, and all patients with hormone receptor–negative breast cancer, combination chemotherapy represents the first treatment of choice. After three decades of clinical trials, it appears that the anthracyclines (e.g., doxorubicin) and the taxanes (e.g., paclitaxel and docetaxel) are the most effective antitumor agents against metastatic breast cancer. A chemotherapeutic regimen that includes an anthracycline or an anthracycline and taxane would be an appropriate initial choice.

BREAST CANCER AND PREGNANCY

The incidence of breast cancer detected during pregnancy is 2 per 10,000 gestations, accounting for 2.8% of all breast malignancies. The diagnosis of breast cancer is typically more difficult in a pregnant woman because of several factors, including a low level of suspicion based on generally young patient age, the relative frequency of nodular changes in the breast during pregnancy, and the fact that increased breast density during pregnancy renders mammographic imaging less accurate. For these reasons, the diagnosis of breast cancer during pregnancy is frequently delayed. This feature, rather than specific differences in the biology of breast cancer among pregnant and nonpregnant women, likely explains the relatively poor prognosis for women with breast cancer detected during pregnancy. When matched for tumor stage, pregnant women with breast cancer appear to have a prognosis no worse than that of nonpregnant patients.

Because of the inaccuracy of mammography in this setting, all persistent, suspicious breast masses discovered during pregnancy should undergo evaluation by fine-needle aspiration, core needle biopsy, or excisional biopsy. Excisional biopsy under local anesthesia represents a safe procedure at any time during pregnancy.

Once a diagnosis of malignancy is established, subsequent treatment decisions are influenced by their timing with respect to the specific trimester of pregnancy. For women who want to complete their pregnancies, the goal should be curative treatment of the breast cancer without injury to the fetus. Numerous studies have demonstrated that termination of pregnancy in hopes of minimizing hormonal stimulation of the tumor does not benefit maternal survival.

Surgical treatment of gestational breast cancer is generally conducted in a manner identical to that of nongestational breast cancer. There is no evidence that extraabdominal surgical procedures are associated with premature labor or that the typically used anesthetic agents are teratogenic. For women desiring modified radical mastectomy as primary therapy, this can be undertaken at any point during pregnancy without undue risk to mother or fetus. For cancer detected during the third trimester, delays in primary treatment of up to 4 weeks to allow for delivery before surgery are acceptable. If modified radical mastectomy is undertaken during pregnancy, breast reconstruction should not be performed simultaneously; a symmetric result is impossible until the postpartum appearance of the contralateral breast is known.

For women desiring breast conservation, treatment is complicated by the fact that radiation therapy is contraindicated during pregnancy. For cancers detected during the third trimester, lumpectomy and axillary dissection can safely be performed using general anesthesia, with radiation therapy delayed until after delivery. Longer delays may be detrimental to maternal outcome, although the time limit within which radiation therapy must be carried out to minimize the risk of local recurrence is unknown.

It may be necessary to administer cytotoxic adjuvant chemotherapy during pregnancy, raising fears of congenital malformations. Most series have demonstrated no increased risk of fetal malformation for chemotherapy administered during the second and third trimesters. In contrast, chemotherapy administration during the first trimester is associated with an increased incidence of spontaneous abortion and congenital malformation, especially when methotrexate is used.

CYSTOSARCOMA PHYLLODES

Cystosarcoma phyllodes represents an uncommon fibroepithelial breast neoplasm, accounting for only 0.5% to 1% of all female breast carcinomas. These tumors can occur in women of all ages, including adolescents and the elderly, with the majority arising in women between 35 and 55 years. Cystosarcoma phyllodes are typically quite large, with a mean diameter of 4 to 5 cm. Given the fact that phyllodes tumors are mammographically indistinguishable from fibroadenomas, the decision to perform excisional biopsy is usually based on large tumor size, a history of rapid growth, and the age of the patient. The ability to predict the behavior of these tumors based on histopathologic features such as histiotype (benign vs. indeterminate vs. malignant), margin status, stromal overgrowth, and size has been difficult due to, in part, their rarity. When metastases from cystosarcoma phyllodes do occur, common sites include the lung, bone, and mediastinum.

Appropriate treatment for phyllodes tumors is complete surgical excision. Breast conservation surgery with appropriate margins is the preferred primary therapy. Depending on the series, the incidence of local recurrence ranges from 5% to15% for benign tumors and 20% to 30% for malignant tumors. Local recurrences are typically salvageable with total mastectomy and have no impact on overall survival. For all phyllodes tumors, the incidence of axillary nodal metastases is less than 1%, obviating lymphadenectomy. The reported rates of distant metastasis for patients with malignant tumors range from 25% to 40%, and the presence of stromal overgrowth may be the strongest predictor of distant metastasis and ultimate outcome. To date, no role for radiation therapy, chemotherapy, or hormonal therapy has been established for this disease.

RECOMMENDED READING

Anonymous. Polychemotherapy for early breast cancer: an overview of the randomized trials. Early Breast Cancer Trialists' Collaborative Group. *Lancet* 1998;352:930.

Anonymous. Tamoxifen for early breast cancer: an overview of the randomized trials. Early Breast Cancer Trialists' Collaborative Group. *Lancet* 1998;351:1451.

Barnovon Y, Wallack MK. Management of the pregnant patient with carcinoma of the breast. *Surg Gynecol Obstet* 1990;171:347.

Braun S, Pantel K, Muller P, et al. Cytokeratin-positive cells in the bone marrow and survival of patients with stage I, II, or III breast cancer. *N Engl J Med* 2000;342:525.

Cady B. A contemporary view of axillary dissection. *Breast Dis Year Book Q* 2001;12:22.

Chaney AW, Pollack A, McNeese MD, et al. Primary treatment of cystosarcoma phyllodes of the breast. *Cancer* 2000;89:1502.

Fisher B, Redmond C, Fisher ER, et al. Ten-year results of a randomized clinical trial comparing radical mastectomy and total mastectomy with or without radiation. *N Engl J Med* 1985;312:674.

Fisher B, Anderson S, Redmond CK, et al. Reanalysis and results after 12 years of follow-up in a randomized clinical trial comparing total mastectomy with lumpectomy with or without irradiation in the treatment of breast cancer. *N Engl J Med* 1995;333:1456.

Fisher B, Bryant J, Wolmark N, et al. Effect of preoperative chemotherapy on the outcome of women with operable breast cancer. *J Clin Oncol* 1998;16:2672.

Greco M, Agresti R, Cascinelli N, et al. Breast cancer patients treated without axillary surgery: clinical implications and biologic analysis. *Ann Surg* 2000;232:1.

Grodstein F, Meir S, Graham C, et al. Postmenopausal hormone therapy and mortality. *N Engl J Med* 1997;336:1769.

Giuliano AE. Sentinel lymph node dissection in breast cancer. *Proc Am Soc Clin Oncol* 2001;530.

Harris JR, Lippman ME, Veronesi U, et al. Breast cancer. *N Engl J Med* 1992;327:319,390,473.

Henderson IC. Risk factors for breast cancer development. *Cancer* 1993;71[suppl6]:2128.

Hortobagyi GN. Treatment of breast cancer. *N Engl J Med* 1998;339:974.

Krag D, Weaver D, Ashikaga T, et al. The sentinel node in breast cancer: a multicenter validation study. *N Engl J Med* 1998;339:941.

Kuerer HM, Hunt KK, Newman LA, et al. Neoadjuvant chemotherapy in women with invasive breast carcinoma: conceptual basis and fundamental surgical issues. *J Am Coll Surg* 2000;190:350.

McGuire WL, Clark GM. Prognostic factors and treatment decisions in axillary node-negative breast cancer. *N Engl J Med* 1992;326: 1756.

Morrow M, Harris JR, Schnitt SJ. Local control following breast-conserving surgery for invasive cancer: results of clinical trials. *J Natl Cancer Inst* 1995;87:1669.

Overgaard M, Hansen PS, Overgaard J, et al. Postoperative radio-therapy in high-risk premenopausal women with breast cancer who receive adjuvant chemotherapy. Danish Breast Cancer Cooperative Group 82b Trial. *N Engl J Med* 1997;337:949.

Singletary SE. Systemic treatment after sentinel lymph node biopsy in breast cancer: who, what, and why? *J Am Coll Surg* 2001;192: 220.

Melanoma

Carlton C. Barnett, Jr., Jeffrey J. Sussman,
and Jeffrey E. Gershenwald

EPIDEMIOLOGY

Although melanoma is a relatively uncommon malignancy world-wide, its incidence is increasing dramatically, representing a significant and growing public health burden. An estimated 51,000 cases of invasive melanoma will be diagnosed in the United States in 2001. The current estimated lifetime risk of an American for developing melanoma is 1 in 74; an estimated 7,700 people will die of melanoma in 2001. Overall, the incidence of melanoma is now increasing faster than that of any other cancer. Melanoma is the most common cancer in American women 25 to 29 years old, and the second most common cancer in American women aged 30 to 34 years (second only to breast cancer). The standardized incidence of melanoma continues to increase in fair-skinned populations throughout the world. The major environmental factor, ultraviolet (UV) radiation (UV-B), is reflected in latitudinal and ethnic patterns of melanoma rates. Although the increase may have abated very recently—possibly as a result of increased early detection, changes in recreational behavior, and increased sun protection—it is unclear when the melanoma epidemic will peak and how geographic patterns will change over time. There have been changes in the distribution and stage of melanoma at diagnosis over the past 30 years, with an increase in thinner lesions. Many melanomas seen at many institutions now measure less than 1 mm in thickness.

RISK FACTORS

1. *Previous melanoma*: The risk of developing a second melanoma in a patient who has had a melanoma is 3% to 7%; this represents a 900-fold higher risk than that of the general population.
2. *Fair complexion*: Fair or red hair, light skin, blue eyes, and a propensity to sunburn are associated with an increased risk of melanoma.
3. *Sunlight exposure*: Occasional or recreational exposure to sunlight, especially a history of severe blistering sunburn, has been associated with increased risk of melanoma. The effects of sunlight have been attributed to exposure to UV-B radiation, which based on hypothetical mechanisms of melanoma induction, may account for approximately two-thirds of melanomas.
4. *Benign nevi*: Although a benign nevus is most likely not a precursor of melanoma, the presence of large numbers of nevi has been consistently associated with an increased risk of melanoma.

5. *Family history*: See the next item, *Genetic predisposition*.
6. *Genetic predisposition*: Specific genetic alterations have been implicated in the pathogenesis of melanoma. At least four distinct genes—located on chromosomes 1p, 6q, 7, and 9—may play a role in melanoma. A tumor suppressor gene located on chromosome 9p21 is probably involved in familial and sporadic cutaneous melanoma. Deletions or rearrangements of chromosomes 10 and 11 are also well documented in cutaneous melanoma. More recently, genetic research has identified specific variants that confer susceptibility to cutaneous malignant melanoma. Variants outside the coding region of the *CDKN2A* gene are associated with melanoma predisposition. A mutation in the 5′ untranslated end of *CDKN2A* generates a novel upstream initiation codon that abrogates expression of p16, which is necessary for tumor suppression.
7. *Atypical mole and melanoma syndrome (AMS)*: Previously known as dysplastic nevus syndrome, AMS is characterized by the presence of large numbers of atypical moles (dysplastic nevi) that represent a distinct clinicopathologic type of melanocytic lesion. They can be precursors of melanoma as well as markers of increased melanoma risk. The actual frequency of an atypical mole progressing to melanoma is small. Patients who are identified as having AMS should be observed closely, and family members should be screened.

PATHOLOGY

The four major melanoma growth patterns are as follows:

1. *Superficial spreading melanoma* constitutes the majority of melanomas (approximately 70%) and generally arises in a preexisting nevus.
2. *Nodular melanoma* is the second most common growth pattern (15%–30%). Nodular melanomas are more aggressive tumors and usually develop more rapidly than superficial spreading melanomas.
3. *Lentigo maligna melanoma* does not have the same propensity to metastasize as do other histologic types. Lentigo maligna melanomas constitute a small percentage of melanomas (4%–10%) and are typically located on the faces of older white women. They are usually large (>3 cm at diagnosis), flat lesions and are uncommon in individuals younger than 50.
4. *Acral lentiginous melanoma* occurs on the palms (palmar) or soles (plantar) or beneath the nail beds (subungual), although not all palmar, plantar, and subungual melanomas are acral lentiginous melanomas. These melanomas account for only 2% to 8% of melanomas in white patients but for a substantially higher proportion of melanomas (35%–60%) in darker-skinned patients. Acral lentiginous melanomas are the most aggressive histologic type. They are often large, with an average diameter of approximately 3 cm.

CLINICAL PRESENTATION

Clinical features of melanoma include (a) variegated color, (b) irregular raised surface, (c) irregular perimeter, and (d) surface ulceration. A biopsy should be performed on any pigmented lesion that undergoes a change in size, configuration, or color. The **ABCDs** of early diagnosis provide an easy way by which physicians and individuals may become familiar with the early signs of malignant melanoma. *A* denotes lesion asymmetry; *B,* border irregularity; *C,* color variegation; and *D,* diameter greater than 6 mm.

When a patient presents with a lesion suggestive of melanoma, a thorough physical examination must be performed, with particular emphasis on the skin, all nodal basins, and subcutaneous tissues. Chest radiograph and liver function studies should be obtained. Further evaluation is based on pathologic findings. We discourage routine extensive evaluation with computed tomography or bone scan because their yield in the absence of symptoms, abnormal laboratory findings, or an abnormal chest radiograph is very low in patients with primary melanoma.

STAGING

A limitation of the current (1997) staging system is that it does not utilize many of the prognostic factors that are currently used in the management of patients with melanoma. The American Joint Committee on Cancer (AJCC) Melanoma Task Force recently completed a comprehensive multivariate analysis of clinicopathologic and survival data for over 17,000 patients with melanoma. Based on these new data, the newly revised staging system for melanoma incorporates several essential factors now utilized in clinical practice yet omitted from the current system; these changes will become effective after the publication of the 6th edition of the *AJCC Staging Manual* in 2002 (Tables 3-1 and 3-2).

The current AJCC classification of the primary lesion is based on microscopic assessment of Breslow tumor thickness and Clark level of invasion. Breslow microstaging determines the thickness of the lesion, measured in millimeters, using an ocular micrometer to measure the total vertical height of the melanoma from the granular layer to the area of deepest penetration. Clark microstaging defines levels of invasion according to depth of penetration into the dermis. While the majority of this pathologic analysis is performed by using hematoxylin and eosin (H&E)–stained tumor, several melanocytic cell markers may be useful in confirming the diagnosis of melanoma. Two widely used antibodies used in immunohistochemical evaluations are S-100 and HMB-45. S-100 is expressed by more than 90% of melanomas but also by several other tumors and some normal tissues, including dendritic cells. In contrast, the monoclonal antibody HMB-45 is relatively specific (yet not as sensitive) for proliferative melanocytic cells and melanoma. It is therefore an excellent confirmatory stain for neoplastic cells when the diagnosis of melanoma is being considered. Recently, anti-MART-1 staining has also been shown to be useful in the diagnosis of melanoma.

T Classification

Consistent and uniform data now support the conclusion that thickness, rather than level of invasion, is more accurate, quantitative, and reproducible in determining outcome. Moreover, the

Table 3-1.   2002 AJCC melanoma TNM classification

T Classification	Thickness	Ulceration Status	
T1	≤ 1.0 mm	a: Without ulceration and level II/III	
		b: With ulceration or level IV/V	
T2	1.01–2.0 mm	a: Without ulceration	
		b: With ulceration	
T3	2.01–4.0 mm	a: Without ulceration	
		b: With ulceration	
T4	> 4.0 mm	a: Without ulceration	
		b: With ulceration	

N Classification	No. of Metastatic Nodes	Nodal Metastatic Mass
N1	1 node	a: Micrometastasis[a]
		b: Macrometastasis[b]
N2	2–3 nodes	a: Micrometastasis
		b: Macrometastasis
		c: In-transit met(s)/ satellite(s) without metastatic nodes
N3	4 or more metastatic nodes, or matted nodes, or in-transit met(s)/satellite(s) with metastatic node(s)	

M Classification	Site	Serum Lactate Dehydrogenase
M1a	Distant skin, subcutaneous, or nodal mets	Normal
M1b	Lung metastases	Normal
M1c	All other visceral metastases	Normal
	Any distant metastasis	Elevated

[a] Micrometastases are diagnosed after sentinel or elective lymphadenectomy.
[b] Macrometastases are defined as clinically detectable nodal metastases confirmed by therapeutic lymphadenectomy or nodal metastasis that exhibits gross extracapsular extension.
Modified from Balch CM, Buzaid AC, Soong SJ, et al. Final version of the American Joint Committee on Cancer staging system for cutaneous melanoma. *J Clin Oncol* 2001;19:3635–3648.

Table 3-2.   2002 AJCC stage groupings for cutaneous melanoma

	Clinical Staging[a]			Pathologic Staging[b]		
	T	N	M	T	N	M
0	Tis	N0	M0	Tis	N0	M0
IA	T1a	N0	M0	T1a	N0	M0
IB	T1b	N0	M0	T1b	N0	M0
	T2a	N0	M0	T2a	N0	M0
IIA	T2b	N0	M0	T2b	N0	M0
	T3a	N0	M0	T3a	N0	M0
IIB	T3b	N0	M0	T3b	N0	M0
	T4a	N0	M0	T4a	N0	M0
IIC	T4b	N0	M0	T4b	N0	M0
III[c]	Any T	N1	M0	—	—	—
		N2				
		N3				
IIIA	—	—	—	T1–4a	N1a	M0
				T1–4a	N2a	M0
IIIB	—	—	—	T1–4b	N1a	M0
				T1–4b	N2a	M0
				T1–4a	N1b	M0
				T1–4a	N2b	M0
				T1–4a/b	N2c	M0
IIIC	—	—	—	T1–4b	N1b	M0
				T1–4b	N2b	M0
				Any T	N3	M0
IV	Any T	Any N	Any M1	Any T	Any N	Any M1

[a] Clinical staging includes microstaging of the primary melanoma and clinical/radiologic evaluation for metastases. By convention, it should be used after complete excision of the primary melanoma with clinical assessment for regional and distant metastases.
[b] Pathologic staging includes microstaging of the primary melanoma and pathologic information about the regional lymph nodes after partial or complete lymphadenectomy. Pathologic stage 0 or stage 1A are the exception; patients do not require pathologic evaluation of the lymph nodes.
[c] There are no stage III subgroups for clinical staging.
Modified from Balch CM, Buzaid AC, Soong SJ, et al. Final version of the American Joint Committee on Cancer staging system for cutaneous melanoma. *J Clin Oncol* 2001;19:3635–3648.

AJCC Melanoma Task Force has adopted the integer values of 1 mm, 2 mm, and 4 mm as cutoffs for the T categories (Table 3-1). Primary tumor ulceration is histopathologically defined as the absence of an intact epidermis overlying a portion of the primary tumor. Importantly, this feature portends a significantly worse prognosis than nonulcerated melanomas of the same thickness. The letter *a* will signify a nonulcerated lesion, while *b* will represent an ulcerated primary. As such, ulcerated primary melanomas will be classified with nonulcerated lesions of the next higher T category (e.g., T1b and T2a), and this is reflected in the new T-stage groupings (Table 3-2). In summary, tumor thickness and ulceration will serve as the dominant prognostic factors in the

T classification. Clark level of invasion will remain a prognostic factor only for patients with T1 primary lesions.

N Classification

Although the 1997 staging system utilizes nodal size as the dominant prognostic factor with respect to N classification, multiple studies have demonstrated that the number of pathologically involved lymph nodes is a dominant and independent predictor of outcome and have provided little support for using gross dimensions of metastatic lymph nodes as a prognostic factor. On the basis of the AJCC analysis, lymph node involvement will be categorized as one, two to three, or four or more nodes involved.

The secondary criterion for the N classification relates to tumor burden as reflected in the designations of microscopic and macroscopic disease. Microscopic disease is defined as disease identified by either sentinel or elective lymphadenectomy (designated a), whereas macroscopic disease is defined as disease identified by clinical examination or radiologic imaging (designated b). This has become particularly relevant in view of the widespread use of intraoperative lymphatic mapping and selective lymphadenectomy. Moreover, recent data from the World Health Organization (WHO) Melanoma Program revealed that, compared to patients who underwent wide local excision of their primary melanoma followed by therapeutic lymphadenectomy when nodal disease was clinically evident, patients who had wide excision and concomitant elective regional lymph node dissection (and had pathologic evidence of microscopic nodal disease) fared significantly better (5-year survival rates, 48.2% vs. 26.6%, $p = 0.04$).

Interestingly, the presence of tumor ulceration, a dominant prognostic factor within the T classification system, has also been shown to be an independent adverse prognostic factor in patients with regional nodal disease. As such, patients with an ulcerated primary lesion will be upstaged within the N category as well as the T category compared to patients with similar nodal tumor burden with a nonulcerated primary lesion.

The presence of clinical or microscopic satellites around a primary melanoma and in-transit metastases between the primary tumor and regional lymph nodes represent various forms of intralymphatic metastases (i.e., similar biology) and portend a poor prognosis. In recognition of this important concept and in view of the similar survival rates among patients with one of these two entities, the AJCC Melanoma Task Force has omitted "satellitosis" from the T category (in which it is currently included) and has recommended that such patients be assigned a separate (N2c) classification. Further, the presence of microsatellites or in-transit metastases with concomitant lymph node metastases is associated with worse outcome than either event alone, leading these patients to be classified as N3 regardless of the number of synchronous metastatic lymph nodes.

M Classification

The number of metastatic sites and increased serum lactate dehydrogenase (LDH) levels are most predictive of poor prognosis.

Furthermore, patients who have distant metastases in soft tissues (skin, subcutaneous tissue and lymph nodes) fare better than patients with metastases to other sites and are designated as having Mla disease. Patients with metastases to the lung have an "intermediate" prognosis, and thus are designated as having Mlb disease. Patients with visceral metastases have "worse prognoses" and are designated as having Mlc disease. However, in view of the relatively poor prognosis associated with distant metastases, there are no stage IV groupings.

BIOPSY

The choice of biopsy technique varies according to the anatomic site, size, and shape of the lesion. Definitive therapy must be considered in choosing a biopsy technique. Either an excisional biopsy or an incisional biopsy using a scalpel or punch is acceptable. An excisional biopsy allows the pathologist to most accurately determine the thickness of the lesion. For excisional biopsies, a narrow margin of normal-appearing skin (1–3 mm) is taken with the specimen. An elliptical incision is used to facilitate closure. The biopsy incision should be oriented to facilitate later wide local excision (e.g., longitudinally on extremities) and minimize the need for a skin graft to provide wound closure. We reserve punch biopsy for lesions that are large, are located on anatomic areas where maximum preservation of surrounding skin is important, or can be completely excised with a 6-mm punch. Punch biopsies should be performed at the most raised or darkest area of the lesion. Full-thickness biopsy into the subcutaneous tissue must be performed to properly microstage the lesion.

Shave biopsies are contraindicated if a diagnosis of melanoma is being considered. Fine-needle aspiration biopsy may be used to document nodal and extranodal melanoma metastases but should not be used to diagnose primary melanomas. We send all pigmented lesions for permanent-section examination and perform definitive surgery at a later time.

MANAGEMENT OF LOCAL DISEASE

Local control of a primary melanoma requires wide excision of the tumor or biopsy site down to the deep fascia with a margin of normal-appearing skin. Risk of local recurrence correlates more with tumor thickness than with margins of surgical excision. It is rational to excise melanomas using surgical margins that vary according to tumor thickness.

Margins

The first randomized study involving surgical margins for melanomas less than 2 mm thick was reported by the WHO Melanoma Group. In an update of the study of 612 evaluable patients randomly assigned to receive a 1-cm or 3-cm margin of excision, there were no local recurrences among patients whose primary melanomas were thinner than 1 mm. There were four local recurrences in the 100 patients with melanomas 1- to 2-mm thick, and all four patients had received 1-cm margin excisions. There was no statistically significant difference in survival between the 1-cm and the 3-cm surgical margin groups.

These results demonstrate that a narrow excision margin for thin (<1 mm) melanomas is safe.

A multiinstitutional prospective randomized trial from France compared a 5-cm margin with a 2-cm margin in 319 patients with melanomas greater than or equal to 2 mm thick. There were no differences in local recurrence rate or survival.

A randomized prospective study conducted by the Intergroup Melanoma Committee compared 2-cm and 4-cm radial margins of excision for intermediate-thickness melanomas (1–4 mm). There was no difference in local recurrence rate between the 2-cm and the 4-cm margin groups. Forty-six percent of the 4-cm group required skin grafts, whereas only 11% of the 2-cm group did ($p < 0.001$). These data strongly support the use of a 2-cm margin for intermediate-thickness lesions.

Although these randomized prospective trials demonstrated the efficacy of 1-cm and 2-cm excision margins for thin and intermediate-thickness melanomas, respectively, the optimal management of thick melanomas (>4 mm thick) is still unknown. A retrospective review of 278 patients with thick primary melanomas demonstrated that the width of the excision margin (≤ 2 cm vs. >2 cm) did not significantly affect local recurrence, disease-free survival, or overall survival rates after a median follow-up of 27 months.

General recommendations for margins are as follows:

1. *Thin melanomas* (<1 mm) have a minimal risk of local recurrence. Wide excision with a 1-cm margin of normal-appearing skin is recommended.
2. *Intermediate-thickness melanomas* (1–4 mm) have an increased risk of local recurrence. A 2-cm margin can safely be used.
3. *Thick melanomas* (>4 mm) have a risk of local recurrence that may exceed 10% to 20%. A 2-cm margin is probably safe, although no prospective randomized trials have specifically addressed this thickness group.

Closure

If there is any question about the ability to achieve suitable wound closure, a plastic or reconstructive surgeon should be consulted. Options for closure include primary closure, skin grafting, and local and distant flaps.

Primary closure is the method of choice for most lesions, but it should be avoided when it will distort the appearance of a mobile facial feature or interfere with function. Many defects can be closed using an advancement flap, undermining the skin and subcutaneous tissues to permit primary closure. Primary closure usually requires that the longitudinal axis of an elliptical incision be at least three times longer than the short axis. Closure of the wound edges is usually performed in two layers. This may consist of a dermal layer of 3-0 or 4-0 undyed absorbable sutures, and either interrupted skin closure using 3-0 or 4-0 nonabsorbable sutures or a running subcuticular skin closure using 4-0 monofilament absorbable sutures.

Application of a *skin graft* is one of the simplest reconstructive methods. Split-thickness skin grafts are used most commonly. For lower-extremity primary lesions, split-thickness grafts should be harvested from the extremity opposite the melanoma. In general, skin grafts should be harvested from an area remote from the primary melanoma and outside the zone of potential in-transit metastasis. A full-thickness skin graft can provide a result that is both durable and of high aesthetic quality. The most common use of the full-thickness graft has been on the face, where aesthetic considerations are most significant. Donor sites for full-thickness skin graft to the face should be chosen from locations that are likely to match the color of the face, such as the postauricular or preauricular skin or the supraclavicular portion of the neck.

Local flaps offer a number of advantages for reconstruction of defects that cannot be closed primarily, especially on the distal extremities and on the head and neck. Color match is excellent, durability of the skin is essentially normal, and normal sensation is usually preserved. Transposition flaps and rotation flaps of many varieties have been used successfully.

Distant flaps should be used when sufficient tissue for a local flap is not available and when a skin graft would not provide adequate wound coverage. Myocutaneous flaps and free flaps can be used. Discussion of such complex methods is beyond the scope of this chapter, but these techniques are familiar to plastic and reconstructive surgeons.

Special Anatomic Sites

Fingers and Toes

More than three-fourths of subungual melanomas involve either the great toe or the thumb. A melanoma located on the skin of a digit or beneath the fingernail should be removed by a digital amputation, saving as much of the digit as possible. In general, amputations are performed at the middle interphalangeal joint of the fingers or proximal to the distal joint of the thumb. More proximal amputations are not associated with prolongation of survival. For a melanoma located on a toe, an amputation of the entire digit at the metatarsal-phalangeal joint is indicated; for melanomas of the great toe, the amputation can be performed proximal to the interphalangeal joint. Lesions arising between two toes often require amputation of both surrounding toes.

Sole of the Foot

Excision of a melanoma on the plantar surface often produces a sizable defect in a weight-bearing area. If possible, a portion of the heel or ball of the plantar surface should be retained to bear the greatest burden of pressure. Where possible, deep fascia over the extensor tendons should be preserved as a base for skin coverage. A plantar flap, which can be raised either laterally or medially, can provide well-vascularized local tissue for weight-bearing areas while also providing some sensation.

Face

Facial lesions usually cannot be excised with more than a 1-cm margin because of adjacent vital structures. The tumor diameter, thickness of the melanoma, and its exact location on the face must all be considered when determining margin width.

Breast

Wide local excision with primary closure is the treatment of choice for melanoma on the skin of the breast; mastectomy is not generally recommended. As with any trunk lesion, lymphoscintigraphy should be done before selective lymphadenectomy (see later) if this is indicated based on the basis of primary tumor factors.

Special Clinical Situations

Giant Congenital Nevi

Decisions about the management of giant congenital nevi are difficult because such lesions are often so extensive that prophylactic surgical excision is impossible. When the location and size of a lesion permit prophylactic excision, excision should be done before the age of 2 years.

Mucosal Melanoma

Patients with true mucosal melanoma—including melanoma of the mucosa of the head and neck, vagina, and anal canal—have, in general, a poor prognosis regardless of surgical therapy. We generally do not recommend an aggressive surgical approach to patients with clinically localized disease. We reserve extended resection for bulky or recurrent tumors and favor therapeutic over elective lymph node dissection (ELND) (see later). In particular, we recommend local excision of anal melanomas over abdominoperineal resection. Abdominoperineal resection is associated with a much higher morbidity, leaves the patient with a permanent colostomy, offers no survival advantage, and does not treat at-risk inguinal nodes unless combined with groin dissection. Adjuvant radiation therapy may be considered for patients with mucosal melanoma in an attempt to decrease the risk of locoregional recurrence.

Desmoplastic Melanoma

Desmoplastic or neurotropic melanoma is a rare variant of melanoma. Desmoplastic melanomas have a propensity for perineural invasion and infiltration of the blood vessel adventitia. These tumors often recur locally. Frozen-section examination is sometimes performed to ensure that excision margins are free of tumor. Adjuvant radiation therapy may decrease the risk of local recurrence.

Pregnancy

The precise influence of pregnancy or hormonal manipulation on the clinical course of malignant melanoma has not been defined. There is no conclusive evidence that concurrent pregnancy has an adverse effect on the disease course. Several large studies report no difference in outcome between gravid and nongravid patients with primary melanoma. Surgery is the treatment of choice in pregnant patients with early stage melanoma. There is no proof that abortion of the pregnancy protects the mother from subsequent development of metastases. Although opinions differ on planning a pregnancy after a diagnosis of melanoma, the weight of evidence does not demonstrate an increased risk of developing metastatic disease with pregnancy. Furthermore, several studies have found no association between oral contraceptive use and survival in melanoma.

General recommendations for managing melanoma during pregnancy are as follows:

1. The ultimate decision about continuing or terminating a pregnancy should be left to the patient and family.
2. A patient who presents with a primary melanoma during pregnancy should be evaluated with the minimum number of diagnostic tests.
3. The primary melanoma should be excised under appropriate anesthesia. ELND should not be performed. However, therapeutic dissection of regional lymph nodes should be considered, if warranted.
4. In pregnant patients with systemic metastases, the decision to abort or continue the pregnancy must be made on a case-by-case basis. Systemic chemotherapy during the second and third trimesters does not usually cause abnormalities in fetal development, unless alkylating agents are used.
5. If the mother had melanoma during pregnancy, the placenta should be examined histologically for evidence of metastasis at the time of delivery. Additionally, the child should be monitored carefully for metastatic disease during the first 6 to 12 months of life.
6. Women of childbearing age who have melanoma should probably not become pregnant or take oral contraceptives for 2 years after their treatment. Those 2 years represent the period of greatest risk for relapse with metastases. Conversely, however, should pregnancy occur during this time, abortion of the pregnancy is not necessary.

MANAGEMENT OF LOCAL RECURRENCE AND IN-TRANSIT DISEASE

The overall risk of local recurrence is low—3% in a collected series of 3,520 patients.

Local recurrence usually develops within 5 years after primary melanoma excision. Local recurrence implies a poor prognosis and often portends distant metastases. In a study of 95 patients with local recurrences, the median survival duration was 3 years, with a 10-year survival rate of only 20%.

In-transit metastases are located between the primary melanoma and the first major regional nodal basin. Overall, the incidence of in-transit metastases is 2% to 3%, but it may be higher in certain subsets of patients. Regional nodal metastases occur in about two thirds of patients with in-transit metastases and, if present, are associated with lower survival rates. Patients with few in-transit metastases have better prognoses than those with multiple lesions.

Comparison studies of treatment alternatives for local recurrences and in-transit disease have not been performed. Options include surgical excision, regional chemotherapy using isolated limb perfusion, and radiation therapy.

A single local recurrence in a patient whose primary melanoma had favorable prognostic features can be excised and no further treatment given. Alternatively, adjuvant treatment can be considered, for example, in the form of high-dose interferon-α (IFN-α). Patients with multiple local recurrences, with local recurrence and poor prognostic features of the primary melanoma, or with in-transit metastases may be considered for regional treatment. Regional treatment options include isolated limb perfusion and radiation therapy using a high-dose-per-fraction technique. More recently, the technique of isolated limb infusion has been used in some centers as a minimally invasive form of regional therapy. Rarely, amputation may be necessary for extensive or deeply infiltrative lesions involving the foot, hand, arm, or leg.

Isolated Hyperthermic Limb Perfusion

Melphalan is the most active single agent for use in hyperthermic isolated limb perfusion. Complete response rates average 40% in patients with measurable disease. Recent nonrandomized studies of hyperthermic limb perfusion by Leinard et al. (1992) have reported a high complete response rate (90%) using a combination of melphalan, tumor necrosis factor-α (TNF-α), and IFN gamma, and a somewhat lower rate with melphalan alone (52%). The durability of these responses has not yet been reported. Fraker et al. (1996) reported a 100% response rate in patients treated with melphalan alone and a 90% response rate in patients perfused with melphalan, IFN gamma, and TNF-α, although the latter combination resulted in a higher complete response rate (80% vs. 61%). Significant palliation of regional symptoms (e.g., pain, edema, bleeding, and ulceration) has also been achieved at the National Institutes of Health using multiagent perfusion regimens in patients with locally advanced melanoma in an extremity. A multicenter randomized trial sponsored by the American College of Surgeons Oncology Group (ACOSOG) is currently underway comparing perfusion of melphalan alone with perfusion with a combination of melphalan and TNF-α for patients with in-transit melanoma metastases.

Role of Adjuvant Hyperthermic Limb Perfusion

Hyperthermic isolated limb perfusion has been shown to benefit only small subgroups of patients in the adjuvant setting. Although a recent randomized multicenter phase III trial showed an increased disease-free interval in patients with in-transit metastases and regional lymph node metastasis, this effect was transient and predominantly occurred in patients with a more favorable prognosis (thickness 1.5–2.99 mm). This study showed no benefit of isolated limb perfusion with respect to time to distant metastasis or survival duration.

Toxicity

Isolated limb perfusion is associated with potentially significant regional toxicity, including myonecrosis, nerve injury, and arterial thrombosis, sometimes requiring major amputation. Systemic toxicity, including hypotension and adult respiratory distress syndrome, is sometimes seen with the addition of TNF-α to the regimen. The treatment requires a high degree of technical expertise and carries a significant risk of major complications, including limb loss. The procedure should therefore be performed only in centers that have experience with the technique, preferably in the setting of a clinical trial. At present, there is little evidence to justify the use of prophylactic perfusion except as part of a clinical trial.

Isolated Limb Infusion

The technique of isolated limb infusion has been utilized in some centers as a minimally invasive form of regional therapy that can spare the significant potential morbidity of isolated limb perfusion. Although long-term results are not available, early results are promising.

MANAGEMENT OF REGIONAL DISEASE

Regional lymph nodes are the most common site of metastatic melanoma. Effective palliation and sometimes cure can be achieved in patients with regional metastases. Fine-needle aspiration or core biopsy can often yield a diagnosis in patients who develop clinically enlarged regional nodes. Open biopsy is rarely warranted.

Surgical excision of nodal metastases is the only treatment effective in achieving local disease control and cure. Incomplete lymph node dissection is unacceptable. Historically, some surgeons preferred to perform lymphadenectomy only for clinically demonstrable nodal metastases. This type of excision has been termed *delayed* or *therapeutic lymph node dissection* (TLND). Other surgeons choose to excise the nodes even when they appear normal in patients who are at increased risk of developing nodal metastases. This excision has been termed *immediate, prophylactic,* or *elective lymph node dissection (ELND)*. More recently, many surgeons have adopted a selective approach to regional lymphadenectomy based on the technique of intraoperative lymphatic mapping and sentinel lymph node (SLN) identification developed by Morton et al. (1992).

ELND has the theoretical advantage of treating melanoma nodal metastases at a relatively early stage in the natural history of the disease. Its disadvantage is that many patients undergo surgery when they do not have nodal metastases. Thus an advantage of TLND is that only patients with demonstrable metastases undergo major operations; this reduces the number of potentially unnecessary lymphadenectomies while not necessarily reducing the chance for cure. The disadvantage of TLND is that delaying treatment until lymph node metastases are clinically palpable may result in many patients having distant micrometastases at the time of lymphadenectomy. Chances for cure may therefore be diminished. The technique of lymphatic mapping and SLN biopsy offers a selective approach to ELND that satisfies many proponents both of ELND and of TLND.

Elective Lymph Node Dissection

The role of ELND in the management of clinically localized (stage I and II) primary melanoma has been the focus of great debates. Although ELND does not offer a survival benefit to all patients, recently completed prospective randomized trials have shown that ELND confers benefit in prospectively defined subgroups of melanoma patients.

An international cooperative study conducted by the WHO Melanoma Group to examine the efficacy of immediate regional node dissection in patients with melanomas of the trunk at least 1.5-mm thick demonstrated that routine use of immediate ELND had no impact. However, compared with patients who had immediate lymph node dissection and microscopic regional node metastasis identified only after pathologic analysis of the surgical specimen, patients in whom node dissection was delayed until the regional nodes became clinically and histologically positive during observation had the poorer prognosis. This suggests that the dissection of clinically undetectable regional node metastasis leads to prolonged long-term survival.

More recently, the long-term results of the Intergroup Melanoma Surgical Trial have been reported. This trial examined 10- to 15-year survival rates in patients with intermediate thickness melanomas (1.0–4.0 mm) who underwent concomitant ELND in a similar group of patients who underwent wide excision alone, and in a group of patients who were observed. Additional prognostic factors, including stratified tumor thickness, anatomic site, age, gender, and the presence or absence of ulceration, were examined. Although this trial did not demonstrate a difference in overall 10-year survival rates, four prospectively selected subgroups were found to have significantly better outcomes with ELND than with nodal observation. First, there was significant improvement in the 10-year survival rate after ELND in patients whose primary tumors were without ulceration, (84% vs. 77%; $p = 0.03$). Second, the 10-year survival rate was significantly better in patients who had primary tumors with a thickness between 1.0 and 2.0 mm than in patients with thicker tumors (86% vs. 80%; $p = 0.03$). Third, the 10-year survival rate following ELND was significantly higher in patients with extremity melanoma than in those with truncal melanomas (84% vs. 78%; $p = 0.05$). Fourth, age younger than 60 years was a significant predictor of improved survival following ELND versus nodal observation (81% vs. 74%; $p = 0.03$). The survival benefit of ELND revealed by this surgical trial provides the impetus to support SLN dissection to allow early surgical intervention if micrometastasis is present.

Intraoperative Lymphatic Mapping and Sentinel Lymph Node Biopsy

A rational alternative or adjunct to ELND has emerged that has already significantly altered the surgical approach to primary melanoma in most large cancer centers, including M.D. Anderson Cancer Center. This approach, termed *selective lymphadenectomy,* includes lymphatic mapping and SLN biopsy and relies on the concept that finite regions of the skin drain first to specific lymph nodes—sentinel lymph nodes—within the regional basin via an organized system of afferent lymphatic channels. At the time of wide excision, a vital blue dye (patent blue V or isosulfan blue) is injected intradermally at the primary melanoma or biopsy site. Exploration of the draining nodal basin (identified by prior lymphoscintigraphy) allows the lymphatic channels and the first draining (i.e., sentinel) lymph node to be identified by their uptake of the blue dye. Using this technique, Morton et al. (1992) proved that (a) the SLN is the first node to which a cutaneous primary melanoma is likely to metastasize, and (b) the histologic status of the SLN reflects the histologic status of the remainder of the regional nodal basin. This approach spares patients with a histologically negative SLN the morbidity and expense of an unnecessary procedure, because ELND is offered only to patients in whom metastatic melanoma is identified in the SLN. Two subsequent series confirmed the results of the original trial: the SLN was identified in 85% or greater of patients, and in 8% or fewer of patients was metastatic melanoma identified elsewhere in the regional nodal basins (by concomitant lymphadenectomy at the time of SLN biopsy) when the SLN was histopathologically free of tumor.

It is imperative that the surgeon contemplating the use of these techniques in his or her practice have adequate pathology and nuclear medicine support; close collaboration is essential to perform these procedures accurately.

Technique

To improve SLN localization, two techniques—preoperative lymphoscintigraphy and intraoperative lymphatic mapping accompanied by use of a handheld gamma probe—have been incorporated into our treatment strategy for patients with clinically node-negative primary melanoma.

Lymphoscintigraphy is an essential adjunct to determining which regional basins are at risk in patients with primary melanomas located in ambiguous drainage sites (e.g., trunk, head, and neck), because historical lymphatic drainage guidelines are often inaccurate. The test involves the intradermal injection of a radiocolloid such as technetium Tc 99m sulfur colloid around the primary tumor site and subsequent nuclear scanning of regional nodal basins. This technique can also be used to localize potential SLNs, before surgical exploration, within epitrochlear or popliteal nodal regions in patients with primary tumors distal to the elbow or knee, respectively. This technique may occasionally identify a SLN present outside typical lymphatic drainage basins, especially in patients with truncal primaries, and may sometimes represent the only evidence of nodal disease. Therefore, failure to accurately identify these nodes may result in understaging of the patient's disease. Moreover, it is not uncommon for two or more nodal basins to be identified by these scans. Because patients with multiple nodal basin drainage patterns may harbor occult metastases in one or more nodal basins, and because the pathologic status of a nodal basin does not necessarily correlate with that of the other regional nodal basins, it is imperative to perform sentinel lymphadenectomy on all regional nodal basins at risk for metastatic disease.

Following the intradermal injection of 0.5 to 1.0 mCi of unfiltered Tc 99m sulfur colloid 1 to 4 hours before surgery, lymphatic mapping is subsequently performed with the aid of a handheld gamma probe. This device, designed for intraoperative use, permits the surgeon to identify the region or regions of greatest radiotracer uptake, which correspond to the sites of the SLNs.

This technology is based on the principle that the radiolabeled colloid is actively incorporated into the draining SLN. Accurate localization can therefore be obtained before incision, resulting in better-directed and smaller incisions as well as rapid intraoperative identification of the node. Although a few groups rely on only one of these techniques (vital blue dye or intraoperative lymphoscintigraphy with use of a handheld gamma probe), we strongly believe that these two techniques are complementary and have incorporated both into our current practice. Our experience with the combination has yielded an SLN identification rate of greater than 99%.

Prognostic Value of Sentinel Lymph Node Status

Following the demonstration that the histologic status of the SLN accurately reflects the histologic status of the nodal basin, several major centers incorporated selective lymphadenectomy into their approach for patients with primary melanoma who have clinically negative regional nodal basins. The experience at M.D. Anderson Cancer Center and H. Lee Moffitt Cancer Center has recently been analyzed. Lymphatic mapping and SLN biopsy were successful in 580 of 612 patients (95%) who underwent the procedure. SLN status was the most significant prognostic factor with respect to disease-free and disease-specific survival rates by univariate and multivariate analyses (Fig. 3-1).

A National Cancer Institute–sponsored international, multicenter prospective randomized trial of SLN biopsy known as the Multicenter Selective Lymphadenectomy Trial (MSLT) is currently accruing patients with stage I or II disease whose melanomas are thicker than 1 mm (principal investigator of this trial is Donald Morton, M.D.). Patients are randomized in a 2:1 fashion to receive either wide local excision and SLN biopsy or wide local excision alone. Completion lymphadenectomy will be performed for those patients with pathologic evidence of metastatic melanoma in at least one SLN. This trial will address the following issues: (a) What is the long-term false-negative rate for SLN biopsy? (b) What, if any, survival benefit is achieved with selective node dissection in patients with micrometastatic regional nodal involvement? (c) What is the therapeutic benefit, if any, of removing a histologically negative SLN that actually harbors submicroscopic disease?

Pathologic Evaluation of the Sentinel Lymph Node

The reported survival benefit for patients with nodal metastases who are treated systemically with high-dose IFN alfa-2b provides at least one impetus for accurate assessment of nodal status in patients with clinically negative nodal basins. Several investigators have demonstrated that SLN biopsy is an accurate way to detect disease in the nodal basin without complete lymphadenectomy. However, conventional histologic techniques for evaluating lymph nodes (i.e., bisection of lymph nodes followed by H&E staining) may underestimate disease, primarily because of sampling error. The combination of serial sectioning and immunostaining improves the detection of microscopic metastases in examined nodes.

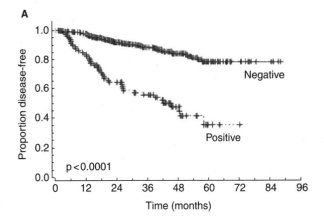

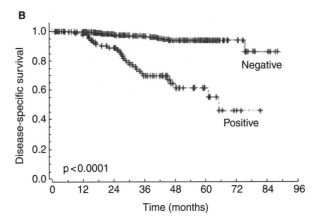

Fig. 3-1.   Kaplan-Meier survival data for patients undergoing successful lymphatic mapping and sentinel lymph node (SLN) biopsy stratified by SLN status. Disease-free survival (A) and disease-specific survival (B) rates were significantly better for patients with a negative SLN biopsy (each $p < 0.0001$). (From Gershenwald JE, Thompson W, Mansfield PF, et al. Multi-institutional melanoma lymphatic mapping experience: the prognostic value of sentinel lymph node status in 612 stage I or II melanoma patients. *J Clin Oncol* 1999;17(3):976–983, with permission.)

In a cohort of 243 consecutive patients who underwent lymphatic mapping at M.D. Anderson had a negative SLN biopsy, and were then followed up expectantly with the remaining lymph nodes intact, local recurrences, in-transit metastases, regional nodal metastases, and/or distant metastases developed in 11% during a median follow-up of 3 years. Although failure in the regional nodal basin was rare, the regional nodes represented the most common site of first recurrence in this population: a nodal metastasis in the previously mapped basin developed in 4%, alone or at the same time as recurrence elsewhere. Three potential mechanisms can be offered to explain these false-negative findings: (a) technical failure—the true SLN was not identified; (b) pathologic failure—the appropriate lymph node was removed but routine histologic evaluation failed to identify microscopic disease; and (c) biologic failure—recurrence occurred in a nodal basin as a result of residual microscopic satellite or in-transit disease that persisted after wide excision of the primary tumor. Therefore, paraffin blocks of the SLN specimens from patients in whom recurrent melanoma developed were reevaluated using a combination of serial sectioning and immunohistochemical staining (S-100 and HMB-45). The SLNs demonstrated evidence of occult disease in 80% of the patients in whom nodal metastasis developed. In contrast, no evidence of micrometastatic nodal disease was demonstrated by any of these techniques in patients who had only local, in-transit, or distant recurrence.

Recently, the molecular biologic technique of reverse transcriptase-polymerase chain reaction (RT-PCR) to detect tyrosinase mRNA has been reported to increase detection of occult disease. The obvious potential advantage of RT-PCR is that the entire node can be evaluated, minimizing sampling error. A potential drawback of this technique is that disease found at this submicroscopic level may not be clinically relevant in patients whose SLNs are negative by other pathologic techniques. A recent study from the H. Lee Moffitt Cancer Center examined RT-PCR, H&E staining, and immunohistochemical staining against S-100 in the evaluation of sentinel lymph nodes. H&E staining revealed metastatic disease in 36 of 233 patients, while S-100 immunostaining revealed metastatic disease in 52 of 233 patients. Significantly, however, RT-PCR for tyrosinase was positive in 114 (63%) of 181 histologically negative nodes. Despite a relatively short median follow-up interval, the recurrence rate in patients with H&E-negative/PCR-negative nodes was 1.6%, while it was 10.1% in the group whose nodes were H&E-negative/PCR-positive ($p = 0.06$). Although recent data suggest that PCR-based prognostic evaluations may be clinically relevant, longer follow-up intervals are required before such evaluations become a standard of care.

The relative clinical importance of conventional histology, serial sectioning, and molecular staging in patients undergoing lymphatic mapping and SLN biopsy is being evaluated in a large, multicenter, randomized, prospective trial known as the Sunbelt Melanoma Trial.

Current Practice Guidelines

In general, we offer selective lymphadenectomy (lymphatic mapping and SLN biopsy) to patients with stage I or II melanoma. Specifically, all patients diagnosed with primary cutaneous melanoma are offered the procedure if the primary melanoma is at least 1.0 mm thick or, if less than 1.0 mm, is at least Clark's level IV, is ulcerated, or demonstrates evidence of regression and if the patient has no evidence of metastatic melanoma in regional lymph nodes and distant sites by physical examination and staging evaluation (chest radiograph and measurement of LDH levels). Recently, we also have offered this procedure to patients whose primary tumor demonstrates evidence of vertical growth phase, a pathologic feature that has been associated with an increased risk of lymphatic metastases.

Patients in whom the primary tumor arises in areas of ambiguous drainage (for example, the trunk) or the distal extremity undergo preoperative lymphoscintigraphy. Technetium 99m sulfur colloid is administered intradermally to establish lymphatic drainage patterns and identify those basins at risk for metastatic melanoma. Patients receive an intradermal injection of 0.5 to 1.0 mCi of unfiltered Tc 99m–labeled sulfur colloid 1 to 4 hours before surgery. In addition, 1 to 3 mL of isosulfan blue dye is injected intradermally around the intact tumor or biopsy site immediately before surgery. Lymphatic mapping is subsequently performed with the aid of a handheld gamma probe. In patients undergoing mapping of more than one basin, the basin with predominant drainage by preoperative lymphoscintigraphy is explored first. An SLN is defined as one that localizes blue dye or concentrates radiolabeled colloid and is located within or, more recently, near a regional nodal basin. All patients also undergo wide local excision of the primary melanoma with margins appropriate for tumor thickness.

Excised SLNs are analyzed by conventional histologic staining (H&E) of grossly sectioned specimens. Histologic serial sectioning is performed on all nonpositive SLNs. Immunohistochemical staining using antisera to the S-100 protein or the melanoma antigen HMB-45 and/or MART1 is performed if suspicious cells are seen to clarify equivocal H&E findings or if the initial pathologic examination is negative. Frozen-section analysis is used only to confirm the presence of metastatic melanoma in SLNs that are grossly suggestive of metastasis and for patients with whom concomitant lymph node dissection has been discussed.

When the SLN is negative, no further surgery is done; the remaining regional nodes are left intact. For patients in whom the SLN or SLNs contain evidence of metastatic melanoma, TLND of the affected basins is recommended.

Postoperative follow-up consists of physical examination, chest x-ray, and determinations of LDH levels. Further investigations, including computed tomography or magnetic resonance imaging, are also performed selectively to confirm abnormal findings suggestive of metastatic melanoma. A routine program of postoperative surveillance can be based on tumor thickness and results of SLN biopsy; one standard follow-up schedule for patients treated at M.D. Anderson consists of evaluation every 3 to 4 months for the first 2 years, every 6 months in years 3 to 5, and annually thereafter.

In centers where a selective approach to ELND is not feasible, the results of the Intergroup Melanoma Committee trial can be incorporated into surgical strategies for patients. ELND should be offered to improve survival benefit in patients younger than 60 years, in patients with primary tumors that are 1.1 to 2.0 mm thick and nonulcerated, and for primary tumors on the extremities.

Technical Considerations

Axillary Lymph Node Dissection

GENERAL. Axillary dissection must be complete and include the level III lymph nodes (Fig. 3-2). The arm, shoulder, and chest are prepared and included in the surgical field.

INCISION. We use a horizontal, slightly S-shaped incision beginning anteriorly along the superior portion of the pectoralis

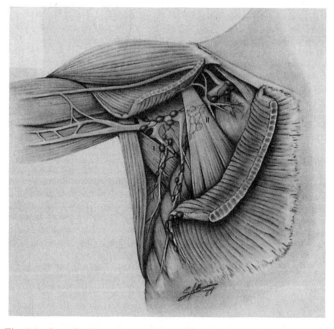

Fig. 3-2. Lymphatic anatomy of the axilla demonstrating the three groups of axillary lymph nodes defined by their relationship to the pectoralis minor muscle. The highest axillary nodes (level III) medial to the pectoralis minor muscle should be included in an axillary lymph node dissection for melanoma. (From Balch CM, Milton GW, Shaw HM, et al., eds. *Cutaneous melanoma.* Philadelphia: Lippincott, 1985.)

major muscle, traversing the axilla over the fourth rib, and extending inferiorly along the anterior border of the latissimus dorsi muscle.

SKIN FLAPS. Skin flaps are raised anteriorly to the midclavicular line, inferiorly to the sixth rib, posteriorly to the anterior border of the latissimus dorsi muscle, and superiorly to just below the pectoralis major insertion. The medial side of the latissimus dorsi muscle is dissected free from the specimen, exposing the thoracodorsal vessels and nerve. The lateral edge of the dissection then proceeds cephalad beneath the axillary vein. These maneuvers allow the remainder of the dissection to proceed from medial to lateral. The fatty and lymphatic tissue over the pectoralis major muscle is dissected free around to its undersurface, where the pectoralis minor muscle is encountered. The interpectoral groove is exposed.

LYMPH NODE DISSECTION. The medial pectoral nerve is preserved. The interpectoral nodes are dissected free. Exposure of the upper axilla is obtained by bringing the patient's arm over the chest by adduction and internal rotation. If nodes are bulky, the pectoralis minor muscle may need to be divided. Dissection proceeds from the apex of the axilla inferolaterally. Dissection of the upper axillary lymph nodes should be sufficiently complete that the thoracic outlet beneath the clavicle, Halsted's ligament, and the subclavius muscle are seen (Fig. 3-3). Fatty and lymphatic tissues are dissected downward over the brachial plexus and axillary artery until the axillary vein is exposed. The apex of the dissected specimen is tagged. Dissection then continues until the thoracodorsal vessels and the long thoracic and thoracodorsal nerves are identified. The fatty tissue between the two nerves is separated from the subscapularis muscle. The specimen is removed from the lateral chest wall. Intercostobrachial nerves traversing the specimen are sacrificed. The specimen is swept off the latissimus dorsi and the serratus anterior muscles.

WOUND CLOSURE. One 15 F closed-suction catheter is placed percutaneously through the inferior flap into the axilla. An additional catheter may be inserted through the inferior flap and placed over the pectoralis major muscle. The skin is closed with interrupted 3-0 undyed absorbable sutures and running 4-0 subcuticular undyed absorbable sutures.

POSTOPERATIVE MANAGEMENT. Suction drainage is continued until output is less than 30 mL per day. By approximately 3 weeks, the suction catheters are removed, regardless of the amount of drainage, to avoid infection. Any subsequent collections of serum are treated by needle aspiration. Mobilization of the arm is discouraged during the first 7 to 10 days after surgery. Over the ensuing 4 weeks, gradual mobilization of the arm is encouraged. The complication rate for axillary lymph node dissection is low. The most frequent complication is wound seroma.

Groin Dissection

For groin dissection, the patient is placed in a slight frog-leg position.

INCISION. A reverse lazy S incision is made from superomedial to the anterior superior iliac spine, vertically down to the inguinal

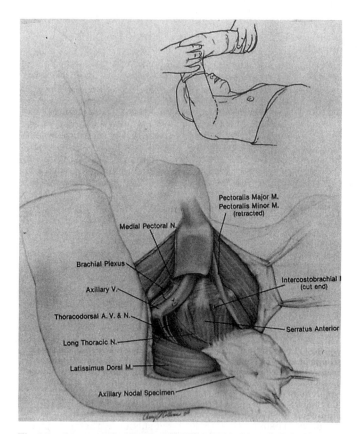

Fig. 3-3. Access to the upper axilla. The arm is draped so that it can be brought over the chest wall during the operation. This facilitates retraction of the pectoralis muscles upward to reveal level III axillary lymph nodes. (From Balch CM, Milton GW, Shaw HM, et al., eds. *Cutaneous melanoma*. Philadelphia: Lippincott, 1985.)

crease, obliquely across the crease, and then vertically down to the apex of the femoral triangle.

SKIN FLAPS. The limits of the skin flaps are medially to the pubic tubercle and the midbody of the adductor magnus muscle, laterally to the lateral edge of the sartorius muscle, superiorly to above the inguinal ligament, and inferiorly to the apex of the femoral triangle. We sometimes incorporate an ellipse of skin with the specimen.

LYMPH NODE DISSECTION. Dissection is carried down to the muscular fascia superiorly (Fig. 3-4). All fatty, node-bearing tissue is swept down to the inguinal ligament and off the external oblique fascia. Medially, the spermatic cord or round ligament is exposed

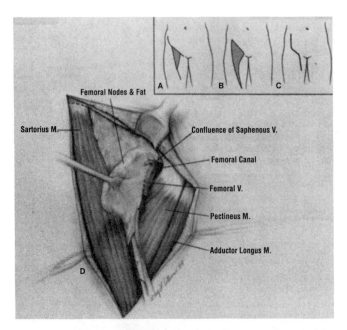

Fig. 3-4. Technique of inguinal lymph node dissection. (From Balch CM, Milton GW, Shaw HM, et al., eds. *Cutaneous melanoma.* Philadelphia: Lippincott, 1985.)

and nodal tissue is swept laterally. Nodal tissue is swept off the adductor fascia to the femoral vein. At the apex of the femoral triangle, the saphenous vein is divided. Laterally, nodal tissue is dissected off the sartorius muscle and the femoral nerve. With dissection in the plane of the femoral vessels, the nodal tissue is elevated up to the level of the fossa ovalis, where the saphenous vein is suture-ligated at the saphenofemoral junction. The specimen is dissected to beneath the inguinal ligament, where it is divided. Cloquet's node (the lowest iliac node) is sent as a separate specimen for frozen-section examination (Fig. 3-5).

SARTORIUS MUSCLE TRANSPOSITION. The sartorius muscle is divided at its insertion on the anterior superior iliac spine (Fig. 3-6). The lateral femoral cutaneous nerve is preserved. The proximal two or three neurovascular bundles going to the sartorius muscle are divided to facilitate transposition. The muscle is placed over the femoral vessels and tacked to the inguinal ligament, fascia of the adductor, and vastus muscle groups.

WOUND CLOSURE. The skin edges are examined for viability and trimmed back to healthy skin, if necessary. Intravenous administration of fluorescein and the Wood's lamp may be used to identify poorly perfused skin edges. Two closed-suction drains are placed through separate stab wounds inferiorly. One is laid medially and the other is laid laterally within the operative wound. The wound

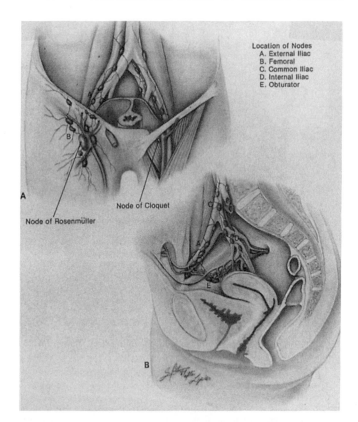

Location of Nodes
A. External Iliac
B. Femoral
C. Common Iliac
D. Internal Iliac
E. Obturator

Node of Cloquet

Node of Rosenmüller

Fig. 3-5. A: Lymphatic anatomy of the inguinal area demonstrating the superficial and deep lymphatic chains. The node of
Cloquet lies at the transition between the superficial and deep
inguinal nodes. It is located beneath the inguinal ligament in the
femoral canal. B: The iliac nodes include those on the common and
superficial iliac vessels and the obturator nodes. Obturator nodes
should be excised as part of an iliac nodal dissection. (From Balch
CM, Milton GW, Shaw HM, et al., eds. *Cutaneous melanoma.*
Philadelphia: Lippincott, 1985.)

is closed with interrupted 3-0 undyed absorbable sutures in the
dermis and skin staples.

POSTOPERATIVE MANAGEMENT. The patient begins ambulating
the day following surgery and is measured for a custom-fit elastic stocking to be used during the day for 6 months. After this
period, the stocking may be discontinued if no leg swelling occurs. We use a mild diuretic, such as hydrochlorothiazide, on an
individual basis.

DISSECTION OF THE ILIAC AND OBTURATOR NODES. We perform
deep (iliac) dissection for the following indications: (a) known

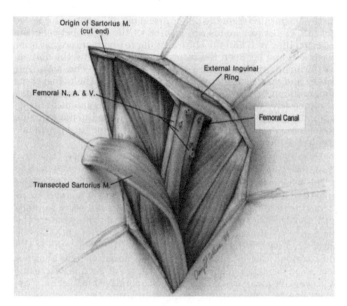

Fig. 3-6. Transection of the sartorius muscle at its origin on the anterior superior iliac spine in preparation for transposition over the femoral vessels and nerves. (From Balch CM, Milton GW, Shaw HM, et al., eds. *Cutaneous melanoma.* Philadelphia: Lippincott, 1985.)

involvement (revealed by preoperative mapping studies), (b) more than three grossly positive nodes in the superficial specimen, or (c) metastatic disease in Cloquet's node by frozen-section examination. To gain access to the deep nodes, we extend the skin incision superiorly. The external oblique muscle is split from a point superomedial to the anterior superior iliac spine to the lateral border of the rectus sheath. The internal oblique and transversus abdominis muscles are divided, and the peritoneum is retracted superiorly. An alternative approach is to split the inguinal ligament vertically, medial to the femoral vein. The ureter is exposed as it courses over the iliac artery. Dissection continues in front of the external iliac artery to separate the external iliac nodes. The inferior epigastric artery and vein are divided if necessary. Dissection of the lymph nodes continues to the common iliac artery. Nodes in front of the external iliac vein are dissected to the point at which the latter proceeds under the internal iliac artery. The plane of the peritoneum is traced along the wall of the bladder, and the fatty tissues and lymph nodes are dissected off the perivesical fat starting at the internal iliac artery. Dissection is completed on the medial wall of the external iliac vein, and the nodal chain is further separated from the pelvic fascia until the obturator nerve is seen. Obturator nodes are located in the space between the external iliac vein and the obturator nerve (in an anteroposterior direction) and between the internal iliac artery and the obturator foramen (in a cephalad-caudad direction). The obturator artery and vein usually need not be disturbed. The transversus abdominis, internal oblique, and external oblique muscles may be closed with running sutures. The inguinal ligament, if previously divided, is approximated with interrupted nonabsorbable sutures to Cooper's ligament medially and to the iliac fascia lateral to the femoral vessels.

COMPLICATIONS. The most common acute postoperative complication is wound infection. Rates range from 5% to 19%. The rate of lymphocele or seroma formation is 3% to 23%. Leaving suction catheters in place until the drainage decreases to 30 to 40 mL per day may reduce the incidence of seroma. However, prolonged stay of catheters is associated with a higher rate of infection. Lymphedema is the most serious long-term complication. Three series have shown that the incidence of leg edema after groin dissection can be decreased by preventive measures, including perioperative antibiotics, elastic stockings, leg elevation exercises, and diuretics. Prophylactic measures are important because reversing the progression of edema is difficult. Skin flap problems occur with some frequency. Expectant management of ischemic edges often results in full-thickness necrosis and prolonged hospitalization. If edges are of questionable viability, therefore, the patient is returned to the operating room early for flap revision. Clinically detectable deep vein thrombosis is uncommon.

Neck Dissection

Metastases to lymph nodes from primary melanomas in the head and neck were previously believed to follow a predictable pattern. However, lymphatic drainage from primary melanomas of the head and neck can be multidirectional and unpredictable; preoperative lymphoscintigraphy is needed to identify the basins at risk for metastases. ELND or SLN biopsy (see later) may be misdirected in as many as 59% of patients if the operation is based on classic anatomic studies without such preoperative evaluation. These findings strongly support the use of lymphoscintigraphy in these patients.

Wide local excision of the primary lesion with either modified radical neck dissection or selective neck dissection, followed by elective-adjunctive radiation therapy, is the treatment of choice at our institution for patients with clinically involved nodes. In patients with lesions 1.5 mm thick or greater who have undergone selective neck dissection or patients with nodal relapse, adjunctive radiation therapy gives a locoregional control rate of 88%.

Melanomas arising on the scalp or face anterior to the pinna of the ear and superior to the commissure of the lip are at risk of metastasizing to intraparotid lymph nodes, because these nodes are contiguous with the cervical nodes. It is advisable to combine neck dissection with parotid lymph node dissection when parotid nodes are clinically involved, followed by radiation therapy.

Adjuvant Therapy

Biologic Therapy

High-dose IFN alfa-2b has been approved by the U.S. Food and Drug Administration as adjuvant treatment for patients who have melanoma with a high risk of recurrence. Approval was based on the results of the Eastern Cooperative Oncology Group (EST 1684) prospective randomized trial for such patients. The majority (75%) of patients had clinically palpable nodal disease. A regimen of adjuvant high-dose IFN alfa-2b (20 million units/m^2/day intravenously for 4 weeks followed by 10 million units/m^2 subcutaneously thrice weekly for the next 48 weeks) resulted in higher relapse-free and overall survival rates in patients with high-risk (especially stage III) disease than in similar patients who did not receive this therapy (Fig. 3-7). For the overall trial, the median relapse-free survival interval was improved from 1.0 to 1.7 years (survival rates, 26% vs. 37% at 5 years) and overall survival interval from 2.8 to 3.8 years (survival rates, 37% vs. 46% at 5 years). Although the absolute improvement in overall survival rates was low (9%) and the rate of toxic effects was high (two deaths; 67% of patients experienced grade 3 toxicity; 50% of patients either stopped treatment early or required dose reduction), interferon alfa-2b currently represents the only adjuvant therapy with efficacy.

Data from the Eastern Cooperative Oncology Group trial E1690 have recently been analyzed. This prospective, randomized, three-arm intergroup trial to evaluate the efficacy of high-dose IFN alfa-2b (HDI) for 1 year, low-dose IFN alfa-2b (LDI) for 2 years, and observation in 642 patients with high-risk (stage IIb or III) melanoma. Relapse-free survival and overall survival endpoints were used. Most patients (75%) had nodal metastases (50% had nodal recurrence). Unlike E1684, E1690 allowed entry of patients with T4 primary tumors regardless of whether node dissection was performed, and 25% of the patients entered onto this trial had deep primary tumors (compared with 11% in E1684). At 52 months median follow-up, HDI demonstrated a relapse-free survival benefit exceeding that of LDI or observation. The 5-year estimated relapse-free survival rates for the HDI, LDI , and observation arms were 44%, 40%, and 35%, respectively ($p = 0.03$). The relapse-free survival benefit was equivalent for node-negative and node-positive patients. Neither HDI nor LDI has demonstrated an overall survived benefit compared with observation at this time. An analysis of salvage therapy for patients whose disease relapsed on E1690 demonstrated that a significantly larger proportion of patients in the observation arm versus the HDI arm received IFN α–containing salvage therapy, this therapy was unavailable to patients during E1684, and patients with undissected regional nodes were not included in E1684. Analysis of treatments received at recurrence demonstrated significantly more frequent use of IFN alfa-2b at relapse from observation than from HDI, which may have confounded the interpretation of the survival benefit of assigned treatments in E1690.

More recently, an Eastern Cooperative Oncology Group (ECOG) trial E1694 compared the effect of immunization with the ganglioside vaccine GM2-KLK/QS-21 to high dose IFN alfa-2b on relapse-free survival and overall survival. The 776 participating patients were randomized to receive either immunization or IFN alfa-2b. Patients were either T4N0M0 or had evidence of regional nodal disease at the time of presentation of the primary melanoma or at first recurrence and had undergone adequate wide excision of

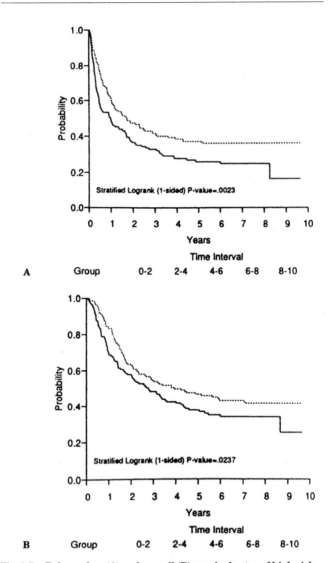

Fig. 3-7. **Relapse-free (A) and overall (B) survival rates of high-risk stage III patients participating in EST 1684. (From Kirkwood JM, Strawderman MH, Ernstoff MS, et al. Interferon-alpha-2b adjuvant therapy of high risk resected cutaneous melanoma: the Eastern Cooperative Oncology Group trial EST 1684. *J Clin Oncol* 1996;14:7, with permission.)**

the primary lesion. An interim analysis performed by ECOG indicated that the relapse-free and overall survival rates for patients receiving the GM2 vaccine were lower than those for patients receiving high-dose IFN. Based on these data, this trial was subsequently closed.

A large body of updated IFN data was presented in two studies at the 2001 Annual Meeting of the American Society of Clinical Oncology. These two studies consisted of a meta-analysis of randomized trials (n = 3,700) and a pooled analysis of primary data from the four ECOG/Intergroup trials of high-dose IFN (n = 1,916). The meta-analysis noted clear benefit for high-dose IFN in terms of relapse-free survival, while the advantage was more modest for overall survival (odds ratio = 0.9, $p = 0.05$) Data from the ECOG database at an updated overall median follow-up of 3.5 years demonstrated that (a) the survival impact of IFN was confined to regimens that incorporated both high-dose induction and high-dose subcutaneous maintenance; (b) reduction of hazard was observed early; and (c) relapse-free survival was sustained off treatment in contrast to the more limited relapse-free survival prolongation reported by the low-dose trials.

The meta-analysis presented at the American Society of Clinical Oncology (ASCO) revealed that low-dose IFN regimens are thought to be ineffective because they have neither convincingly nor consistently achieved disease-free survival and overall survival gains. However, Kirkwood et al. (2001) have presented strong data supporting a sustained survival impact for patients receiving high-dose IFN in at least two randomized trials, E1684 and E1690, and for improved disease-free survival in all four ECOG high-dose IFN studies. The observation that other studies have been unable to consistently confirm the overall survival benefits suggests that the advantage may be modest. It is also important to recognize that data from patients enrolled in other IFN trials at various dosing levels remain immature. Additional follow-up is warranted from these important trials, including E1694 (median follow-up 2.1 years), EORTC 18952 (median follow-up 1.9 years), and the AIM-High study (median follow-up 1.33 years). Further trials are needed to clarify dosing schedules, compare IFN with other therapies, and evaluate IFN's efficacy in patients with minimal nodal disease (i.e., SLN microscopically positive or PCR positive). Some of these questions will be addressed in the multicenter Sunbelt Melanoma Trial.

Current candidates for adjuvant IFN include patients with locally recurrent, nodal, in-transit, or satellite disease. Optimally, eligible patients should be entered into available trials.

Radiation Therapy

The role of radiation therapy as adjuvant treatment after TLND or as an alternative to ELND in the regional treatment of patients with intermediate to thick melanomas has not been clearly defined. Adjuvant radiation therapy, either alone in clinically node-negative patients or in conjunction with surgery in pathologically node-positive patients, has resulted in a locoregional control rate in excess of 85%. Proof of a therapeutic benefit from adjuvant radiation therapy can be obtained only from a prospective randomized trial. In general, patients with head and neck primary tumors, with multiple involved or matted regional nodes, or with extracapsular extension of regional lymphatic metastases should be considered for adjuvant radiation therapy.

Chemotherapy

No confirmed studies have demonstrated a benefit of adjuvant chemotherapy in patients with melanoma who are at high risk for relapse. On the contrary, a randomized trial of adjuvant dacarbazine (DTIC) versus no adjuvant treatment resulted in a statistically significant decrease in survival in the adjuvant treatment arm. Adjuvant systemic therapy should be considered only in the context of a clinical trial.

MANAGEMENT OF DISTANT METASTATIC DISEASE

Common sites of distant metastasis in melanoma patients are, in order of decreasing frequency, skin and subcutaneous tissues, lung, liver, and brain. Patients with systemic metastases have poor prognoses. Mean survival duration is about 6 months. General guidelines for choosing treatment modalities follow, but no treatment for metastatic melanoma has been proven to prolong survival. Experimental treatments are an option for most patients in whom distant metastases are diagnosed.

Surgery

Surgery is a very effective palliative treatment for isolated accessible metastases. Examples of accessible lesions include isolated visceral metastases, isolated brain metastases, and occasionally isolated lung metastases. Some melanoma patients with a solitary pulmonary lesion have potentially curable primary lung cancer. Gastrointestinal tract obstruction from metastatic melanoma is usually due to large polypoid lesions that mechanically obstruct the bowel or that act as a lead point for intussusception. These submucosal lesions are generally removed by bowel resection. Liver metastases are associated with such a short survival time (i.e., 2-4 months) that surgical excision is generally not indicated.

Melanoma ranks only behind small-cell carcinoma of the lung as the most common tumor that metastasizes to the brain. An unusual feature of cerebral metastases is their propensity for hemorrhage, which occurs much more frequently than with other histologic types of metastases. Hemorrhage occurs in 33% to 50% of patients with melanoma metastases to the brain. Surgical excision (followed in selected cases by cranial irradiation) is the treatment of choice in the case of a solitary, surgically accessible metastasis. Tumor excision is relatively safe; it alleviates symptoms in most patients and prevents further neurologic damage. Although long-term disease-free survival is uncommon, a few patients live more than 5 years after surgery. Radiation therapy is preferred when the lesions are numerous or are located in areas that preclude a safe operation.

Radiation Therapy

In the treatment of cutaneous and lymph node metastases with radiation, most authors have observed improved response rates with higher fractional doses of radiation. The appropriate dose fractionation should be based on considerations of normal tissue tolerance. Multiple or recurrent skin or subcutaneous lesions may be treated successfully by hypofractionated radiation therapy. Symptomatic bony metastases from melanoma also respond to this treatment.

Chemotherapy

A number of single agents have limited activity against metastatic melanoma, generally producing overall response rates of 10% to 20% and complete remissions in less than 5% of patients. DTIC is the only drug approved for use in melanoma, but some antitumor activity has been found with the nitrosoureas (e.g., carmustine [BCNU]), carboplatin, and high-dose cisplatin. Based on the principle of combining active agents against melanoma to attain at least an additive antitumor effect, the "Dartmouth regimen," or CBDT, includes cisplatin, BCNU, DTIC, and tamoxifen. Although the initial overall response rate of 55% and complete response rate of 20% were promising when first published in 1984, subsequent studies, including a large multicenter trial sponsored by the National Cancer Institute of Canada, showed no statistically significant difference in response rate or survival when tamoxifen was omitted from the regimen. Median durations of response have been short, in the range of 3 to 6 months. If the tumor has no objective response after two or three courses of a particular chemotherapy regimen, it is usually best to discontinue that therapy and consider other approaches.

Biologic Therapy

In patients with localized superficial skin metastases and no evidence of bulky disease or visceral metastases, bacille Calmette-Guerin (BCG) can induce regression of most lesions into which it is injected. Interferon also has local activity when injected intradermally or subcutaneously.

The demonstration that IFN-α and interleukin-2 (IL-2) are active against melanoma has enabled some new strategies for systemic therapy. Both agents elicit response rates in the range of 10% to 20%. Although these response rates are not significantly different from those for single-agent chemotherapy, some responses can be dramatic. However, large doses of IL-2 can be highly toxic.

Monoclonal antibody therapy is generally well tolerated and has shown activity in phase I trials. Monoclonal antibodies have been used to target radiation and potent plant toxins to tumors in patients with metastatic melanoma, and anti-idiotype antibodies have been used to stimulate immune responses.

The use of tumor vaccines is being evaluated in the treatment of advanced disease and as adjuvant therapy for patients with high-risk disease. These vaccines may contain (a) irradiated tumor cells, usually obtained from the patient; (b) partially or completely purified melanoma antigens; or (c) tumor cell membranes from melanoma cells infected with virus (viral oncolysates). Synthetic vaccines containing genes that encode for tumor antigens or the peptide antigens themselves are also being evaluated, as are vaccines containing genes encoding for immune co-stimulation signal proteins.

In patients without preexisting antibodies against the melanoma antigen GM2 ganglioside, a 23% increase in disease-free survival has been demonstrated with GM2/BCG vaccine in patients with stage III disease. An Eastern Cooperative Oncology Group trial (E1694) comparing the effect of immunization with GM2-KLH/QS-21 to high-dose IFN α-2b on relapse-free and overall survival rates was recently reported. The 776 participating patients were randomized to receive either immunization or IFN α-2b. Patients were either T4N0M0 or had evidence of regional nodal disease at the time of presentation of the primary melanoma or at first recurrence and had undergone adequate wide excision of the primary lesion. An interim analysis performed by ECOG indicated that the relapse-free and overall survival rates for patients receiving the GM2 vaccine were lower than those for patients receiving high-dose IFN. This trial was subsequently closed.

Novel vaccine strategies under investigation include administration of synthetic peptides based on known melanoma T-cell antigens, genetic vaccines, and combinations of vaccines with delivery of cytokines or co-stimulatory molecules, in some cases using gene therapy (transfection) technology. Morton and colleagues (1992) reported encouraging results using a polyvalent melanoma vaccine (Cancervax) in nonrandomized studies of patients with stage III or IV disease. This vaccine is currently being tested in prospective randomized trials for patients with stage III or stage IV disease. For patients with stage III disease, a double-blinded phase III trial is ongoing to determine whether adjuvant BCG plus Cancervax will effectively prolong overall and disease-free survival compared to BCG plus placebo. These patients must be rendered surgically free of disease within 4 months of diagnosis of stage III melanoma. For stage IV patients a phase III double-blinded trial is ongoing to determine whether adjuvant Cancervax plus BCG will effectively prolong disease-free and overall survival compared to placebo plus BCG. These patients must be rendered surgically free of disease and be within 6 months of the diagnosis of stage IV melanoma. Additionally, eligible patients must have no more than two involved organ sites and no more than five individual metastases.

Cellular therapies also exhibit some promise. Rosenberg and colleagues at the U.S. National Cancer Institute and others have reported their experiences with adoptive immunotherapy using tumor-infiltrating lymphocytes and, more recently, dendritic cells. An overall response rate of 37% was seen in patients with stage IV disease. Newer forms of cellular-based therapy are being developed, including effector cells from tumor vaccine-primed lymph nodes. Current trials using in vitro pulsed dendritic cell infusion are ongoing. Additionally, new work examining the preferential induction of apoptosis by sequential 5-Aza-2 deoxycytidine-depsipeptide FR901228 treatment in melanoma cells to improve recognition of specific targets by cytolytic T lymphocytes may serve as a useful adjunct to immunotherapy.

Biochemotherapy

Phase I and II studies have evaluated combinations of IL-2, IFN, and chemotherapy (cisplatin, DTIC, or cyclophosphamide). Preliminary results from a series of small studies using combinations of IL-2, IFN α, and cisplatin have indicated overall response rates of 40%. Recently, a phase III trial comparing in-patient sequential biochemotherapy (BC) with traditional out-patient chemotherapy with respect to response, time to progression, overall survival rate and toxicity has been completed at M.D. Anderson. All patients had either stage IV or inoperable stage III disease, with an ECOG performance status of 0 to 3, no symptomatic brain metastases, no prior chemotherapy, and adequate cardiac, hematologic, and renal reserves. The response rate for BC was 48%, while it was 25% with standard chemotherapy ($p = 0.0001$). The time to progression with BC was 4.6 months, while in patients who received standard chemotherapy was 2.4 months ($p = 0.0007$). The median survival was 11.8 months for BC and 9.5 months for standard chemotherapy ($p = 0.055$). BC did induce severe constitutional toxic effects, myelosuppression, infections, and hypotension, but all of these were found to be manageable on the general ward. In a more recent phase II trial by this group, the addition of IFN alfa-2a to IL-2 BC was examined. Although the response rate for this regimen was low, durable responses with median survival durations of 30+ months were seen in selected patients. This would support consideration of this form of treatment in patients with advanced disease who have otherwise limited treatment options.

FOLLOW-UP

Melanoma can have a more variable and unpredictable clinical course than almost any other human cancer. The schedule of follow-up evaluation at M.D. Anderson for patients with high-risk melanoma without clinical evidence of recurrence is as follows: year 1 to 2, every 3 to 4 months; years 3 to 5, every 6 months; and annually thereafter. At each visit the patient undergoes a physical examination, a chest radiograph, and measurement of LDH. Abnormal findings may prompt further workup. Particular attention should be given to signs or symptoms of central nervous system involvement. Extensive radiographic evaluation of patients with AJCC stage I, II, or III melanoma who are clinically free of disease rarely reveals metastases.

RECOMMENDED READING

Albertini JJ, Cruse CW, Rapaport D, et al. Intraoperative radiolymphoscintigraphy improves sentinel lymph node identification for patients with melanoma. *Ann Surg* 1996;223:217.

Ang KK, Peters LJ, Weber RS, et al. Postoperative radiotherapy for cutaneous melanoma of the head and neck region. *Int J Radiat Oncol Biol Phys* 1994;30:795.

Balch CM, Buzaid AC, Atkins M, et al. A new American Joint Committee on Cancer staging system for cutaneous melanoma. *Cancer* 2000;88:1484.

Balch CM, Buzaid AC, Soong SJ, et al. Final version of the

American Joint Committee on Cancer staging system for cutaneous melanoma. *J Clin Oncol* 2001;19:3635–3648.

Balch CM, Houghton AN, Milton GW, et al., eds. *Cutaneous melanoma*, 2nd ed. Philadelphia: Lippincott, 1992.

Balch CM, Soong S-J, Bartolucci AA, et al. Efficacy of an elective regional lymph node dissection of 1 to 4 mm thick melanomas for patients 60 years of age and younger. *Ann Surg* 1996;224:255.

Balch CM, Soong S-J, Milton GW, et al. A comparison of prognostic factors and surgical results in 1,786 patients with localized (stage I) melanoma treated in Alabama, USA, and New South Wales, Australia. *Ann Surg* 1982;196:677.

Balch CM, Soong S-J, Murad TM, et al. A multifactorial analysis of melanoma. II. Prognostic factors in patients with stage I (localized) melanoma. *Surgery* 1979;86:343.

Balch CM, Soong S-J, Ross MI, et al. Long-term results of a multi-institutional randomized trial comparing prognostic factors and surgical results for intermediate thickness melanomas (1.0 to 4.0 mm). *Ann Surg Oncol* 2000;7:87.

Balch CM, Soong SJ, Gershenwald JE, et al. Prognostic factors analysis of 17,600 melanoma patients: validation of the new American Joint Committee on Cancer melanoma staging system. *J Clin Oncol* 2001;19:3622–3634.

Balch CM. The role of elective lymph node dissection in melanoma: rationale, results and controversies. *J Clin Oncol* 1988;6:163.

Bedrosian I, Faries MB, Guerry D 4th, et al. Incidence of sentinel node metastasis in patients with thin primary melanoma (≤ 1 mm) with vertical growth phase. *Ann Surg Oncol* 2000;7:251.

Buzaid AC, Ross MI, Balch CM, et al. Critical analysis of the current American Joint Committee on Cancer staging system for cutaneous melanoma and proposal of a new staging system. *J Clin Oncol* 1997;15:1039.

Cannon-Albright LA, Goldgar DE, Meyer LJ, et al. Assignment of a locus for familial melanoma, MLM, to chromosome 9p 13-p22. *Science* 1992;258:1148.

Cascinelli N, Morabito A, Santinami M, et al. Immediate or delayed dissection of regional nodes in patients with melanoma of the trunk: a randomised trial. WHO melanoma programme. *Lancet* 1998;14:793.

Clary BM, Brady MS, Lewis JJ, et al. Sentinel lymph node biopsy in the management of patients with primary cutaneous melanoma: review of a large single-institutional experience with an emphasis on recurrence. *Ann Surg* 2001;233:250.

Elder DE, Guerry D, Van Horn M, et al. The role of lymph node dissection for clinical stage I malignant melanoma of intermediate thickness (1.51-3.99 mm). *Cancer* 1985;56:413.

Essner R, Bostick PJ, Glass EC, et al. Standardized probe-directed sentinel node dissection in melanoma. *Surgery* 2000;127:26.

Eton O, Buzaid AC, Bedikian AY, et al. A phase II study of "decrescendo" interleukin-2 plus interferon-α-2a in patients with progressive metastatic melanoma after chemotherapy. *Cancer* 2000;88:1703.

Eton O, Legha S, Bedekian A, et al. Sequential biochemotherapy versus chemotherapy for metastatic melanoma: results from a Phase III randomized trial. *J Clin Oncol* 2002;20:2045–2052.

Evans GRD, Friedman J, Shenaq J, et al. Plantar flap reconstruction for acral lentiginous melanoma. *Ann Surg Oncol* 1997;4:575.

Fleming ID, Cooper JS, Henson DE, et al., eds. *AJCC cancer staging manual*, 5th ed. Philadelphia: Lippincott, 1997.

Fraker DL, Alexander HR, Andrich M, et al. Palliation of regional symptoms of advanced extremity melanoma by isolated limb perfusion with melphalan and high dose tumor necrosis factor. *Cancer J Sci Am* 1995;1:122.

Fraker DL, Alexander HR, Andrich M, et al. Treatment of extremity melanoma using hyperthermic isolated limb perfusion with melphalan, tumor necrosis factor and interferon-gamma: result of TNF dose escalation study. *J Clin Oncol* 1996;14:479.

Gershenwald JE, Berman RS, Porter G, et al. Regional nodal basin control is not compromised by prior sentinel lymph node biopsy in patients with melanoma. *Ann Surg Oncol* 2000;7(3):226–231.

Gershenwald JE, Buzaid AC, Ross MI. Classification and staging of melanoma. *Hematol Oncol Clin North Am* 1998;12:737.

Gershenwald JE, Colome-Grimmer MI, Lee JE, et al. Patterns of recurrence following a negative sentinel lymph node biopsy in 243 patients with stage I or II melanoma. *J Clin Oncol* 1998;16:2253.

Gershenwald JE, Colome-Grimmer MI, Lee JE, et al. Routine histologic examination of the sentinel lymph node understages the nodal basin in stage I and II melanoma patients. *Proc Am Soc Clin Oncol* 1997;16:493a.

Gershenwald JE, Mansfield PF, Lee JE, et al. The role for lymphatic mapping and sentinel lymph node biopsy in patients with thick (>4 mm) primary melanoma. *Ann Surg Oncol* 2000;7(2):160–165.

Gershenwald JE, Prieto V, Colome-Grimmer MI, et al. The prognostic significance of microscopic tumor burden in 945 melanoma patients undergoing sentinel lymph node biopsy [abstract]. Presented at the 36th annual meeting of the American Society of Clinical Oncology, New Orleans, LA, May 20–23, 2000. *Proc Am Soc Clin Oncol* 2000;19:551a.

Gershenwald JE, Schacherer C, Emerson M, et al. Patterns of failure and survival analysis in sentinel lymph node positive melanoma patients. Presented at the 37th annual meeting of the American Society of Clinical Oncology, San Francisco, CA, May 12–15, 2001.

Gershenwald JE, Sumner W, Porter G, et al. Role of sentinel lymph node biopsy in patients with thin (<1mm) cutaneous melanoma [abstract]. Presented at the 53rd Annual Meeting of the American Society of Surgical Oncology, New Orleans, LA, March 16–19, 2000.

Gershenwald JE, Thompson W, Mansfield PF, et al. Multi-institutional melanoma lymphatic mapping experience: the prognostic value of sentinel lymph node status in 612 stage I or II melanoma patients. *J Clin Oncol* 1999;17(3):976–983.

Gershenwald JE, Tseng C-H. Thompson W, et al. Improved sentinel lymph node localization in patients with primary melanoma with the use of radiolabeled colloid. *Surgery* 1998;124:203.

Gershenwald JE. Melanoma. *Oncologist* 2001;6(5):402–406.

Hancock BW, Harris S, Wheatley K, Gore M. Adjuvant interferon-alpha in malignant melanoma: current status. *Cancer Treat Rev* 2000;26:81–89.

Hayward N. New developments in melanoma genetics. *Curr Oncol Rep* 2000;2:300.

Heaton KM, Sussman JJ, Gershenwald JE, et al. Surgical margins and prognostic factors in patients with thick (>4 mm) primary melanoma. *Ann Surg Oncol* 1998;5:322.

Jemal A, Devesa SS, Fears TR, et al. Cancer surveillance series: changing patterns of cutaneous malignant melanoma mortality rates among whites in the United States. *J Natl Cancer Inst* 2000; 92:811.

Kirkwood JM, Ibrahim JG, Sondak VK, et al. High- and low-dose interferon alfa-2b in high-risk melanoma: first analysis of intergroup trial E1690/S9111/C9190. *J Clin Oncol* 2000;18:2444–2458.

Kirkwood JM, Ibrahim JG, Sosman JA, et al. High-dose interferon alfa-2b significantly prolongs relapse-free and overall survival compared with the GM2-KLH/QS-21 vaccine in patients with resected stage IIB-III melanoma: results of intergroup trial E1694/S9512/C509801. *J Clin Oncol* 2001;19:2370–2380.

Kirkwood JM, Manola J, Ibrahim J, et al. Pooled-analysis of four ECOG/intergroup trials of high-dose interferon alfa-2b (HDI) in 1916 patients with high-risk resected cutaneous melanoma [abstract]. Presented at the 38th annual meeting of the American Society of Clinical Oncology, Orlando, FL, May 18–21, 2002.

Kirkwood JM, Strawderman MH, Ernstoff MS, et al. Interferon-alpha-2b adjuvant therapy of high risk resected cutaneous melanoma: the eastern cooperative oncology group trial EST 1684. *J Clin Oncol* 1996;14:7.

Koops HM, Vaglini M, Suciu S, et al. Prophylactic isolated limb perfusion for localized high-risk limb melanomas: results of a multicenter randomized phase III trial. *J Clin Oncol* 1998;16:2906.

Krag DN, Meijer SJ, Weaver DL, et al. Minimal-access surgery for staging of melanoma. *Arch Surg* 1995;130:654.

Leinard D, Ewalenko P, Delmotte JJ, et al. High dose recombinant tumor necrosis factor alpha in combination with interferon gamma and melphalan in isolation perfusion of the limbs for melanoma and sarcoma. *J Clin Oncol* 1992;10:52.

Livingston PO, Wong GYC, Adluri S, et al. Improved survival in stage III melanoma patients with GM2 antibodies: a randomized trial of adjuvant vaccination with GM2 ganglioside. *J Clin Oncol* 1994;12:1036.

Mansfield PF, Lee JE, Balch CM. Melanoma: surgical controversies and current practice. *Curr Probl Surg* 1994;31:253.

McCarthy WH, Shaw HM, Milton GW. Efficacy of elective lymph node dissection in 2,347 patients with clinical stage I malignant melanoma. *Surg Gynecol Obstet* 1985;161:575.

McMasters KM, Reintgen DS, Ross MI, et al. Sentinel lymph node biopsy for melanoma: how many radioactive nodes should be removed? *Ann Surg Oncol* 2001;8(3):192–197.

Milton GW, Shaw HM, McCarthy WH, et al. Prophylactic lymph node dissection in clinical stage I cutaneous malignant melanoma: results of surgical treatment in 1319 patients. *Br J Surg* 1982; 69:108.

Morton DL, Foshag LJ, Hoon DSB, et al. Prolongation of survival in metastatic melanoma after active specific immunotherapy with a new polyvalent melanoma vaccine. *Ann Surg* 1992;216: 463.

Morton DL, Wen DR, Wong JH, et al. Technical details of intraoperative lymphatic mapping for early stage melanoma. *Arch Surg* 1992;127:392.

Norman J, Cruse CW, Espinoza C, et al. Redefinition of cutaneous lymphatic drainage with the use of lymphoscintigraphy for malignant melanoma. *Am J Surg* 1991;162:432.

Porter GA, Ross MI, Berman RS, et al. Significance of multiple nodal basin drainage in truncal melanoma patients undergoing sentinel lymph node biopsy. *Ann Surg Oncol* 200;7:256.

Porter GA, Ross MI, Berman RS, et al. How many lymph nodes are enough during sentinel lymphadenectomy for primary melanoma? *Surgery* 2000;128(2):306–311.

Reintgen D, Cruse CW, Berman C, et al. The orderly progression of melanoma nodal metastases. *Ann Surg* 1994;220:759.

Reintgen DS, Balch CM, Kirkwood J, et al. Recent advances in the care of the patient with malignant melanoma. *Ann Surg* 1997;225:1.

Reintgen DS, Cox EB, McCarty KM Jr, et al. Efficacy of elective lymph node dissection in patients with intermediate thickness primary melanoma. *Ann Surg* 1983;198:379.

Rigel DS, Carucci JH. Malignant melanoma: prevention, early detection, and treatment in the 21st century. *CA Cancer J Clin* 2000; 50:215.

Rosenberg SA, Yannelli JR, Yang JC, et al. Treatment of patients with metastatic melanoma with autologous tumor infiltrating lymphocytes and interleukin-2. *J Natl Cancer Inst* 1994;86:1159.

Ross M, Reintgen DS, Balch C. Selective lymphadenectomy: emerging role of lymphatic mapping and sentinel node biopsy in the management of early stage melanoma. *Semin Surg Oncol* 1993;9:219, 1993.

Ross MI, Gershenwald JE. Melanoma lymphatic mapping: scientific support for the sentinel lymph node concept and biologic significance of the sentinel node. In: Whitman ED, Reintgen D, eds. *Radioguided surgery Georgetown,* TX: Landes Bioscience, 1999: 48–63.

Ross MI. Surgical management of stage I and II melanoma patients: approach to the regional lymph node basin. *Semin Surg Oncol* 1996;12:394.

Shivers S, Wang X, Li W, et al. Molecular staging of malignant melanoma. *JAMA* 1998;280:1410.

Sim FH, Taylor WF, Pritchard DJ, et al. Lymphadenectomy in the management of stage I malignant melanoma: a prospective randomized study. *Mayo Clin Proc* 1986;61:697.

Sumner W 3rd, Ross MI, Mansfield PF, et al. Implications of lymphatic drainage to unusual sentinel lymph node sites in patients with primary cutaneous melanoma. *Cancer* 2002:95:354–360.

Sumner WE, Ross MI, Prieto VG, et al. Patterns of failure in patients with thick (≥ 4 mm) melanoma undergoing sentinel node biopsy [abstract]. Presented at the Fifth World Conference on Melanoma, Venice, Italy, February 28–March 3, 2001. *Melanoma Res* 2001;11[suppl 1]:S109–S110.

Thompson JF, Kam PC, Waugh RC, et al. Isolated limb infusion with cytotoxic agents: a simple alternative to isolated limb perfusion. *Semin Surg Oncol* 1998;14:238.

Thompson JF, McCarthy WH, Bosch CMJ, et al. Sentinel lymph node status as an indicator of the presence of metastatic melanoma in regional lymph nodes. *Melanoma Res* 1995;5:255.

Travis J. Closing in on melanoma susceptibility gene(s). *Science* 1992;258:1080.

Veronesi U, Adamus J. Bandiera DC, et al. Delayed regional lymph node dissection in stage I melanoma of the skin of the lower extremities. *Cancer* 1982;49:2420.

Veronesi U, Adamus J, Bandiera DC, et al. Inefficacy of immediate node dissection in stage I melanoma of the limbs. *N Engl J Med* 1977;297:627.

Veronesi U, Cascinelli N, Adamus J, et al. Primary cutaneous melanoma 2 mm or less in thickness: results of a randomized study comparing wide with narrow surgical excision. A preliminary report. *N Engl J Med* 1988;318:1159.

Wang X, Heller R, Van Voorhis N, et al. Detection of submicroscopic metastases with polymerase chain reaction in patients with malignant melanoma. *Ann Surg* 1994;220:768.

Wayne JD, Albo D, Hunt K, et al. Anaphylactic reaction to isosulfan blue dye (IBD) during sentinel lymph node biopsy (SLNB) is more common in breast cancer than in melanoma [abstract]. Presented at the 37th annual meeting of the American Society of Clinical Oncology, San Francisco, May 12–15, 2001.

Weiguo L, Stall A, Shivers SC, et al. Clinical relevance of molecular staging for melanoma. Comparison of RT-PCR and immunohistochemistry staining in sentinel lymph nodes of patients with melanoma. *Ann Surg* 2000;231:795.

Nonmelanoma Skin Cancer

Nestor F. Esnaola and Keith M. Heaton

EPIDEMIOLOGY AND ETIOLOGY

Basal cell carcinoma (BCC) and squamous cell carcinoma (SCC) of the skin are the most common malignancies in the white population. The male:female ratio for nonmelanoma skin cancers (NMSCs) is 3:1, and BCCs occur four times more frequently than SCCs. NMSCs account for almost one third of all cancers in the United States, with more than 600,000 new cases reported each year, and an annual cost of $500 million. These figures may underestimate the true incidence of NMSC, however, because most cases are diagnosed and treated on an outpatient basis and often not recorded in tumor registries. Despite their significant morbidity and cost, NMSCs account for only 2,500 deaths each year, mostly from metastatic SCC.

Exposure to ultraviolet radiation (UVR) in sunlight, and in particular ultraviolet B (UVB; in the range of 280–320 nm) is accepted to be the dominant risk factor for NMSC, although both BCC and SCC can also occur at unexposed sites. Recent studies suggest that severe sun exposure during childhood and adolescence is associated with an increased risk of BCC, while increasing chronic sun exposure in the 10 years before diagnosis is more likely to be associated with SCC. Skin pigmentation is protective and is associated with a lower rate of skin cancers and inversion of the BCC:SCC ratio. Other risk factors for NMSC include photochemotherapy (PUVA) for psoriasis, ionizing radiation, human papillomavirus, chemical carcinogens (e.g., arsenic, mineral oils), cigarette smoking, and chronic irritation or ulceration (e.g., burn scars, chronic fistulas). Patients who are chronically immunosuppressed following organ transplantation have an 18-fold increase in SCC, particularly in sun-exposed areas.

DIFFERENTIAL DIAGNOSIS

Benign Epidermal Tumors

Seborrheic keratoses (warts) present as pigmented verrucous plaques on the face and trunk of elderly individuals. They are often itchy, and can be distinguished from melanomas and pigmented actinic keratoses by their dull, crumbling surface. Although easily treated with excision or curettage, these lesions tend to recur.

Tricholemmal (pilar) cysts present as smooth, mobile nodules on the scalp, particularly in middle-aged women. Infected cysts tend to rupture and proliferate and can mimic SCC. Uncomplicated cysts can be enucleated, while proliferating cysts require excision with an adequate margin to prevent recurrence.

Keratoacanthoma is a benign tumor that usually presents in elderly people as a single, raised 1 to 2 cm lesion in the center of the face with a characteristic horn-filled crater. These tumors can be distinguished from SCC by their rapid growth phase over a few weeks. Although most lesions involute spontaneously over 3 to 6 months, excision or curettage can rule out SCC and results in a better cosmetic outcome.

Premalignant Conditions

Actinic (solar) keratoses present as dry, scaly plaques on the scalp, face, and backs of the hands of fair-skinned elderly persons and affect up to 50% of the population in some areas. Although these lesions are usually asymptomatic and have a low risk of progressing to SCC, increasing size, erosion, and tenderness can signal malignant evolution. Regular use of sunscreen preparations has been shown to prevent the development of new actinic keratoses and the remission of existing lesions. Cryotherapy or topical 5-fluorouracil (5-FU) are the standard treatments for these lesions. Indurated or persistent lesions are best excised with adequate surgical margins to rule out the possibility of SCC.

Bowen's disease represents SCC in situ, and its incidence increases rapidly in individuals over age 60. It mimics psoriasis and lichen simplex, and presents as small, red, scaly areas on sun-exposed skin that eventually enlarge into well-demarcated scaly plaques. Histologic characteristics include atypical squamous cells proliferating throughout the epidermis. The transformation rate of Bowen's disease to invasive SCC has been estimated at 4% to 6%. Although freezing and cauterization are often effective, tumor extension into untreated appendage ducts can result in recurrences, which are best treated with excision. Topical 5-FU has also been shown to be effective.

There is no known precursor lesion for BCC.

BASAL CELL CARCINOMA

BCCs are slow-growing, malignant neoplasms that usually arise de novo from the epidermal basal cell layer of the skin and its appendages. They are more common in men, and 95% of cases occur in patients older than 40. BCC develops on hair-bearing skin, most commonly on sun-exposed areas, and approximately 85% of lesions are found on the head (particularly the upper central part of the face) and neck.

Histologically, most tumors are well-differentiated and characterized by dark cells with scant cytoplasm arranged into palisading lobules that extend three-dimensionally into the surrounding dermis. BCCs can behave in nonaggressive and aggressive fashions depending on their histologic growth pattern:

Non-Aggressive Types

1. *Nodular-ulcerative* BCC has the classic appearance of a waxy, skin-colored nodule with rolled edges and overlying telangiectasias. These tumors tend to ulcerate to form so-called rodent ulcers. Patients often present with lesions that heal and bleed again with minor trauma.
2. *Superficial* BCC is less common than nodular-ulcerative BCC and occurs on unexposed skin (i.e., trunk). It can resemble dermatitis, although it is usually redder and more well-defined.

Aggressive, Diffuse Types

1. *Sclerosing* or *morpheic* BCC appears almost exclusively on the face as a flat, yellow, indurated plaque. Although erosions are common, ulceration is rare. Histologic analysis of these lesions reveals narrow strands of basaloid cells embedded in dense dermal stroma similar to metastatic breast carcinoma and desmoplastic epithelioma.

2. *Infiltrating* BCC has a predilection for the trunk and presents as subtle, flesh-colored papules. There is no fibrotic response, and therefore, no palpable induration associated with these lesions.

Nodular-ulcerative and superficial BCCs can present as pigmented lesions that can be difficult to distinguish from seborrheic keratoses and nodular melanomas. Superficial BCCs and some nodular-ulcerative BCCs can have an indolent course. The typical BCC grows slowly; however, if untreated it can eventually invade surrounding structures (including muscle, cartilage, and bone) by direct extension. If neglected, massive tumor invasion can lead to destruction of vital organs and even death. Sclerosing BCC is particularly difficult to treat because of its indistinct margins and deep infiltration. Metastases from BCC are extremely rare (0.0028%–0.5% of cases). Large, invasive lesions located on the head or neck, persistent or recurrent tumors, and basisquamous tumors (which have histologic features of both BCC and SCC) are more likely to metastasize. Although most metastases are to regional lymph nodes, distant sites may also be involved.

SQUAMOUS CELL CARCINOMA

Approximately 80% of UVR-induced SCCs develop on the head, neck, or arms, often from precursor lesions of actinic keratosis. SCCs arise from basal keratinocytes and typically present as firm, keratotic nodules on an erythematous base. The lesion may be raised, with central ulceration, crusting, and raised margins. Histologically, SCC is characterized by nests of atypical keratinocytes that extend beyond the dermoepidermal junction into the dermis. Grading is based on the degree of cell differentiation. Poorly differentiated tumors lack keratinization and exhibit marked cellular atypia, making them difficult to distinguish from anaplastic melanoma, lymphoma, and mesenchymal tumors.

SCC may metastasize to regional lymph nodes and distant sites, including bone, brain, and lungs. The overall rate of metastases with SCC has been estimated at 2% to 3%, and varies according to prognostic factors such as the anatomic site (i.e., lip), depth of invasion, and degree of differentiation. For example, SCCs arising from actinic keratoses have a low propensity to metastasize (0.5%), whereas tumors arising from old burns, irradiated sites, and chronic sinus tracts or ulcers metastasize much more frequently (18%, 20%, and 31%, respectively). Patients receiving immunosuppressive therapy and patients with leukemia or lymphoma also have an increased risk of metastases.

KAPOSI'S SARCOMA

Before 1981, about 100 cases of Kaposi's sarcoma (KS) were diagnosed in the United States each year. With the advent of the acquired immunodeficiency syndrome (AIDS) epidemic, the incidence of this tumor has increased dramatically. KS is a neoplasm of vascular endothelial cells characterized by the presence of bluish-red nodules, edema, and hemosiderin deposition. KS lesions often begin as soft, red patches that darken and harden with time and occasionally erode and ulcerate. Although initially unilateral, lesions eventually appear in a disseminated, centripetal fashion as the disease progresses. Classic KS is typically seen on the ankles and soles of elderly men of Jewish or Italian descent. Mucosal (i.e., oral palate) and visceral lesions are more common in iatrogenic (immunosuppression-induced) and AIDS-related KS. Isolated KS lesions can usually be treated with excision or cryotherapy. Other options include radiation therapy and intralesional cytotoxic chemotherapy. Cessation of immunosuppressive therapy can induce tumor regression in patients with iatrogenic KS.

SYNDROMES ASSOCIATED WITH NONMELANOMA SKIN CANCERS

Xeroderma pigmentosum is an autosomal recessive disease that occurs in approximately 1 in 250,000 individuals and is characterized by photophobia, severe sun sensitivity, and advanced sun damage. Malignant skin cancers are 1,000 times more common in these patients and appear 40 years earlier than they do in the general population.

Nevoid basal cell carcinoma (Gorlin's) syndrome is an autosomal dominant disorder characterized by multiple BCCs. The lesions can appear during childhood but tend to proliferate between puberty and 35 years of age. Despite their large number, few lesions become locally invasive.

Sebaceous nevus of Jadassohn usually manifests as a single, oval, orange-yellow, alopecic plaque on the scalp of a child. During puberty, this lesion becomes verrucous. In adult life, both benign and malignant skin tumors (particularly BCC) may develop.

BIOPSY TECHNIQUES

Four principal biopsy techniques are used for cutaneous lesions. A *shave biopsy* is performed by slicing a superficial portion of the tumor with a scalpel. A *punch biopsy* obtains a deeper specimen by introducing a sharp, cylindrical instrument into the reticular dermis or subcutaneous tissue. An *incisional biopsy* removes a portion of the tumor, whereas an *excisional biopsy* removes the entire tumor. To facilitate an accurate diagnosis, the biopsy technique selected should be the one that yields the optimal pathologic specimen. For example, a shave biopsy may be done in cases of suspected nodular-ulcerative or superficial BCC, but an invasive SCC may be missed. One of the other techniques is indicated in suspected cases of pigmented or sclerosing BCC or to confirm the diagnosis of benign keratoacanthoma.

STAGING

The current American Joint Committee on Cancer staging system for BCC and SCC of the skin is shown in Table 4-1.

Table 4-1. TNM staging for basal cell carcinoma and squamous cell carcinoma of the skin

Primary tumor (T)

Tx	Primary tumor cannot be assessed
T0	No evidence of primary tumor
Tis	Carcinoma *in situ*
T1	Tumor ≤ 2 cm in greatest dimension
T2	Tumor > 2 cm but ≤ 5 cm in greatest dimension
T3	Tumor > 5 cm in greatest dimension
T4	Tumor invades deep extradermal structures (i.e., cartilage, skeletal muscle, or bone)

Nodal involvement (N)

Nx	Regional lymph nodes cannot be assessed
N0	No regional lymph node metastasis
N1	Regional lymph node metastasis

Distant metastasis (M)

Mx	Presence of distant metastasis cannot be assessed
M0	No distant metastasis
M1	Distant metastasis

Stage grouping

Stage 0	Tis	N0	M0
Stage I	T1	N0	M0
Stage II	T2	N0	M0
	T3	N0	M0
Stage III	T4	N0	M0
	Any T	N1	M0
Stage IV	Any T	Any N	M1

Adapted from Fleming ID, Cooper JS, Henson DE, et al., eds. *AJCC manual for staging of cancer,* 5th ed. Philadelphia: Lippincott-Raven, 1997.

TREATMENT

Once a histologic diagnosis has been made, numerous factors must be considered in selecting the appropriate therapy. These factors include the location and size of the tumor, the histopathologic type of the tumor, and the age and general medical condition of the patient. Patient preference and the cost of the treatment should also be considered. Commonly used treatments are divided into surgical (excisional and destructive) and nonsurgical therapies.

Excisional Surgical Techniques

Excisional surgery is a mainstay of therapy and is effective for all NMSCs. Complete excision of a tumor has the advantage of allowing optimal evaluation of tumor margins.

Excisions with predetermined margins are ideally performed along Langer's lines to ensure a good cosmetic result. Elliptical excisions are usually performed on the scalp, forehead, cheeks, chin, trunk, and extremities. When dealing with lesions on the eyelids, alar rim of the nose, lips, and ears, however, wedge-shaped excisions may minimize distortion. Although there is no uniform recommendation regarding surgical margins, many surgeons use a margin of 3 to 5 mm for small, well-defined lesions and at least 1 cm for larger, histologically aggressive, or recurrent tumors. Surgical defects can be closed using primary closure techniques, local flaps, skin grafts, and rarely, healing by secondary intention. For NMSCs with metastatic potential, clinical evaluation of regional lymph nodes is mandatory. Lymph node dissection should only be performed, however, if there is clinically palpable lymphadenopathy or biopsy-proven disease.

Mohs micrographic surgery is a specialized technique in which serial horizontal sections of excised tissue are systematically mapped and microscopically evaluated using frozen sections. Because margins are checked thoroughly at the time of surgery, this technique allows the complete removal of difficult lesions with maximal preservation of the surrounding tissues. As a result, Mohs surgery is the preferred treatment for tumors at critical sites, aggressive tumors, and recurrent tumors. However, this is a specialized technique that is both time-consuming and expensive. The reconstructive choices after Mohs surgery are similar to those available after traditional excision.

Destructive Surgical Techniques

Curettage and cautery/electrodesiccation is often used by dermatologists to treat low-risk BCCs (i.e., small, non-aggressive histologic type at a noncritical site) and superficial SCCs. In this technique, a curette is first used to enucleate the tumor (which is often soft and friable) from the firm underlying stroma. The base is then charred with cautery or electrodesiccated with a carbon dioxide laser, and the cycle is repeated two or three times. Several visits may be required, and healing usually occurs over 2 to 6 weeks, with minimal scarring in most cases. The recurrence rate increases with increasing tumor size, and the 5-year cure rate for recurrent BCC treated with this technique is only 60%. Because of wound contracture, distortion is especially likely to occur around the eyes and lips. Curettage and cautery/electrodesiccation are particularly useful for lower extremity tumors or when optimal cosmetic results are not essential.

Cryosurgery involves freezing the lesion, often with local anesthesia, using liquid nitrogen delivered by a spray apparatus or a cryoprobe. Before the procedure, a biopsy is performed to confirm the diagnosis and evaluate the depth of the tumor. After treatment, patients may experience pain and blistering, and abnormal pigmentation develops in some patients at the treated site. Although cryosurgery is effective in the treatment of premalignant lesions and superficial tumors, it should not be used for large, aggressive, or recurrent tumors. Favorable anatomic sites for cryosurgery include the eyelids, ears, face, neck, and trunk. Particular care must be taken when treating tumors of the inner canthi of the eyes, alare nasi, nasolabial folds, and periauricular areas. These sites are usually associated with deep infiltration by tumor and require wider margins to minimize the chance of recurrence.

Nonsurgical Therapy

Radiation therapy is the therapy of choice for elderly patients with extensive lesions who are poor surgical candidates. It is particularly useful for lesions on the eyelids, inner and lateral canthi of the eyes, pinnae of the ears, alare nasi, nasolabial folds, and lips. Although radiation therapy can also be used to treat small skin cancers at other sites, the cosmetic results are inferior to those after surgical excision. Radiation therapy can also be used to treat incompletely excised or recurrent BCCs, unless the primary tumor was initially treated with radiation. Although radiation therapy is painless and well tolerated, it requires several sessions, a healing period of up to 8 weeks, and is somewhat more costly. Furthermore, histologic evidence of adequacy of treatment cannot be assessed.

Topical therapy usually involves application of creams or lotions containing 1% to 5% 5-FU twice daily for 4 to 6 weeks. This treatment causes oozing, crusting, and ulceration, and lesions may require an additional 3 to 6 weeks to heal. Because the recurrence rate after treatment with topical 5-FU is higher than that with other therapies, this treatment is usually reserved for patients with multiple, superficial lesions or bedridden patients with limited life expectancy.

Intralesional interferon therapy is currently being investigated for the treatment of nodular-ulcerative and superficial BCC and SCC. Several recent studies have reported failure rates ranging from 20% to 45% at 3 months after treatment. This technique is time-consuming and extremely expensive. In light of the fact that data on long-term cure rates are not yet available, use of interferon therapy should be considered investigational at this time.

Photodynamic therapy, another investigational treatment, usually involves the use of a topical or systemic photosensitizer that is allowed to accumulate within tumor tissues before being activated by the application of visible light. Although systemic photosensitizers are cleared from most organs after 48 to 72 hours, they are retained by tumors, skin, and the reticuloendothelial system. As a result, patients experience photosensitivity and must be shielded from sunlight for the duration of the therapy. Exposure to light at 620 to 630 nm results in the local release of oxygen-free radicals and the selective killing of tumor cells. Preliminary results are variable, showing success rates of 54% to 100%. The recurrence rates for aggressive and thick tumors treated with this technique are high, however, likely due to limited penetration and activation by the light source.

Systemic chemotherapy with cisplatinum-based regimens has been used in patients with uncontrolled local disease and disseminated BCC, a rapidly fatal condition.

SCREENING AND PREVENTION

Recent evidence suggests that the incidence of NMSCs is increasing rapidly. Because it is easy to implement, screening for skin cancer is theoretically promising, but few reports have demonstrated its effectiveness. Nevertheless, monthly self-examinations of all areas of the body using full-length and hand-held mirrors are useful for detecting potential lesions. Any change in an existing lesion or the appearance of a new lesion should be brought to the attention of a physician.

The key to preventing sun damage and skin cancer is to reduce exposure to UVR in sunlight. People of all ages should protect their skin by avoiding direct sunlight, particularly between 10 a.m. to 4 p.m., by wearing protective clothing, and by applying sunscreens with a sun protection factor of 15 or higher to all exposed areas. Although most chemical sunscreens (p-aminobenzoic acid, benzophenones, cinnamates, salicylates, and anthranilates) absorb and filter out UVB radiation, only the benzophenones and anthranilates absorb UVA radiation. Recent studies have shown that regular use of sunscreen can reduce the incidence of actinic keratosis and SCCs, but not BCCs, likely because the index skin damage associated with BCC occurs during childhood and adolescence.

Because the protection provided by topical sunscreens is incomplete, other chemoprevention strategies have been investigated. However, several large trials involving chemoprophylaxis with beta-carotene and 13-*cis*-retinoic acid have failed to show efficacy in preventing NMSC.

RECOMMENDED READING

Chu AC, Edelson RL, eds. *Malignant tumors of the skin.* London: Arnold Publishers, 1999.

Champion RH, Burton JL, Burns DA, Breathnach SM, eds. *Rook/Wilkinson/Ebling textbook of dermatology,* 6th ed. Oxford: Blackwell Science, 1998.

Gallagher RP, Hill GB, Bajdik CD, et al. Sunlight exposure, pigmentary factors, and risk of nonmelanocytic skin cancer: I. basal cell carcinoma, II. squamous cell carcinoma. *Arch Dermatol* 1995;131:157–169.

Green A, Williams G, Neale R, et al. Daily sunscreen application and beta carotene supplementation in prevention of basal-cell and squamous-cell carcinomas of the skin: a randomized controlled trial. *Lancet* 1999;354:723–729.

Levine N, Moon TE, Cartmel B, et al. Trial of retinol and isotretinoin in skin cancer prevention: a randomized, double-blind, controlled trial: Southwest Skin Cancer Prevention Study Group. *Cancer Epidemiol Biomarkers Prev* 1997;6:957–961.

Miller PK, Roenigk RK, Brodland DG, et al. Cutaneous micrographic surgery: Mohs procedure. *Mayo Clin Proc* 1992;67:971–980.

Milroy CJ, Richman PI, Wilson GD, et al. Reporting basal cell carcinoma: a survey of the attitudes of histopathologists. *J Clin Pathol* 1999;52:867–869.

Telfer NR, Colver GB, Bowers PW. Guidelines for the management of basal cell carcinoma. *Br J Dermatol* 1999;141:415–423.

Thompson SC, Damien J, Marks R. Reduction of solar keratoses by regular sunscreen use. *N Engl J Med* 1993;329:1147–1151.

Bone and Soft Tissue Sarcoma

Janice N. Cormier, A. Scott Pearson, Sarkis H. Meterissian, and Kenneth K. Tanabe

EPIDEMIOLOGY

In the year 2000, approximately 8,000 new cases of sarcoma were diagnosed in the United States. These rare tumors account for less than 1% of all newly diagnosed adult cancers and represent 7% of malignancies diagnosed in children. Several distinct groups of sarcomas have been recognized: soft tissue sarcomas, bone sarcomas (osteosarcomas/chondrosarcomas), Ewing's sarcomas, and peripheral primitive neuroectodermal tumors.

Soft tissue sarcomas can occur at any site throughout the body, and they encompass more than 50 histiotypes. The majority of primary soft tissue sarcomas originate in an extremity (59%), with the next most frequent anatomic site of origin being the trunk (19%), followed by the retroperitoneum (13%), and the head/neck region (9%). The most common histologic types of soft tissue sarcoma in adults (excluding Kaposi's sarcoma) are malignant fibrous histiocytoma (24%), leiomyosarcoma (21%), liposarcoma (19%), synovial sarcoma (12%), and malignant peripheral nerve sheath tumors (6%). Rhabdomyosarcoma is the most common soft tissue sarcoma of childhood and accounts for approximately 250 cases annually.

Over the past two decades, a multimodality treatment approach has been successfully applied to patients with extremity sarcomas improving survival and quality of life. However, patients with abdominal sarcomas continue to have high rates of recurrence and poor overall survival. The overall 5-year survival rate for patients with all stages of soft tissue sarcoma is 50% to 60%. Most patients die of metastatic disease, which becomes evident within 2 to 3 years of initial diagnosis in 80% of cases. The following are factors that increase a patient's risk for soft tissue sarcoma.

Environmental Factors

Although patients with sarcoma frequently report a history of trauma in the tumor area, a causal relationship has not been established. More often, a minor injury calls attention to a preexisting tumor that may be accentuated by edema or a hematoma.

Occupational Chemicals

Exposure to some herbicides such as phenoxyacetic acids and wood preservatives containing chlorophenols has been linked to an increased risk for the development of soft tissue sarcoma. Several chemical carcinogens including thorotrast, vinyl chloride, and arsenic have been associated with hepatic angiosarcoma. Exposure to asbestos has been associated with the development of mesotheliomas.

Previous Radiation Exposure

External radiation therapy is a rare but well-established cause of soft tissue sarcoma. An eight- to 50-fold increase in the incidence of sarcomas has been reported among patients treated for cancers of the breast, cervix, ovary, testes, and lymphatic system. In a review of 160 patients with postirradiation sarcomas, the most common histologic types were osteogenic sarcoma, malignant fibrous histiocytoma, angiosarcoma, and lymphangiosarcoma. The risk for sarcomas after radiation therapy increases with increasing dosage. The interval between irradiation and the development of sarcoma is usually at least 10 years. Postirradiation sarcomas are often diagnosed at a more advanced stage and therefore, have a poorer prognosis compared with other sarcomas.

Chronic Lymphedema

Stewart and Treves first described the association of chronic lymphedema following axillary dissection and subsequent lymphangiosarcoma in 1948. Lymphangiosarcoma has also been described in patients following filarial infections and in the lower extremities of patients with congenital or heritable lymphedema.

Genetic Predisposition

Specific inherited genetic alterations have been associated with an increased risk of bone and soft tissue sarcomas. For example, patients with Gardner's syndrome (familial polyposis) have a higher than normal incidence of desmoids; patients with germ line mutations in the tumor suppressor gene *p53* (Li-Fraumeni syndrome) have a high incidence of sarcomas; and patients with von Recklinghausen's disease who have abnormalities in the neurofibromatosis type 1 gene (NF1) have an increased risk of neurofibrosarcomas. Soft tissue sarcomas can occur in patients with hereditary retinoblastoma as a second primary malignancy.

Oncogene Activation

Oncogenes are genes that are capable of inducing malignant transformation and tend to drive cells toward proliferation. Several oncogenes have been identified in association with soft tissue sarcomas including MDM2, N-myc, c-erB2, and members of the *ras* family. Amplification of these genes has been shown to correlate with adverse outcome in a variety of soft tissue sarcomas.

Cytogenetic analysis of soft tissue tumors has led to the identification of distinct chromosomal translocations that appear to encode for oncogenes associated with certain histologic subtypes. The gene rearrangements best characterized to date are found in Ewing's sarcoma, clear cell sarcoma, myxoid liposarcoma, alveolar rhabdomyosarcoma, desmoplastic small round cell tumors, and synovial sarcoma.

Tumor Suppressor Genes

Tumor suppressor genes play a critical role in growth inhibition within the cell and are capable of suppressing growth in cancer cells. Inactivation of tumor suppressor genes can occur through hereditary or sporadic mechanisms. The two genes that are most relevant to soft tissue tumors are the retinoblastoma (*Rb*) tumor suppressor gene and the *p53* tumor suppressor gene. Mutations or deletions in *Rb* can lead to the development of retinoblastoma as well as sarcomas of soft tissue and bone. Mutations in the *p53* tumor suppressor gene are the most common mutations in human solid tumors and have been reported in 30% to 60% of cases of soft tissue sarcomas.

PATHOLOGY

Sarcomas are a heterogeneous group of tumors that arise predominantly from the embryonic mesoderm but can also arise from the ectoderm (e.g., peripheral nervous sheath tumors). Mesodermal cells give rise to the connective tissues distributed throughout the body, including pericardium, pleura, blood vessel endothelium, smooth and striated muscle, bone, cartilage, and synovium. These are the cells from which nearly all sarcomas originate. Consequently, sarcomas develop in a wide variety of anatomic sites.

Despite the variety of histologic subtypes, sarcomas have many common clinical and pathologic features. The overall clinical behavior of most types of sarcoma is similar and determined by anatomic location (depth), grade, and size. The dominant pattern of metastasis is hematogenous. Lymph node metastasis is rare (<5%) except in a few histologic subtypes such as epithelioid sarcoma, rhabdomyosarcoma, clear cell sarcoma, and angiosarcoma.

Tumor grade has been firmly established to have prognostic significance and has been incorporated into the staging of soft tissue sarcomas. However, some experts have suggested that pathologic classification is far more important than grade when other pretreatment variables are taken into account. Table 5-1 characterizes the relationship between histiotype and tumor aggressiveness. Tumors with little or no metastatic potential include desmoids, atypical lipomatous tumors (also called well-differentiated liposarcoma), dermatofibrosarcoma protuberans, and hemangiopericytomas. Those subtypes with an intermediate risk of metastatic spread include myxoid liposarcoma, myxoid malignant fibrous histiocytoma, and extraskeletal chondrosarcoma. Among the highly aggressive tumors that have a substantial metastatic potential are angiosarcoma, clear cell sarcoma, pleomorphic and dedifferentiated liposarcoma, leiomyosarcoma, rhabdomyosarcoma, and synovial sarcoma.

Approximately 15% of all soft tissue sarcomas occur in the retroperitoneum. Of tumors that occur in the retroperitoneum, approximately 80% are malignant, with liposarcoma, fibrosarcoma, leiomyosarcoma, and malignant fibrous histiocytoma accounting for the vast majority of histologic types identified.

It is not uncommon for expert sarcoma pathologists to disagree about specific histologic diagnoses or criteria for defining tumor grade in 25% to 40% of individual cases. Few pathologists have the opportunity to study many of these rare tumors during their careers, and this lack of experience may contribute to the relatively low concordance rate. The high rate of pathologic discordance among pathologists emphasizes the need for more objective molecular and biochemical markers to improve conventional histologic assessment.

Table 5-1.   Relationship of sarcoma histiotype and tumor aggressiveness

Low metastatic potential

Desmoid tumor
Atypical lipomatous tumor
Dermatofibrosarcoma protuberans
Hemangiopericytoma

Intermediate metastatic potential

Myxoid liposarcoma
Myxoid malignant fibrous histiocytoma
Extraskeletal chondrosarcoma

High metastatic potential

Alveolar soft part sarcoma
Angiosarcoma
Clear cell sarcoma ("melanoma of soft parts")
Epithelioid sarcoma
Extraskeletal Ewing's sarcoma
Extraskeletal osteosarcoma
Malignant fibrous histiocytoma
Liposarcoma (pleomorphic and dedifferentiated)
Leiomyosarcoma
Neurogenic sarcoma (malignant schwannoma)
Rhabdomyosarcoma
Synovial sarcoma

STAGING

The current version of the American Joint Committee on Cancer (AJCC) staging criteria for soft tissue sarcomas relies on histopathologic grade (G), tumor size and depth (T), as well as the presence of metastases (distant [M] or nodal [N]) (Table 5-2). This sytem does not apply to visceral sarcomas, Kaposi's sarcoma, dermatofibrosarcoma, or desmoid tumors.

Histopathologic Grade

Histopathologic grade remains the most important prognostic factor available for determining disease-free and overall survival rate. To accurately determine tumor grade, an adequate tissue sample must be well-fixed and well-stained and available for review by an experienced sarcoma pathologist. The pathologic features that define grade include cellularity, differentiation, pleomorphism, necrosis, and the number of mitoses. Tumor grade has been shown to predict the development of metastases with a 5% to 10% metastatic potential for low-grade lesions, 25% to 30% for intermediate-grade lesions, and 50% to 60% for high-grade tumors.

Tumor Size

Tumor size at presentation is also an important determinant of outcome. Sarcomas have classically been stratified into two groups based on size: T1 lesions ($\leq$5 cm) or T2 lesions (>5 cm).

Table 5-2. American Joint Committee on Cancer staging criteria for soft tissue sarcomas

Primary tumor (T)

TX	Primary tumor cannot be assessed	
T0	No evidence of primary tumor	
T1	Tumor ≤ 5 cm in greatest dimension	
	T1a	Tumor above superficial fascia
	T1b	Tumor invading or deep to superficial fascia
T2	Tumor > 5 cm in greatest dimension	
	T2a	Tumor above superficial fascia
	T2b	Tumor invading or deep to superficial fascia

Regional lymph nodes (N)

NX	Regional lymph nodes cannot be assessed
N0	No regional lymph node metastasis
N1	Regional lymph node metastasis

Distant metastasis (M)

MX	Distant metastasis cannot be assessed
M0	No distant metastasis
M1	Distant metastasis

Histopathologic grade (G)

GX	Grade cannot be assessed
G1	Well differentiated
G2	Moderately differentiated
G3	Poorly differentiated
G4	Undifferentiated

Stage grouping

Stage I			
	A	G1–2, T1a–1b, N0, M0	(low grade, small, superficial and deep)
	B	G1–2, T2a, N0, M0	(low grade, large, superficial)
Stage II			
	A	G1–2, T2b, N0, M0	(low grade, large, deep)
	B	G3–4, T1a–1b, N0, M0	(high grade, small, superficial, deep)
	C	G3–4, T2a, N0, M0	(high grade, large, superficial)
Stage III		G3–4, T2b, N0, M0	(high grade, large, deep)
Stage IV		Any G, any T, N1, M0	(any metastasis)
		Any G, any T, N0, M1	

Adapted from Fleming ID, Cooper JS, Henson DE, et al., eds. *AJCC manual for staging of cancer,* 5th ed. Philadelphia: Lippincott-Raven, 1997.

The 1997 AJCC staging system defines more accurately the effect of size on prognosis according to its association with a superficial or deep tumor location. Tumors that are superficial to the superficial investing muscular fascia in extremity soft tissue sarcoma are designated *a* lesions in the T score (Ta) whereas tumors deep to the fascia and all retroperitoneal and visceral lesions are designated *b* (Tb).

Nodal Metastasis

Lymph node metastasis is rare. Less than 5% of soft tissue sarcomas metastasize to the nodes. In the 1997 AJCC staging manual, nodal disease is designated stage IV disease, which portends a poor prognosis. A few histologic subtypes such as epithelioid sarcoma, rhabdomyosarcoma, clear cell sarcoma, and angiosarcoma, have been found to have a higher incidence of nodal involvement.

Distant Metastasis

Distant metastases occur most frequently in the lung. Selected patients with pulmonary metastases may become long-term survivors with resection and chemotherapy. Other potential sites of metastasis include bone, brain, and liver. Visceral and retroperitoneal sarcomas have a higher incidence of liver and peritoneal metastases.

EXTREMITY SOFT TISSUE SARCOMAS

More than 50% of soft tissue sarcomas originate in an extremity. The most common subtypes include malignant fibrous histiocytoma, liposarcoma, synovial sarcoma, and fibrosarcoma, although a variety of other histologic types are also seen.

Clinical Presentation

Most extremity soft tissue sarcomas present as an asymptomatic mass, and therefore the size at presentation usually depends on the anatomic site of the tumor. For example, although a 2- to 3-cm tumor may become readily apparent on the back of the hand, a tumor in the thigh may grow to 10 to 15 cm in diameter before it becomes apparent. Frequently, a traumatic event to the affected area will call attention to the preexisting lesion. Some patients present with pain; however, there appear to be no signs or symptoms that reliably distinguish between benign and malignant soft tissue tumors. Small lesions that by clinical history have been unchanged for several years may be closely observed without biopsy. However, a biopsy should be performed for all other tumors.

Biopsy

Accurate preoperative histologic diagnosis is a critical step in determining the primary treatment of soft tissue sarcomas. The biopsy should yield enough tissue to make a pathologic diagnosis without causing complications.

Core-needle biopsies and fine-needle aspirations have been demonstrated to be accurate diagnostic tools, particularly when the diagnosis correlates closely with clinical findings and imaging. Ultrasound and computed tomography (CT) guidance can enhance the positive yield rate by ensuring more accurate localization of the tumor, particularly in deeply located extremity or retroperitoneal tumors.

In some cases, however, tissue samples larger than those provided by needle biopsy may be necessary to obtain sections of viable tissue adequate for determination of grade and histologic type. Excisional biopsy is indicated for lesions smaller than 3 cm. Soft tissue tumors larger than 3 cm in diameter should be assessed by incisional biopsy, regardless of whether malignancy is suspected. This technique should be ideally performed in a designated treatment center and by the surgeon who will be responsible for the definitive surgery.

The biopsy incision should be oriented longitudinally along the extremity, to allow subsequent wide local excision to encompass the biopsy site, scar, and tumor *en bloc*. A poorly oriented biopsy incision often mandates an excessively large surgical defect for wide local excision. This may then result in a larger postoperative radiation therapy field to encompass all tissues at risk. Hemostasis must be achieved at the time of biopsy to prevent dissemination of tumor cells into adjacent tissue planes by hematoma.

Evaluation

The goals of pretreatment radiologic imaging are to accurately define the local extent of a tumor, and evaluate for the presence of malignant disease. Magnetic resonance imaging (MRI) has supplanted CT scans as the imaging technique of choice in the evaluation of soft tissue sarcomas of the extremity. MRI provides accurate delineation of muscle groups and distinction between bone, vascular structures, and tumor. In addition, sagittal and coronal views allow three-dimensional evaluation of anatomic compartments.

The CT scan remains the imaging technique of choice for evaluating retroperitoneal sarcomas. The current generation of CT scanners have the ability to rapidly provide a detailed survey of the abdomen and pelvis with delineation of adjacent organs and vascular structures. For extremity sarcoma, CT may be of importance in instances when the patient has limited access or a contraindication to MRI. A CT scan of the abdomen and pelvis should be obtained when the histologic assessment of an extremity sarcoma reveals myxoid liposarcoma, because this histologic subtype is known to metastasize to the abdomen.

CT is more sensitive than conventional radiographs in the detection of lung, pleural, and mediastinal metastases. Chest CT is used most often in patients with high-grade lesions. Searches for bone and brain metastases are rarely indicated, unless symptoms of metastases to these sites are present.

Management of Local Disease

The success of local tumor control depends on several tumor-related and treatment-related prognostic factors. In multivariate analyses, tumors with high histologic grade, large tumor size (>5 cm), positive surgical margins, or intraoperative violation of the tumor capsule have been associated with a high local recurrence rate. Histologic grade and tumor size are the most significant risk factors for distant metastasis and tumor-related mortality.

Surgery

The type of surgical resection selected is determined by a number of factors, including tumor location, tumor size, depth of invasion, involvement of nearby structures, necessity for skin grafting or autogenous tissue reconstruction, and the patient's performance status.

In the 1970s, 50% of patients presenting with extremity sarcomas were treated with amputation for local control of their tumors. Despite a local recurrence rate of less than 10% following radical surgery, large numbers of patients continued to die from metastatic disease. This realization led to more modern methods of local therapy using conservative surgical excision combined with postoperative radiation therapy with local control rates of 78% to 91%.

Wide local excision is the primary treatment modality for patients with extremity sarcomas. A zone of compressed reactive tissue that forms a pseudocapsule generally surrounds the tumors. The pseudocapsule may mistakenly guide resection by the inexperienced surgeon. Extensions of tumor that go beyond the pseudocapsule must be considered in planning surgery and radiotherapy. The goal of local therapy is to resect the tumor with a 2-cm margin of surrounding normal soft tissue. In some anatomic areas, these margins are not attainable because of the proximity of vital structures. The biopsy site or tract should also be included en bloc with the resected specimen when possible.

Elective regional lymphadenectomy is rarely indicated in patients with soft tissue sarcomas. However, in patients with rhabdomyosarcoma or epithelioid sarcoma with suspicious clinical or radiologic findings, fine-needle aspiration of lymph nodes should be considered. In these rare cases, a lymph node dissection may be indicated for regional control of disease. A prospective trial is currently under way to evaluate the role of lymphatic mapping and sentinel lymph node biopsy in pediatric patients with extremity rhabdomyosarcomas.

There have been several studies reporting favorable local control rates for extremity tumors treated with conservative resection combined with radiation therapy. In a small study from the National Cancer Institute, there was no difference in survival among patients treated with conservative surgery plus radiation therapy compared with patients treated with amputation. In 1985, based on the limited data available, the National Institutes of Health developed a consensus statement recommending limb-sparing surgery for the majority of patients with high-grade extremity sarcomas. However, for patients whose tumor cannot be grossly resected with a limb-sparing procedure and function preservation ($<5\%$), amputation remains the treatment of choice.

Radiation Therapy

The primary goal of radiation therapy is to optimize local tumor control after conservative surgical resection. The optimal mode or timing of delivery, preoperative versus postoperative versus intraoperative versus brachytherapy, has not yet been defined.

The evidence for adjunctive radiation therapy in patients eligible for conservative surgical resection comes from two randomized trials and a number of large single institution reports. In the randomized trial from the National Cancer Institute, 91 patients with high-grade extremity tumors were treated with limb-sparing surgery followed by chemotherapy alone or radiation therapy plus adjuvant chemotherapy. A second group of 50 patients with low-grade tumors were treated with resection alone versus resection with radiation therapy. The 10-year local control rate for all patients receiving radiation therapy was 98% compared with 70% for those not receiving radiation therapy.

In another randomized trial performed at Memorial Sloan Kettering Cancer Center, 164 patients were randomized to observation or brachytherapy following conservative surgery. The 5-year local control rate for patients with high-grade tumors was 66% in the observation group and 89% in the group treated with brachytherapy. There was no significant difference between the groups with low-grade tumors.

Until recently, the policy at M.D. Anderson Cancer Center was to administer radiation therapy as an adjunct to surgery for all patients with intermediate and highly aggressive tumors of any size. However, several groups have stated that all small soft tissue sarcomas (≤ 5 cm) should be considered favorable tumors for which postoperative radiation therapy does not improve 5-year survival or local-recurrence-free survival. The use of radiation therapy should be strongly considered after excision of tumors 5 cm or smaller when margins are close, positive, or uncertain, and in instances when reexcision in this group of patients is not practical.

Preoperative Versus Postoperative External-Beam Radiation Therapy

There is no consensus as to the optimal sequence of radiation therapy and surgery. The available data are based largely on single institution, nonrandomized studies. At M.D. Anderson, radiation therapy is preferentially used preoperatively. There are several advantages to preoperative radiation therapy. First, multidisciplinary planning with the radiation oncologist, medical oncologist, and surgeon is facilitated early in the course of therapy with the tumor in place. Also, preoperative radiation therapy allows the delivery of lower doses of radiation to an undisturbed tissue bed with potentially improved tissue oxygenation. In addition, the size of the preoperative radiation fields and the number of joints included in the fields is significantly smaller than that of postoperative radiation fields, which may result in improved functional outcome.

Critics of preoperative radiation therapy cite the difficulty with the pathologic assessment of margins, and the increased rate of wound complication as deterrents to preoperative radiation therapy. However, plastic surgery techniques with advanced tissue transfer procedures are being used more frequently in these high-risk wounds with better outcomes. Results are encouraging, with a high success rate (>90%) of healed wounds in a single-stage operation.

Brachytherapy

Brachytherapy has been reported to achieve local control rates comparable with those achieved with external-beam radiation therapy. Brachytherapy involves the placement of multiple catheters in the tumor resection bed. Guidelines have been established that recommend placing the after-loading catheters at 1-cm increments with a 2-cm margin around the surgical bed. After adequate wound healing is established, usually after the fifth postoperative day, the catheters are loaded with radioactive wires (iridium-192) delivering 42 to 45 Gy to the tumor bed over 4 to 6 days. The frequency of wound complications with brachytherapy is similar to that seen with postoperative radiation therapy (approximately 10%).

The primary benefit to brachytherapy is the shorter overall treatment time of 4 to 6 days compared with preoperative or postoperative regimens that generally take 4 to 6 weeks. Brachytherapy also produces less radiation scatter in critical anatomic regions (e.g., gonads and joints) with potentially improved function. Cost-analysis comparison of brachytherapy versus external beam radiation therapy found lower charges for patients undergoing adjuvant irradiation with brachytherapy for soft tissue sarcoma.

Systemic Chemotherapy

Despite improvements in the rate of local control, metastasis and death remain significant problems for patients with high-risk soft tissue sarcomas. Patients considered at high risk for death from sarcoma include patients presenting with metastatic disease as well as patients presenting with localized sarcomas arising in nonextremity sites or demonstrating intermediate- or high-grade histology or large (T2) tumor size. The treatment regimen for patients with high-risk localized disease, metastatic disease, or both often includes chemotherapy.

As a group, sarcomas include histologic subtypes that are very responsive to cytotoxic chemotherapy as well as subtypes that are universally resistant to current agents. Only three drugs, doxorubicin, dacarbazine, and ifosfamide, have consistently demonstrated response rates of 20% in advanced soft tissue sarcomas. The majority of active chemotherapeutic trials have included doxorubicin as part of the treatment regimen. Response to ifosfamide has been reported to vary from 20% to 60% in single-institution series using higher dose regimens or when combined with doxorubicin.

Adjuvant (Postoperative) Chemotherapy

Individual randomized trials of adjuvant chemotherapy have failed to demonstrate improvement in disease-free and overall survival in patients with soft tissue sarcomas. However, there are several criticisms of these individual trials that may explain why they failed to demonstrate improvement in survival.

First, the chemotherapy regimens utilized were suboptimal with single-agent drugs (most commonly doxorubicin) and less intensive dosing schedules. Second, the sample sizes in these trials were not large enough to detect clinically significant differences in survival. Additionally, the majority of patients that did not respond to the initial treatment regimen were started on other chemotherapeutic regimens that potentially affected disease-free and overall survival. Lastly, most studies included patients at low risk for metastasis and death, that is, those with small (<5 cm) and low-grade tumors.

Hence, adjuvant chemotherapy for patients with soft tissue sarcomas remains controversial. To address this question, a formal meta-analysis was performed in 1997. The Sarcoma Meta-Analysis Collaboration reported on 1,568 patients from 14 trials of doxorubicin-based adjuvant chemotherapy to evaluate the effect of adjuvant chemotherapy on localized, resectable soft tissue sarcomas. With a median follow-up of 9.4 years, doxorubicin-based chemotherapy significantly improved the time to local and distant recurrence and overall recurrence-free survival. However, the absolute benefit in overall survival for the entire group was only 4%, which was not statistically significant. In examining subsets, those patients with extremity tumors did show a 7% benefit in survival.

Neoadjuvant (Preoperative) Chemotherapy

The basis of neoadjuvant/preoperative chemotherapy for soft tissue sarcomas is based on the belief that only 30% to 50% of patients will respond to standard chemotherapeutic regimens. Neoadjuvant chemotherapy enables the oncologist to identify those select patients whose disease is responsive to chemotherapy by measuring response with the primary tumor in situ. Patients who respond with tumor shrinkage after two or four courses undergo local treatment with surgery, radiation therapy, or a combination followed by postoperative chemotherapy with the same agents. Patients who are unresponsive to short courses of preoperative chemotherapy are spared the toxic effects of prolonged postoperative chemotherapy with agents to which they have demonstrated insensitivity. In a retrospective review of this approach at M.D. Anderson, marked improvement in overall, disease-free, and distant disease-free survival rates were seen in patients who responded to neoadjuvant therapy.

Regional Chemotherapy/Isolated Limb Perfusion

Isolated limb perfusion (ILP) is an investigational approach for treating extremity sarcomas. There are approximately 10% of patients that present with extremity sarcomas for which amputation is the only option for local treatment. The regional administration of high-dose chemotherapy via ILP has been attempted mainly as a limb-sparing alternative in these patients.

The technique of ILP involves isolation of the main artery and vein of the perfused limb from the systemic circulation. The specific tumor site determines the choice of the specific anatomic approach. External iliac vessels are used for thigh tumors, femoral or popliteal vessels for calf tumors, and axillary vessels for upper extremity tumors. The vessels are dissected, and all collateral vessels are ligated. The vessels are then cannulated and connected to a pump oxygenator similar to that used in cardiopulmonary bypass. A tourniquet or Esmarch band is applied to the limb to achieve complete vascular isolation. The chemotherapeutic agents are then added to the perfusion circuit and recirculated for 90 minutes. The temperature of the perfused limb is maintained during the entire procedure by both external heating and warming of the perfusates. At the end of the procedure, the drugs are washed out of the limb, the cannulas are removed, and the blood vessels repaired.

Several problems are evident when trying to interpret the studies published to date including the heterogeneous nature of patients treated and the wide variety of chemotherapeutic agents used in the perfusion circuit. Despite these problems, favorable response rates ranging from 18% to 80% with overall 5-year survival rates of 50% to 70% have been reported.

Management of Local Recurrence

Recurrent disease will develop in up to 20% of patients with extremity sarcoma. There continues to be controversy regarding the impact of local failures on survival and distant disease-free survival. Many believe recurrence represents a harbinger of distant metastatic disease. The adequacy of surgical resection clearly can play a role in the development of local recurrences. Patients with microscopically positive surgical margins are at increased risk for local recurrence.

An isolated local recurrence should be treated aggressively with margin-negative re-resection (possibly amputation) with the addition of radiation therapy. Patients previously treated with external beam radiation therapy may be considered for brachytherapy or intraoperative radiation therapy. Several small studies have shown that patients with isolated local recurrences may be successfully re-treated with local-recurrence-free survival rates approaching 72%.

Management of Distant Disease

The majority of patients with soft tissue sarcomas present without evidence of distant metastases. The incidence of metastases is 40% to 50% in patients with intermediate- and high-grade extremity sarcomas, compared with only 5% in patients with low-grade sarcomas. Most metastases to distant sites occur within 2 years of initial diagnosis. For primary extremity sarcomas, the predominant site of distant metastasis is the lung in 73% of cases.

In the absence of extrapulmonary metastases, lung metastases should be resected if the patient is medically fit to withstand a thoracotomy and the lesions are amenable to resection. Large series have reported 3-year survival rates of 40% to 50% in patients with completely resectable pulmonary metastases. A disease-free interval of more than 12 months, the ability to resect all metastatic disease, age less than 50 years, and absence of preceding local recurrence were found to be independent prognostic factors in multivariate analysis of patients undergoing resection of pulmonary metastases.

General Recommendations

General recommendations for management of extremity soft tissue sarcomas are as follows:

1. Soft tissue tumors smaller than 3 cm should be evaluated by excisional biopsy with 1- to 2-cm margins.
2. Soft tissue tumors larger than 3 cm should be evaluated with radiologic imaging and tissue diagnosis by fine needle aspiration or core needle biopsy.
3. Evaluate for metastatic disease once sarcoma diagnosis is established: chest radiograph for low- or intermediate-grade lesions and T1 tumors and chest CT for high-grade or T2 tumors.
4. Wide local excision with 2-cm margins is adequate therapy for low-grade lesions and T1 tumors.
5. Radiation therapy plays a critical role in the management of T2 tumors.
6. Patients with high-grade sarcomas should be considered for preoperative (neoadjuvant) or postoperative (adjuvant) chemotherapy.
7. An aggressive surgical approach should be taken in the treatment of patients with an isolated local recurrence or resectable distant metastases.

RETROPERITONEAL SARCOMAS

Fifteen percent of soft tissue sarcomas in adults occur in the retroperitoneum. Most retroperitoneal tumors are malignant, and approximately one-third are soft tissue sarcomas. The differential diagnosis of a patient presenting with a retroperitoneal tumor includes lymphoma, germ cell tumors, and undifferentiated carcinomas. The most common sarcomas occurring in the retroperitoneum are liposarcomas, malignant fibrous histiocytomas, and leiomyosarcomas.

Although significant advances in the understanding of extremity soft tissue sarcomas have resulted in improved treatments and outcomes, similar progress has not been achieved in the understanding and treatment of retroperitoneal soft tissue sarcomas. Patients with retroperitoneal soft tissue sarcomas generally have a worse prognosis than those with extremity sarcomas. This is because retroperitoneal soft tissue sarcomas commonly grow to larger sizes before they become clinically apparent, and they often involve important vital structures that preclude surgical resection. Furthermore, the surgical margins that can be obtained around these sarcomas are often inadequate because of anatomic constraints.

Clinical Presentation

Retroperitoneal sarcomas generally present as large masses; nearly 50% are larger than 20 cm at the time of diagnosis. They typically do not produce symptoms until they grow large enough to compress or invade contiguous structures. On occasion, patients may present with neurologic symptoms from compression of lumbar or pelvic nerves or obstructive gastrointestinal symptoms related to displacement or direct tumor involvement of an intestinal organ.

Evaluation

The workup of a retroperitoneal mass begins with an accurate history that should exclude signs and symptoms associated with lymphoma (e.g., fever and night sweats). Complete physical examination with particular attention to all nodal basins and a testicular examination for males is critically important. Laboratory assessment can be helpful; an increased lactate dehydrogenase concentration can be suggestive of lymphoma, whereas an increased β-human chorionic gonadotropin level, alpha-fetoprotein level, or both can indicate a germ cell tumor.

Radiologic assessment should include a CT scan of the abdomen and pelvis to define the extent of the tumor and its relationship to surrounding structures, particularly vascular structures. Imaging should also evaluate the liver for the presence of metastases, discontinuous abdominal disease, and bilateral renal function. Thoracic CT is indicated to evaluate for the presence of lung metastases. In patients presenting with an equivocal history, unusual appearance of the mass, unresectability, or distant metastasis or who are potentially eligible for a neoadjuvant protocol, a CT-guided core-needle biopsy is appropriate for obtaining a tissue diagnosis.

Management

Complete surgical resection is the most effective treatment for primary or recurrent retroperitoneal sarcomas. These tumors often involve vital structures precluding surgical resection. Even if surgical resection can be performed, margins are often compromised because of anatomic constraints. In several retrospective assessments of patients with retroperitoneal sarcoma, complete surgical excision was achieved in only 40% to 60% of patients. In an analysis of 500 patients with retroperitoneal soft tissue sarcomas treated at Memorial Sloan Kettering Cancer Center, the median survival duration of patients who underwent complete resection was 103 months versus 18 months for patients undergoing incomplete resection, which was no different than observation without resection.

Surgical resection should not be offered to patients unless radiographic evidence indicates the potential for full resection. Palliative surgical procedures may be performed to address symptoms of intestinal obstruction or bleeding. In particular, patients with atypical lipomatous tumors, also termed well-differentiated liposarcomas may benefit symptomatically by repeated debulking.

Adjuvant Therapy

Chemotherapy has not been shown to be effective treatment for retroperitoneal sarcomas. Several centers have ongoing protocols to determine the role of preoperative chemotherapy and radiation therapy for these tumors.

Management of Recurrent Disease

Retroperitoneal sarcomas will recur in two-thirds of patients. In addition to recurring locally in the tumor bed and metastasizing to the lungs, retroperitoneal leiomyosarcomas frequently spread to the liver. Also, retroperitoneal sarcomas can recur diffusely throughout the peritoneal cavity (sarcomatosis). The approach to resectable recurrent disease after treatment of a retroperitoneal sarcoma is similar to the approach taken after the recurrence of an extremity sarcoma. In a large series at Memorial Sloan Kettering Cancer Center, the authors were able to resect recurrent tumors in 57% of patients with a first recurrence. However, the resection rate fell to 20% after a second recurrence and to 10% after a third. Isolated liver metastases, if stable over several months, may be amenable to resection.

Well-differentiated liposarcoma may recur in a poorly differentiated form. This dedifferentiated retroperitoneal liposarcoma is more aggressive with greater propensity for distant metastasis than its well-differentiated precursor.

Follow-Up

The goal of follow-up strategies for detection of any type of cancer recurrence is based on the premise that early recognition and treatment of recurrent, local, or distant disease can prolong survival. The ideal follow-up strategy should be easy to implement, accurate and cost-effective.

The primary determinant of survival in patients with soft tissue sarcoma is the development of distant metastases. The pattern of recurrence is related to the anatomic site of the primary tumor. Patients with extremity sarcomas generally experience recurrence with distant pulmonary metastases, whereas patients with retroperitoneal or intraabdominal sarcomas tend to have local recurrences as frequently as pulmonary metastases.

The ability of early detection of recurrence to improve overall survival depends on the availability of effective therapeutic interventions. A few reports involving small numbers of patients have reported on the ability to salvage patients with recurrent local disease with radical reexcision with or without radiation therapy. Similarly, several groups have reported on patients with prolonged survival following resection of pulmonary metastases. These limited data form the basis of aggressive surveillance strategies for patients with soft tissue sarcoma.

The majority of recurrent soft tissue sarcomas occur within the first 2 years after completion of therapy. Patients should be evaluated with a complete history and physical examination every 3 months and a chest radiograph every 6 months during this high-risk period. If the chest radiograph reveals a suspicious nodule, a CT scan of the chest should be obtained for further assessment. Most experts recommend that the tumor site be evaluated every 6 months with either an MRI for an extremity tumor or a CT scan for intraabdominal or retroperitoneal tumors. In some circumstances, ultrasound can be used to assess for extremity tumor recurrence. Follow-up intervals may be lengthened to every 6 months with annual imaging for years 2 through 5. After 5 years, patients should be assessed annually and a chest radiograph should be obtained.

OTHER SOFT TISSUE LESIONS

Sarcoma of the Breast

Sarcomas in the breast are rare tumors, accounting for less than 1% of all breast malignancies and less than 5% of all soft tissue sarcomas. A variety of histologic subtypes have been reported to occur within the breast, including angiosarcoma, stromal sarcoma, fibrosarcoma, and malignant fibrous histiocytoma. Cystosarcoma phyllodes is generally excluded from other soft tissue sarcomas because these tumors are thought to originate from hormonally responsive stromal cells of the breast and the majority are benign tumors.

As in patients with sarcomas of other anatomic sites, histopathologic grade and tumor size are important prognostic factors. Local recurrences increase as the tumor size increases and tumors smaller than 5 cm are associated with better overall survival. Local and distant recurrence is more common in high-grade lesions. Complete excision with negative margins is the primary therapy. Mastectomy carries no additional benefit if complete excision can be accomplished by wide local excision. Because of low rates of regional lymphatic spread, axillary dissection is not routinely indicated. Neoadjuvant chemotherapy or radiation therapy may be considered for patients with large, higher-risk tumors.

Desmoids

Desmoid tumors do not metastasize and are considered low-grade sarcomas. Approximately half of these tumors arise in the extremity, with the remaining lesions located on the trunk or in the retroperitoneal position. Abdominal wall desmoids are associated with pregnancy and are thought to be under hormonal influence. Patients with Gardner's syndrome may have retroperitoneal desmoids as an extracolonic manifestation of the disease. Surgical resection with wide local excision should be the primary therapy of desmoid tumors. Local recurrence may occur in up to one-third of patients. Adjuvant radiation therapy has been associated with reduced local recurrence.

Dermatofibrosarcoma Protuberans

Dermatofibrosarcoma protuberans is a neoplasm arising in the dermis that may occur anywhere in the body. Approximately 40% arise on the trunk, with most of the remaining tumors distributed between the head and neck and extremities. The lesion presents as a nodular, cutaneous mass with slow and persistent growth. Satellite lesions may be found with larger tumors. Wide local excision is recommended, although recurrence rates are as high as 30% to 50%.

BONE SARCOMAS

Epidemiology

Malignant tumors of the musculoskeletal system constitute 10% of newly diagnosed cancers in the population less than 30 years of age and account for 1,000 cases annually in the United States.

However, malignant tumors arising from the skeletal systems represent only 0.2% of all primary cancers.

Osteosarcoma and Ewing's sarcoma are the two most common malignant conditions of bone.

Osteosarcoma has a peak frequency during adolescent growth. Ewing's sarcoma occurs most frequently in the second decade of life.

Clinical Presentation

The most common presentation of bone sarcomas (Ewing's or osteosarcoma) is pain or swelling in a bone or joint. As with soft tissue sarcomas in adults, often a traumatic event draws attention to the swelling and can delay diagnosis. Osteosarcoma most commonly involves the metaphysis of long bones especially the distal femur, proximal tibia, or humerus. Ewing's sarcoma may involve flat bones or the diaphysis of tubular bones such as the femur, pelvis, tibia, and fibula. Ewing's sarcoma may also occur in soft tissues. Chondrosarcoma occurs most commonly in the pelvis, proximal femur, and shoulder girdle.

Up to 25% of patients presenting with osteosarcoma or Ewing's sarcoma have metastatic disease at presentation. The most frequent metastatic sites for osteosarcoma include the lung (90% of cases) and the bone (10%), whereas Ewing's sarcoma metastases occur in the lung (50%), bone (25%), and bone marrow (25%).

Staging

As with soft tissue sarcomas, histopathologic grade is a crucial component of staging bone sarcomas. The surgical staging system for musculoskeletal sarcoma is based on the system by Enneking and includes prognostic variables such as histopathologic grade (G), location of the tumor (T), and the presence or absence of metastases (M). The three stages are stage I, low grade (G1); stage II, high grade (G2); and stage III, G1 or G2 with the presence of metastases (M1). Each stage is subdivided into *a* if the lesion is anatomically confined within well-delineated surgical compartments (T1) or *b* if the lesion is located beyond such compartments in ill-defined fascial planes and spaces (T2).

Diagnosis

The evaluation of patients with a suspected bone tumor should include a thorough history and physical examination, plain radiographs, and MRI of the entire affected bone. Bone scanning and CT of the chest are also necessary.

On plain radiographs, malignant bone tumors demonstrate irregular borders often with evidence of bone destruction and periosteal reaction. Soft tissue extension is also frequently seen.

Biopsy

In the evaluation of a patient suspected of harboring an osteosarcoma, a core-needle biopsy is the diagnostic procedure of choice. A core-needle biopsy performed under radiographic guidance may be up to 100% diagnostic for osteosarcoma.

Treatment

Effective multimodality therapy has dramatically improved 5-year survival rates from 10% to 20% in 1970 to the current 60% to 70% for childhood musculoskeletal tumors. Limb salvage is standard treatment for most patients with osteosarcoma.

Surgery

Limb salvage is the standard surgical approach to bone sarcomas whenever feasible. Successful limb-sparing surgery consists of three phases: tumor resection, bone reconstruction, and soft tissue coverage. Complete surgical extirpation of the primary tumor and any metastases is essential for osteosarcoma because this tumor is relatively resistant to radiation therapy.

If possible, resection of Ewing's sarcoma is also desirable. If surgical removal with a wide surgical margin can be achieved, the prognosis is favorable (12-year relapse-free survival of 60%). However, Ewing's sarcoma most typically involves the pelvis with extensive soft tissue mass invading the pelvic cavity that makes it difficult to carry out radical surgery.

Surgical resection is usually the only treatment modality indicated for the management of chondrosarcomas, because this type of tumor is unresponsive to existing adjuvant therapies.

Chemotherapy

Chemotherapy has revolutionized the approach to most bone sarcomas and is considered standard care for osteosarcoma and Ewing's sarcoma. The bleak 15% to 20% survival rate with surgery alone during the 1960s has improved to 55% to 80% with the combination of chemotherapy to surgical resection. The timing of chemotherapy, the mode of delivery, and the drug combinations continue to be studied in multiinstitutional trials. Effective agents include doxorubicin, cisplatin, methotrexate, ifosfamide, and cyclophosphamide. Randomized clinical trials of patients with osteosarcoma have demonstrated that the use of combination chemotherapy in addition to surgery results in cure rates of 58% to 76%. Preoperative chemotherapy is an attractive option because of its potential to downstage tumors, thus allowing for the maximal application of limb-sparing surgery. Additionally, tumor necrosis following preoperative chemotherapy has been shown to be the most important prognostic variable determining survival.

Multiagent chemotherapy has also been demonstrated to be essential in the treatment of Ewing's sarcoma. Trials spanning over 20 years performed by the Intergroup Study of Ewing's sarcoma have established the efficacy of multi-drug regimens (i.e., regimens that involve combinations of vincristine, doxorubicin, cyclophosphamide, ifosfamide, and etoposide) in improving 5-year relapse-free survival rates up to 70% in patients with nonmetastatic disease.

Radiation Therapy

Because osteosarcomas are generally radiation-resistant, the major role of radiation therapy is for the palliation of large, unresectable tumors. In contrast, radiation therapy is the primary mode of treatment for most localized Ewing's sarcomas. Preoperative irradiation may also be considered to reduce tumor volume before attempted surgical resection.

Recurrent Disease

Bone tumors disseminate through the bloodstream and commonly metastasize to the lungs and bony skeleton. In the past, only 10% to 30% of patients presenting with detectable metastatic osteosarcoma became long-term disease-free survivors. More recent studies have shown that combined modality approaches consisting of surgical resection of the primary tumor and metastatic deposits in conjunction with multiagent chemotherapy can improve 5-year disease-free survival rates to 47%.

Patients with Ewing's sarcoma may recur with distant disease as long as 15 years after initial diagnosis. In a retrospective analysis of 241 patients with Ewing's sarcoma of the pelvis, tumor volume, responsiveness to chemotherapy, and adequate surgical margins were the major factors that influenced prognosis.

Patients with suspected tumor recurrence should undergo a complete evaluation to determine the extent of the disease. Pulmonary metastasectomy has become the mainstay of treatment for patients with osteosarcoma. Prognosis can generally be determined by response to previous therapy, duration of remission, and extent of metastases. Multimodality therapy, including chemotherapeutic agents not previously used, is the general recommendation for treatment.

Sacrococcygeal Chordoma

The notochordal remnant is the origin of this rare tumor. Chordomas are locally aggressive tumors with high recurrence rates. Vague symptoms often result in delayed presentation. Surgical resection should involve a multidisciplinary approach involving the surgical oncologist, neurosurgeon, and reconstructive plastic surgeon. A two-part procedure is used at our institution. The first part involves an anterior approach during which blood supply to the tumor, arising from the iliac vessels, is controlled. Several days later, a posterior approach is used to resect the tumor. Radiation therapy should be considered because of high rates of local recurrence.

RECOMMENDED READING

American Joint Committee on Cancer. *AJCC cancer staging manual.* Philadelphia: Lippincott-Raven, 1997.

Arndt CA, Crist WM. Common musculoskeletal tumors of childhood and adolescence. *N Engl J Med* 1999;341:342.

Ayala AG, Ro JY, Fanning CV, et al. Core needle biopsy and fine-needle aspiration in the diagnosis of bone and soft tissue lesions. *Hematol Oncol Clin North Am* 1995;9:633.

Baldini EH, Goldberg J, Jenner C, et al. Long-term outcomes after function-sparing surgery without radiotherapy for soft tissue sarcoma of the extremities and trunk. *J Clin Oncol* 1999;17:3252.

Barkley HT, Martin RG, Romsdahl MM, et al. Treatment of soft tissue sarcomas by preoperative irradiation and conservative surgical resection. *Int J Radiat Oncol Biol Phys* 1988;14:693.

Billingsley KG, Burt ME, Jara E, et al. Pulmonary metastases from soft tissue sarcoma: analysis of patterns of disease and postmetastasis survival. *Ann Surg* 1999;229:602.

Billingsley KG, Lewis JJ, Leung DH, et al. Multifactorial analysis of the survival of patients with distant metastasis arising from primary extremity sarcoma. *Cancer* 1999;85:389.

Brady MS, Gaynor JJ, Brennan MF. Radiation-associated sarcoma of bone and soft tissue. *Arch Surg* 1992;127:1379.

Brennan MF, Casper ES, Harrison LB, et al. The role of multimodality therapy in soft tissue sarcoma. *Ann Surg* 1991;214:328.

Casson AG, Putnam JB, Natarajan G, et al. Five year survival after pulmonary metastasectomy for adult soft tissue sarcoma. *Cancer* 1992;69:662.

Chang AE, Kinsella T, Glatstein E, et al. Adjuvant chemotherapy for patients with high-grade soft tissue sarcomas of the extremity. *J Clin Oncol* 1988;6:1491.

Chang AE, Matory YL, Dwyer AJ, et al. Magnetic resonance imaging versus computed tomography in the evaluation of soft tissue tumors of the extremities. *Ann Surg* 1997;205:340.

Davis AM, Bell RS, Goodwin PJ. Prognostic factors in osteosarcoma: a critical review. *J Clin Oncol* 1994;12:423.

Eggermont AM, Schrafford T, Koops H, et al. Isolated limb perfusion with tumor necrosis factor and melphalan for limb salvage in 186 patients with locally advanced soft tissue extremity sarcoma. The cumulative multicenter European experience. *Ann Surg* 1996;224:756.

Eilber FR, Eckardt J. Surgical management of soft tissue sarcomas. *Semin Oncol* 1997;24:526.

Fong Y, Coit DG, Woodruff JM, Brennan MF. Lymph node metastasis from soft tissue sarcoma in adults. Analysis of data from a prospective database of 1772 sarcoma patients. *Ann Surg* 1993;217:72.

Geer RJ, Woodruff J, Casper ES, et al. Management of small soft tissue sarcomas of the extremity in adults. *Arch Surg* 1992;127:1285.

Glenn J, Sindelar WF, Kinsella T, et al. Results of multimodality therapy of resectable soft tissue sarcomas of the retroperitoneum. *Surgery* 1985;97:316.

Gutman H, Pollock RE, Benjamin RS, et al. Sarcoma of the breast: implications for extent of therapy. The M. D. Anderson experience. *Surgery* 1994;116:505.

Heslin MJ, Smith JK. Imaging of soft tissue sarcomas. *Surg Oncol Clin North Am* 1999;8:91.

Hoffmann C, Ahrens S, Dunst J, et al. Pelvic Ewing sarcoma: a retrospective analysis of 241 cases. *Cancer* 1999;85:869.

Huth JF, Eilber FR. Patterns of metastatic spread following resection of extremity soft tissue sarcomas and strategies for treatment. *Semin Surg Oncol* 1988;4:20.

Jaques DP, Coit DG, Hajdu SI, et al. Management of primary and recurrent soft tissue sarcoma of the retroperitoneum. *Ann Surg* 1990;212:51.

Karakousis CP, Proimakis C, Rao U, et al. Local recurrence and survival in soft tissue sarcomas. *Ann Surg Oncol* 1996;3:255.

Lawrence W Jr., Donegan WL, Natarajan N, et al. Adult soft tissue sarcomas. A pattern of care survey of the American College of Surgeons. *Ann Surg* 1987;205:349.

Levine EA. Prognostic factors in soft tissue sarcoma. *Semin Surg Oncol* 1999;17:23.

Lewis JJ, Leung D, Woodruff JM, Brennan MF. Retroperitoneal soft tissue sarcoma: analysis of 500 patients treated and followed at a single institution. *Ann Surg* 1998;228:355.

Lienard D, Ewalenko P, Delmotte JJ, et al. High-dose recombinant tumor necrosis factor alpha in combination with interferon gamma and melphalan in isolation perfusion of the limbs for melanoma and sarcoma. *J Clin Oncol* 1992;10:52.

Lindberg RD, Martin RG, Romsdahl MM, et al. Conservative surgery and postoperative radiotherapy in 300 adults with soft tissue sarcomas. *Cancer* 1981;47:2391.

Localio AS, Eng K, Ranson JHC. Abdominosacral approach for retrorectal tumors. *Am Surg* 1980;179:555.

Mazanet R, Antman KH. Adjuvant therapy for sarcomas. *Semin Oncol* 1991;18:603.

Midis GP, Pollock RE, Chen NP, et al. Locally recurrent soft tissue sarcoma of the extremities. *Surgery* 1998;123:666.

National Institutes of Health consensus development panel on limb-sparing treatment of adult soft tissue sarcoma and osteosarcomas. 1985;3:1.

Patel SR, Benjamin RS. New chemotherapeutic strategies for soft tissue sarcomas. *Semin Surg Oncol* 1999;17:47.

Pezzi CM, Pollock RE, Evans HL, et al. Preoperative chemotherapy for soft tissue sarcoma of the extremities. *Ann Surg* 1990;211:476.

Pisters PW, Harrison LB, Leung DH, et al. Long-term results of a prospective randomized trial of adjuvant brachytherapy in soft tissue sarcoma. *J Clin Oncol* 1996;14:859.

Pisters PWT, Harrison LB, Woodruff JM, et al. A prospective randomized trial of adjuvant brachytherapy in the management of low grade soft tissue sarcomas of the extremity and superficial trunk. *J Clin Oncol* 1994;12:1150.

Pisters PW, Leung DH, Woodruff J, et al. Analysis of prognostic factors in 1,041 patients with localized soft tissue sarcomas of the extremities. *J Clin Oncol* 1996;14:1679.

Pollock RE, Karnell LH, Menck HR, et al. The National Cancer Data Base report on soft tissue sarcoma. *Cancer* 1996;78:2247.

Potter DA, Kinsella T, Glatstein E, et al. High-grade soft tissue sarcomas of the extremities. *Cancer* 1986;58:190.

Ramanathan RC, A'Hern R, Fisher C, et al. Modified staging system for extremity soft tissue sarcomas. *Ann Surg Oncol* 1999;5:57.

Razek A, Perez C, Tefft M, et al. Intergroup Ewing's sarcoma study: local control related to radiation dose, volume and site of primary lesion in Ewing's sarcoma. *Cancer* 1980;46:516.

Rosenberg SA, Tepper J, Glatstein E, et al. The treatment of soft tissue sarcomas of the extremities: prospective randomized evaluations of (1) limb-sparing surgery plus radiation therapy compared with amputation and (2) the role of adjuvant chemotherapy. *Ann Surg* 1982;196:305.

Sarcoma Meta-analysis Collaboration. Adjuvant chemotherapy for localized resectable soft tissue sarcoma of adults: meta-analysis of individual data. *Lancet* 1997;350:1647.

Singer S. New diagnostic modalities in soft tissue sarcoma. *Semin Surg Oncol* 1999;17:11.

Singer S, Corson JM, Demetri GD, et al. Prognostic factors predictive of survival for truncal and retroperitoneal soft tissue sarcoma. *Ann Surg* 1995;221:185.

Storm FK, Mahvi DM. Diagnosis and management of retroperitoneal soft tissue sarcoma. *Ann Surg* 1991;214:2.

Suit HD, Mankin HJ, Wood WC, et al. Treatment of the patient with stage M0 soft tissue sarcoma. *J Clin Oncol* 1988;6:854.

Tanabe KK, Pollock RE, Ellis LM, et al. Influence of surgical margins on outcome in patients with preoperatively irradiated extremity soft tissue sarcomas. *Cancer* 1994;73:1652.

Van Geel AN, Pastorino U, Jauch KW, et al. Surgical treatment of lung metastases: the European Organization for Research and Treatment of Cancer-soft tissue and bone sarcoma group study of 255 patients. *Cancer* 1996;77:675.

Varma DG. Optimal radiologic imaging of soft tissue sarcomas. *Semin Surg Oncol* 1999;17:2.

Verweij A, van Oosterom A, Somers R, et al. Chemotherapy in the multidisciplinary approach to soft tissue sarcomas: EORTC soft tissue and bone sarcoma group studies in perspective. *Ann Oncol* 1992;3[suppl 2]:75.

Whooley BP, Mooney MM, Gibbs JF, et al. Effective follow-up strategies in soft tissue sarcoma. *Semin Surg Oncol* 1999;17:83.

Yang JC, Chang AE, Baker AR, et al. Randomized prospective study of the benefit of adjuvant radiation therapy in the treatment of soft tissue sarcomas of the extremity. *J Clin Oncol* 1998;16:197.

Zahm SH, Fraumeni JR Jr. The epidemiology of soft tissue sarcoma. *Semin Oncol* 1997;24:504.

Carcinoma of the Head and Neck

Kresimira M. Milas

EPIDEMIOLOGY

This chapter focuses on squamous cell carcinomas (SCCs) of the head and neck and on salivary gland tumors; thyroid and parathyroid tumors are discussed in Chapter 16.

Approximately 67,000 cancers of the head and neck are diagnosed in the United States each year, accounting for 2% to 3% of all cancers. The relative frequencies of primary head and neck tumors by site are 40% in the oral cavity, 25% in the larynx, 15% in the oropharynx, 7% in the major salivary glands, and 13% at other sites. The male-to-female ratio is 3:1, and the average age at onset is approximately 50 years.

There is an increased incidence of SCC in patients with heavy tobacco and alcohol exposure. Some studies have shown an association between SCC and syphilis, viruses (Epstein-Barr virus, herpes simplex virus, human papillomavirus), occupational exposure (sawdust, metal dust), ultraviolet light exposure, and neglect of oral hygiene.

PATHOLOGY

SCC is by far the most common tumor encountered, comprising greater than 90% of all head and neck cancers. The cancer may be intraepithelial (in situ) or invasive, in which case it is classified as well differentiated, moderately differentiated, poorly differentiated, or undifferentiated based on decreasing amounts of keratinization. This histologic grading has not consistently predicted clinical behavior. There are four morphologic growth patterns: exophytic, ulcerative, infiltrative, and verrucous. The ulcerative type is most common and portends a poor prognosis. Premalignant lesions include leukoplakia (white plaque), hyperplasia (thickened mucosa), erythroplakia (velvety red area), and dysplasia; the last two have the highest propensity for malignant transformation. Regional metastasis to cervical lymph nodes is common and related to size and thickness of the primary tumor. The most frequent sites for distant metastases are the lungs, liver, and bone.

CLINICAL PRESENTATION AND EVALUATION

SCC of the mucous membranes of the head and neck can arise from any of the premalignant lesions or an ulcer, spread in area and depth, and eventually invade adjacent structures. Signs and symptoms of SCC of the head and neck include a nonhealing ulcer, neck mass, bleeding, otalgia, unexplained facial pain, dysphagia, odynophagia, and hoarseness.

The presence of such symptoms necessitates a detailed clinical examination. Bimanual palpation of the neck, oral cavity, tonsils, and base of the tongue is required in every patient. In addition, the nasal cavity, nasopharynx, oropharynx, hypopharynx, and larynx should be examined; in skillful hands, these examinations can all be done with a mirror, but flexible endoscopy can also provide valuable clinical information. Approximately 5% of patients with head and neck cancer will have a second primary SCC of the head and neck, esophagus, or lung, which can best be evaluated by panendoscopy (direct laryngoscopy, esophagoscopy, and bronchoscopy with directed biopsy). A computed tomography (CT) scan from the skull base to the clavicle is an extremely informative test and should be part of the clinical workup before panendoscopy and biopsy. The CT scan is useful for identification of occult tumors, local tumor extension, and lymph node disease. In a patient with a clinically apparent primary tumor, a biopsy specimen can be obtained with a scalpel, punch forceps, or fine needle in an outpatient setting. A chest radiograph and liver function studies are adequate screening examinations for distant metastatic disease. An isolated pulmonary nodule seen on chest radiograph in a patient with a known SCC of the head and neck more likely represents a primary lung cancer (second primary) than metastatic disease from the head and neck primary tumor. A diagnostic biopsy of the lung lesion is necessary before treatment of the head and neck cancer is undertaken.

Two mistakes commonly made in the evaluation of patients with head and neck tumors can lead to treatment delays. First, an incomplete examination of the upper aerodigestive system can allow one to miss small lesions. It is imperative that patients who present with symptoms suggestive of head and neck cancer be evaluated by a physician experienced in performing a thorough head and neck examination. The second common mistake occurs when patients with a cervical mass experience delays in referral for biopsy while extended courses of antibiotic therapy are tried. A patient with persistent adenopathy after a 2-week course of antibiotics should be evaluated with a fine-needle aspiration (FNA) biopsy.

STAGING

Head and neck cancers are staged according to the TNM system of the American Joint Committee on Cancer Staging (Table 6-1). The T staging is based on the location of the primary tumor and thus varies for each site in the head and neck. Prognosis correlates strongly with stage at diagnosis. For many head and neck cancer sites, survival exceeds 80% in patients with stage I disease. Most patients, however, have stage III or IV disease at diagnosis and a survival rate of less than 40%.

GENERAL PRINCIPLES OF TREATMENT

Surgery, radiation therapy, or both are the conventional treatment modalities used in the management of head and neck tumors. In general, chemotherapy and immunotherapy are appropriate only as part of clinical protocols, as palliative measures in patients with incurable disease, or for tumors that persist after conventional therapy.

Table 6-1.   AJCC staging system for head and neck cancers

Stage grouping

Stage I	T1, N0, M0
Stage II	T2, N0, M0
Stage III	T3, N0, M0
	T1–3, N1, M0
Stage IV	T4, N0 or N1, M0
	Any T, N2 or N3, M0
	Any T, any N, M1

Primary tumor (T) dependent on anatomic location

Regional lymph nodes (N)

N0	No regional lymph node metastasis
N2a	Metastasis in single ipsilateral lymph node > 3 cm but < 6 cm
N2b	Metastasis in multiple ipsilateral lymph nodes, none > 6 cm
N2c	Metastasis in bilateral or contralateral lymph nodes, none > 6 cm
N3	Metastasis in a lymph node > 6 cm

Metastatic disease

M0	No evidence of distant metastasis
M1	Evidence of distant metastasis

Adapted from Beahrs OH, Henson DE, Hutter RVP, et al., eds. *Manual for staging of cancer,* 4th ed. Philadelphia: Lippincott, 1992.

Surgical resection generally offers the best chance for complete tumor cure and provides a specimen that can be used to verify the adequacy of excision margins. Morbidity is minimal when the tumor is small and accessible, but significant cosmetic and functional deficits are not unusual after resection of large tumors; disabilities can be minimized with appropriate reconstructive techniques.

Radiation therapy is effective in the treatment of head and neck tumors. The advantage of radiation therapy is that anatomic structures can be preserved while local tumor control is achieved. However, irradiation of the head and neck produces acute mucositis and, over the long term, xerostomia, fibrosis of the skin and soft tissue, and altered pituitary and thyroid function.

Surgery and radiation therapy are often combined to achieve local control of head and neck cancer. Most surgeons prefer that radiation be administered postoperatively, where it seems to lead to better response rates than before surgery. The main indications for postoperative radiation are high risk of local and regional failure (stage III and IV disease), residual tumor at surgical margins, and histopathologic features that suggest unusual tumor aggressiveness (i.e., vessel invasion, perineural invasion, anaplastic appearance, multiple positive nodes, or extracapsular nodal spread).

Rehabilitation is important during and after treatment, and includes physical and occupational therapy, speech and swallowing rehabilitation, and nutritional support. A novel and still experimental strategy of chemoprevention is currently being evaluated in clinical trials, which administer retinoid-derived compounds to decrease the incidence of second primary tumors and to induce regression of premalignant lesions. Similarly, clinical trials are currently in place to evaluate the usefulness of gene therapy (e.g., restoration of the normal p53 gene) in the treatment of head and neck malignancies.

NECK DISSECTION

There are several approaches to the treatment of lymph node metastases in patients with head and neck cancer. Metastatic SCC to a single small neck node without extracapsular tumor spread can be controlled with either radiation alone or neck dissection. When disease in the neck is more extensive (≥N2, extranodal spread), combined surgery and radiation therapy treatment is important because neither modality alone leads to successful tumor control.

Surgical treatment of the neck relies on three major types of neck dissection: radical neck dissection, modified radical neck dissection, or selective neck dissection. The classical *radical neck dissection* refers to removal of all ipsilateral cervical lymph nodes in levels I–V (Fig. 6-1). The dissection extends from the inferior border of the mandible to the clavicle, posteriorly to the anterior border of the trapezius muscle, and anteriorly to the lateral border of the sternohyoid muscle. The depth of dissection extends to the fascia overlying the anterior scalene and levator scapulae muscles. The spinal accessory nerve, internal jugular vein, and sternocleidomastoid muscle are removed.

Modified radical neck dissection was developed to reduce the morbidity of the classical operation. The modified dissection still removes all lymph nodes routinely excised in a radical neck dissection. However, at minimum the spinal accessory nerve is preserved, as are frequently also the internal jugular vein and sternocleidomastoid muscle.

Selective neck dissection is the term reserved for less extensive lymph node dissections. The most common selective dissection is the supraomohyoid neck dissection, in which submental, submandibular, and upper and middle jugular lymph nodes (levels I–III) are removed. Such procedures are used to remove lymph nodes corresponding to the most significant drainage basins of specific head and neck tumor sites, and are usually used for staging a patient with nonpalpable neck nodes. Another common selective neck dissection, used to treat patients with posterior scalp melanoma, is the posterolateral neck dissection. In this procedure, the suboccipital, retroauricular, upper jugular, middle jugular, and lower jugular lymph nodes (levels II–V) are removed. Finding nodal disease may warrant progression to a more extensive neck dissection.

At the University of Texas M.D. Anderson Cancer Center, the neck dissection most commonly performed for a primary cancer of the head and neck is a modified radical neck dissection. It is used to treat neck metastases when they are identified and electively for conclusive staging of cervical lymph node disease. The radical neck dissection is reserved for treatment of disease that has extended into the sternocleidomastoid muscle, jugular vein, or spinal accessory nerve.

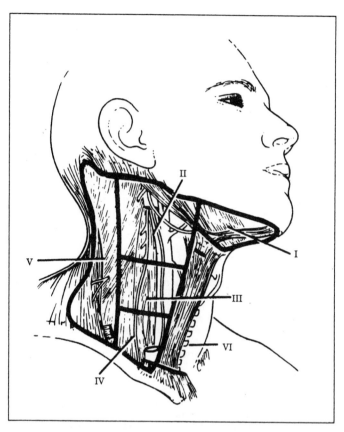

Fig. 6-1. **Lymph node groups. Level I, submental and submandibular lymph node groups; level II, upper jugular group; level III, middle jugular groups; level IV, lower jugular group; level V, posterior triangle group; level VI, anterior compartment group.**

CARCINOMA OF THE ORAL CAVITY

In the United States, cancer of the oral cavity develops in approximately 30,000 people and causes approximately 10,000 deaths annually. The incidence is twice as high in males as in females. The oral cavity extends from the vermillion border of the lips to the plane between the junction of the hard and soft palates. It includes the lips, buccal mucosa, gingiva, retromolar trigone, floor of the mouth, hard palate, and anterior two-thirds of the tongue.

The staging system for tumors of the oral cavity is shown in Table 6-2. The treatment for carcinoma of the oral cavity is determined by location and stage of the primary tumor. For small stage T1 and some stage T2 tumors, radiation or surgery yield similar results. Surgical treatment for stage T1 oral cancer is accomplished by excising the primary tumor with an adequate margin

Table 6-2.   Staging system for oral cavity tumors

Tis	Carcinoma *in situ*
T1	Tumor ≥ 2 cm at greatest dimension
T2	Tumor > 2 cm but not 4 cm at greatest dimension
T3	Tumor > 4 cm at greatest dimension
T4	Tumor invades adjacent structures (e.g., cortical bone, deep extrinsic muscle of tongue, maxillary sinus, or skin)

Adapted from Beahrs OH, Henson DE, Hutter RVP, et al., eds. *Manual for staging of cancer,* 4th ed. Philadelphia: Lippincott, 1992.

(approximately 1 cm) and repairing the defect by primary closure, local advancement flaps, or split-thickness skin grafts. Stage T2 disease can be treated in the same way, but a flap closure is almost always necessary for larger defects.

Radiation therapy as a primary treatment modality for cancers of the oral cavity may involve interstitial radioactive implants, external beam therapy, or both. Small superficial cancers can be treated with interstitial implants: local control rates of 80% to 95% can be achieved for T1 to T2 lesions of the oral tongue and floor of the mouth. Cancers arising at other sites are usually best treated with surgical excision. Postoperative adjuvant external beam radiation therapy is effective in improving local control rates for tumors likely to recur (T3 and T4).

Lymph nodes that are clinically involved with tumor are always treated with a neck dissection. However, treatment of the clinically uninvolved neck is still controversial, with three options available: observation, elective neck dissection, or elective irradiation. Most clinicians believe treatment is indicated when there is greater than 20% chance of nodal metastases. At M.D. Anderson Cancer Center, most, if not all, stage T1 and T2 oral cavity carcinomas are treated with primary surgical excision and a supraomohyoid neck dissection. If there is no nodal involvement or if only a single node is involved, without evidence of extracapsular extension, postoperative radiation therapy is not given. If there are multiple positive nodes or extranodal extension, postoperative radiation therapy to the neck is used to lower the incidence of disease recurrence. Radiation therapy for clinically negative cervical nodes is reserved for patients whose primary tumor is to be treated by radiation therapy as well.

Early lesions have a reasonably good prognosis, but the 5-year disease-free survival rate for patients with advanced oral cavity cancers has remained at approximately 30% to 40% over the past 20 years. Adverse prognostic factors include site of the lesion, depth of invasion, and presence of nodal metastases.

Lip

Small lesions of the lip can be cured with either radiation or surgical excision. Most T1 lesions are best treated by surgery alone, with a greater than 90% 5-year survival rate. However, T1 lesions of the commissure are best treated by radiation therapy. Lesions larger than 2 cm should be treated by surgical excision with immediate reconstruction and postoperative radiation therapy.

Invasion of the mental nerve is associated with an 80% incidence of node involvement and only a 35% 5-year survival rate.

Floor of the Mouth

Small lesions confined to the floor of the mouth can be treated by intraoral excision with tumor-free surgical margins or radiation therapy. Floor-of-the-mouth lesions frequently involve adjacent structures, such as the deep muscles of the tongue and mandible. In most cases, a cheek flap with marginal or segmental mandibulectomy is required to obtain adequate margins.

Tongue

Carcinoma of the tongue is the most common intraoral malignancy. An intraoral glossectomy can be performed for patients with lesions limited to the anterior or middle third of the oral tongue. Tumor thickness is the most accurate predictor of lymph node involvement. Lesions thinner than 1 cm have a minimal incidence of lymph node involvement. Thicker lesions have a greater than 20% chance of lymph node positivity; therefore, a supraomohyoid neck dissection should be included in the treatment of patients with a tongue carcinoma 1 cm or thicker and a clinically uninvolved neck. The lower jugular nodes are typically involved in patients with clinically positive cervical nodes; therefore, a complete modified radical neck dissection is required. Tumors of the posterior oral tongue with extension into the base of the tongue are best treated by a transcervical excision combined with an en bloc neck dissection. Smaller surgical defects can be allowed to heal by primary intention, while larger ones may require split-thickness skin grafting; in some instances, the edge of the tongue can be approximated upon itself.

Hard Palate

Most SCCs of the upper gum and hard palate begin on the gingiva and can be excised with negative margins. Large lesions of the palate that have invaded the bone will require a partial maxillectomy. Reconstruction for maxillary defects of the oral cavity is best achieved using a prosthetic dental appliance.

CARCINOMA OF THE LARYNX

The incidence of carcinoma of the larynx in the United States is approximately 13,000 cases per year, with a male-to-female ratio of 9:1. Most patients are middle-aged or older men who smoke tobacco and drink alcohol. There is also a risk associated with exposure to the human papillomavirus.

The larynx has three subsites: the glottis (true vocal cords), the supraglottis (false cords, epiglottis, aryepiglottic folds, arytenoids, and ventricles), and the subglottis (inferior border of vocal cords to inferior border of cricoid cartilage). The lymphatics of the larynx are numerous, except over the vocal cords, where the mucosa is thin, adheres tightly to the vocal ligament, and lacks lymphatic channels. Above the level of the ventricles, the efferent lymphatics of the superior portion of the larynx extend to the pyriform sinus upward to join the jugular chain. From the inferior larynx, the efferent lymphatics drain into the pretracheal, para-tracheal, and deep cervical lymph nodes. The lymphatic drainage of the larynx is usually bilateral, and any laryngeal tumor, except a lesion of the true vocal cords, should be considered a midline cancer with the propensity to metastasize to bilateral neck nodes.

Glottic carcinomas are those that involve the upper surface of the vocal cords and continue down to 1 cm below this plane. Glottic cancers account for 65% of cancers of the larynx. They usually are well differentiated, grow slowly, and metastasize late. Metastasis occurs only after the disease has infiltrated muscle or has spread beyond the limits of the true vocal cords into the paraglottic space or from the anterior commissure into the pretracheal region.

Supraglottic cancers account for 35% of laryngeal tumors. They are usually aggressive tumors causing both local extension and lymph node metastasis. The lymphatic channels of the supraglottis drain to the jugulodigastric and middle and inferior internal jugular chains. Supraglottic tumors have a high risk of bilateral nodal involvement.

Subglottic cancers are rare. They commonly produce extension into the lymph nodes of the prelaryngeal area, inferior internal jugular chain, and thyroid gland, and have a high risk of bilateral cervical metastasis.

The staging system for tumors of the larynx is summarized in Table 6-3.

Patient Evaluation

The initial presenting symptoms of cancer of the larynx depend on the site and stage of the disease. Only lesions of the true vocal cords produce early symptoms and facilitate early intervention.

Table 6-3.   Staging system for cancers of the larynx

Supraglottis

T1	Tumor confined to site of origin
T2	Tumor involving adjacent supraglottic sites, without glottic fixation
T3	Tumor limited to the larynx, with fixation and/or extension to the postericoid medial wall of the pyriform sinus or pre-epiglottic space
T4	Massive tumor extending beyond the larynx to involve the oropharynx, soft tissues of the neck, or destruction of thyroid cartilage

Glottis

T1	Tumor confined to vocal folds, with normal vocal cord mobility
T2	Tumor extension to supraglottis and/or subglottis with normal or impaired vocal cord mobility
T3	Tumor confined to larynx, with fixation of the vocal cords
T4	Massive tumor, with thyroid cartilage destruction and/or extension beyond the confines of the larynx

Adapted from Beahrs OH, Henson DE, Hutter RVP, et al., eds. *Manual for staging of cancer,* 4th ed. Philadelphia: Lippincott, 1992.

Supraglottic lesions are usually discovered at a much later stage upon development of dysphagia, odynophagia, hemoptysis, or referred otalgia. Often supraglottic tumors produce a large lesion that can eventually impair motion of the vocal cord and cause hoarseness. Physical examination usually reveals either an exophytic or a submucosal lesion. CT is very useful for determining paraglottic, subglottic, pyriform sinus, and extralaryngeal involvement, and for revealing clinically occult lymph node disease.

Treatment

The goal of treatment for laryngeal carcinoma is tumor extirpation while preserving voice function if possible. Mucosal stripping of the cord can be effective treatment for patients with carcinoma in situ, but repeated attempts at stripping leave the cord difficult to examine for the development of a malignant lesion. Therefore radiation therapy is recommended for patients with recurrent premalignant vocal cord lesions. In general, radiation therapy can also satisfy treatment goals for patients with T1 and T2 lesions, although some surgeons still choose to operate on early laryngeal cancers. More advanced cancer usually requires removal of all or part of the larynx and postoperative irradiation.

The local control rate for T1 and T2 lesions treated by radiation therapy is 71% to 100%. Salvage laryngectomy improves the local control rate to 88% to 100%. The local control rate for patients with T3 laryngeal carcinomas treated by surgery and radiation therapy is 85%, with a 67% 5-year survival rate. Patients with T4 lesions treated by surgery and radiation therapy can anticipate a 30% to 50% 5-year survival rate.

Surgery

A vertical laryngectomy (hemilaryngectomy) is used for patients with T1 or T2 vocal cord tumors who are not candidates for radiation therapy (usually due to prior irradiation). Hemilaryngectomy can also be used in select patients with persistent or recurrent disease after radiation therapy. It preserves voice function with some hoarseness. A supraglottic laryngectomy is used for patients with early (T1 or T2) supraglottic cancers. It is often associated with aspiration and is contraindicated in patients with poor pulmonary function. Total laryngectomy is the procedure of choice for patients with stage T3 or T4 cancers of the larynx. This procedure is seldom performed when patients have normal vocal cord mobility. A wide-field laryngectomy includes the paralaryngeal soft tissue, which extends between the internal jugular veins and the lymph nodes in levels II to V (Fig. 6-1). In some instances, portions of the hypopharynx will also need to be removed, in which case a 1-cm mucosal margin is desirable because of the risk of submucosal microscopic disease. An ipsilateral thyroid lobectomy is indicated when the tumor involves the subglottis, pyriform apex, or paratracheal nodes, or when the tumor extends through the thyroid cartilage on the same side as the lesion.

Radiation Therapy

Early (stage T1 or T2) glottic and supraglottic cancers respond to external beam radiation therapy, and tumor control is usually achieved with a 65- to 70-Gy dose. Glottic tumors, which have a low incidence of lymph node involvement, can be treated through small portals that encompass only the larynx. With careful treatment, there is minimal damage to normal tissues, and the patient can retain a normal voice. Supraglottic tumors, because of their higher incidence of lymph node involvement, require larger fields that encompass the lymphatic drainage of the neck. Lymph nodes in the primary drainage basin, if clinically uninvolved, should be treated with a 50-Gy dose.

Postoperative radiation therapy to the primary site or the regional lymph nodes is indicated for patients who have undergone a total laryngectomy and who have multiple positive lymph nodes, extranodal disease, close or positive surgical margins, T4 disease, or subglottic extension of tumor. Patients who have undergone a tracheotomy to achieve airway control before laryngectomy also require postoperative radiation therapy to control disease at the tracheostoma.

CARCINOMA OF THE OROPHARYNX, NASOPHARYNX, AND HYPOPHARYNX

The oropharynx begins at the ring bounded by the anterior tonsillar pillars, uvula, and base of tongue. Superiorly, the soft palate separates it from the nasopharynx, and inferiorly, the epiglottis divides it from the hypopharynx. Pain, dysphagia, and a neck mass are the most common presenting symptoms in patients with oropharyngeal cancer. External beam or interstitial radiation therapy has been used for curative treatment and results in overall local control rates for all primary sites ranging from 90% (T1) to 55% (T4). Cancers of the tonsillar fossa respond best to radiation therapy. Surgical excision of all but the smallest palatal and tonsillar lesions is generally inadequate. Larger lesions most frequently involve the supraglottic pharynx and are treated as described earlier.

Nasopharyngeal carcinoma is uncommon in most of the world, with highest incidence in China and Africa, where it seems related to risk factors in the diet and viral agents (Epstein-Barr virus). A neck mass is the presenting complaint in 90% of patients; other symptoms include nasal obstruction and abnormalities of hearing. One-fourth of patients have invasion of tumor into the base of skull and cranial nerve deficits. Treatment usually involves radiation therapy of the primary tumor and draining lymph nodes. Surgical resection, even of small tumors, is limited because of high associated morbidity. Overall 5-year survival is 50%.

The hypopharynx is the region of entrance to the esophagus and includes the pyriform sinuses, posterior pharyngeal wall, and postcricoid area. Seventy percent of cancers occur in the pyriform sinus and produce few symptoms until they are advanced. Diffuse local spread and lymph node metastases are common. Combined modality treatment is usually required, as is total laryngectomy in most patients. Hypopharyngeal cancer is difficult to control and has poor 5-year survival rates: 25% without nodal disease and 10% in presence of nodal metastases.

CERVICAL LYMPH NODE METASTASIS FROM AN UNKNOWN PRIMARY TUMOR

Benign conditions, inflammatory and infectious diseases, and primary and metastatic cancer can lead to the development of an enlarged cervical lymph node. A complete history and physical examination, as well as FNA biopsy, are helpful in diagnosing the correct etiology. Among malignancies, SCC of the head and neck is by far the most common reason for enlarged cervical lymph nodes, followed by lymphoma and solid tumor metastases, including those from lung, breast, and thyroid cancer. Management of biopsy-proven malignancy in a cervical lymph node when no primary tumor is apparent can be very challenging.

A thorough search for a primary tumor is essential and should be the first priority of management. Knowledge of lymphatic drainage patterns and the metastatic propensity of various cancers can provide some clues. Metastatic SCC in a cervical node may have originated in many different sites. The location of the node can provide valuable diagnostic information as to the possible origin of the primary tumor. A valuable diagnostic strategy, however, is to consider whether the lymph node malignancy is of squamous or nonsquamous origin. The clinical management then becomes organized according to a very specific course in each case.

Most patients with metastatic SCC to lymph nodes in zones II or III have a primary tumor in the nasopharynx, tonsil, or tongue base (Waldeyer's ring). They should undergo careful clinical examination with panendoscopy. In the absence of overt anomalies, a CT or magnetic resonance imaging scan of the head and neck may be a useful next step. The patient should also be scheduled for an examination under anesthesia in the operating room for the purpose of obtaining biopsies. How to perform the biopsy is debatable. One approach advocates blind biopsies of the ipsilateral nasopharynx, tonsil, base of tongue, pyriform sinus, and even postcricoid area. Alternatively, only sites of mucosal abnormalities, however minor, are biopsied. If the primary tumor is identified, an appropriate treatment decision can be made that incorporates both the primary tumor and the cervical node. If the primary tumor remains unidentified, the neck is treated with a modified or radical neck dissection, depending on the extent of lymph node disease, and radiation therapy is administered to Waldeyer's ring and both sides of the neck. An ipsilateral tonsillectomy is also recommended.

A patient with a cervical lymph node metastasis and a small tumor of the head and neck that is detected only by an examination under general anesthesia can usually be treated with radiation therapy alone. The cervical lymphatics can be adequately treated with radiation therapy if the involved lymph node is small (<3 cm) based on physical examination and CT scan, although some surgeons advocate a neck dissection in all patients to determine the extent of regional disease. A modified radical neck dissection should be performed if the enlarged lymph node is larger than 3 cm or if residual disease persists after radiation therapy.

For cervical lymph node metastases that are adenocarcinoma or other nonsquamous carcinomas, the strategy is completely different. These tumors most likely originate below the level of the clavicles. Extensive workup consisting of CT of the chest and abdomen, imaging of the bowel, and bone scan to exclude other sites of distant metastasis should be made before the neck is treated. Again, if the primary is not identified, the neck is treated with surgery and radiation therapy as described for squamous metastases.

The finding of metastatic thyroid carcinoma in a cervical lymph node is sufficient information to proceed with neck exploration and thyroidectomy. Lymphoma can be diagnosed by FNA but cannot be subtyped; therefore, an accessible lymph node should be removed. The diagnosis of adenocarcinoma requires an evaluation of the salivary glands if the node is cephalad in the neck. Needle biopsy evidence of adenocarcinoma in inferior neck nodes should prompt an evaluation of the lungs, breasts, pancreas, and colon.

Five-year survival rates of 50% have been reported for patients with cervical metastases from an unknown primary tumor. Close follow-up is mandatory, as the primary site will become evident in 15% to 20% of patients over 5 years. The 5-year survival rate for patients with metastatic adenocarcinoma to the cervical lymph nodes is less than 5%.

CARCINOMA OF THE SALIVARY GLANDS

The parotid, submandibular, and submaxillary glands are the major salivary glands and together account for more than 95% of salivary gland tumors. The remaining tumors involve minor salivary glands, which are small foci of glandular tissue found in submucosa throughout the oral cavity with highest density on the palate. Salivary gland tumors appear sporadically (5%–10% of all head and neck tumors) and are not associated with smoking, alcohol use, or other environmental factors.

Neoplasms of the parotid gland account for 90% of all tumors of the three major salivary glands. Submandibular gland tumors are less common (10%), and submaxillary ones are exceedingly rare (<1%). The smaller the size of a salivary gland, the greater the likelihood that a tumor will be malignant. Three-fourths of parotid tumors will be benign, whereas 50% of submandibular and virtually all sublingual tumors are malignant.

The most common benign tumors are pleomorphic adenomas and benign cystic lymphomatosum (Warthin's tumor, which is almost exclusive to the parotid gland). The most common malignant histologic types are mucoepidermoid, adenoid cystic carcinoma, and adenocarcinoma. The parotid gland may be the site of metastatic disease (cutaneous head tumors, bronchogenic, and breast cancer) or lymphoma.

The superficial portion of the parotid gland is the largest and rests lateral to the facial nerve. The deep lobe is medial to the facial nerve and extends to the retromandibular and parapharyngeal spaces. Drainage to the mouth is via Stensen's duct. There are numerous lymph nodes within the parotid gland itself; lymphatic drainage then goes to preauricular, infra-auricular, and deep upper jugular lymph nodes.

The submandibular glands are paired glands located medial to the body of the mandible and thus adjacent to all structures within the submandibular triangle: the facial vessels, the marginal mandibular branch of the facial nerve, the lingual vessels and nerve, and the hypoglossal nerve. Wharton's duct opens into the floor of the mouth. The submandibular gland is invested with the superficial layer of cervical fascia and has lymphatic drainage into the deep jugular chain.

The sublingual glands are located on the paramedian floor of the mouth just deep to the mucosa and superficial to the mylohyoid muscle.

Patient Evaluation

Asymptomatic swelling is the initial complaint in the overwhelming majority of patients with salivary gland tumors. Facial paralysis (especially if associated with a small mass), enlarged regional lymph nodes, and fixation to skin or adjacent tissues are very strong indications of malignancy. Episodic swelling associated with meals suggests an obstructive or inflammatory process. Diffuse submandibular gland enlargement is benign in 90% of patients, but duct obstruction by an underlying malignancy needs to be excluded in all cases. Other symptoms, such as pain and rapid growth, do not distinguish infiltrative from inflammatory disease consistently well. Differentiation from collagen vascular diseases, such as Wegener's granulomatosis and Sjögren's syndrome, that affect the parotid gland is necessary. Any mass in the preauricular area or the angle of the mandible should be presumed to arise from the parotid gland.

Fine-needle aspiration, which has a sensitivity greater than 95%, is a useful biopsy technique. It is used often to distinguish inflammatory and neoplastic enlargements of the submandibular gland. Use of FNA or open biopsy for diagnosing parotid lesions is more controversial. Most parotid neoplasms will require surgical removal. Therefore the usefulness of FNA must be weighed against whether the decision to proceed with surgery will be changed. FNA is rarely indicated for minor salivary glands; biopsy with cup forceps is performed instead.

The role of CT in the evaluation of salivary tumors is limited to patients with symptoms suspicious of malignancy or when distinction between inflammatory and neoplastic disease remains unclear. A CT scan is valuable to identify tumor extension into the deep parotid lobe and parapharyngeal space.

Treatment

Surgery is the treatment of choice for salivary gland neoplasms. Many surgeons rely on intraoperative frozen-section biopsy to determine the extent of surgical procedure.

Benign neoplasms can be cured if completely excised, which usually is accomplished by superficial parotidectomy or submandibular excision. The facial nerve can be peeled off benign tumors without risk of recurrence. Violating the capsule of pleomorphic adenomas predisposes to recurrence.

Current treatment of malignant salivary tumors mainly involves surgery and radiation. The extent of surgery is dictated by tumor size and degree of local extension, and should include a rim of normal tissue. In the case of the parotid gland, the minimum operation is a superficial parotidectomy. For lesions of the submandibular gland, adequate surgical excision includes removal of the gland and the associated investing fascia and lymph nodes. In some instances, resection of part or all of the mandible, floor of the mouth, lingual and hypoglossal nerves, and a supraomohyoid neck dissection will be necessary. No chemotherapy regimen has proved to be effective, and immunotherapy is in the clinical trial phase.

Every effort should be made to preserve facial nerve function, even when dealing with malignancy, unless the tumor has adhered to or directly invaded the nerve. If the facial nerve must be sacrificed, it should be immediately reconstructed with either a nerve graft or a cranial nerve XII to VII anastomosis. Postoperative radiation therapy should be planned. There is no evidence that this approach compromises local and regional control.

Only node-positive necks, where malignancy in lymph nodes was detected either before or during surgery, require neck dissection. Postoperative radiation to the neck is indicated in almost all cases of cervical metastatic disease.

Postoperative radiation therapy to the surgical area for malignant tumors is indicated in almost all cases except for small, low-grade tumors. Typically, radiation therapy is given for high-grade mucoepidermoid carcinoma, adenoid cystic carcinoma, adenocarcinoma, malignant mixed tumor, SCC, multicentric recurrent pleomorphic adenoma, and highly cellular acinic cell carcinoma. Radiation therapy is also beneficial for patients with perineural invasion, positive nodes, skin involvement, or microscopic residual disease.

Overall, 20% of patients will develop distant metastasis. The 5-year survival rates for patients with malignant salivary gland tumors vary from 95% for low-grade mucoepidermoid carcinoma to 75% for adenoid cystic carcinoma and 50% for high-grade mucoepidermoid carcinoma and malignant mixed tumors.

SURVEILLANCE

Following curative treatment of head and neck cancers, patients must be observed closely for the development of local as well as distant recurrences. Physical examination performed by someone skilled in examination of the head and neck is the most important part of the postoperative follow-up. At M.D. Anderson, follow-up of patients occurs every 3 months for the first 2 years postoperatively, then every 6 months for the next 3 years, and yearly thereafter. A chest radiograph and liver function studies are performed yearly.

RECOMMENDED READING

Byers RM. The role of a modified neck dissection. In: Jacobs C, ed. Cancers of the head and neck Boston: Martinus Nijhoff, 1987.

Byers RM, Wolf PF, Ballantyne AJ. Rationale for elective modified neck dissection. *Head Neck* 1988;10:160.

Clayman GL. Gene therapy for head and neck cancer. *Head Neck* 1995;17:535.

Crissman JD, Gluckman J, Whiteley J, et al. Squamous cell carcinoma of the floor of mouth. *Head Neck* 1980;3:2.

Eiband JD, Elias GE, Suter CM, et al. Prognostic factors in squamous cell carcinoma of the larynx. *Am J Surg* 1989;158:314.

Forastiere A, Koch W, Trotti A, Sidransky D. Head and neck cancer [review]. *N Engl J Med* 2001;345(26):1890–1900.

Frankenthaler RA, Luna MA, Lee SS, et al. Prognostic variables in parotid gland cancer. *Arch Otolaryngol Head Neck Surg* 1991;117:1251.

Gluckman J, Gullane P, Johnson J. Practical approach to head and neck tumors New York: Raven Press, 1994.

Khuri FR, Lippman SM, Spitz MR, et al. Molecular epidemiology and retinoid chemoprevention of head and neck cancer. *JNCI* 1997;89:199.

Kim KB, Khuri FR, Shin DM. Recent advances in the management of squamous cell carcinoma of the head and neck [review]. *Expert Rev Anticancer Ther* 2001;1(1):99–110.

Lefebvre JL, Degueant C, Castelain B, et al. Interstitial brachytherapy and early tongue squamous cell carcinoma management. *Head Neck* 1990;12:232.

Mendenhall WM, Million RR, Sharkey DE, et al. Stage T3 squamous cell carcinoma of the glottic larynx treated with surgery and/or radiation therapy. *Int J Radiat Oncol Biol Phys* 1984;10:357.

Mendenhall WM, Parsons JT, Stringer SP, et al. T1–T2 vocal cord carcinoma: a basis for comparing the results of irradiation and surgery. *Head Neck Surg* 1988;10:373.

Murphy BA, Cmelak A, Burkey B, et al. Topoisomerase I inhibitors in the treatment of head and neck cancer [review]. *Oncology (Huntington)* 2001;15(7 suppl 8):47–52.

Myers EN, Suen JC, eds. *Cancer of the head and neck.* Philadelphia: Saunders, 1996.

Rice DM, Spiro RH, eds. *Current concepts in head and neck cancer* Atlanta: American Cancer Society, 1989.

Ridge JA, Hooks MA, Lee R, Benner SE. Head and neck tumors. In: Pazdur R, Coia L, Hoskins W, et al., eds. *Cancer management: a multidisciplinary approach.* Huntington, NY: PRR, Inc, 1996.

Robbins KT, Medina JE, Wolfe GT, et al. Standardizing neck dissection terminology. Official report of the Academy's Committee for Head and Neck Surgery and Oncology. *Arch Otolaryngol Head Neck Surg* 1991;117:601.

Rudat V, Wannenmacher M. Role of multimodal treatment in oropharynx, larynx, and hypopharynx cancer [review]. *Semin Surg Oncol* 2001;20(1):66–74.

Taylor SG 4th. Head and neck cancer [review]. *Cancer Chemother Biol Response Modif* 2001;19:465–483.

Wang RC, Goepfert H, Barber A, et al. Squamous cell carcinoma, metastatic to the neck from an unknown primary site. In: Larson DL, Ballantyne AJ, Guillamondegui OM, eds. Cancer in the neck New York: Macmillan, 1986.

Weber RS, Byers RM, Petit B, et al. Submandibular gland tumors. *Arch Otolaryngol Head Neck Surg* 1990;116:1055.

Weber RS, Callender DL. Laryngeal conservation. *Semin Radiat Oncol* 1992;2:149.

Thoracic Malignancies

Ara A. Vaporciyan and Stephen G. Swisher

PRIMARY NEOPLASMS OF THE LUNG

In 1997, lung cancer will account for an estimated 160,000 deaths and 170,000 new cases of cancer in the United States. Although less publicized than breast or prostate cancer, lung cancer is the most common cause of cancer-related death in both men and women. Approximately 25% of all cancer deaths are attributable to lung cancer. However, as seen in Fig. 7-1, the overall age-adjusted death rates for lung cancer have begun to level off (although they continue to increase in women). This leveling off is attributable to an overall decrease in the number of males who smoke. Unfortunately, this good news is countered by a disturbing increase in smoking among certain minority and adolescent age groups. The overall 5-year survival rate for lung cancer is only 14%, primarily because the disease is usually advanced at presentation. If the disease is found at an early stage, the 5-year survival rate approaches 60% to 70%.

Epidemiology

Smoking is the primary etiology in more than 80% of lung cancers, and secondhand smoke increases the risk of lung cancer by 30%. Despite the strong association of lung cancer with smoking, such cancers develop in only 15% of heavy smokers. Giant bullous emphysema and airway obstructive disease can act synergistically with smoking to induce lung cancer, perhaps because of poor clearance and trapping of carcinogens. Industrial and environmental carcinogens have been implicated, including residential radon gas, asbestos, uranium, cadmium, arsenic, and terpenes.

Pathology

Lung cancer can be broadly separated into two groups: non–small cell lung cancers (NSCLC) and small cell lung cancers (SCLC). This is a popular division because, for the most part, NSCLC is often managed with surgery when the tumor is localized, whereas SCLC is almost always managed nonsurgically with chemotherapy and radiation therapy. The three major types of NSCLC are adenocarcinoma, squamous cell carcinoma, and large cell carcinoma (Table 7-1).

Non–small Cell Lung Carcinoma

Adenocarcinoma is the most common type of NSCLC and accounts for more than 40% of cases. It is the most common lung cancer found in nonsmokers and women. The lesions tend to be located in the periphery and to develop systemic metastases even in the face of small primary tumors.

Bronchoalveolar cell carcinoma is a subset of adenocarcinoma, whose incidence appears to be increasing with time. This tumor is

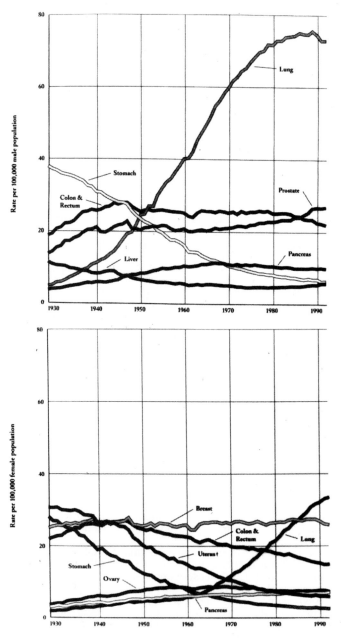

Fig. 7-1. The age-adjusted cancer death rate continues to rise in females but appears to have leveled off in males.

Table 7-1. Frequency of histologic subtypes of primary lung cancer

Cell Type	Estimated Frequency (%)
Non-small–cell lung cancer	
Adenocarcinoma	40
Bronchoalveolar	2
Squamous cell carcinoma	25
Large-cell carcinoma	7
Small-cell lung cancer	
Small-cell carcinoma	20
Neuroendocrine, well differentiated	1
Carcinoids	5

also associated with women and nonsmokers and can present as a single mass, multiple nodules, or an infiltrate. The clinical course can vary from indolent progression to rapid diffuse dissemination.

Squamous cell carcinoma accounts for approximately 25% of all lung cancers. Most (66%) present as central lesions and are associated with cavitation in 7% to 10% of cases. Unlike adenocarcinoma, the tumor often remains localized, tending to spread initially to regional lymph nodes rather than systemically.

Large cell carcinoma accounts for approximately 7% to 10% of all lung cancers. Clinically, large cell carcinomas behave aggressively, with early metastases to the regional nodes in the mediastinum and distant sites such as the brain.

Small Cell Lung Carcinoma

Small cell carcinoma is associated with neuroendocrine carcinoma because of ultrastructural and immunohistochemical similarities. Some pathologists think small cell carcinomas represent a spectrum of disease beginning with the well-differentiated, benign carcinoid tumor (Kulchitsky I), including the less differentiated atypical carcinoids (Kulchitsky II) or neuroendocrine carcinomas, and ending with the undifferentiated small cell carcinomas (Kulchitsky III). Small cell carcinomas tend to present with metastatic and regional spread and are usually treated with chemotherapy with or without radiation therapy. Surgery is only used to remove the occasional localized peripheral nodule.

Carcinoids tend to arise from major bronchi and are central tumors. Metastasis is rare. Immunohistochemically, carcinoids express neuron-specific enolase, chromogranin, and synaptophysin virtually without exception.

Neuroendocrine carcinomas or *atypical carcinoids* occur more peripherally than carcinoids and have a more aggressive course, although surgery should still be considered according to clinical stage. Without appropriate immunostaining, they may inadvertently be classified as large cell carcinomas.

Diagnosis

Signs and symptoms occur in 90% to 95% of patients at the time of diagnosis. Intraparenchymal tumors cause cough, hemoptysis, dyspnea, wheezing, and fever (often due to infection from proximal bronchial tumor obstruction). Regional spread of the tumor within the thorax can lead to pleural effusions or chest wall pain. Less common symptoms are superior vena cava syndrome, Pancoast's tumor, Horner's syndrome, and involvement of the recurrent laryngeal nerve, the phrenic nerve, the vagus nerve, or the esophagus. Paraneoplastic syndromes are found in 10% of patients with lung cancer, most commonly those with SCLC. These syndromes are numerous and can affect endocrine, neurologic, skeletal, hematologic, and cutaneous systems.

A standard chest radiograph (CXR) is the initial diagnostic study for the evaluation of suspected lung cancer. The limit of detection of a lung mass is approximately 7 mm. Computed tomography (CT) can provide additional information and should include imaging of the liver and adrenal glands to rule out two common sites for intra-abdominal metastases. CT helps assess local extension to other thoracic structures as well as the presence of mediastinal adenopathy. Unfortunately, CT cannot definitively predict mediastinal nodal involvement because not all malignant lymph nodes are enlarged and many enlarged nodes are simply larger because of proximal infection. Lymph nodes larger than 1 cm have a 30% chance of being benign, whereas lymph nodes smaller than 1 cm still have a 15% chance of containing tumor. Because of this uncertainty, histologic confirmation is required to confirm the presence of mediastinal adenopathy. Histologic confirmation can be obtained by CT-guided fine-needle aspiration (FNA), bronchoscopy-directed Wang needle aspiration, or mediastinoscopy. At present, magnetic resonance imaging (MRI) adds little to the information gained by CT imaging, and other modalities such as positron emission tomography are still being evaluated. Because of their low yield, bone scans and MRI or CT of the brain should only be obtained when symptoms of metastatic disease are present (i.e., bone pain, headaches, or visual disturbances).

Histologic diagnosis of a lung tumor can be obtained by sputum cytology and bronchoscopy (central lesions) or by fluoroscopic FNA, or CT-guided biopsy (peripheral lesions). In certain patients whose probability of having cancer is high, the diagnosis can be obtained at the time of surgery (thoracotomy or video-assisted thoracic surgery [VATS]) with frozen-section analysis of a wedge resection.

Staging

The primary goal of pretreatment staging is to determine the extent of disease so that prognosis and treatment can be determined. In SCLC, most patients present with metastatic or advanced locoregional disease. A simple two-stage system classifies the SCLC as limited or extensive disease. Limited disease is confined to one hemithorax, ipsilateral or contralateral hilar or mediastinal nodes, and ipsilateral supraclavicular lymph nodes.

Extensive disease has spread to the contralateral supraclavicular nodes or distant sites such as the contralateral lung, liver, brain, or bone marrow. Staging for SCLC requires a bone scan, bone marrow biopsy, and CT scans of the abdomen, brain, and chest.

Staging of NSCLC has most recently involved a system proposed in 1985: the International Lung Cancer Staging System or International Staging System (ISS). This system is based on TNM classifications as shown in Table 7-2. Survival rates for patients with NSCLC by stage of disease are shown in Fig. 7-2. Because of heterogeneity within groups, further modifications to the ISS have been proposed that involve splitting stage I into IA (T1N0) and IB (T2N0) and stage II into IIA (T1N0) and IIB (T2N0) and moving the good-prognosis T3N0 patients (chest wall involvement without nodal spread) into IIB. Staging of NSCLC involves a thorough history and physical examination, CXR, and CT scans of the chest and upper abdomen. Because of the low yield in asymptomatic patients, a bone scan or CT or MRI of the brain should only be obtained when suspected by history.

Treatment

Pretreatment Assessment

Once a patient has been staged clinically with noninvasive tests, a physiologic assessment should be performed to determine the patient's ability to tolerate different therapeutic modalities. In addition to a general evaluation of the patient's overall medical status, specific attention should be paid to the cardiovascular and respiratory systems. Cardiovascular screening should include a history and physical examination as well as a CXR and electrocardiography. Patients with signs and symptoms of significant cardiac disease should undergo further noninvasive testing, including either exercise testing, echocardiography, or nuclear perfusion scans. Significant reversible cardiac problems should be addressed before therapy (i.e., chemotherapy, radiation therapy, or surgery).

The pulmonary reserve of patients with lung cancer is commonly diminished as a result of tobacco abuse. Simple spirometry is an excellent initial screening test to quantify a patient's pulmonary reserve and ability to tolerate surgical resection. A postoperative forced expiratory volume in 1 second (FEV_1) of less than 0.8 L or less than 35% of predicted postoperative FEV_1 is associated with an increased risk of perioperative complications, respiratory insufficiency, and death. The predicted postoperative FEV_1 is estimated by subtracting the contribution of the lung to be resected from the preoperative FEV_1. In certain instances, the lung to be resected does not contribute much to the preoperative FEV_1 because of tumor, atelectasis, or pneumonitis. Thus more accurate determination of predicted postoperative FEV_1 can be obtained by performing a ventilation-perfusion scan and subtracting the exact contribution of the lung to be resected. In patients who fail spirometry criteria but are still thought to be operative candidates, oxygen consumption studies can be obtained that measure both respiratory and cardiac capacity. A maximum oxygen consumption (VO_2 max) of greater than 15 mL min^{-1} kg^{-1} indicates low risk, whereas a VO_2

Table 7-2. TNM descriptors

Primary tumor (T)

Tx   Primary tumor cannot be assessed or tumor proven by the presence of malignant cells in sputum or bronchial washings but not visualized by imaging or bronchoscopy

T0   No evidence of primary tumor

Tis   Carcinoma *in situ*

T1   Tumor ≤ 3 cm in greatest dimension, surrounded by lung or visceral pleura, without bronchoscopic evidence of invasion more proximal than the lobar bronchus[a] (i.e., not in the main bronchus)

T2   Tumor with any of the following features of size or extent:
> 3 cm in greatest dimension
Involving main bronchus, ≥ 2 cm distal to the carina
Invading the visceral pleura
Associated with atelectasis or obstructive pneumonitis that extends to the hilar region but does not involve the entire lung

T3   Tumor of any size that directly invades any of the following: chest wall (including superior sulcus tumors), diaphragm, mediastinal pleura, parietal pericardium; or tumor in the main bronchus < 2 cm distal to the carina but without involvement of the carina; or associated atelectasis or obstructive pneumonitis of the entire lung

T4   Tumor of any size that invades any of the following: mediastinum, heart, great vessels, trachea, esophagus, vertebral body, carina; or tumor with a malignant pleural or pericardial effusion,[b] or with satellite tumor nodule(s) within the ipsilateral primary-tumor lobe of the lung

Regional lymph nodes (N)

Nx   Regional lymph nodes cannot be assessed

N0   No regional lymph node metastasis

N1   Metastasis to ipsilateral peribronchial and/or ipsilateral hilar lymph nodes, and intrapulmonary nodes involved by direct extension of the primary tumor

N2   Metastasis to ipsilateral mediastinal, and/or subcarinal lymph nodes(s)

N3   Metastasis to contralateral mediastinal, contralateral hilar, ipsilateral or contralateral scalene, or supraclavicular lymph node(s)

Distant metastasis (M)

Mx   Presence of distant metastasis cannot be assessed

M0   No distant metastasis

M1   Distant metastasis present[c]

---

[a] The uncommon superficial tumor of any size with its invasive component limited to the bronchial wall, which may extend proximally to the main bronchus, is also classified T1.

[b] Most pleural effusions associated with lung cancer are due to tumor. However, there are a few patients in whom multiple cytopathologic examinations of pleural fluid show no tumor. In these cases, the fluid is nonbloody and is not an exudate. When these elements and clinical judgment dictate that the effusion is not related to the tumor, the effusion should be excluded as a staging element and the patient's disease should be staged T1, T2, or T3. Pericardial effusion is classified according to the same rules.

[c] Separate metastatic tumor nodule(s) in the ipsilateral nonprimary-tumor lobe(s) of the lung also are classified M1.

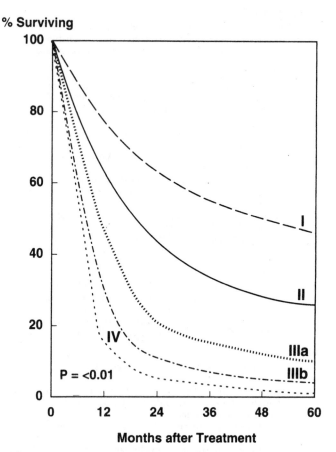

% Surviving

Months after Treatment

Fig. 7-2. **Cumulative survival according to clinical stage of non–small cell lung cancer.**

max of less than 10 mL min^{-1} kg^{-1} is associated with high risk (a mortality rate of more than 30% in some series). Additional risk factors for lung resection include a predicted postoperative diffusing capacity (DLCO) or maximum ventilatory ventilation (MVV) of less than 40% and hypercarbia (>45 mm CO_2) or hypoxemia (<60 mm O_2) on preoperative arterial blood gases. In conjunction with clinical assessment, these tests can help identify those patients at high risk for complications during and after surgical resection.

Preoperative training with an incentive spirometer, initiation of bronchodilators, weight reduction, good nutrition, and cessation of smoking for at least 2 weeks before surgery can help minimize complications and improve performance on spirometry for patients with marginal pulmonary reserve.

Non–small Cell Lung Carcinoma

In early-stage NSCLC, surgery is a critical part of treatment. Unfortunately, more than 50% to 70% of NSCLC patients present with advanced disease for which surgery alone is not an option. An algorithm for treatment based on clinical stage is presented in Fig. 7-3. Physiologically fit patients with early stage lesions (stage I or II) are treated with surgery. Definitive radiation therapy is indicated if surgery cannot be tolerated. Five-year survival rates of 60% to 70% and 39% to 43% can be achieved for patients with stage I and II disease, respectively. Chest wall involvement without nodal spread (T3N0) was formally considered stage IIIa, but because survival rates of 33% to 60% have been achieved with surgery, they are now considered as early stage lesion (stage IIa). If these patients cannot tolerate surgery because of poor medical status, definitive radiation can result in survival rates of 15% to 35%.

The remainder of patients with stage IIIa disease (N2 disease or chest wall with nodal involvement) classically have a poor response to surgery, with 5-year survival rates of less than 15%. The standard treatment for these patients and those with stage IIIb or IV includes chemotherapy (VP-16 and cisplatin) and definitive radiation therapy for local palliation. Some reports have demonstrated improved survival when chemotherapy is combined with radiation therapy as opposed to radiation therapy alone.

A small subset of stage IIIb tumors can be approached surgically. These tumors are considered stage IIIb because of local extension (T4N0) into adjacent structures rather than systemic spread (nodes, hematogenous metastases) and may benefit from aggressive surgical resection of the atrium, carina, or vertebrae. Survival rates of up to 30% have been reported. Metastatic disease is only treated surgically in the unusual circumstance of an isolated brain metastasis with a node-negative lung primary. Several reports have documented better local control (in the brain and lung) with surgery and a subset of long-term survivors. The presence of mediastinal nodes, however, contraindicates surgical resection and mandates radiation therapy for the lung primary.

SURGERY

Pneumonectomy. The removal of the whole lung was previously the most commonly performed operation for NSCLC; it now accounts for only 20% of all resections. Although a more complete resection is accomplished using pneumonectomy versus parenchyma-conserving techniques (lobectomy), it comes at the cost of higher mortality (4%–10%) and morbidity without clear survival benefits.

Lobectomy. The similar survival of patients treated by lobectomy versus pneumonectomy, along with the lower morbidity and mortality associated with lobectomy, make lobectomy the preferred method of resection. Sleeve lobectomies and bronchoplasty procedures in which portions of the main bronchus are removed without loss of the distal lung have further decreased the need for pneumonectomies.

Lesser Resections. Segmentectomies and nonanatomic resections (wedge resection and lumpectomy) are associated with

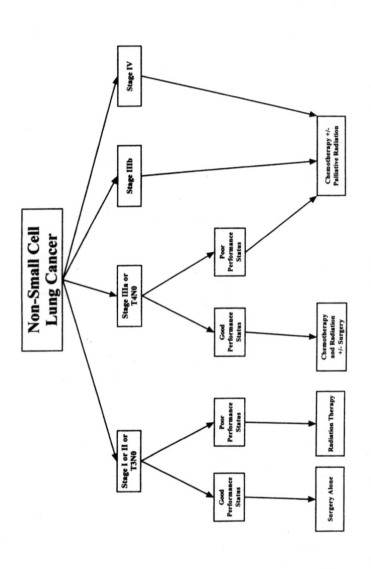

increased local recurrence when compared with lobectomy. The general consensus remains that these procedures should be performed only in high-risk patients with minimal pulmonary reserve who could not tolerate a lobectomy.

Extended Operations.   Recent improvements in surgery and critical care have allowed certain tumors, previously considered unresectable, to be removed with acceptable morbidity and mortality. Carinal sleeve resections and extended resections for superior sulcus tumors with hemivertebrectomy and instrumentation of the spine can now be performed in a small subset of patients whose tumors were previously considered surgically unresectable. These procedures should only be performed in patients without mediastinal nodal involvement because 5-year survival rates are less than 5% for patients with extended resections in the presence of nodal involvement.

Mediastinal Lymph Node Dissection.   Complete mediastinal lymph node dissection is controversial because survival benefits have not been clearly demonstrated. It allows more accurate staging and determination of prognosis and may improve local control but at the cost of slightly increased operative time (20 minutes) and morbidity.

CHEMOTHERAPY

Almost 50% of patients present with extrathoracic spread, and an additional 15% are unresectable because of locally advanced tumor. In addition, the long-term survival for resectable stage II and IIIa tumors remains poor. Therefore the use of adjuvant chemotherapy to treat patients with unresectable tumors and improve the results of surgery is an area of intense investigation. Agents with proven response rates include cisplatin and other platinum analogs, ifosfamide, vinca alkaloids, mitomycin C, and etoposide. Promising new agents include edatrexate, gemcitabine, taxanes, and navelbine. Response rates are higher with combination chemotherapy than with single-agent chemotherapy. Overall response rates as high as 80% have been reported, but complete responses are seen in only 10% to 15% of patients with localized disease and less than 5% of patients with hematogenous metastases.

Small Cell Lung Carcinoma

Unlike NSCLC, SCLC tends to be disseminated at presentation and is therefore not amenable to cure with surgery or thoracic radiation therapy alone. Without treatment, the disease is rapidly fatal, with few patients surviving more than 6 months. Fortunately, SCLC is very sensitive to chemotherapy, and more than two-thirds of patients achieve a partial response after systemic therapy with multidrug regimens. Treatment of SCLC therefore revolves around systemic chemotherapy. An algorithm based on the extent of disease is presented in Fig. 7-4. Complete response is seen in as many as 20% to 50% of patients with limited disease, but these responses are not durable, and the 5-year survival rate is still less than 10%.

←

Fig. 7-3.   Algorithm for treatment of non–small cell lung cancer.

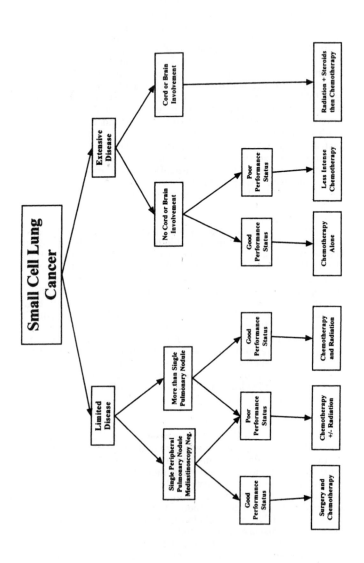

Chemotherapeutic regimens for SCLC most commonly include combinations of cyclophosphamide, cisplatin, etoposide, doxorubicin, and vincristine. Thoracic radiation therapy has been shown to improve local control of the primary tumor and is often included as part of the treatment for limited SCLC. In addition, because brain metastases are noted in 80% of patients with SCLC during the course of their disease, patients who show no evidence of brain metastases on CT scans and who achieve a good response from therapy are usually treated with prophylactic brain irradiation to minimize the chances of developing this morbid site of treatment failure.

There does exist a small role for surgical resection of SCLC. Solitary peripheral pulmonary nodules with no evidence of metastatic disease after evaluation with bone scan, bone marrow biopsy, and CT of the abdomen, brain, and chest can be treated with lobectomy and postoperative chemotherapy if mediastinoscopy is negative. In these select patients, a 5-year survival rate of 50% has been achieved for T1N0, T2N0, and completely resected N1 disease. Surgery for more central lesions, however, has not been demonstrated to improve survival over that achieved with chemotherapy and radiation therapy alone.

Surveillance

The few treatment options for tumor recurrence in NSLC have limited the cost-effectiveness of aggressive radiologic surveillance following surgical resection. Nevertheless, there is an increased incidence of second primary lung cancers (3% per year), and annual or semiannual CXR may help detect these lesions. Any patient who experiences symptoms in the interim should also be evaluated aggressively for recurrence or a new primary.

METASTATIC NEOPLASMS TO THE LUNG

The lung and liver are the most common sites of metastases. Patients with isolated lung metastases can achieve survival rates of 25% to 40% if complete surgical resection is obtained. Because metastases can recur, resection involves nonanatomic wedge or laser resections to preserve the lung parenchyma.

Pathology

The biology of the underlying primary malignancy determines the behavior of its metastases. Metastases may occur via hematogenous, lymphatic, direct, or aerogenous routes. Thirty percent of patients with lung cancer die with isolated pulmonary metastases.

Diagnosis

Because of their predominantly peripheral localization, most pulmonary metastases remain asymptomatic, with fewer than 5% showing symptoms at presentation. Diagnosis is commonly made

Fig. 7-4. Algorithm for treatment of small cell lung cancer.

during radiographic follow-up after treatment of the primary malignancy.

Routine CXR during surveillance after cancer treatment is an effective means of screening patients for pulmonary metastases. Indeed, several studies have demonstrated the increased sensitivity of CT over standard CXR. However, the cost-effectiveness of CT for screening remains low, and no data as yet suggest that early detection with CT leads to improved survival. Planning of surgical interventions, however, should be based on CT findings, even though CT scanning still misses approximately 30% of the nodules found at surgery.

When multiple pulmonary nodules are present in patients with a known previous malignancy, the likelihood of metastatic disease approaches 100%. New solitary lesions, however, often represent primary lung cancers because many of the risk factors are similar.

Staging

No valid staging system exists for pulmonary metastases. The International Registry of Lung Metastases (IRLM) has identified three parameters of prognostic significance: resectability, disease-free interval, and number of metastases. The present criteria for resectability include resectable pulmonary nodules, control of the primary tumor, adequate predicted postoperative pulmonary reserve, and no extrathoracic metastases. Favorable histologies for long-term survival following resection include sarcoma, breast, colon, and genitourinary metastases. Unfavorable histologies include melanomas, esophageal, pancreatic, and gastric cancers.

Treatment

Surgery

Preoperative evaluation for resection of pulmonary metastases is similar to that of any other pulmonary resection. Because of the increased risk of recurrent metastases and need for future thoracotomies, parenchyma-conserving procedures are favored (wedge resection, laser or cautery excision). The various surgical approaches include the following:

Median sternotomy allows bilateral exploration with one incision. Lesions located near the hilum can be difficult to reach, and exposure of the left lower lobe—especially in patients with obesity, cardiomegaly, or an elevated left hemidiaphragm is poor.

Bilateral anterothoracosternotomy (clamshell procedure) allows excellent exposure of both hemithoraces, including the left lower lobe, although some surgeons think the incision increases postoperative pain.

Posterolateral thoracotomy is a more common incision for access to the lung. The limitation to one hemithorax, however, necessitates a second staged operation for removing bilateral metastases.

Thoracoscopic resection allows visualization of both hemithoraces during the same anesthetic. Pleural-based lesions are therefore easily visualized and excised. Unfortunately, the ability to carefully evaluate the parenchyma for deeper or smaller nonvisualized lesions is poor, and some reports suggest an increased risk of local recurrence with thoracoscopy.

At surgery, wedge resections with a 1-cm margin are preferred. If multiple nodules within one segment, lobe, or lung preclude resection of multiple wedges, then laser resections can be performed.

Adjuvant Therapy

The role of radiation therapy in the treatment of pulmonary metastases is limited to the palliation of symptoms of advanced lesions with extensive pleural, bony, or neural involvement. The value of chemotherapy preoperatively or postoperatively remains controversial. There are many isolated reports of the benefit of chemotherapy, especially when the primary tumor is sensitive (e.g., osteosarcoma, teratoma, and other germ cell tumors). However, improvements in survival are more difficult to achieve when the primary is of other types.

Surveillance

The frequency and intensity of follow-up after resection are determined by the primary tumor but usually involve annual or biannual CXR. CT scans should be reserved for evaluations subsequent to abnormal CXR findings or evaluation of adjuvant therapies.

NEOPLASMS OF THE MEDIASTINUM

The mediastinal compartment can harbor a number of lesions of congenital, infectious, developmental, traumatic, or neoplastic origin. Earlier recommendations advocated a direct surgical approach to all mediastinal tumors, with biopsy or debulking of unresectable lesions. However, recent advances in imaging and noninvasive diagnostic techniques, as well as improvements in chemotherapy and radiation therapy, have led to a more conservative approach, with management decisions based on better preoperative evaluation.

Pathology

A recent study combining nine previous series was performed to better approximate the true incidence of mediastinal lesions (Table 7-3). In adults, neurogenic and thymic tumors contribute 23% and 19%, respectively, to the overall incidence, whereas in

Table 7-3. Overall incidence of mediastinal tumors

Thymic	19 (3)*
Neurogenic	23 (39)*
Lymphoma	12
Germ cell	12
Cysts	18
Mesenchymal	8
Miscellaneous	8

*( ) incidence in children.

children they contribute 39% and 3%, respectively. This section will not attempt to describe the myriad of cystic and other rare miscellaneous lesions but will concentrate on the more common diagnoses.

Neurogenic tumors include schwannoma, neurofibroma, ganglioneuroblastoma, neuroblastoma, pheochromocytoma, and paraganglioma. They are the most common tumors arising in the posterior compartment.

Thymoma arises from thymic epithelium, although its microscopic appearance is a mixture of lymphocytes and epithelial cells. Thymomas are classified as lymphocytic (30% of cases), epithelial (16%), mixed (30%), and spindle cell (24%). Histologic evidence of malignancy is difficult to obtain, as benign and malignant lesions can have similar histologic and cytologic features. Surgical evidence of invasion at the time of resection is the most reliable method of differentiating between malignant and benign thymomas.

Lymphomas comprise approximately 50% of childhood and 20% of adult anterior mediastinal malignancies. They are treated nonsurgically but may require surgery to secure a diagnosis.

Germ cell tumors are comprised of teratomas, seminomas, and nonseminomatous germ cell tumors. Teratomas are the most common and are mostly benign. Malignant teratomas are very rare and often widely metastatic at the time of diagnosis. Seminomas progress in a locally aggressive fashion. Nonseminomatous malignant tumors include embryonal carcinoma and choriocarcinoma, both of which carry a poor prognosis, and the more favorable endodermal sinus tumor.

Miscellaneous cysts and mesenchymal tumors include thyroid goiters, thyroid malignancies, mediastinal parathyroid adenomas, bronchogenic cysts, pericardial cysts, duplications, diverticula, and aneurysms.

Diagnosis

Mediastinal lesions are most commonly asymptomatic. When symptoms do occur, they result from compression of adjacent structures or systemic endocrine or autoimmune effects of the tumors. Children, with their smaller chest cavities, tend to have symptoms at presentation (two-thirds of children vs. only one-third of adults) and more commonly have malignant lesions (greater than 50%). Symptoms can include cough, stridor, and dyspnea (more common in children) as well as symptoms of local invasion such as chest pain, pleural effusion, hoarseness, Homer's syndrome, upper-extremity and back pain, paraplegia, and diaphragmatic paralysis.

Chest radiography remains a mainstay of diagnosis. Fifty percent of lesions are diagnosed by CXR. The position of the tumor within the mediastinum on lateral projection can help tailor the differential diagnosis (Fig. 7-5, Table 7-4). The standard for further assessment of the lesion is CT, specifically with contrast enhancement. Certain tumors and benign conditions can be diagnosed or strongly suggested by their appearance on CT scans. Angiography or MRI may be required if a major resective procedure is planned and vascular involvement suspected. Nuclear imaging such as thyroid and parathyroid scanning,

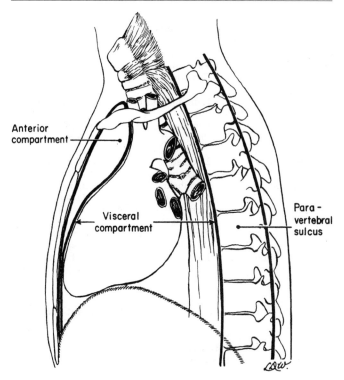

Fig. 7-5. Anatomic boundaries of mediastinal masses according to one commonly used classification.

gallium scanning for lymphoma, and metaiodobenzylguanidine scanning for pheochromocytomas may also be indicated.

The use of serum markers can be of some assistance in the diagnosis of some germ cell and neuroendocrine tumors. In addition, the association of myasthenia gravis with thymoma can also assist in the diagnosis.

Because many mediastinal tumors are treated without surgery, a determined effort should be made to achieve a tissue diagnosis noninvasively. FNA, with its reasonable sensitivity, is an excellent starting point, but the diagnosis of lymphoma can be difficult because only a limited number of cells are retrieved. Bronchoscopy and esophagoscopy can also be useful if symptoms or imaging studies suggest tumor involvement.

If these procedures cannot facilitate a diagnosis then a mediastinoscopy to access paratracheal lesions can be performed. Although the risk of vascular or tracheobronchial injury is present, the incidence of complications is very low in experienced hands. If more invasive procedures are required to make the diagnosis, an anterior or parasternal mediastinotomy (Chamberlain procedure) or thoracoscopy can be performed. Rarely, a sternotomy or thoracotomy will be required to obtain a tissue diagnosis.

Table 7-4.   Usual location of the common primary tumors and cysts of the mediastinum

Anterior Compartment	Visceral Compartment	Paravertebral Sulci
Thymoma	Enterogenous cyst	Neurilemoma: (schwannoma)
Germ cell tumors	Lymphoma	Neurofibroma
Lymphoma	Pleuropericardial cyst	Malignant schwannoma
Lymphangioma	Mediastinal granuloma	Ganglioneuroma
Hemangioma	Lymphoid hamartoma	Ganglioneuro-blastoma
Lipoma	Mesothelial cyst	Neuroblastoma
Fibroma	Neuroenteric cyst	Paraganglioma
Fibrosarcoma	Paraganglioma	Pheochromocytoma
Thymic cyst	Pheochromocytoma	Fibrosarcoma
Parathyroid adenoma	Thoracic duct cyst	Lymphoma
Aberrant thyroid		

Table 7-5.   Frequency and treatment of malignant chest wall tumors

Cell Type	Estimated Frequency (%)	Standard Therapy
Chondrosarcoma	35	Surgical resection
Plasmacytoma	25	Radiation + chemotherapy
Ewing's sarcoma	15	Surgery + chemotherapy
Osteosarcoma	15	Surgery + chemotherapy
Lymphoma	10	Chemotherapy ± radiation

Staging
Staging is determined by the specific histologic characteristics and its extent at the time of diagnosis.

Treatment
Therapy, like staging, is determined by the type of tumor and its histologic characteristics (Table 7-5). The primary determination to be made is whether the lesion will require resection as part of its treatment or whether chemotherapy or radiation therapy is sufficient. Thymomas should all be resected, with the possibility of postoperative radiation therapy. Benign neurogenic tumors are sometimes observed in older debilitated patients; however, if the patient is otherwise healthy or if malignant potential is suspected, then resection should be pursued. Germ cell tumors should be treated on the basis of their histologic characteristics. In particular, benign teratomas should be resected, seminomas should be treated with radiation therapy, and nonseminomatous tumors should be treated initially with chemotherapy. In the

subset of nonseminomatous tumors that have a residual mass but negative markers, surgical resection should be performed to rule out residual tumor. Lymphomas should not be resected and should be treated with radiation therapy or chemotherapy on the basis of their stage and histologic appearance (i.e., Hodgkin's vs. non-Hodgkin's).

Surveillance

The frequency and intensity of follow-up after resection are determined by the primary tumor. CXR remains the mainstay of surveillance, with CT scanning reserved for evaluation subsequent to abnormal CXR findings.

NEOPLASMS OF THE CHEST WALL

Primary chest wall malignancies account for less than 1% of all tumors and include a wide variety of bone and soft-tissue lesions. The absence of large series makes the prospective evaluation of treatment options difficult. As more patients with these tumors are treated at large referral institutions, the initiation of multi-institutional trials will help settle some of the more controversial aspects of therapy.

Pathology

Primary chest wall tumors include chondrosarcoma (20%), Ewing's sarcoma (8%–22%), osteosarcoma (10%), plasmacytoma (10%–30%), and infrequently, soft-tissue sarcoma. Chondrosarcomas arise from the ribs in 80% of cases and from the sternum in the remaining 20%. They are related to prior chest wall trauma in 12.5% of cases and are very resistant to radiation and chemotherapeutic agents. Ewing's sarcoma is part of a spectrum of disease having primitive neuroectodermal tumors at one end and Ewing's sarcoma at the other. Multimodality therapy, including both radiation therapy and chemotherapy, has been shown to be beneficial for this tumor. Osteosarcomas are best treated with neoadjuvant therapy, with prognosis being predicted by the tumor's response to chemotherapy. Plasmacytoma confined to the chest must be confirmed by evaluating the remaining skeletal system. Surgery can then be used to confirm the diagnosis. If radiation therapy is unable to achieve local control, then resection may be indicated. Soft-tissue sarcomas are rare and are primarily resected. Adjuvant therapy is based on tumor histologic findings.

Diagnosis

Chest wall tumors are asymptomatic in 20% of patients, whereas the remaining 80% have an enlarging mass. Fifty percent to 60% of these patients will have associated pain. Radiographic assessment usually includes CXR and CT; however, MRI is being used instead with increasing frequency because of its ability to image in multiple planes with superior anatomic distinction, which can better reveal the extent of disease than CT or plain radiography. Pathologic diagnosis is made with FNA (64% accuracy) or core cutting biopsy (96% accuracy).

Staging

Chest wall lesions are staged according to the primary tumor identified. Most progress to pulmonary or hepatic metastases without lymphatic involvement.

Treatment

As outlined earlier, the treatment of chest wall lesions is determined by the diagnosis. Most, with few exceptions, require resection as part of the treatment. Posterior lesions reaching deep to the scapula or lesions that require resection of less than two ribs do not require reconstruction of the chest wall. However, all other lesions require some form of stable reconstructive technique. A simple mesh closure using Marlex or Proline mesh is acceptable as long as the material is secured in position under tension. Some surgeons think there is a loss of tensile strength over time. A more rigid prosthesis is methyl methacrylate sandwiched between two layers of Marlex mesh. Long-term seroma formation plagues all types of repair, particularly this latter repair technique.

If the chest wall lesion involves the overlying muscle or the skin, a large defect may be present after resection. This may require a muscle flap for final reconstruction, especially if postoperative radiation therapy is considered. Although description of the techniques available is beyond the scope of this manual, a combination of muscle flap with primary skin closure, muscle flap with skin grafting, or myocutaneous flap coverage can be used.

Surveillance

Once treated and in remission, chest wall tumors tend to recur locally or with pulmonary or hepatic metastases. Regular follow-up with careful examination and a CXR should suffice to detect all significant sites of recurrence.

NEOPLASMS OF THE PLEURA

There are two main types of pleural neoplasms. Malignant pleural mesothelioma remains an uncommon and highly lethal tumor with no adequate method of treatment. It behaves primarily as a locally aggressive tumor with locally invasive failure after therapy and only metastasizes late in its course. Its relationship with asbestos exposure was suggested in the 1940s and 1950s, and clearly established in 1960. A more localized pleural tumor, known as localized fibrous tumor of the pleura, can also occur; when malignant, it is frequently classified as a localized mesothelioma.

Pathology

Localized mesotheliomas and malignant localized fibrous tumors of the pleura are very rare. There is some controversy as to whether these lesions are even mesothelial at all because no epithelial component may be identifiable. More commonly, a benign localized fibrous tumor of the pleura is found. On the other hand, diffuse pleural mesothelioma is always a malignant process. There is a 20-year latency for development of this disease after exposure to asbestos. A recent surge in the incidence of

Table 7-6. Staging of mesothelioma

Stage	Characteristic
I	Within the capsule of the parietal pleura: ipsilateral pleura, lung, pericardium, or diaphragm
II	Tumor involving the chest wall or mediastinum: esophagus, trachea, or great vessels
	Positive lymph nodes within the chest
III	Tumor penetrating the diaphragmatic muscle to involve the peritoneum or the retroperitoneal space; tumor penetrating the pericardium to involve its internal surface or the heart
	Involvement of the opposite pleura
	Positive lymph nodes outside the chest
IV	Distant bloodborne metastases

this disease reflects the widespread use of asbestos in the 1940s and 1950s, and this surge should continue because mechanisms for limiting occupational asbestos exposure were not instituted until the 1970s. Mesothelioma almost always exhibits an epithelial component, which can be combined with sarcomatoid features. Thus it can be hard to differentiate this lesion from metastatic adenocarcinoma. Immunohistochemistry and electron microscopy, however, have aided in establishing the diagnosis.

Diagnosis

The presentation of mesothelioma is often vague and nonspecific, with dyspnea and pain common in 90% of patients. Radiographic diagnosis in the early stage is often difficult, with the findings limited to a pleural effusion in many cases. Even CT may fail to identify any other abnormalities at this stage. The classic finding of a thick, restrictive pleural rind is a late finding. Thoracentesis is diagnostic in 50% of patients, and pleural biopsy is positive in 33%. If the diagnosis remains elusive, thoracoscopy is diagnostic in 80% of patients.

Staging

A staging system for mesothelioma has been proposed by Butchart and is shown in Table 7-6.

Treatment

The treatment of mesothelioma is still evolving. Attempts at radical resections, such as extrapleural pneumonectomy, have led to some improvements in local control but only limited impact on survival at the cost of a significantly increased operative risk. Likewise, chemotherapy and radiation therapy have had only limited effects, with less impact on palliation. Institutional trials are under way to examine new methods of treatment, such as intrapleural instillation of new chemotherapeutic agents.

Surveillance

Mesotheliomas tend to recur locally. CT scans are required to detect recurrences or follow residual disease. Unfortunately, treatment options are limited, but they do include radiation therapy and chemotherapy.

RECOMMENDED READING

Anderson BO, Burt ME. Chest wall neoplasms and their management. *Ann Thorac Surg* 1994;58:1774.

Dartevelle PG. Extended operations for the treatment of lung cancer. *Ann Thorac Surg* 1997;63:12.

Ginsberg RJ, Rubinstein LV. Randomized trial of lobectomy versus limited resection for T1 N0 non–small cell lung cancer: lung cancer study group. *Ann Thorac Surg* 1995;60:615.

Moreno de la Santa P, Butchart EG. Therapeutic options in malignant mesothelioma. *Curr Opin Oncol* 1995;7:134.

Mountain CF. Revisions in the international system for staging lung cancer. *Chest* 1997;111:1710.

Nesbitt JC, Putnam JB, Walsh GL, et al. Survival in early-stage non–small cell lung cancer. *Ann Thorac Surg* 1995;60:466.

Parker SL, Tong T, Bolden S, et al. Cancer statistics, 1997. *CA Cancer J Clin* 1997;47:5.

Pastorino U, Buyse M, Friedel G, et al. Long-term results of lung metastasectomy: prognostic analyses based on 5206 cases. *J Thorac Cardiovasc Surg* 1997;113:37.

Roth JA, Fossella F, Komaki R, et al. A randomized trial comparing perioperative chemotherapy and surgery with surgery alone in resectable stage III non–small cell lung cancer. *J Natl Cancer Inst* 1994;86:673.

Shields TW. Primary mediastinal tumors and cysts and their diagnostic investigation. In: Shields TW, eds. *Mediastinal surgery.* Philadelphia: Lea & Febiger, 1991.

Sugarbaker DJ, Jaklitsch MT, Liptay MJ. Mesothelioma and radical multimodality therapy: who benefits? *Chest* 1995;107:3455.

Walsh GL, Morice RC, Putnam JB, et al. Resection of lung cancer is justified in high-risk patients selected by exercise oxygen consumption. *Ann Thorac Surg* 1994;58:704.

Walsh GL, O'Connor M, Willis KM, et al. Is follow-up of lung cancer patients after resection medically indicated and cost effective? *Ann Thorac Surg* 1995;60:1563.

Esophageal Carcinoma

Alexander A. Parikh, Ara A. Vaporciyan,
and Stephen G. Swisher

Cancer of the esophagus is uncommon, thought to represent approximately 1.5% of newly diagnosed invasive malignancies in the United States; it's the ninth most common malignancy worldwide. It is highly virulent, however, and causes 2% of all cancer-related deaths. Surgical resection is the mainstay of therapy, although most cases are diagnosed at a late stage. In the past 30 years, the overall 5-year survival rate has improved from 3% to only 15%. Recent treatment strategies have included multi-modality approaches that combine surgery, radiation therapy, and chemotherapy. These approaches have resulted in 5-year survival rates of 40% to 75% in the subset of patients who have a complete histologic response after preoperative therapy.

EPIDEMIOLOGY

Carcinoma of the esophagus accounts for approximately 12,000 to 13,000 new cases and 11,000 to 12,000 deaths in the United States each year. In the past, squamous cell carcinomas (SCC) accounted for more than 95% of cases, but in recent years, adenocarcinoma arising in the background of Barrett's esophagus has become increasingly common, and it now accounts for more than 50% of the esophageal cancers at many major centers. Esophageal carcinoma, particularly SCC, has substantial geographic variation, from 1.5 to 7 cases per 100,000 people in most parts of the world, including the United States, to 100 to 500 per 100,000 people in its endemic areas such as northern China, South Africa, Iran, Russia, and India. Males have a two to three times higher risk than women, and a seven to ten times higher risk for the development of adenocarcinoma. Furthermore, in the United States, SCC is approximately five times more common among African Americans than it is among whites, whereas adenocarcinoma occurs approximately three to four times more often in whites, particularly in men. Both types are rare in patients younger than 40 years, but the incidence increases thereafter.

ETIOLOGY AND RISK FACTORS

Several different environmental and genetic risk factors have been identified as potential causes of esophageal cancers, particularly SCC. In geographic areas where esophageal cancer is endemic, for example, diets are deficient in vitamins A, C, riboflavin, and protein and have excessive nitrates and nitrosamines. Fungal contamination of foodstuffs and the associated aflatoxin production may be another important risk factor.

The combination of smoking and alcohol consumption has a deadly synergistic effect on the development of SCC, increasing the risk by as much as 44 times. Other causes and risk factors include SCC of the head and neck (presumably because of the risk associated with alcohol and smoking), achalasia (as high as 30 times increased risk), strictures resulting from ingestion of caustic agents such as lye, Zenker's diverticula, esophageal webs in Plummer-Vinson syndrome, prior radiation, and familial diseases such as tylosis (50% have cancer by age 45 years). For adenocarcinoma, the primary etiologic factor is Barrett's esophagus, with an estimated annual incidence of malignant transformation of 1% to 2%, representing a 125 times greater risk than that in the general population. The role of tobacco and alcohol in the absence of gastroesophageal reflux disease and Barrett's esophagus is less clear.

PATHOLOGY

Esophageal cancer has two histologic types: SCC and adenocarcinoma. In the United States, approximately 20% of cases of SCC involve the upper third of the esophagus, 50% involve the middle third, and the remaining 30% extend from the distal part of the esophagus to the gastroesophageal junction. SCC rarely invades the stomach, and there is usually a discrete segment of normal mucosa between the cancer and the gastric cardia. In contrast, nearly 90% of adenocarcinomas develop in the distal esophagus, and many extend into the stomach if they are located near the gastroesophageal junction. Fewer cases develop in the middle third and the proximal esophagus. Adenocarcinomas arising in Barrett's esophagus are thought to comprise 20% to 50% of all adenocarcinomas involving the gastroesophageal junction. They vary from 1 to 10 cm and range from flat, infiltrative lesions to fungating polypoid masses. Ulceration is often present and may even be deep enough to cause perforation. Microscopically, adenocarcinomas resemble those in the gastric cardia, and most are well or moderately differentiated and advanced at the time of diagnosis.

CLINICAL FEATURES

Clinical presentation is generally insidious, and typical symptoms occur late in the course of the disease, usually precluding early intervention. Most patients experience symptoms for 2 to 6 months before they seek medical attention. The most common symptom is progressive dysphagia, which occurs in as many as 80% to 90% of patients. This is usually a late sign because 50% to 75% (approximately 13 mm) of the esophageal lumen must be reduced before patients experience this symptom. Weight loss is also common, with an estimated mean weight loss of 10 kg from the onset of symptoms. Weight loss of more than 10% of normal body weight is associated with decreased long-term survival. Other symptoms include varying degrees of odynophagia (in approximately 50%) as well as emesis, cough, regurgitation, and aspiration pneumonia. Hoarseness is usually due to invasion of the recurrent laryngeal nerve, and Horner's syndrome indicates invasion of the sympathetic trunk. Hematemesis and melena usually indicates friability of the tumor or its invasion into major vessels. Erosion into the aorta resulting in exsanguinating hemorrhage has been reported. Bleeding from the tumor mass can occur in 4% to 7% of patients.

DIAGNOSTIC EVALUATION

Results of the physical examination depend in large part on the degree of weight loss and cachexia. Enlarged cervical or supraclavicular lymph nodes can be biopsied with fine-needle aspiration, and bone pain should be evaluated with a bone scan to exclude distant metastases. All neurologic symptoms (e.g., headaches, visual disturbances) should also be assessed with computed tomography (CT) or magnetic resonance imaging (MRI) of the brain.

Plain posteroanterior and lateral chest radiographs provide assessment of the status of the pulmonary parenchyma (i.e., metastasis, coexisting bronchogenic carcinoma, and pneumonia). A double-contrast barium esophagogram provides information about the location, length, and anatomic configuration of the lesion as well as an evaluation of the stomach for evidence of disease or abnormalities that would preclude its use as a conduit. The esophagogram is also useful in showing the degree of luminal compromise or stricture and the presence of a tumor-related tracheoesophageal fistula. CT scans of the chest and abdomen should also be obtained to evaluate local invasion of mediastinal structures and any notable adenopathy.

Upper endoscopy is currently the most widely used technique for the diagnosis of esophageal cancer. Flexible endoscopy allows magnified visual observation and histologic sampling of the esophagus and observation of the stomach, pylorus, and duodenum in search of coexisting disease. Biopsy and brush cytology can produce diagnostic accuracy of nearly 100% with adequate sampling, and endoscopic dilation of tight strictures can be performed to allow passage of the endoscope beyond the tumor. Involvement of the upper or middle third of the esophagus mandates bronchoscopy to rule out tracheobronchial involvement.

STAGING

The staging system of the American Joint Commission on Cancer uses the TNM classification and is the most commonly used system in the United States (Table 8-1). Although CT scanning is probably the most widely used noninvasive staging modality, its accuracy is still limited because the ability to predict invasion of surrounding structures depends on the presence of periesophageal and mediastinal fat, which is often scarce in the typical cachectic patient. Overall accuracy in determining resectability and T stage have been estimated at 60% to 70%, whereas accuracy in determining N stage is generally less than 60%. Accuracy in detection of metastatic disease is somewhat better, estimated at 70% to 90% for lesions larger than 1 cm. The use of MRI adds relatively little to the evaluation and staging of esophageal cancer because it suffers the same limitations as CT but newer techniques such as positron emission tomography appear more promising. Recent studies with this technique have found an improved ability to detect both locoregional nodal metastases and distant disease with overall levels of accuracy of nearly 60% and 90%, respectively. Further studies confirming these results are needed.

Endoscopic ultrasonography (EUS) is probably the most accurate means currently available for T and N staging. Reported

Table 8-1. TNM staging for esophageal cancer

Primary tumor (T)

Tx	Primary tumor cannot be assessed
T0	No evidence of primary tumor
Tis	Carcinoma *in situ*
T1	Tumor invades lamina propria or submucosa
T2	Tumor invades muscularis propria
T3	Tumor invades adventitia
T4	Tumor invades adjacent structures

Regional lymph nodes (N)

Nx	Regional nodes cannot be assessed
N0	No regional node metastasis
N1	Regional node metastasis

Distant metastasis (M)

Mx	Presence of distant metastasis cannot be assessed
M0	No distant metastases
M1	Distant metastasis

Tumors of the lower thoracic esophagus
- M1a Metastasis in celiac lymph nodes
- M1b Other distant metastasis

Tumors of the mid-thoracic esophagus
- M1a Not applicable
- M1b Nonregional lymph nodes or other distant metastasis

Tumors of the upper thoracic esophagus
- M1a Metastasis in cervical nodes
- M1b Other distant metastasis

Stage grouping

Stage 0	Tis	N0	M0
Stage I	T1	N0	M0
Stage IIA	T2	N0	M0
	T3	N0	M0
Stage IIB	T1	N1	M0
	T2	N1	M0
Stage III	T3	N1	M0
	T4	Any N	M0
Stage IV	Any T	Any N	M1
Stage IVA	Any T	Any N	M1a
Stage IVB	Any T	Any N	M1b

Adapted from Fleming ID, Cooper JS, Henson DE, et al., eds. *AJCC manual for staging of cancer,* 5th ed. Philadelphia: Lippincott-Raven, 1997.

overall accuracy for T staging is 76% to 90%; overall accuracy in predicting resectability is approximately 90% to 100% for adenocarcinoma, but decreases to 75% to 80% for SCC. Studies comparing EUS and CT scanning generally agree that EUS is superior in overall T staging and assessment of regional lymph nodes (70%–86% accuracy). The precise differentiation between benign and malignant nodes occasionally remains problematic, however, because of micrometastases that are undetectable by EUS and enlarged inflammatory lymph nodes that are incorrectly classified as metastatic. Another limitation of EUS is that stenosis caused by the tumor, which is usually associated with advanced lesions, prevents the endoscope from passing, thus preventing visualization of the entire tumor and the surrounding nodes. Smaller-caliber probes are being introduced and may decrease the incidence of this problem. EUS is generally not helpful in detecting metastatic disease (M stage) because of the limited depth of the transducer field.

Minimally invasive techniques such as thoracoscopy and laparoscopy are increasingly important in the staging of esophageal cancer. Thoracoscopy allows visualization of the entire thoracic esophagus and the periesophageal nodes (N1) when performed through the right hemithorax, and of the aortopulmonary and periesophageal nodes and the lower esophagus, when performed through the left chest. Lymph nodes can be sampled for histologic evaluation, the pleura can be examined, and adjacent organ invasion (T4) can be confirmed. The overall accuracy for detecting lymph node involvement has been reported to be as high as 81% to 95%. Laparoscopy and laparoscopic ultrasonography (LUS) are useful in evaluating the peritoneum, liver, gastrohepatic ligament, gastric wall, diaphragm, and the perigastric and celiac lymph nodes. Biopsies and peritoneal washings can be performed to confirm N1 and M1 disease. In addition, a feeding jejunostomy can be placed for nutritional support before treatment begins. Studies have suggested that the overall accuracy in staging and determination of resectability in esophageal cancer is as high as 90% to 100%, and that laparoscopy and LUS may prevent unnecessary surgical resection in as many as 20% of patients. Prospective comparisons against CT and EUS have suggested that laparoscopy and LUS have superior overall accuracy in staging, particularly for lymph nodes and metastatic disease.

Other important staging modalities include bronchoscopy, which should be used in patients with midesophageal or supracarinal lesions to determine invasion of the trachea and mainstem bronchi (T4 lesion) and mediastinoscopy, which is used occasionally to assess regional lymph nodes (N1) at the right and left peritracheal lymph node stations, along the mainstem bronchi, and around the subcarina.

TREATMENT

Patients should be approached with the intent of performing a surgical resection because it affords the best chance for cure (Fig. 8-1). Because accurate clinical staging is so difficult, all patients who can physiologically tolerate resection and have no clinically evident distant metastases should generally undergo surgical exploration, at least with minimally invasive techniques. If

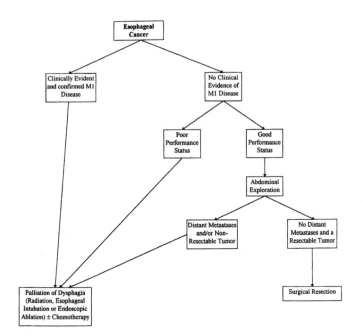

Fig. 8-1. Algorithm for treatment of esophageal cancer.

distant metastases or advanced locoregional disease are found at exploration, nonoperative palliation should be undertaken because of the high perioperative mortality rate (approximately 20%) associated with surgical bypass.

Although it is generally agreed that surgical resection is the primary form of therapy for local and locoregional disease, great controversy remains over the extent of the resection necessary and over the value and extent of lymphadenectomy. There is a belief, particularly among Western surgeons, that lymph node metastases are markers for systemic disease and that removal of involved nodes is therefore of no benefit. On the other hand, many Japanese and other Eastern surgeons believe that some patients with affected lymph nodes can be successfully cured with an aggressive surgical approach that focuses on wide peritumoral excision and extended lymphadenectomies using a transthoracic/thoracoabdominal and cervical approach.

Operative Techniques

Evaluation of pulmonary reserve and cardiac status is warranted for most patients. Specific considerations in patients with esophageal cancer include the presence and severity of nutritional depletion, dehydration, and anemia. If present, these conditions should be corrected as expeditiously as possible.

All operations begin with a thorough abdominal exploration for evidence of metastatic disease. The two most common sites of metastases are the liver and the celiac nodes. If metastatic disease is identified, surgical resection should be performed only if nonsurgical palliation of dysphagia is not possible. After a complete abdominal exploration, the stomach is mobilized by dividing the gastrocolic ligament caudally and short gastric vessels proximally with preservation of the right gastric and gastroepiploic arteries. The lesser omentum is divided close to the liver, and the left gastric artery is identified and ligated. A pyloroplasty or pyloromyotomy is also performed to avoid gastric stasis, which can accompany the division of the vagus nerves during esophageal transection.

Subtotal Esophagectomy

Distal esophageal tumors located at the gastroesophageal junction can be managed by subtotal esophagectomy with adequate local control. Known as an Ivor-Lewis (or Tanner-Lewis modification) esophagectomy, this requires a right thoracotomy to complete the mobilization of the esophagus and create an intrathoracic esophagogastric anastomosis, usually at the level of the azygos vein. The proximal esophageal margin should be examined for the presence of cancer; if cancer is found, a total esophagectomy should be performed. A cervical anastomosis is preferred in this situation because a greater level of risk is associated with a high intrathoracic anastomosis.

Total Esophagectomy

Proximally located (e.g., cervical or upper esophageal) tumors require a total esophagectomy because it is difficult to achieve negative margins with segmental resections (e.g., Ivor-Lewis esophagectomy). The two most popular methods differ according to whether thoracotomy is used for esophageal mobilization. The esophagus can be mobilized using a right thoracotomy with the conduit brought either substernally or through the posterior mediastinum to the neck for anastomosis. Alternatively, a transhiatal esophagectomy can be performed with mobilization of the intrathoracic esophagus from the esophageal hiatus to the thoracic inlet without the need for thoracotomy. The advantage of the transhiatal technique is that it avoids thoracotomy while achieving a complete removal of the esophagus. The potential disadvantages of this technique include less complete periesophageal lymphadenectomy and the risk of causing tracheobronchial or vascular injury during blunt dissection of the esophagus. In addition, the use of a cervical anastomosis is associated with a higher rate of anastomotic leakage than is an intrathoracic anastomosis (12% vs. 5%, respectively) although the mortality is much less with a cervical leak than it is with a thoracic leak (2% vs. 50%, respectively).

Reconstruction after Resection

The stomach, colon, and jejunum have all been used successfully as replacement conduits after esophagectomy. The stomach is preferred because of the ease of its mobilization and its excellent blood supply. Pyloroplasty or pyloromyotomy is required to avoid gastric stasis secondary to the division of the vagus nerves during esophagectomy. No difference has been seen in the leak rate or in the development of strictures between stapled and hand-sewn anastomoses.

The colon is the most commonly used alternative when the stomach cannot be used as a replacement conduit. Either the right or the left colon can be used, although the segment of left and transverse colon that is supplied by the left colic artery is generally longer and therefore may be preferable. The colonic arterial anatomy should be evaluated preoperatively by arteriography, and the colonic mucosa by colonoscopy to rule out any pathologic conditions. Free jejunal grafts, which have been used successfully after resection of hypopharyngeal or upper-cervical esophageal tumors, are another alternative to gastric or colonic conduits. In this case, the mesenteric vessels are usually anastomosed to the external carotid artery and the internal jugular vein.

Few prospective studies have been performed to evaluate the use of different surgical techniques, but evidence from several nonrandomized and small randomized trials is that overall survival is unchanged regardless of the technique used. Proponents of radical resection have reported increased survival rates with more extensive surgical procedures in studies from Japan, but most of these comparisons have been retrospective. Furthermore, it is unclear whether more extensive dissection actually leads to improved survival or whether these superior results are a function of more accurate staging. It is also unclear whether the cancer in the East differs biologically from that in the West and has an inherently better prognosis. Recent prospective randomized studies in the United States and Western Europe have also failed to show any significant difference in morbidity, mortality, or recurrence rates or in the overall survival rate when comparing transhiatal esophagectomy with transthoracic or total thoracic esophagectomy or when comparing the number of lymph nodes resected. Either technique is acceptable, and until prospective randomized trials conclusively prove an advantage in overall survival rate with a particular type of surgery, the choice among surgical resection techniques should be left to the preference of the surgeon and the particular characteristics of the patient.

Mortality rates for transhiatal or transthoracic esophagectomies are now less than 5%, and morbidity rates range from 10% to 27%. Overall survival rates after surgical resection correspond to the stage of the disease and vary from 5% to 50%. The 5-year survival rates have been reported to be 60% to 90% for stage I, 30% to 60% for stage II, 5% to 30% for stage III, and 0% to 20% for stage IV (Fig. 8-2). Unfortunately, the vast majority (70%) of patients already have stage III or IV disease at diagnosis.

When examining the pattern of failure after surgical resection, one finds that most patients experience either distant metastasis or both localized and distant disease, and only a small minority experience solely a recurrence of localized disease. Because even extensive resections fail to cure these patients, other treatment modalities, such as radiation therapy and chemotherapy, have been investigated.

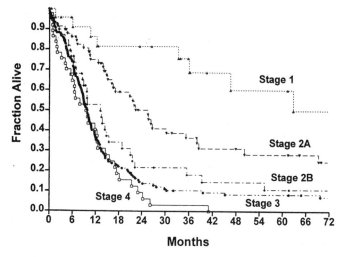

Fig. 8-2. Survival curves for patients with esophageal cancer.

Adjuvant Therapy

Results of several randomized prospective trials on the use of adjuvant radiation therapy (45–56 Gy) after resection have been published. Although reductions in local recurrences have been noted, no significant survival advantage has been found; because treatment-related toxicity can be severe, radiotherapy is now generally recommended only in cases of positive margins or residual disease.

Postoperative chemotherapy with various agents and combinations, including 5-fluorouracil (5-FU), cisplatin, mitomycin C, and vindesine, also has no proven role in the treatment of resectable lesions according to the results of prospective randomized trials. Furthermore, chemotherapy after esophagectomy is generally not well tolerated and many patients fail to complete their treatment regimen. Adjuvant chemotherapy, therefore, cannot be recommended outside the setting of clinical trials. Several newer agents including paclitaxel have shown activity against esophageal cancer in preliminary studies, however, and we await the results of further clinical trials.

The combination of these forms of adjuvant therapy–postoperative chemoradiation therapy, has the potential for benefit by affecting both distant and local disease in hopes of improving overall survival, but only preliminary phase II and nonrandomized studies have been performed so far. Although postoperative chemoradiation therapy has seemed to offer promise when compared with historical controls, compliance with treatment has not been ideal and formal prospective, randomized phase III trials are needed before a final determination and recommendations can be made.

Neoadjuvant Therapy

Largely because of the disappointing results of trials with adjuvant chemotherapy and radiation therapy, researchers have
turned their attention toward the use of preoperative or neoadjuvant therapy. Preoperative radiation therapy has been investigated in several prospective randomized trials; the results have
been subjected to meta-analysis. Despite some initial response,
the results of these trials have shown little or no overall benefit in terms of survival rate. Preoperative radiation therapy
alone is therefore not generally recommended even in the face
of clinical trials. Although results of phase II studies of induction
chemotherapy had been promising, those of prospective randomized trials of different agents and combinations, particularly regimens that included 5-FU and cisplatin have also failed to show
any advantage in survival rate. Although responders seemed to
have better survival rates, non-responders fared worse than controls, thereby abolishing any overall benefit. Currently, patients
are being recruited for two randomized trials in Europe (one for
SCC, the other for adenocarcinoma) that will compare the use
of 5-FU plus cisplatin with surgery, although a large U.S. Intergroup randomized trial recently failed to find any advantage in
survival rate with the same agents.

Most recently, attention has been directed toward evaluating
the effect of neoadjuvant chemoradiation therapy on esophageal
carcinoma with the hope of applying the theoretical advantages
of neoadjuvant therapy to *both* local and systemic disease. A
prospective randomized study conducted at the University of
Dublin with 113 patients with adenocarcinoma evaluated neoadjuvant cisplatin plus 5-FU and 40 Gy of radiation with surgery
alone. The investigators reported a 25% complete pathologic response and a significant increase in median survival (16 vs.
11 months) and 5-year survival rate (32% vs. 6%) for the patients
receiving the neoadjuvant treatment. A European multicenter
randomized trial compared surgery alone with preoperative cisplatin plus radiation therapy (37 Gy) in 282 patients with stages I
and II SCC. Although a 26% complete response rate and T and
N downstaging were noted in the neoadjuvant arm as well as a
longer disease-free survival, median survival (18.6 months) and
3-year survival rate (37% vs. 34%) did not differ between groups.
Only single-agent chemotherapy was used, however, and the improved cancer-free survival in the multimodality-treated arm was
offset by an increased postoperative mortality rate, most likely
related to the large-fraction radiation treatment.

Another randomized study conducted at the University of
Michigan included 100 patients with adenocarcinoma or SCC
who were treated with surgery alone or with cisplatin, 5-FU, and
vinblastine plus radiation therapy (45 Gy) followed by resection.
A 28% complete-response rate was noted in the patients given
neoadjuvant therapy, but the median length of survival was no
different, and although there was a trend toward an improved
3-year survival rate in the patients given neoadjuvant therapy
(30% vs. 16%), the difference was not statistically significant.
Complete pathologic response to therapy, however, was significantly associated with improved survival. Largely because of

these results, a large randomized U.S. Intergroup trial was designed to randomize patients with resectable SCC or adenocarcinoma to either preoperative combination 5-FU, cisplatin, and 50.4 Gy radiation, or surgery alone. Enrollment in this trial was stopped in 2000 because of poor accrual, which was thought to be secondary to the general perception that it is no longer valid to use surgery alone as a control.

Definitive Radiation Therapy and Chemoradiation Therapy

Although surgical resection remains the preferred therapy for esophageal cancer, definitive radiation therapy and chemoradiation therapy have been used in patients who are not candidates for surgical resection. Local control rates ranged between 40% and 75%, and median and 5-year survival rates ranged from 9 to 24 months, and from 18% to 40%, respectively. Several prospective randomized trials have shown that definitive chemoradiation therapy is superior to radiation therapy alone in the treatment of esophageal cancer. Although direct comparisons against surgical therapy (with or without neoadjuvant therapy) have been attempted in the United States and Europe, both trials have failed to recruit patients, largely because of physicians' reluctance to accept a nonsurgical approach in patients who are operative candidates. At this time, therefore, definitive chemoradiation therapy should be reserved for those patients who are poor surgical candidates.

Other Therapeutic Modalities

In certain parts of the world, particularly in areas where esophageal cancer is endemic, mass screening and advances in diagnostic techniques have led to increased numbers of superficial esophageal cancers. Studies from Japan have suggested that for lesions confined to the epithelium and lamina propria, lymphatic spread is rare. In some of these patients, endoscopic mucosal resection is a feasible option, although experience with this technique is still limited. Laser therapy and argon-beam coagulation therapy are primarily used for palliation, but in patients who are not candidates for surgery with superficial cancers and carcinoma in situ, these methods can also be useful. Although experience with these techniques is limited, investigators have reported tumor-free survival for several months after therapy, although recurrence rates after about 1 year can be significant. Similarly, photodynamic therapy has been used in non-surgical candidates and results of preliminary studies in patients with early stage tumors have suggested that tumor-free survival can last several months and that complete remission is possible in some patients (at a 2-year follow up). Long-term studies are still needed, however.

Palliation for Unresectable Tumors

Common indications for palliation in patients with advanced disease include dysphagia, presence of esophagorespiratory fistula, recurrent bleeding, and prolongation of survival. Tumor debulking surgery has been performed, and although survival duration seems somewhat improved relative to that in patients who did not undergo resection, few randomized trials have been performed, and morbidity can be significant. Other options for palliation include (a) dilation, which is a safe and effective method to relieve dysphagia, although it usually requires multiple procedures; (b) stents, both rigid and expandable, that have become very popular in recent years for relieving dysphagia as well as for treating fistulas and bleeding; (c) laser therapy, which has been effective in relieving dysphagia from shorter strictures and those with intraluminal rather than infiltrative growth; (d) photodynamic therapy, which results in fewer perforations than do dilations or laser therapy and is tolerated better but requires more frequent sessions; (e) bipolar electrocautery and coagulation with tumor probes that use heat to destroy tumor cells and cause circumferential injury; and (f) brachytherapy, which delivers radioactive seeds intraluminally.

All of these techniques have advantages and disadvantages, and short-term success rates of 80% to 100% have been reported. If these treatment options fail, an endoscopic prosthesis can often be placed with good results. These techniques are not without complications, however, and ulceration, obstruction, dislocation, and aspiration have all been reported. Recently, improvements in definitive radiation therapy and chemotherapy have also provided excellent means for short-term palliation. With nonoperative treatment, however, long-term local control is still poor (40% locoregional failure). Which method to use therefore depends on the experience of the physician and the particular needs and condition of the patient.

Surveillance

A barium swallow study should be obtained in the first preoperative month as a baseline study. Asymptomatic patients can be assessed with yearly physical examinations and chest radiography. Any symptoms (e.g., pain, dysphagia, weight loss) should be evaluated aggressively with CT scanning, barium studies, or endoscopy. Benign strictures at the anastomosis should be treated with dilation. Unfortunately, treatment options are limited for locoregional or distant recurrences. If radiation therapy was not given preoperatively or postoperatively, it can be used along with the previously mentioned nonoperative methods of palliation (i.e., dilation, stenting, laser, photodynamic or thermal resection).

RECOMMENDED READING

Ajani JA. Current status of new drugs and multidisciplinary approaches in patients with carcinoma of the esophagus. *Chest* 1998;113[suppl 1]:112S.

Akiyama H, Tsurumaru M, Udagawa H, et al. Esophageal cancer. *Curr Probl Surg* 1997;34:767.

Bosset JF, Gignoux M, Triboulet JP, et al. Chemoradiotherapy followed by surgery compared with surgery alone in squamous-cell cancer of the esophagus. *N Engl J Med* 1997;337:161.

Goldminc M, Maddern G, LePrise E, et al. Oesophagectomy by transhiatal approach or thoracotomy: a prospective randomized controlled trial. *Br J Surg* 1993;80:367.

Gore RM. Esophageal cancer: clinical and pathologic features. *Radiol Clin North Am* 1997;35:243.

Herskovic A, Martz K, Al-Sarraf M, et al. Combined chemotherapy and radiotherapy compared with radiotherapy alone in patients with cancer of the esophagus. *N Engl J Med* 1992;326:1593.

Kelsen DP, Ginsberg R, Pajak TF, et al. Chemotherapy followed by surgery compared with surgery alone for localized esophageal cancer. *N Engl J Med* 1998;339:1979.

Knyrim K, Wagner HJ, Bethge N, et al. A controlled trial of an expansile metal stent for palliation of esophageal obstruction due to inoperable cancer. *N Engl J Med* 1993;329:1302.

Orringer MB, Marshall B, Iannettoni MD. Transhiatal esophagectomy: clinical experience and refinements. *Ann Surg* 1999;230: 392.

Roth JA, Pass HI, Flanagan MM, et al. Randomized clinical trial of preoperative and postoperative adjuvant chemotherapy with cisplatin, vindesine and bleomycin for carcinoma of the esophagus. *J Thorac Cardiovasc Surg* 1988;96:242.

Swisher SG, Holmes EC, Hunt KK, et al. The role of neoadjuvant therapy in surgically resectable esophageal cancer. 1996;131:819.

Swisher SG, Hunt KK, Holmes EC, et al. Changes in the surgical management of esophageal cancer from 1970 to 1993. *Am J Surg* 1995;169:609.

Urba SG, Orringer MB, Turrisi A, et al. Randomized trial of preoperative chemoradiation versus surgery alone in patients with locoregional esophageal carcinoma. *J Clin Oncol* 2001;19:305.

Walsh TN, Noonan N, Hollywood D, et al. A comparison of multimodal therapy and surgery for esophageal adenocarcinoma. *N Engl J Med* 1996;335:462.

Gastric Cancer

Eddie K. Abdalla, Syed Arif Ahmad,
David B. Pearlstone, and Charles A. Staley

INTRODUCTION

The majority (95%) of gastric cancers are adenocarcinomas. Evolution in the evaluation and treatment of gastric adenocarcinoma
has led to a shift in the management of this disease over the
past 5 years. Laparoscopy has become an essential component
of pretreatment staging for resectable gastric adenocarcinoma.
The American Joint Committee on Cancer (AJCC) staging system has been altered to reflect the number rather than location
of nodes involved with metastatic tumor, an approach that has
been shown to better stratify patients with regard to prognosis
for this disease. Finally, evidence that the addition of chemoradiation therapy to potentially curative surgical resection increases
disease-free and overall survival has led to the recommendation
by many investigators for multimodality treatment of most resectable gastric adenocarcinomas. This chapter details the epidemiology, preoperative evaluation, surgical treatment, and adjuvant treatment of gastric cancer and discusses the management
of advanced disease. A brief discussion of gastric lymphoma, a
rare type of gastric cancer, is also included.

EPIDEMIOLOGY

In the United States in 2001, 21,700 new cases of adenocarcinoma
of the stomach and 12,800 deaths due to this disease are expected,
which will make gastric cancer the tenth most common cancer in
the United States. There has been a decrease in incidence since
the 1930s, when gastric adenocarcinoma was the most commonly
reported malignancy in the country, although the reasons for the
decreasing incidence are not clear. The approximate incidence in
the United States is ten cases per 100,000 people, compared with
78 cases per 100,000 people in Japan (the country with one of the
highest incidences of this disease). Survival of patients with gastric cancer remains poor, with virtually no change in the overall
5-year survival rates ranging from 53% in Japan to 10% in Eastern Europe. Recent analysis of the National Cancer Data Base
in the United States reveals a 6% to 12% better 5-year survival
for females compared with males, for patients with distal tumors
compared with patients with proximal tumors, and for Japanese
or Japanese-Americans compared with members of other ethnic
groups.

RISK FACTORS

Many factors have been associated with an increased risk of
gastric adenocarcinoma. Diet is thought to play a major role.
Geographic regions with diets high in salt and smoked foods
tend to have high incidences of gastric carcinoma, whereas

diets high in raw vegetables, vitamin C, and antioxidants may be protective. Animal studies have shown that polycyclic hydrocarbons and dimethylnitrosamines, substances produced after prolonged smoking of fish and meat, can induce malignant gastric tumors.

In the United States, male gender, black race, and low socioeconomic class are associated with a higher risk of gastric carcinoma. A specific occupational hazard may exist for metal workers, miners, and rubber workers and for workers exposed to dust from wood and asbestos. Cigarette smoking poses a clear risk, possibly as a result of decreased vitamin C levels, but alcohol consumption has not been as consistently correlated with the development of gastric carcinoma. An association between gastric carcinoma and blood group A was described in 1953, but the relative risk was only 1.2. Familial clustering of gastric adenocarcinoma, although rare, has been reported.

Helicobacter pylori, a gram-negative microaerophilic bacterium living within the mucous layer in the gastric pits, has been implicated in the genesis of gastric carcinoma. The incidence of *H. pylori* infection is increased in areas where there is a high rate of gastric cancer and is also increased among patients with gastric cancer in the United States. Further, nearly 90% of patients with intestinal-type gastric cancer have *H. pylori* detected in adjacent, histologically normal mucosa whereas only 32% of patients with diffuse-type gastric cancer have this finding. (Intestinal- and diffuse-type gastric cancers are discussed in the Pathology section below.) Finally, the risk of adenocarcinoma appears to increase with serologic evidence of immunoglobulin G antibody to *H. pylori* bacterial proteins and with infection of greater than 10 years duration.

Gastric polyps are rarely precursors of gastric cancer. Hyperplastic polyps, the polyps most commonly found in the stomach, are benign lesions. Villous adenomas do indicate an increased risk of malignancy not only within the polyp itself, but also elsewhere in the stomach. However, villous adenomas represent only 2% of all gastric polyps. Pernicious anemia is associated with a 10% incidence of gastric cancer, a risk that is about three to five times that of the normal population. The risk of developing carcinoma in a chronic gastric ulcer is small; however, up to 10% of patients with gastric carcinoma are misdiagnosed as having a benign gastric ulcer on evaluation with only a double-contrast examination of the upper gastrointestinal tract. Operations for benign peptic ulcers also appear to be associated with an increased risk of subsequent stomach cancer. Typically appearing 15 or more years after gastrectomy, gastric stump cancer has been variously reported to occur from zero to five times as often in patients who have had gastrectomy as in individuals without previous gastric resection. Chronic atrophic gastritis and the intestinal metaplasia that often results are also risk factors for gastric carcinoma but may not be direct precursor conditions. To date, no association has been demonstrated between long-term H2 blockade and gastric cancer incidence.

Most recently, several genetic alterations have been found to be associated with gastric cancer. A study of *p53* expression in 418 patients with gastric cancer revealed *p53* expression in more than 55% of tumors; however, there was no correlation between *p53* expression and depth of invasion, lymph node involvement, or survival.

PATHOLOGY

Ninety-five percent of gastric cancers are adenocarcinomas, which arise almost exclusively from the mucus-producing rather than the acid-producing cells of the gastric mucosa. Lymphoma, carcinoid, leiomyosarcoma, and squamous cell carcinoma make up the remaining 5% of gastric cancers. In the United States, gastric cancer is divided into ulcerative (75%), polypoid (10%), scirrhous (10%), and superficial (5%) subtypes on the basis of findings on macroscopic examination. Adenocarcinoma of the stomach is an aggressive tumor, often metastasizing early by both lymphatic and hematogenous routes and directly extending into adjacent structures. Extension through the serosal surface can lead to peritoneal spread of tumor.

Two histologic types of gastric adenocarcinoma are recognized: intestinal and diffuse. Each type has distinct clinical and pathologic features. The intestinal type is found in geographic regions with a high incidence of gastric cancer and is characterized pathologically by the tendency of malignant cells to form glands. The tumors are usually well differentiated, consisting of papillary, glandular, and tubular variants, and are associated with metaplasia or chronic gastritis. They occur more commonly in older patients and tend to spread hematologically to distant organs. The diffuse type is identified by the lack of organized gland formation, is usually poorly differentiated, and is composed of signet ring cells. This type of tumor is more common in younger patients with no history of gastritis and spreads by transmural extension and through lymphatic invasion. The incidence of diffuse-type tumors varies little from country to country and appears to be increasing worldwide.

In the past, most gastric carcinomas (60%–70%) were found in the antrum. Between 1980 and 1990, the proportion of gastric carcinomas arising in the antrum decreased, and the proportion arising in the cardia increased. Nine percent of patients have tumor involvement of the entire stomach, known as linitis plastica; this entity portends a dismal prognosis. In general, gastric tumors are more common on the lesser curve of the stomach than on the greater curve. In the United States, the incidence of synchronous lesions is 2.2%, compared with an incidence of up to 10% in Japanese patients with pernicious anemia.

CLINICAL PRESENTATION

Gastric adenocarcinoma usually lacks specific symptoms early in the course of the disease. Patients often ignore vague epigastric discomfort and indigestion and may be treated presumptively for benign disease for 6 to 12 months before diagnostic studies are performed. Rapid weight loss, anorexia, and vomiting are more common with advanced disease than with early stage disease. The most frequent presenting symptoms of 1,121 patients at Memorial Sloan-Kettering Cancer Center were weight loss, pain, vomiting, and anorexia. The epigastric pain is usually similar to the pain caused by benign ulcers, can mimic angina, and often is relieved by eating food. Dysphagia is usually associated with tumors of the cardia or gastroesophageal junction. Antral tumors may cause symptoms of gastric outlet obstruction. Although very rare, large tumors that directly invade the transverse colon may present with colonic obstruction. Physical examination will reveal a palpable mass in up to 30% of patients.

Approximately 10% of patients will present with one or more signs of metastatic disease. The most common indications of metastasis are a palpable supraclavicular lymph node (Virchow's node), a mass palpable on rectal examination (Blumer's shelf), a palpable periumbilical lymph node (Sister Mary Joseph's node), ascites, jaundice, a liver mass, or a pelvic mass. The most common site of hematogenous spread is the liver; tumor also frequently spreads directly to the lining of the peritoneal cavity.

Gastric tumors may be associated with chronic blood loss, which can be detected with fecal occult blood tests, but massive upper gastrointestinal bleeding is rare. In Japan, the high incidence of gastric cancer has led to the institution of routine endoscopic screening; as a result, in that country the disease is most commonly detected before symptoms occur.

Recent analysis at the University of Texas M.D. Anderson Cancer Center has revealed that patients with gastric adenocarcinoma younger than 35 years of age have a consistently aggressive phenotype and poor prognosis regardless of stage.

PREOPERATIVE EVALUATION

National Comprehensive Cancer Network Guidelines for Initial Evaluation

The National Comprehensive Cancer Network has developed consensus guidelines for the clinical evaluation and staging of patients suspected of having gastric adenocarcinoma. The recommended initial evaluation includes a complete history and physical examination, laboratory studies (complete blood cell count and platelet counts and measurement of electrolytes, creatinine, and liver function), chest radiography, and computed tomography (CT) of the abdomen and pelvis. Upper gastrointestinal contrast studies are not mandatory. Esophagogastroduodenoscopy is necessary, and provides a tissue diagnosis and anatomic localization of the primary tumor. This initial workup enables stratification of patients into two clinical stage groups: those with locoregional disease (AJCC stage I–III) and those with systemic disease (AJCC stage IV) (Table 9-1). Patients with systemic disease are considered for palliative therapy depending on symptoms and functional status. Patients with locoregional disease are further stratified on the basis of functional status and comorbid conditions; further studies in patients with localized disease may include laparoscopy and pulmonary function tests. Patients with locoregional disease who are considered candidates for surgery proceed to definitive (frequently multimodality) therapy including laparotomy and resection. Patients with occult M1 disease found at laparoscopy are considered for palliative therapy.

Table 9-1. TNM classification of carcinoma of the stomach

Category	Criteria
Primary tumor (T)	
Tx	Primary tumor cannot be assessed
T0	No evidence of primary tumor
Tis	Carcinoma *in situ*
T1	Tumor invades lamina propria or submucosa
T2	Tumor invades muscularis propria or subserosa
T3	Tumor penetrates serosa (visceral peritoneum) without invasion of adjacent structures
T4	Tumor invades adjacent structures
Regional lymph nodes (N)	
Nx	Regional lymph nodes cannot be assessed
N0	No regional lymph node metastasis
N1	Metastases in 1–6 lymph nodes
N2	Metastases in 7–15 lymph nodes
N3	Metastases in > 15 lymph nodes
Distant metastasis (M)	
Mx	Distant metastasis cannot be assessed
M0	No distant metastasis
M1	Distant metastasis

Stage grouping			
Stage 0	Tis	N0	M0
Stage IA	T1	N0	M0
Stage IB	T1	N1	M0
	T2	N0	M0
Stage II	T1	N2	M0
	T2	N1	M0
	T3	N0	M0
Stage IIIA	T2	N2	M0
	T3	N1	M0
	T4	N0	M0
Stage IIIB	T3	N2	M0
Stage IV	T4	N1-3	M0
	T1–3	N3	M0
	Any T	Any N	M1

Adapted from Stomach. In: Fleming ID, Cooper JS, Henson DE, et al., eds. *AJCC Cancer Staging Manual,* 5th ed. Philadelphia: Lippincott-Raven, 1998: 71–75.

Upper Gastrointestinal Endoscopy and Endoscopic Ultrasonography

Upper gastrointestinal endoscopy with biopsy is essential for diagnosis of gastric tumors and enables anatomic assessment of the proximal extent of the tumor, tumor size, and often, provided that luminal obstruction does not prevent passage of the gastroscope beyond the tumor, the distal extent of the tumor. Tumor location (gastroesophageal junction, cardia, corpus, or antrum) guides surgical or palliative treatment planning. In selected patients with

advanced disease, esophagogastroduodenoscopy enables palliative treatment with laser ablation, dilation, or tumor stenting. In
more than 90% of patients, four to six tissue biopsies and cytologic
brushings are sufficient for accurate diagnosis.

In the case of adenocarcinoma, depth of tumor invasion is a
major determinant of stage and directly correlates with prognosis. Gastric mural endoscopic ultrasonography (EUS) can achieve
spatial resolution of 0.1 mm, which allows for reasonably accurate assessment of the degree of tumor penetration through the
layers of the gastric wall. However, because EUS cannot reliably
distinguish between tumor and fibrosis (either treatment-related
or secondary to peptic ulceration), EUS is used primarily for initial staging rather than assessing response to therapy.

Pathologic confirmation of the findings on preoperative staging
with EUS has demonstrated overall staging accuracy to be 75%.
Correct assignment of tumor stage is poor on the basis of EUS
for T2 lesions (38.5%) but better for T1 (80%) and T3 (90%) lesions. The accuracy of nodal staging with EUS is as low as 50%,
but technical improvements and experience have improved the
accuracy of nodal evaluation to about 65% for N1 disease. EUS-
guided fine-needle aspiration may further improve the accuracy
of nodal staging but this technique is technically challenging. As
a result, the optimal use of EUS is largely confined to regional
referral centers.

Computed Tomography

CT is the standard imaging study used to stage intra-abdominal
malignancies. Abdominal and pelvic CT is performed early in the
overall staging evaluation of patients with newly diagnosed gastric cancer. This allows patients with visceral metastatic disease
or malignant ascites to avoid unnecessary laparotomy. CT of the
chest may be required for complete staging of proximal gastric
tumors.

The major limitations of CT as a staging study are in the evaluation of early gastric tumors and small (<5 mm) metastases
on peritoneal or liver surfaces. Specific techniques such as spiral CT with an intravenous contrast agent plus an oral positive
contrast agent (barium) or negative contrast agent (water) may
significantly improve the sensitivity of CT. The overall accuracy
of CT in assessing tumor stage is reported to be 66% to 77%. CT
accurately assigns nodal stage in only 25% to 86% of patients.

Laparoscopy and Laparoscopic Ultrasonography

The value of further staging with laparoscopy is apparent upon
recognition of the low sensitivity of CT—even high quality spiral
CT performed with gastric-specific protocols in the detection of
small (<5 mm) macrometastases on the peritoneal surface, and in
or on the liver. Laparoscopic inspection of the peritoneal surfaces
and the liver enables easy detection and pathologic confirmation
of metastases not revealed on CT. Identification of advanced disease allows patients to be spared non-therapeutic laparotomy and
other local therapies, such as radiation therapy, that may not be
justified in the setting of advanced disease. Patients with small-
volume metastatic disease in the peritoneum or liver identified

at laparotomy have a life expectancy of only 3 to 9 months and thus rarely benefit from palliative resection.

Researchers from Memorial Sloan-Kettering Cancer Center and M.D. Anderson Cancer Center have evaluated the feasibility, yield, and clinical benefit of laparoscopic staging after high-quality abdominal CT staging. They found that laparoscopy identified CT-occult metastatic disease in 23% to 37% of patients. Moreover, fewer than 2% of the patients in whom CT-occult metastases were identified on laparoscopy required subsequent laparotomy for palliation. Thus, with the use of laparoscopic inspection of the peritoneal cavity, approximately one-fourth of patients presumed to have localized high-risk gastric cancer can be spared a non-therapeutic laparotomy. On the basis of the available data, the National Comprehensive Cancer Network has integrated laparoscopy into the recommended routine staging algorithm for patients with locoregional and selected advanced gastric cancers.

Simple laparoscopy has limitations in the staging of gastric cancer—specifically, it does not provide a means for three-dimensional evaluation of the liver and peritoneal cavity, palpation of structures to enable identification of small intra-parenchymal hepatic metastases and involved perigastric lymph nodes, or assessment of critical tumor-vessel relationships. Laparoscopic ultrasonography (LUS) has been proposed as a means to overcome some of these limitations and to improve the diagnostic yield. The majority of studies of LUS in the staging of gastric cancer are difficult to interpret because the use of state-of-the-art prelaparoscopy staging (particularly CT) varied and results were reported in a manner that makes it difficult to determine the specific added benefit of LUS over high-quality CT plus laparoscopy alone. Given the limitations of the available data, the significant financial expense associated with the equipment required for LUS, and the operator-dependent nature of the technique, LUS is best regarded as a technique that requires further investigation to define its role in the staging of gastric cancer.

Peritoneal Cytology

Cytologic analysis of peritoneal fluid or fluid obtained by peritoneal lavage may identify patients with occult carcinomatosis. Peritoneal dissemination of gastric carcinoma can occur with transmural penetration of the tumor to the gastric serosa. Many institutions have adopted cytologic assessment of peritoneal fluid as part of the preoperative staging procedure; the fluid is usually obtained by percutaneous or laparoscopic aspiration (with or without peritoneal lavage) performed at the time of staging laparoscopy. Peritoneal cytologic analysis is relatively simple and fast and is therefore feasible in an intraoperative setting.

Patients with positive findings on peritoneal cytology have a prognosis similar to that of patients with macroscopic visceral or peritoneal disease. The primary concerns regarding the use of peritoneal cytology are the possibility of false-positive results and the fact that some reports do not confirm the prognostic significance of positive findings on peritoneal cytology. For these reasons, efforts are ongoing to develop more sensitive and specific techniques for identifying peritoneal dissemination, including immunostaining and reverse transcriptase-polymerase chain reaction testing for carcinoembryonic antigen (CEA) mRNA.

Other Studies

Positron emission tomography (PET), which allows estimation of tumor metabolism by measurement of the uptake of a radiotracer—most commonly fluorodeoxyglucose—is currently being evaluated as a staging tool for gastric cancer. This technique may reveal CT-occult metastases (particularly extra-abdominal disease) and may be used to assess response to neoadjuvant therapy. The cost of PET is high, availability is limited, and the additional yield of PET over standard staging studies is under investigation.

Investigation of a potential role for sentinel lymph node biopsy for gastric carcinoma is ongoing. The procedure can be technically challenging, as the lymphatic drainage from different anatomic regions of the stomach is quite variable. Skip metastases (involvement of nodes in N2 or N3 stations without involvement of N1 nodes) are relatively uncommon, occurring in 13% to 16% of patients. Questions regarding the appropriate extent of pathologic evaluation of sentinel lymph nodes have not yet been investigated thoroughly. Currently, sentinel node biopsy for staging of gastric cancer is strictly investigational.

Increased levels of CEA are seen in only 30% of patients with gastric carcinoma. Because the CEA level is usually normal in early gastric cancer, CEA is not a useful screening marker. Serial determinations of CEA level may be helpful in detecting tumor recurrence or in patients who present with an increased CEA level, in monitoring response to treatment.

STAGING SYSTEMS

Many staging systems for gastric adenocarcinoma have been proposed over time. Overlapping and confusing systems persist, so a basic understanding of the older systems is necessary to discuss and to understand the literature. The pathologic staging system currently in use worldwide is the AJCC TNM staging system. Additionally, the term *R status* is used to describe the residual disease remaining after resection. Several other largely abandoned systems arose in an attempt to describe both the extent of *disease* and the extent of *resection* or *lymphadenectomy* necessary based on the disease in a given patient. Subsequent sections explain the various staging systems in use in the literature.

American Joint Committee on Cancer Staging System

Staging of gastric adenocarcinoma has changed significantly over the past 5 years. In 1997, the AJCC published a revised TNM staging system in which patients are stratified on the basis of the number rather than the location of any involved lymph nodes (Table 9-1). The 1997 revisions were based on data from Japan and later from the West describing outcomes based on the number of involved lymph nodes. Survival is closely linked to the AJCC pathologic stage, particularly the nodal stage.

The validity of the newer TNM staging system is well established. Three important clinicopathological factors have been

Table 9-2.   Current description of completeness of resection based on presence or absence of residual disease following resection and pathologic evaluation of resection margins

Description	Gross or Pathologic Extent of Residual Disease
R0	No residual gross or microscopic disease
R1	Microscopic residual disease only
R2	Gross residual disease

shown to stratify patients into distinct groups with different risks of tumor-related death: the depth of penetration of the primary tumor through the gastric wall, the absence or presence and extent of lymph node involvement, and the absence or presence of distant metastases. Some investigators (such as Roder et al., 1998) argue that survival is also independently predicted by tumor location (cardia compared to distal tumors) and suggest that future AJCC staging systems should reflect the poorer prognosis for proximal tumors seen in their analyses.

Residual Disease: R Status

The term *R status* is commonly used to describe the tumor status in a patient following resection, first described by Hermanek et al. in 1994. The R status is assigned following pathologic evaluation of the margins of resection (Table 9-2). The term R0 resection indicates that microscopic margins are free of tumor and that no gross or microscopic disease remains in the resection bed. R1 indicates that all gross disease is extirpated, but microscopic margins are positive for tumor. R2 indicates that gross residual disease remains. Long-term survival can be expected only in patients who undergo R0 resection for gastric adenocarcinoma, and significant effort is made to avoid R1 or R2 resections.

Japanese R and PNHS Systems

The previously described R status after resection can be confused with an older Japanese classification of gastric resection that also used the letter R. That nomenclature was designed to describe the anatomic echelons of lymph nodes successfully resected upon examination of a *total* gastrectomy specimen: R0, incomplete removal of N1 echelon nodes (regional lymph nodes); R1, complete removal of N1 nodes; R2 complete removal of N2 nodes (N1 plus hepatic, splenic, celiac, and left gastric lymph nodes); R3, complete removal of N3 nodes (N2 plus para-aortic and retroperitoneal lymph nodes). The nodal stations are numbered as shown in Fig. 9-1, with the recommendations for nodal resection based on tumor location as presented in Table 9-3. As previously mentioned, this R designation is no longer widely used because it is easily confused with the more universally accepted system describing the pathologic completeness of resection described in the section above, and because this older system does not predict prognosis as clearly as the AJCC TNM system. Additionally, the description of lymph nodes by anatomic location (such as portal or celiac lymph nodes) is more readily understood. The R1 and R2 lymphadenectomy concept is still occasionally referred to

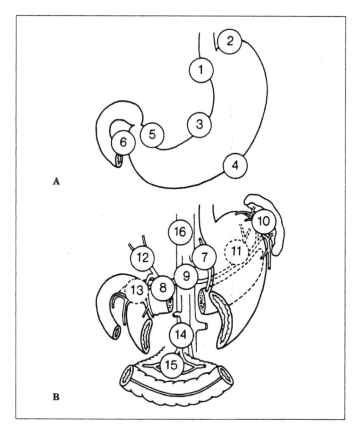

Fig. 9-1.   Japanese classification of regional gastric lymph nodes. A: Perigastric lymph nodes. *1*, right pericardial; *2*, left pericardial; *3*, lesser curvature; *4*, greater curvature; *5*, suprapyloric; *6*, infrapyloric. B: Extraperigastric lymph nodes. *7*, left gastric artery; *8*, common hepatic artery; *9*, celiac artery; *10*, splenic hilus; *11*, splenic artery; *12*, hepatic pedicle; *13*, retropancreatic; *14*, mesenteric root; *15*, middle colic artery; *16*, para-aortic. (Adapted from Kodama Y, Sugimachi K, Soejima K, et al. Evaluation of extensive lymph node dissection for carcinoma of the stomach. *World J Surg* 1981;5:242.)

in the Japanese literature (Fig. 9-2), although the description of the gastrectomy plus D1, D2, or D3 lymphadenectomy may help to avoid the confusion created by the use of the terms R1 or R2, which are better reserved for use as described in the previous section and in Table 9-2.

Another complex Japanese staging system describing serosal invasion (S), nodal involvement (N), peritoneal metastases (P), and hepatic metastasis (H) has also been largely abandoned, as the current AJCC TNM staging system is simpler, and again, stratifies patients into prognostic groups.

Table 9-3.   Japanese definitions of N1, N2, N3 nodal resections by site of tumor[a]

Lymph Node Group	Location of Primary Tumor			
	Entire Stomach	Lower Third	Middle Third	Upper Third
N1	1–6	3–6	1, 3–6	1–4
N2	7–11	1, 7–9	2, 7–11	5–11
N3	12–14	2, 10–14	12–14	12–14

[a] The numbers in the table correspond to the lymph node positions described in Figure 9-1; N1–N3 not to be confused with TNM stage in Table 9–1 (see text). Adapted from Behrns KE, Dalton RR, van Heerden JA, et al. Extended lymph node dissection for gastric cancer. Is it of value? *Surg Clin North Am.* 1992;72:433–443.

Japanese Classification: Results of Resection

The extent of pathologic lymph node involvement relative to the scope of the lymphadenectomy performed is the distinguishing characteristic of this Japanese classification scheme (Table 9-4). This classification scheme is predicated on the unproved assumption that extended lymph node clearance beyond the level of pathologic involvement may result in enhanced survival. In yet another Japanese system (Table 9-5), completeness of nodal dissection is described as D1 (removal of all nodal tissue within 3 cm of the primary tumor), D2 (D1 plus clearance of hepatic, splenic, celiac, and left gastric nodes), or D3 (total gastrectomy, omentectomy, splenectomy, distal pancreatectomy, celiac and portal lymphadenectomy). Although these classifications are not part of the AJCC staging system, the D terminology persists in many discussions and publications.

Recommendations

As previously mentioned, the current recommendations in Japanese centers for nodal resection based on tumor location are presented in Table 9-3. D3 total gastrectomy (resection of N3 echelon nodes) is not recommended in the West based on large series which show that extended lymphadenectomy, especially with splenectomy/pancreatectomy, is associated with higher operative mortality, and does not provide a survival advantage over a D1 lymphadenectomy despite a lower local recurrence rate. The staging system used internationally is the new AJCC TNM system; however, understanding the R status to describe the presence (R1 or R2) or absence (R0) of residual disease, and the D nomenclature to describe the extent of lymphadenectomy is important to be able to critically evaluate and understand discussions in the gastric cancer arena.

SURGICAL TREATMENT

In the absence of documented metastatic disease, aggressive surgical resection of gastric tumors is justified. The appropriate

Lower third lesions

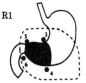

R1

3 Lesser curvature
4 Greater curvature
5 Suprapyloric
6 Infrapyloric

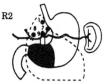

R2

1 R Cardiac
7 L Gastric artery
8 Hepatic
9 Celiac

Middle third lesions

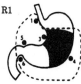

R1

1 R cardiac
3 Lesser curvature
4 Greater curvature
5 Suprapyloric
6 Infrapyloric

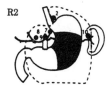

R2

2 L cardiac*
7 L gastric artery
8 Hepatic artery
9 Celiac
10 Splenic hilar
11 Splenic artery

Upper third lesions (includes cardia)

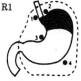

R1

1 R cardiac
2 L cardiac
3 Lesser curvature
4 Greater curvature
and short gastric

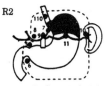

R2

5 Suprapyloric*
6 Infrapyloric*
7 L gastric artery
8 Hepatic artery
9 Celiac
10 Splenic hilar
11 Splenic artery
110 Paraesophageal
(cardia lesions)

Fig. 9-2. Extent of R1 and R2 lymphadenectomy by tumor location.
Dashed line indicates the scope of the lymphadenectomy. An R2
dissection must remove all the R1 lymph nodes as well as the
majority of the R2 lymph nodes. The *asterisk* indicates those nodes
for which removal is optional. (From Smith JW, Shiu MH, Kelsey L,
Brennan MF. Morbidity of radical lymphadenectomy in the curative
resection of gastric carcinoma. *Arch Surg* 1991;126:1469.)

Table 9-4. Japanese classification: results of resection

Absolute curative resection
- One tier of nodes beyond involved nodes is completely resected
- No direct invasion of adjacent organs and
- No involvement of margins of gastric resection

Relative curative resection

As for absolute curative resection except:
- Failure to clear a tier of nodes beyond involved nodes or
- Local peritoneal spread that is completely resected with primary tumor

Noncurative resection
- Failure to meet any above criteria
- Resection in patients who are found to have positive infracolic or periaortic nodes

Relative noncurative resection
- Complete macroscopic resection with microscopically positive margins

Absolute noncurative resection
- Gross residual disease

Adapted from Kajitani T. The general rules for gastric cancer study in surgery and pathology. Part I. Clinical classification. *Jpn J Surg* 1981;11:127.

Table 9-5. "D" nomenclature: extent of surgical resection and lymphadenectomy

Description	Regions Included in Resection
D1	Removal of all nodal tissue within 3 cm of the primary tumor
D2	D1 plus clearance of hepatic, splenic, celiac, and left gastric lymph nodes
D3	D2 plus omentectomy, splenectomy, distal pancrectomy, and clearance of porta hepatis lymph nodes

surgical procedure for a given patient must take into account the location of the lesion and the known pattern of spread.

Proximal Tumors

Proximal tumors account for 35% to 50% of all gastric carcinomas. The optimal surgical management of proximal gastric tumors is controversial. The options include total gastrectomy and proximal subtotal gastrectomy. In general, proximal tumors are more advanced at presentation and have a poorer long-term prognosis than distal cancers. Consequently, palliative rather than curative resections are more likely to be performed in patients with proximal tumors. Because of the advanced stage at diagnosis of most tumors of the cardia, some authors argue that any operation is realistically a palliative procedure and that therefore one should always perform the simpler proximal subtotal gastrectomy, especially because total gastrectomy does not improve prognosis for patients with stage III and IV disease. However, a survival benefit and lower recurrence rate have been shown for patients with stage I and II disease who undergo a total gastrectomy, and some studies show poorer quality of life with proximal subtotal gastrectomy than with total gastrectomy.

At M.D. Anderson, we perform a total gastrectomy with a Rouxen-Y reconstruction and regional lymphadenectomy for proximal gastric lesions. This procedure has the advantage of avoiding the alkaline reflux gastritis often associated with proximal subtotal gastrectomy. There is no significant increase in mortality or morbidity with total gastrectomy compared with proximal subtotal gastrectomy; in fact, several studies have shown the morbidity and mortality to be significantly less after total gastrectomy.

Mid-Body Tumors

Mid-stomach tumors account for 15% to 30% of all gastric cancers. On the basis of the same arguments as those presented for proximal tumors (see the preceding section), we recommend total gastrectomy with regional lymphadenectomy for tumors located in the mid-body of the stomach.

Distal Tumors

Distal tumors account for approximately 35% of all gastric cancers. The standard operation for these lesions is a distal subtotal gastrectomy with regional lymphadenectomy. This procedure entails resection of approximately three-fourths of the stomach, including the majority of the lesser curvature. Studies have shown that microscopic invasion beyond 6 cm from the gross tumor is exceedingly rare. We therefore recommend a 5- to 6-cm luminal resection margin when possible. Even if this distance is achieved, margins should be evaluated with frozen-section techniques.

Splenectomy

Splenectomy is not performed unless there is tumor adherence or invasion of the spleen. Routine splenectomy does not improve survival but does increase the morbidity and mortality of gastrectomy. If a splenectomy is contemplated because of tumor adherence, pneumococcal polysaccharide vaccine should be given before surgery.

Lymphadenectomy

Probably the single greatest current controversy in gastric surgery is the role of extended lymphadenectomy in the treatment of gastric cancer. Radical lymphadenectomy was adopted on the basis of an initial report in 1981 by Kodama et al. that showed a survival benefit for patients with serosal or regional lymph node involvement that underwent an R2 or R3 lymphadenectomy (old Japanese nomenclature) (resection of N2 or N3 echelon nodes, see Table 9-5). Patients undergoing radical lymphadenectomy had a 39% 5-year survival rate, compared with 18% for an R1 lymphadenectomy. Figure 9-2 shows the site-specific extent of dissection for R1 and R2 lymphadenectomies. Many other studies from Japan have shown a similarly significant survival benefit for patients undergoing radical lymphadenectomy. Unfortunately, Western studies have not been able to repeat the

Japanese results, which contributes to this already significant controversy.

The difference in survival between Japanese and Western studies appears to result from several causes. The significant differences in the staging systems between the two countries make it difficult to compare survival rates stage for stage between studies. In addition, the Japanese nodal dissection and pathologic analysis is much more meticulous and extends to the retroperitoneal and periaortic nodes in many cases. Western series, on the other hand, potentially understage patients because in many cases only perigastric nodes are dissected and the involvement of celiac and portal nodes (N2 echelon) and periaortic nodes (N3 echelon) is not evaluated. Mass screening programs in Japan have increased the percentage of cancers diagnosed at an early stage to greater than 40% (vs. <10% in the United States). It is also postulated that there is an inherent difference in the biology of gastric cancer between the two countries, with the Japanese having a less aggressive form of tumor. Furthermore, most of the Japanese data come from comparisons of radical lymphadenectomy with historical controls from previous decades rather than from prospective randomized trials. The higher percentage of early-stage gastric cancers being diagnosed currently in Japan could account in part for this increased survival compared with historical controls.

Wanebo et al. (1996) reviewed outcomes in 18,346 patients with gastric cancer whose records were prospectively gathered in a database that included information from 200 tumor registries in the United States. Compared with patients undergoing D1 dissection, patients undergoing D2 nodal dissection (including lymph nodes ≤3 cm from the primary tumor, see Table 9-4) had no increase in median survival time (D2, 19.7 months; D1, 24.8 months) or in 5-year survival rate (D2, 26.3%; D1, 30%). Similar results have been shown in a prospective randomized study from South Africa. In contrast, in a study from Austria (Jatzko et al., 1995) in which 345 patients with potentially curable gastric cancer were prospectively randomized to extended lymphadenectomy, patients had 5- and 10-year survival rates similar to those of patients in Japanese studies, with no increase in morbidity or mortality. Shiu et al. (1987) retrospectively reviewed 210 patients with gastric cancer treated at Memorial Sloan-Kettering Cancer Center and found that a lymphadenectomy that failed to include the lymph nodes at least one echelon beyond the histologically involved nodes was predictive of a poor prognosis. These researchers also showed that there was not a significant difference in morbidity between R1 and R2 nodal dissections (old Japanese nomenclature). In contrast, in a study from the Netherlands, Bonenkamp et al. (1999) reported on 711 patients prospectively randomized to D1 or D2 nodal dissections. Patients undergoing more extended lymphadenectomy had a significantly higher operative mortality rate (D2, 43%; D1, 25%; $p < 0.001$) and experienced significantly more complications (D2, 10%; D1, 4%; $p = 0.004$). 5-year relapse rates (D1, 43%; D2, 37%) and 5-year survival rates were similar (D1 45%; D2 47%). Similar results have been obtained from the MRC trial (Cuschieri et al., 1999). In this study, 400 patients with gastric adenocarcinoma were prospectively randomized as in the Dutch trial to D1 or D2 nodal resection. Similarly, in this study there was no difference in overall 5-year survival between the 2 groups (D1, 35%; D2, 33%). In this study pancreatico-splenectomy as part of the D2 resection resulted in an increased postoperative morbidity and mortality, as well as a decreased long-term survival. These data do not support the routine use of D2 lymph node dissection in patients with gastric adenocarcinoma.

Current standard recommendations include a D1 dissection (regional lymphadenectomy) though major centers continue to study the potential benefit and morbidity of more extended nodal dissections.

SURGICAL TECHNIQUE

Total Gastrectomy

Once the preoperative workup excludes the presence of distant metastases or an unresectable tumor, the patient should undergo diagnostic laparoscopy. If findings on laparoscopy are negative, an open laparotomy, exploration, and gastrectomy are performed through a midline or bilateral subcostal incision.

For a total gastrectomy, the dissection is begun by separating the omentum from the mesocolon. The right gastroepiploic vessels are ligated at their origin, and the subpyloric nodes are resected with the specimen. The first portion of the duodenum is mobilized and divided 2 cm distal to the pylorus. The gastrohepatic ligament is opened and the left gastric artery is ligated at its origin. It is important to remember that an aberrant or accessory left hepatic artery may originate from the left gastric artery and reside in the lesser omentum. If an extended lymphadenectomy is done, the celiac, hepatic artery, and splenic artery nodes are dissected along with the specimen. The short gastric vessels are ligated sequentially up to the gastroesophageal junction. Dissection around the gastroesophageal junction can free 7 to 8 cm of distal esophagus, which facilitates transection of the esophagus with adequate proximal margins. After the esophagus is divided, the resection margins are evaluated by frozen-section examination. If the tumor is adherent to the spleen, pancreas, liver, diaphragm, colon, or mesocolon, the involved organs are removed en bloc.

There are many types of reconstruction, but the most frequently used is a Roux-en-Y anastomosis. If a significant portion of the distal esophagus is resected, a left thoracoabdominal or right thoracotomy (Ivor-Lewis approach) may be used. Reconstruction with pouches and loops to act as reservoirs provides no benefit over a straight Roux-en-Y reconstruction. Care is taken to ensure that the Roux limb is at least 45 cm long. A feeding jejunostomy tube is placed for postoperative nutritional support.

Subtotal Gastrectomy

The mobilization for subtotal gastrectomy is identical to that described in the preceding section for total gastrectomy except that only approximately 80% of the distal stomach is resected (Fig. 9-3). The dissection of the distal short gastric vessels is performed first to ensure splenic preservation. The small remnant of stomach that is left is supplied by the remaining short gastric vessels. A roux-en-Y reconstruction is strongly recommended for

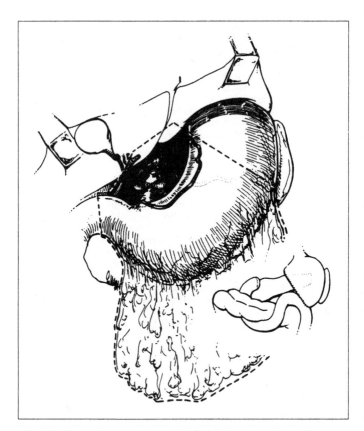

Fig. 9-3.   Resection margins for subtotal gastrectomy. Inset shows
placement of anastomosis. (From MacDonald JS, Steele G, Gunderson
LL. Cancer of the stomach. In: DeVita VT, Hellman S, Rosenberg SA,
eds. *Cancer: Principles and Practice of Oncology*, 4th ed.
Philadelphia: Lippincott Williams & Wilkins, 1993.)

patients left with a small gastric pouch (<20% of the stomach),
although a loop gastrojejunostomy is acceptable for patients with
larger pouches.

Figure 9-4 outlines the M.D. Anderson treatment algorithm for
potentially resectable gastric carcinoma.

Fig. 9-4.   The University of Texas M.D. Anderson Cancer Center
algorithm for the evaluation and treatment of potentially resectable
gastric adenocarcinoma. *Occasionally, at the time of open surgical
exploration for tumors believed to be resectable on the basis of
radiologic and laparoscopic staging, metastatic disease is found. In
this situation, selection of patients for palliative resection is made on
an individualized basis. Patients with metastatic disease have a
dismal prognosis (see text).

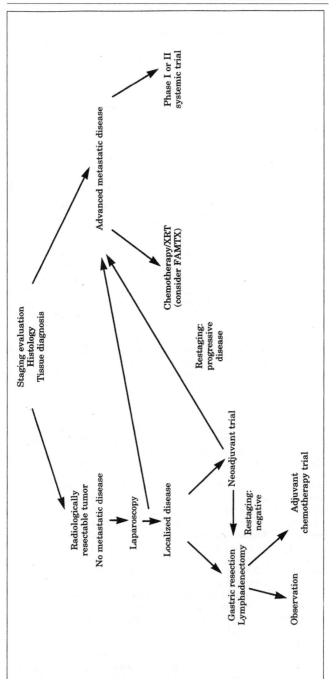

Table 9-6.   Complications of gastric resection

Complication	Patients Affected (%)
Pulmonary	3–55
Infectious	3–22
Anastomotic	3–21
Cardiac	1–10
Renal	1–8
Bleeding	0.3–5
Pulmonary embolus	1–4

COMPLICATIONS OF SURGERY

Complications of gastric resection are listed in Table 9-6. The most devastating complication of a gastric resection is an anastomotic leak, which is seen in 3% to 21% of patients. We no longer routinely obtain a barium upper-gastrointestinal tract study before oral feeding is begun. Leaks can occur late, and an intact anastomosis early in the postoperative period does not guarantee an uncomplicated course. Feeding is begun 5 to 7 days postoperatively if the patient is asymptomatic. Upper gastrointestinal tract contrast studies are performed on the basis of clinical indications (e.g., fever, tachycardia, or tachypnea). Because the food reservoir is gone, many patients must initially change their eating habits to six small meals per day. Many patients require supplemental jejunostomy feedings after discharge until their oral intake is adequate. Within several months, most patients will increase their intestinal capacity and be able to eat larger meals less frequently (three or four meals per day).

OUTCOMES AFTER SURGERY

The overall 5-year survival rate for gastric cancer is 10% to 21% in most Western series, a consequence of the high proportion of tumors that are at an advanced stage at presentation. Patients who undergo potentially curative resection have a slightly better prognosis (5-year survival rate of 24%–57%). Patients who undergo curative resection in Japan are reported to have at least a 50% 5-year survival. Overall 5-year survival rates for Japan and the United States by TNM stage are listed in Table 9-7.

In 1989, Cady et al. reviewed a series of 211 patients with gastric cancer. Eighty-three percent of the patients underwent laparotomy and 17% did not undergo laparotomy because distant metastatic disease or diffuse peritoneal spread was identified before surgery. Among patients who underwent laparotomy, 58% underwent resection. Resection was considered potentially curative in approximately two-thirds of resected patients and palliative in one-third. These patients were treated before the more widespread use of diagnostic laparoscopy. The overall 5-year survival rate for all 211 patients was 21%, but patients who underwent surgical resection had a 5-year survival rate of 36%. This figure increased to 58% for patients treated with curative intent. The rate of curative resection among patients with proximal tumors was half that among patients with distal tumors. Fifteen

Table 9-7. Five-year survival rates after gastrectomy with complete resection and > 15 lymph nodes examined

| | 5-Year Survival Rate(%) | | | |
| | United States[a] | | | |
AJCC Stage	All (n=32,532)	Japanese-Americans (n=697)	Japan[b] (n=587)	Germany[c] (n=1,017)
IA	78	95	95	86
IB	58	75	86	72
II	34	46	71	47
IIIA	20	48	59	34
IIIB	8	18	35	25
IV	7	5	17	16
Overall	28	42	NR	NR

AJCC, American Joint Committee on Cancer Staging; n, number of patients; NR, not reported.

[a]From Hundahl SA, Phillips JL, Menck HR. The National Cancer Data Base Report on poor survival of U.S. gastric carcinoma patients treated with gastrectomy: fifth edition American Joint Committee on Cancer staging, proximal disease, and the "different disease" hypothesis. *Cancer* 2000;88:921–932.

[b]From Ichikura T, Tomimatsu S, Uefuji K, et al. Evaluation of the New American Joint Committee on Cancer/International Union against cancer classification of lymph node metastasis from gastric carcinoma in comparison with the Japanese classification. *Cancer* 1999;86:553–558.

[c]From Roder JO, Bottcher K, Busch R, et al. Classification of regional lymph node metastasis from gastric carcinoma. German Gastric Cancer Study Group. *Cancer* 1998;82:621–631.

percent of the patients had linitis plastica; these patients had a median survival of 12 months with no long-term survivors. Resection should generally be avoided in patients with linitis plastica unless palliation of an obstructing or bleeding tumor is necessary.

Shiu et al. reviewed multiple prognostic variables for gastric cancer in 1989. The five independent variables found to correlate with a poor prognosis were high TNM stage, metastatic involvement of four or more lymph nodes, poorly differentiated tumors, splenectomy, and regional lymphadenectomy not extensive enough relative to the nodal stage. Each of these variables had a negative impact on survival.

Disease recurrence has been analyzed in autopsy, reoperative, and clinical series. Some component of disease failure can be found in up to 80% of patients following gastrectomy. In 1982, Gunderson and Sosin analyzed patterns of failure in a prospective study of 109 patients who underwent gastric resection and subsequent reoperation at the University of Minnesota. Of the 107 evaluable patients, 86 (80%) had recurrent disease. Locoregional failure alone occurred in only 22 (9%) of these 86 patients, but peritoneal seeding was a component of recurrence in 54% of patients with recurrent disease. Isolated distant metastases were uncommon but occurred as some component of failure in 29% of patients with recurrence.

In 1990, Landry et al. from Massachusetts General Hospital reviewed disease recurrence in 130 patients treated by resection with curative intent. The overall locoregional failure rate was 38% (49/130); 21 patients (16%) had locoregional failure alone, 28 patients (22%) had locoregional failure and distant metastasis, and 39 patients (30%) had distant metastasis alone. The risk of locoregional recurrence increased with the degree of tumor penetration through the gastric wall. The most frequent sites of locoregional recurrence were the gastric remnant at the anastomosis, the gastric bed, and the regional nodes. The overall incidence of distant metastases was 52% (67 patients), and the incidence of distant metastases increased with advancing stage of disease. The overall recurrence rate was 68% (88 patients).

EARLY GASTRIC CANCER

In the early 1960s, the Japanese defined early gastric cancer as carcinoma limited to the mucosa and submucosa regardless of the presence or absence of lymph node metastasis. This pathologic classification is based on the high cure rate in this group of patients. The incidence of early gastric cancer has increased in the United States from approximately 5% to 15% of all gastric cancers over the past 20 years. In Japan, aggressive screening during the past 15 years resulted in an even greater increase in incidence in that country, from 5% to greater than 40%. The mean age of patients at diagnosis in Western studies is 63 years, whereas in Japanese patients it is 55 years. Most patients with early gastric cancer present with gastrointestinal symptoms similar to those of peptic ulcer disease, including epigastric pain and dyspepsia. In contrast to patients with advanced gastric cancer, patients with early gastric cancer rarely have significant weight loss at the time of diagnosis.

Endoscopy and biopsy have been instrumental in the increase in the diagnosis of early gastric cancer. In collected Western series, only 22% of early gastric cancers were diagnosed with a barium upper gastrointestinal tract study, whereas 80% were diagnosed with endoscopy. The Japanese have classified early gastric cancer pathologically on the basis of gross endoscopic appearance. They define three basic morphologic types of tumors: type I, protruded or polypoid; type II, superficial (IIa, elevated; IIb flat; IIc, depressed); and type III, excavated or ulcerated. By the TNM classification, early gastric cancer would include all T1 tumors with any stage of nodal disease.

Despite a high potential cure rate, 10% to 15% of early gastric tumors are associated with positive lymph nodes that may extend to the N2 nodal basin. As a result, gastrectomy with D1 or D2 lymphadenectomy generally remains the treatment of choice, even for early lesions. However, recognition that tumor size (mucosal area), morphology, and submucosal invasion are significant predictors of nodal metastases in T1 tumors, has provided the basis for a move toward less aggressive treatment for selected early tumors. In 1994, Takekoshi reported on 343,993 cases of gastric cancer from 104 centers in Japan. Analysis of mucosal resection for early tumors based on the endoscopic appearance (previously described) enabled establishment of specific criteria for mucosal resection of early gastric cancers without submucosal invasion.

Subsequent analyses have refined the criteria necessary for safe endoscopic mucosal resection of AJCC T1 gastric cancers to include only the following: (a) well-differentiated endoscopic type I or IIa, less than 2 cm in area, or (b) well-differentiated endoscopic type IIc, without an ulcer scar, less than 1 cm in area. The incidence of nodal metastases based on these criteria is 0.01%. Close endoscopic follow-up is necessary, but this localized treatment provides a cure rate exceeding 90%. Following any endoscopic mucosal resection, the finding of submucosal invasion on permanent serial sectioning mandates conventional gastrectomy with at least a D1 lymphadenectomy. Recurrence following mucosal resection that meets criteria can be re-resected mucosally; if at any time following mucosal resection gastrectomy is necessary, expected survival is equivalent to survival seen in historical control patients who underwent gastrectomy primarily. This further reiterates the safety of the endoscopic technique in selected patients. Endoscopic mucosal resection is not currently recommended by the AJCC or National Comprehensive Cancer Network (NCCN), although ongoing analysis in Japan and in the West provides the basis for further study of this treatment in the future.

ADJUVANT THERAPY

In the majority of patients who undergo potentially curative resection for gastric cancer (nearly 80%), some form of recurrence develops. Effective adjuvant therapy is needed, but results have been inconsistent at best. Only recently has a survival benefit of adjuvant therapy been convincingly demonstrated, with combined-modality treatment.

Postoperative Chemotherapy

Studies investigating whether chemotherapy alone improves survival after complete resection of gastric adenocarcinoma have produced inconsistent results. Two early studies conducted by the Veterans Administration Surgical Adjuvant Group investigated the use of triethylene thiophosphoramide (thiotepa) and floxuridine (FUDR) following surgical resection. There was no survival benefit seen in either study, and the toxicity of thiotepa was substantial. A meta-analysis by Hermans et al. (1993) reviewed the results of 11 prospective randomized trials of adjuvant chemotherapy involving 2,096 patients and concluded that postoperative chemotherapy offers no survival advantage compared with surgery alone.

Three trials have studied the use of fluorouracil (5-FU) and semustine (methyl-CCNU) as adjuvant therapy. The Gastrointestinal Tumor Study Group randomly assigned patients to receive no additional therapy or 18 months of 5-FU and semustine after complete resection. A survival benefit was noted in patients who received chemotherapy. However, an Eastern Cooperative Oncology Group trial using the same doses and schedules of chemotherapy failed to confirm this survival benefit. A third study by Veterans Administration Surgical Adjuvant Group using the same agents but a different dosing schedule also found no survival benefit. Given the lack of confirmation of a clear survival benefit with adjuvant 5-FU and semustine and given the significant risk of treatment-induced acute nonlymphocytic leukemia, many investigators believe that this adjuvant regimen is inappropriate.

A single study from Spain by Estape et al. (1991) with a follow-up of 10 years has shown a survival benefit with the use of adjuvant mitomycin C. The chemotherapy schedule used in this study was 20 mg/m^2 given intravenously once every 6 weeks for four cycles. Thirty-one of the 37 patients in the control arm died of recurrent disease, compared with 16 of the 33 patients in the treatment arm. The most significant advantage was seen in patients with T3 N0 M0 tumors. The major criticism of this study is the relatively small sample size. Other studies of mitomycin C (at lower doses) in combination with 5-FU and either cyclophosphamide or cytarabine have failed to show a survival benefit from adjuvant chemotherapy.

More recently, chemotherapy regimens that include doxorubicin have been studied. Several groups have reported no survival benefit from the combination of 5-FU, doxorubicin, and mitomycin C in an adjuvant setting. In an addendum to the previously discussed meta-analysis, Hermans et al (1994) recalculated their meta-analysis data with the inclusion of three additional prospective trials. This analysis suggested a slight survival benefit to adjuvant chemotherapy; however, a specific adjuvant regimen could not be recommended based on this data. Thus, other approaches are necessary. Some of these other treatment approaches are discussed below.

Postoperative External-Beam Radiation Therapy

Most studies of radiation therapy for gastric cancer have examined radiation therapy as an adjuvant to surgery or combined with sensitizing chemotherapy (usually 5-FU).

Studies from the Mayo Clinic in the 1960s of low-dose bolus 5-FU with 4,000-cGy external-beam radiation therapy versus radiation therapy alone showed that combination therapy provided improved survival. The data were interpreted to mean that the improvement was related to a radiation-sensitizing effect of the chemotherapy because the 5-FU dose was relatively low.

Two randomized studies have examined patients assigned to receive no additional therapy or radiation therapy with concurrent 5-FU after complete tumor resection. Dent et al. (1979) studied 142 patients but found no benefit with this combined regimen, although some patients may have had incomplete resection, and the radiation therapy dose was only 2,000 cGy. A second study, by Moertel et al. (1984), showed a benefit of chemotherapy plus radiation therapy, but the study results were skewed because ten patients who were randomized to the experimental arm refused treatment. Interest was generated by this study because the 5-year survival rate was slightly longer and the local recurrence rate was lower in the adjuvant-therapy group than in the surgery-only group.

Many investigators believe that the standard of care for resectable gastric cancer has changed in the past 2 years on the basis of the Southwest Oncology Group initiated national intergroup trial (INT-0116) that evaluated two cycles of 5-FU and leucovorin followed by radiation therapy with concurrent chemotherapy following R0 resection of gastric adenocarcinoma (MacDonald et al., 2001). Five hundred fifty-six evaluable patients were randomly assigned to curative resection (275 patients) or curative resection with chemoradiation (281 patients): 4,500 cGy external-beam radiation therapy was delivered concurrently with 5-FU and leucovorin. The first cycle utilized the Mayo Clinic regimen (425 mg/m^2 5-FU and 20 mg/m^2 leucovorin) for 5 consecutive days followed by concurrent chemoradiation. Chemotherapy doses were decreased stepwise during radiation therapy. One month after completion of radiation therapy, two additional cycles of 5-FU and leucovorin were given. Three deaths were attributed to adjuvant therapy (1%), and morbidity was acceptable; however, only 65% of the patients were able to complete the adjuvant treatment. Adjuvant therapy produced significant improvement in disease-free and overall 3-year survival rates. The median survival for the surgery-only group was 26 months, compared to 40 months for the chemoradiation group; 3-year survival rates were 41% and 52%, respectively. This seminal study is largely responsible for the latest recommendations for a combined-modality approach to resectable gastric cancer.

Intraoperative Radiation Therapy

Most of the data available on intraoperative radiation therapy (IORT) for gastric cancer is based on the report of Abe and Takahashi from Japan (1981). In a prospective nonrandomized trial, these authors compared 110 patients treated with surgery alone with 84 patients treated with surgery plus IORT. The 5-year survival rates were similar in patients with stage I disease; however, a suggestion of a survival benefit from IORT was seen in patients with stage II, III, and IV disease. In contrast, a small (<40 patients) randomized study of IORT done at the National Cancer Institute showed neither a disease-free nor an overall survival benefit with IORT despite a marked decrease in locoregional recurrence. Other studies involving IORT have generally been conducted in combination with chemotherapy (see the next section).

Neoadjuvant Chemotherapy

The use of neoadjuvant chemotherapy in the treatment of gastric cancer evolved from preoperative treatment strategies used for esophageal and rectal cancers. There are several potential advantages of neoadjuvant chemotherapy for gastric cancer (Ajani, 1998 and Minsky, 1996). These include biologic advantages (treatment of well-oxygenated tissue and decreased tumor seeding at surgery), mechanical advantages (smaller treatment volume and displacement of contiguous structures by the intact tumor reduce radiation therapy toxicity), and the potential opportunity to assess tumor sensitivity to a chemotherapeutic regimen. If the tumor responds to the neoadjuvant therapy, treatment can be continued postoperatively. Multivariate analysis of the three phase II trials of neoadjuvant therapy at M.D. Anderson (Lowy et al., 1999) revealed that response to neoadjuvant chemoradiation therapy is the single most important predictor of overall survival after such treatment for gastric cancer, which further supports the examination of neoadjuvant approaches to the treatment of this disease.

Another theoretical advantage would be an improved R0 resection rate. Finally, the interval required for neoadjuvant therapy provides a period of time to evaluate for progression of disease, thus improving patient selection for resection. A potential disadvantage of the neoadjuvant approach is the overtreatment of patients with early stage disease; however, improved pretreatment staging minimizes this risk. Further, the combined local and distant failure rate for totally resected gastric cancer remains at 70% in Western series, which argues strongly in favor of any strategy that may reduce the risk of recurrence. Several trials have evaluated the combination of etoposide, cisplatin, and either 5-FU or doxorubicin in the neoadjuvant setting. Clinical response rates have ranged from 21% to 31%, and complete pathologic response rates have ranged from 0% to 15%. Recent work from M.D. Anderson has evaluated the effect of an integrated staging and preoperative-therapy approach on the fraction of patients undergoing potentially curative (R0) resection. Thirty patients whose disease was staged as T2-3 N0-1 M0 on the basis of CT, EUS, and laparoscopy were treated with neoadjuvant chemotherapy consisting of 5-FU, interferon alfa-2b, and cisplatin (median, three preoperative cycles; range, one to five cycles). The overall clinical response rate was 34%; 25 patients (83%) underwent subsequent R0 resection. This favorable resection rate is considerably higher than historical R0 resection rates of approximately 50%, suggesting that the combination of enhanced preoperative staging and induction chemotherapy may indeed improve rates of potentially curative resection.

The approach to adjuvant therapy for gastric adenocarcinoma at M.D. Anderson has been largely to deliver the therapy preoperatively. Multimodality neoadjuvant therapy combining sensitizing chemotherapy with external-beam radiation therapy is under study. A few studies have demonstrated acceptable toxicity for neoadjuvant therapy; these studies are best exemplified by a recent pilot study of preoperative chemoradiotherapy for resectable gastric cancer at our institution (Lowy et al., 2001) in which 24 patients were treated with 4,500-cGy external-beam radiation therapy and concurrent infusional 5-FU (300 mg/m^2). Patients were restaged 4 to 6 weeks after completing treatment and if free of disease, underwent resection and IORT (10 Gy). Several findings were of significant interest. First, 23 (96%) of 24 patients completed chemoradiation therapy, a rate significantly higher than in trials of postoperative adjuvant therapy. Four patients had progression of disease and did not undergo resection; the remaining 19 patients underwent resection with D2 lymphadenectomy and IORT. The morbidity and mortality rates were acceptable (32%, and 15% respectively). Of the patients who underwent resection, 2 (11%) had complete pathologic responses, and 12 (63%) had significant pathologic evidence of treatment effect. The proportion of patients who completed all planned therapy was far greater in this trial than in trials of postoperative adjuvant therapy, most likely since operative complications, which occur in all series, do not delay neoadjuvant therapy. Other studies of neoadjuvant chemoradiation therapy from Russia (Skoropad et al., 2000) and the United States (Weese et al., 2000) demonstrate similarly acceptable morbidity and also demonstrate a survival advantage over surgery alone, consistent with the national intergroup adjuvant therapy trial (INT-0116) described earlier in this chapter in the section Postoperative External-Beam Radiation Therapy.

MANAGEMENT OF ADVANCED DISEASE

Because of the low cure rate for gastric cancer and the advanced disease stage at presentation among most patients with gastric cancer in the West, appropriate use of palliative techniques is essential. Many patients (20% to 30%) present with stage IV disease, and an additional 28% to 37% initially believed to have localized disease are found to have metastatic disease after complete staging. The 5-year survival rate for patients with stage IV disease approaches zero—hence, the majority of newly diagnosed gastric cancers are incurable. Palliation is an essential component of gastric cancer management.

Optimal palliation relieves or abates symptoms while causing minimal morbidity and improving the patient's quality of life. Prolonged survival is generally not a goal of palliative treatment, but palliation may relieve debilitating, potentially life-threatening problems such as gastrointestinal bleeding or gastric outlet obstruction.

Palliative Surgery

Surgical palliation of advanced gastric cancer may include resection or bypass alone or in combination with endoscopic, percutaneous, or radiation therapy interventions. Complete staging is required for determination of the best palliative approach. In patients found to have peritoneal disease, hepatic metastases, extensive nodal metastases, or ascites and patients with problems including bleeding or proximal or distal gastric obstruction, palliation by endoscopic means is most appropriate. Surgical palliation is associated with higher morbidity and mortality than endoscopic palliation—an important factor in patients with short life expectancy. Laser recanalization or simple dilatation with or without stent placement can be used to treat obstruction. Repeat endoscopy may be required at periodic intervals. Patients who undergo stent placement for gastric outlet obstruction are frequently able to eat solid or semisolid food and may not require any further intervention before death.

Selection of patients for palliative resection is complex. Clearly, R2 resection is to be avoided whenever possible as the outcome after such procedures is uniformly poor. In patients with an excellent performance status, experienced surgeons can perform palliative R1 distal gastrectomy with minimal morbidity and acceptable mortality rates. Palliative total gastrectomy and esophagogastrectomy should be approached with greater caution because the morbidity from these procedures is high and there is little evidence that they improve patients' quality of life. Good palliation is obtained with surgery less than 50% of the time. The operative mortality rate for subtotal resection at institutions with extensive experience ranges from 6% to 15%, while the mortality rate for palliative total gastrectomy or esophagogastrectomy ranges from 20% to 40%. Survival after palliative treatment is dismal (mean, 4.2 months; range, 0–13 months).

Specific indications for palliative resection, surgical bypass (open or laparoscopic), and endoscopic palliation remain undefined. However, assessment of morbidity, mortality, and quality of life reveals that carefully selected patients (particularly those without macroscopic metastatic disease) may benefit from palliative resection. Advanced endoscopic techniques, including laser or argon-beam tumor ablation and endoscopic placement of coated metallic stents, provide better palliation of dysphagia than does surgical bypass with lower morbidity. Other techniques utilizing multimodality therapy (radiotherapy, surgery and endoscopy) are likely to lead to continued improvements in quality of life and lower morbidity with palliative therapy. However, earlier diagnosis and advances in curative therapy will ultimately be required to definitively reduce the occurrence and morbidity of advanced disease for patients with gastric adenocarcinoma.

Palliative Chemotherapy

The impact of chemotherapy on advanced gastric carcinoma has been disappointing. Several single-agent drug regimens have been tested, including 5-FU, doxorubicin, and mitomycin C. The response rates have ranged from 17% to 30%; however, the responses have generally been brief and have not significantly improved survival.

Many chemotherapy combinations using agents known to be active against gastric adenocarcinoma have been investigated. The combination of 5-FU, doxorubicin, and mitomycin C (FAM) was studied in the 1980s. Initially, it produced a response rate of 42% and median response duration of 9 months, with no complete responses. Other studies of this regimen have shown similar results. In a single study in which etoposide was used in combination with doxorubicin and cisplatin (EAP), the response rate was 64%. However, other investigators have not reproduced this high response rate and have documented significant morbidity and mortality due to myelosuppression. As a result, combinations of etoposide with other agents, including leucovorin and 5-FU, have been investigated. Results have varied, but these combinations are generally well tolerated by older, high-risk patients. Methotrexate has been combined with doxorubicin and 5-FU in clinical trials to produce a regimen termed FAMTX. Response rates ranging from 33% to 59%, complete response rates as high as 21%, and median survival times as long as 9 months have been reported. No combination chemotherapy regimen has been shown to be decisively superior to single-agent therapy. However, many investigators are encouraged by the initial results with FAMTX. This provides the basis for further studies of this therapeutic combination, perhaps with radiation therapy.

Phase II studies at M.D. Anderson utilizing irinotecan (CPT-11) and cisplatin administered weekly showed a 9-month median survival and median time to progression of 24 weeks. Other trials using intracellular signal inhibitors (such as bryostatin-1, a protein kinase C inhibitor) in combination with traditional chemotherapeutic agents (such as paclitaxel) for stage IV disease and trials with newer, synthetic taxane analogs are also ongoing at many institutions, including M.D. Anderson.

Palliative Radiation Therapy

There are several isolated case reports of the benefit of radiation therapy for palliative treatment of advanced gastric carcinoma. However, no large prospective trial has demonstrated long-term benefit from radiation therapy alone in patients with advanced disease. This modality is most likely best used in combination with chemotherapy as described earlier in this chapter.

Intraperitoneal Hyperthermic Perfusion

The use of intraperitoneal chemotherapy has been investigated for several years, particularly in the treatment of ovarian, appendiceal, and colorectal cancers. Intraperitoneal 5-FU was initially shown to decrease peritoneal recurrence in patients with colorectal cancer. Koga et al. (1988) reviewed their experience with a combination of hyperthermia and mitomycin C used in an adjuvant setting for gastric cancer. The researchers showed that this procedure was technically feasible and safe. Patients who underwent perfusion did not have an increased incidence of postoperative complications. Yonemura et al. (1996) have reported that adjuvant hyperthermic intraperitoneal chemotherapy with mitomycin C, etoposide, and cisplatin after gastric resection in patients with peritoneal seeding resulted in complete responses in eight (19%) of 43 patients and partial responses in nine (21%) of 43 patients. A randomized trial in patients who were treated at the time of complete resection of tumors that penetrated the gastric serosa but had no evidence of peritoneal metastases showed that hyperthermic intraperitoneal chemotherapy with mitomycin C reduced the incidence of peritoneal recurrence and provided a small survival advantage at 3 years. Fujimoto et al. (1990) evaluated 59 patients who underwent gastrectomy and were then randomly assigned to no further therapy or intraperitoneal hyperthermic perfusion. The patients treated with perfusion survived longer than the controls (1-year survival rate of 80% vs. 34%). Patients with peritoneal seeding also had a significant survival benefit when they underwent perfusion with hyperthermic mitomycin C. Other centers have not found such encouraging results and this technique is currently under investigation in several centers in the United States.

Immunotherapy and Hormonal Therapy

A number of investigators have examined the use of immunologic agents alone and in combination with chemotherapy as adjuvant treatment in patients with gastric adenocarcinoma. Maehara et al. (1994) reported that patients randomly assigned to receive standard chemotherapy with intraperitoneal injection of the streptococcal preparation OK-432 had significantly decreased rates of peritoneal recurrence and longer survival times compared with patients who received chemotherapy alone. Similarly, data from Japan and Korea suggest that immunochemotherapy utilizing microbacterium-derived polysaccharides may provide a survival benefit in patients following potentially curative resection. Adjuvant hormonal therapy with tamoxifen has been disappointing. Studies of immunotherapy and hormonal therapy are ongoing. The role of immunomodulators in gastric cancer remains to be defined.

SURVEILLANCE

Patients are examined every 3 months for the first 2 years following curative resection of gastric adenocarcinoma. A careful history and physical examination are performed, along with laboratory studies (complete blood cell count and liver function tests). Chest radiographs are obtained every 6 months. Patients undergo abdominal and pelvic CT scanning 6 months after surgery and yearly thereafter. Yearly endoscopy should be considered in patients who have undergone subtotal gastrectomy. Patients who undergo protocol-based therapy often have more frequent staging studies even though this has never been proven to impact patient survival.

GASTRIC LYMPHOMA

In contrast to the decreasing incidence of gastric adenocarcinoma, the incidence of gastric lymphoma is steadily increasing. *H. pylori* has been implicated in the development of gastric lymphoma. The stomach is the most common site for lymphoma in the gastrointestinal tract, accounting for two-thirds of gastrointestinal lymphomas. Non-Hodgkin's lymphomas are the second most common malignancy of the stomach after adenocarcinoma. The average age of patients with gastric lymphoma is 60 years. The most frequent symptoms at the time of presentation are pain (68%), weight loss (28%), bleeding (28%), and fatigue (16%). Obstruction, perforation, and massive bleeding are uncommon.

Before the advent of endoscopy, the diagnosis of gastric lymphoma was usually made at operation. Endoscopy permits a correct tissue diagnosis in approximately 80% of cases. Most lesions are located in the distal stomach and spread locally by submucosal infiltration. Once the diagnosis has been made, a careful work-up—including a physical examination (with special attention to adenopathy), routine laboratory tests along with lactate dehydrogenase and β2-microglobulin determinations, a bone marrow biopsy, pedal lymphangiogram, chest radiograph, and CT scan of the abdomen—should be done to fully assess the extent of disease. Pathologic examination shows most cases to be B-cell non-Hodgkin's lymphoma, and the diffuse histiocytic subtype is predominant. The disease is staged using the modified Ann Arbor staging system (see Chapter 17). Histologic grade and pathologic stage are two variables that independently predict survival.

The treatment of gastric lymphoma varies among institutions, with some centers advocating surgery alone and others promoting chemotherapy and radiation therapy alone. Surgery is necessary in some cases to confirm the diagnosis. Surgical resection is curative in many patients with localized disease and can prevent the rare complications of bleeding or perforation in patients receiving radiation therapy or chemotherapy. Moreover, more accurate staging is obtained at surgery. If surgery is performed an attempt should be made to resect the entire area involved with lymphoma while leaving grossly uninvolved stomach intact. Negative margins, however, are not necessary for cure. Several studies have shown adjuvant radiotherapy to be of no benefit.

Many patients with gastric lymphoma undergo chemotherapy in addition to resection. Some authors have found no survival benefit with adjuvant chemotherapy. Still other authors believe that patients will benefit from a combination of radiation therapy and chemotherapy without any need for surgery. In fact, cure rates of 70% have been seen in patients with Ann Arbor stage IE and IIE gastric lymphoma treated with chemotherapy alone. Talamonti et al. (1990) reported that in patients with stage I and II disease, surgery alone produced a 5-year survival rate of 82%, whereas radiation therapy produced a 5-year survival rate of only 50%.

At M.D. Anderson, patients with gastric lymphoma are initially treated with a chemotherapeutic regimen based on doxorubicin and cyclophosphamide. A complete response has been documented in more than 80% of patients treated with this aggressive protocol. Radiation therapy and surgery are reserved for patients who do not have a complete response to chemotherapy or who have recurrent disease.

RECOMMENDED READING

Abe M, Takahashi M. Intraoperative radiotherapy: the Japanese experience. *Int J Radiat Oncol Biol Phys* 1981;7:863–868.

Ajani JA, Baker J, Pisters PW, et al. Irinotecan plus cisplatin in advanced gastric or gastroesophageal junction carcinoma. *Oncol (Huntingt)* 2001;15:52–54.

Ajani JA, Mansfield PF, Lynch PM, et al. Enhanced staging and all chemotherapy preoperatively in patients with potentially resectable gastric carcinoma. *J Clin Oncol* 1999;17:2403–2411.

Ajani JA, Ota DM, Jessup JM, et al. Resectable gastric carcinoma. An evaluation of preoperative and postoperative chemotherapy. *Cancer* 1991;68:1501–1506.

Ajani JA. Current status of therapy for advanced gastric carcinoma. *Oncol (Huntingt)* 1998;12:99–102.

Alexander HR, Grem JL, Pass HI, et al. Neoadjuvant chemotherapy for locally advanced gastric adenocarcinoma. *Oncol (Huntingt)* 1993;7:37–42.

Begg CB, Cramer LD, Hoskins WJ, et al. Impact of hospital volume on operative mortality for major cancer surgery. *JAMA* 1998;280:1747–1751.

Behrns KE, Dalton RR, van Heerden, Sarr MG. Extended lymph node dissection for gastric cancer. Is it of value? *Surg Clin North Am* 1992;72:433–443.

Boddie AW, McMurtrey MJ, Giacco GG, et al. Palliative total gastrectomy and esophagogastrectomy. A reevaluation. *Cancer* 1983;51:1195–1200.

Bonenkamp JJ, Hermans J, Sasako M, et al. Extended lymph-node dissection for gastric cancer. Dutch Gastric Cancer Group. *N Engl J Med* 1999;340:908–914.

Bonenkamp JJ, Songun I, Hermans J, et al. Randomised comparison of morbidity after D1 and D2 dissection for gastric cancer in 996 Dutch patients. *Lancet* 1995;345:745–748.

Bozzetti F, Bonfanti G, Bufalino R, et al. Adequacy of margins of resection in gastrectomy for cancer. *Ann Surg* 1982;196:685–690.

Brady MS, Rogatko A, Dent LL, et al. Effect of splenectomy on morbidity and survival following curative gastrectomy for carcinoma. *Arch Surg* 1991;126:359–364.

Burke EC, Karpeh MS, Conlon KC, et al. Laparoscopy in the management of gastric adenocarcinoma. *Ann Surg* 1997;225:262–267.

Burke EC, Karpeh MS, Conlon KC, et al. Peritoneal lavage cytology in gastric cancer: an independent predictor of outcome. *Ann Surg Oncol* 1998;5:411–415.

Cady B, Rossi RL, Silverman ML. Piccione W, Heck TA. Gastric adenocarcinoma. A disease in transition. *Arch Surg* 1989;124:303–308.

Childs DS, Moertel CG, Holbrook MA, et al. Treatment of unresectable adenocarcinomas of the stomach with a combination of 5-fluorouracil and radiation. *Am J Roentgenol Radium Ther Nucl Med* 1968;102:541–544.

Conlon KC, Karpeh MS. Laparoscopy and laparoscopic ultrasound in the staging of gastric cancer. *Semin Oncol* 1996;23:347–351.

Cook AO, Levine BA, Sirinek KR, et al. Evaluation of gastric adenocarcinoma. Abdominal computed tomography does not replace celiotomy. *Arch Surg* 1986;121:603–606.

Correa P, Shiao YH. Phenotypic and genotypic events in gastric carcinogenesis. *Cancer Res* 1994;54:1941s–1943s.

Cuschieri A, Weeden S, Fielding J, et al. Patient survival after D1 and D2 resections for gastric cancer: long-term results of the MRC randomized surgical trial. Surgical Cooperative Group. *Br J Cancer* 1999;79:1522–1530.

Davies J, Chalmers AG, Sue-Ling HM, et al. Spiral computed tomography and operative staging of gastric carcinoma: a comparison with histopathological staging. *Gut* 1997;41:314–319.

Dent DM, Werner ID, Novis B, et al. Prospective randomized trial of combined oncological therapy for gastric carcinoma. *Cancer* 1979;44:385–391.

Dupont JB, Lee JR, Burton GR, et al. Adenocarcinoma of the stomach: review of 1,497 cases. *Cancer* 1978;41(3):941–947.

Earle CC, Maroun JA. Adjuvant chemotherapy after curative resection for gastric cancer in non-Asian patients: revisiting a meta-analysis of randomised trials. *Eur J Cancer* 1999;35:1059–1064.

Ell C, May A. Self-expanding metal stents for palliation of stenosing tumors of the esophagus and cardia: a critical review. *Endoscopy* 1997;29:392–398.

Estape J, Grau JJ, Alcobendas F, et al. Mitomycin C as an adjuvant treatment to resected gastric cancer. A 10-year follow-up. *Ann Surg* 1991;213:219–221.

Fujii K, Isozaki H, Okajima K, et al.. Clinical evaluation of lymph node metastasis in gastric cancer defined by the fifth edition of the TNM classification in comparison with the Japanese system. *Br J Surg* 1999;86:685–689.

Fujimoto S, Shrestha RD, Kokubun M, et al. Positive results of combined therapy of surgery and intraperitoneal hyperthermic perfusion for far-advanced gastric cancer. *Ann Surg* 1990;212:592–596.

Gastrointestinal Tumor Study Group. A comparison of combination chemotherapy and combined modality therapy for locally advanced gastric carcinoma. *Cancer* 1982;49:1771–1777.

Geoghegan JG, Keane TE, Rosenberg IL, et al. Gastric cancer: the case for a more selective policy in surgical management. *J R Coll Surg Edinb* 1993;38(4):208–212.

Goh PM, So JB. Role of laparoscopy in the management of stomach cancer. *Semin Surg Oncol* 1999;16:321–326.

Greenlee RT, Murray T, Bolden S, et al. Cancer statistics, 2000. *CA Cancer J Clin* 2000;50:7–33.

Gunderson LL, Sosin H. Adenocarcinoma of the stomach: areas of failure in a re-operation series (second or symptomatic look) clinicopathologic correlation and implications for adjuvant therapy. *Int J Radiat Oncol Biol Phys* 1982;8:1–11.

Halvorsen RA, Yee J. McCormick VD. Diagnosis and staging of gastric cancer. *Semin Oncol* 1996;23:325–335.

Hamazoe R, Maeta M, Kaibara N. Intraperitoneal thermochemotherapy for prevention of peritoneal recurrence of gastric cancer. Final results of a randomized controlled study. *Cancer* 1994;73:2048–2052.

Hermanek P, Wittekind C. Residual tumor (R) classification and prognosis. *Semin Surg Oncol* 1994;10:12–20.

Hermans J, Bonenkamp JJ, Boon MC, et al. Adjuvant therapy after curative resection for gastric cancer: meta-analysis of randomized trials. *J Clin Oncol* 1993;11:1441–1447.

Hermans J, Bonenkamp JJ. Meta-analysis of adjuvant chemotherapy in gastric cancer: a critical reappraisal [letter]. *J Clin Oncol* 1994;12:877–880.

Hundahl SA, Phillips JL, Menck HR. The National Cancer Data Base Report on poor survival of U.S. gastric carcinoma patients treated with gastrectomy: fifth edition American Joint Committee on Cancer staging, proximal disease, and the "different disease" hypothesis. *Cancer* 2000;88:921–932.

Ichikura T, Tomimatsu S, Uefuji K, et al. Evaluation of the New American Joint Committee on Cancer/International Union against cancer classification of lymph node metastasis from gastric carcinoma in comparison with the Japanese classification. *Cancer* 1999;86:553–558.

Jatzko GR, Lisborg PH, Denk H, et al. A 10-year experience with Japanese-type radical lymph node dissection for gastric cancer outside of Japan. *Cancer* 1995;76:1302–1312.

Jentschura D, Winkler M, Strohmeier N, et al. Quality-of-life after curative surgery for gastric cancer: a comparison between total gastrectomy and subtotal gastric resection. *Hepatogastroenterology* 1997;44:1137–1142.

Kajitani T. The general rules for gastric cancer study in surgery and pathology. Part I. Clinical classification. *Jpn J Surg* 1981;11:127–139.

Karpeh MS, Kelsen DP, Tepper JE. Cancer of the stomach. In: DeVita VT, Hellman S, Rosenberg SA, eds. *Cancer: principles and practice of oncology,* 6th ed. Philadelphia: Lippincott Williams & Wilkins, 2001:1092–1126.

Kelsen D. Adjuvant therapy of upper gastrointestinal tract cancers. *Semin Oncol* 1991;18:543–559.

Kodama Y, Sugimachi K, Soejima K, et al. Evaluation of extensive lymph node dissection for carcinoma of the stomach. *World J Surg* 1981;5:241–248.

Koga S, Hamazoe R, Maeta M, et al. Prophylactic therapy for peritoneal recurrence of gastric cancer by continuous hyperthermic peritoneal perfusion with mitomycin C. *Cancer* 1988;61:232–237.

Kuntz C, Herfarth C. Imaging diagnosis for staging of gastric cancer. *Semin Surg Oncol* 1999;17:96–102.

Landry J, Tepper JE, Wood WC, et al. Patterns of failure following curative resection of gastric carcinoma. *Int J Radiat Oncol Biol Phys* 1990;19:1357–1362.

Lawrence M, Shiu MH. Early gastric cancer. Twenty-eight-year experience. *Ann Surg* 1991;213:327–334.

Lightdale CJ. Endoscopic ultrasonography in the diagnosis, staging and follow-up of esophageal and gastric cancer. *Endoscopy* 1992;24[suppl 1]:297–303.

Lowy AM, Feig BW, Janjan N, et al. A pilot study of preoperative chemoradiotherapy for resectable gastric cancer. *Ann Surg Oncol* 2001;8:519–524.

Lowy AM, Mansfield PF, Leach SD, Ajani J. Laparoscopic staging for gastric cancer. *Surgery* 1996;119:611–614.

Lowy AM, Mansfield PF, Leach SD, et al. Response to neoadjuvant chemotherapy best predicts survival after curative resection of gastric cancer. *Ann Surg* 1999;229:303–308.

MacDonald JS. Gastric cancer: chemotherapy of advanced disease. *Hematol Oncol* 1992;10:3–42.

MacDonald JS, Smalley S, Benedetti J, et al. Chemoradiotherapy after surgery compared with surgery alone for adenocarcinoma of the stomach or gastroesophageal junction. *N Engl J Med* 2001; 345:725–730.

MacDonald JS, Steele G, Gunderson LL. Cancer of the stomach. In: DeVita VT, Hellman S, Rosenberg SA, eds. *Cancer: principles and practice of oncology,* 4th ed. Philadelphia: Lippincott Williams & Wilkins, 1993.

Maehara Y, Okuyama T, Kakeji Y, et al. Postoperative immuno-chemotherapy including streptococcal lysate OK-432 is effective for patients with gastric cancer and serosal invasion. *Am J Surg* 1994;168:36–40.

Makuuchi H, Kise Y, Shimada H, et al. Endoscopic mucosal resection for early gastric cancer. *Semin Surg Oncol* 1999;17:108–116.

Minsky BD. The role of radiation therapy in gastric cancer. *Semin Oncol* 1996;23:390–396.

Moertel CG, Childs DS, O'Fallon JR, et al. Combined 5-fluorouracil and radiation therapy as a surgical adjuvant for poor prognosis gastric carcinoma. *J Clin Oncol* 1984;2:1249–1254.

Monson JR, Donohue JH, McIlrath DC, et al. Total gastrectomy for advanced cancer. A worthwhile palliative procedure. *Cancer* 1991;68:1863–1868.

NCCN practice guidelines for upper gastrointestinal carcinomas. National Comprehensive Cancer Network. *Oncol (Huntingt)* 1998; 12:179–223.

Noguchi Y, Imada T, Matsumoto A, et al. Radical surgery for gastric cancer. A review of the Japanese experience. *Cancer* 1989;64:2053–2062.

Nomura A, Stemmermann GN, Chyou PH, et al. *Helicobacter pylori* infection and gastric carcinoma among Japanese Americans in Hawaii. *N Engl J Med* 1991;325:1132–1136.

Oiwa H, Maehara Y, Ohno S, et al. Growth pattern and *p53* over-expression in patients with early gastric cancer. *Cancer* 1995; 75[suppl]:1454–1459.

Ono H, Kondo H, Gotoda T, et al. Endoscopic mucosal resection for treatment of early gastric cancer. *Gut* 2001;48:225–229.

Parsonnet J, Vandersteen D, Goates J, et al. Helicobacter pylori infection in intestinal- and diffuse-type gastric adenocarcinomas. *J Natl Cancer Inst* 1991;83:640–643.

Roder JD, Bottcher K, Busch R, et al. Classification of regional lymph node metastasis from gastric carcinoma. German Gastric Cancer Study Group. *Cancer* 1998;82:621–631.

Rugge M, Cassaro M, Leandro G, et al. Helicobacter pylori in promotion of gastric carcinogenesis. *Dig Dis Sci* 1996;41:950–955.

Sawyers JL. Gastric carcinoma *Curr Probl Surg* 1995;32:101–178.

Shiu MH, Moore E, Sanders M, et al. Influence of the extent of resection on survival after curative treatment of gastric carcinoma. A retrospective multivariate analysis. *Arch Surg* 1987;122:1347–1351.

Shiu MH, Perrotti M, Brennan MF. Adenocarcinoma of the stomach: a multivariate analysis of clinical, pathologic and treatment factors. *Hepatogastroenterology* 1989;36:7–12.

Skoropad VY, Berdov BA, Mardynski YS, et al. A prospective, randomized trial of preoperative and intraoperative radiotherapy versus surgery alone in resectable gastric cancer. *Eur J Surg Oncol* 2000;26:773–779.

Smith JW, Brennan MF. Surgical treatment of gastric cancer. Proximal, mid, and distal stomach. *Surg Clin North Am* 1992;72:381–399.

Smith JW, Shiu MH, Kelsey L, et al. Morbidity of radical lymphadenectomy in the curative resection of gastric carcinoma. *Arch Surg* 1991;126:1469–1473.

Songun I, Keizer HJ, Hermans J, et al. Chemotherapy for operable gastric cancer: results of the Dutch randomised FAMTX trial. The Dutch Gastric Cancer Group (DGCG). *Eur J Cancer* 1999;35:558–562.

Stomach. In: Fleming ID, Cooper JS, Henson DE et al., eds. *AJCC Cancer Staging Manual,* 5th ed. Philadelphia: Lippincott-Raven, 1998:71–75.

Sugarbaker PH, Yonemura Y. Clinical pathway for the management of resectable gastric cancer with peritoneal seeding: best palliation with a ray of hope for cure. *Oncology* 2000;58:96–107.

Svedlund J, Sullivan M, Liedman B, et al. Quality of life after gastrectomy for gastric carcinoma: controlled study of reconstructive procedures. *World J Surg* 1997;21:422–433.

Tada M, Tanaka Y, Matsuo N, et al. Mucosectomy for gastric cancer: current status in Japan. *J Gastroenterol Hepatol* 2000;15[suppl]:D98–D102.

Tahara E. Genetic alterations in human gastrointestinal cancers. The application to molecular diagnosis. *Cancer* 1995;75:1410–1417.

Takekoshi T. [General view of gastric cancer with depth invasion into muscle layer (m cancer) from a survey of reports of the Japanese Research Society for Gastric Cancer]. *J Gastroenterol Mass Survey* 1994;32:93–132.

Talamonti MS, Dawes LG, Joehl RJ, et al. Gastrointestinal lymphoma. A case for primary surgical resection. *Arch Surg* 1990;125:972–976.

Wanebo HJ, Kennedy BJ, Chmiel J, et al. Cancer of the stomach. A patient care study by the American College of Surgeons. *Ann Surg* 1993;218:583–592.

Wanebo HJ, Kennedy BJ, Winchester DP, et al. Gastric carcinoma: does lymph node dissection alter survival? *J Am Coll Surg* 1996;183:616–624.

Weese JL, Harbison SP, Stiller GD, et al. Neoadjuvant chemotherapy, radical resection with intraoperative radiation therapy (IORT): improved treatment for gastric adenocarcinoma. *Surgery* 2000;128:564–571.

Yim HB, Jacobson BC, Saltzman JR, et al. Clinical outcome of the use of enteral stents for palliation of patients with malignant upper GI obstruction. *Gastrointest Endosc* 2001;53:329–332.

Yonemura Y, Fujimura T, Nishimura G, et al. Effects of intraoperative chemohyperthermia in patients with gastric cancer with peritoneal dissemination. *Surgery* 1996;119:437–444.

Zinniger M. Extent of gastric cancer in the intramural lymphatics and its relation to gastrectomy. *Am Surg* 1954;20:920.

Small-Bowel Malignancies and Carcinoid Tumors

Rosa F. Hwang, Emily K. Robinson,
James C. Cusack, Jr., and Douglas S. Tyler

EPIDEMIOLOGY

Malignancies of the small intestine are rare, with only an estimated 4,600 new cases diagnosed in the United States in 1995. The small intestine represents 75% of the length and 90% of the surface area of the alimentary tract, accounting for only 1% of gastrointestinal (GI) neoplasms. The incidence of this rare malignancy is 0.7 to 1.6 per 100,000 persons, with a slight male predominance. Mean age at presentation is 57 years. Associated conditions include familial polyposis, Gardner's syndrome, Peutz-Jeghers syndrome, adult (nontropical) celiac sprue, von Recklinghausen's neurofibromatosis, and Crohn's disease. In addition, immunosuppressed patients such as those with immunoglobulin A (IgA) deficiency are thought to be at increased risk of small-bowel malignancies. As many as 25% of affected patients have synchronous malignancies, including neoplasms of the colon, endometrium, breast, and prostate gland.

The peak incidence of carcinoid tumors is in the sixth and seventh decades of life, although these tumors have been reported in patients as young as 10 years. The sites of origin of carcinoid tumors are shown in Table 10-1. Approximately 85% of carcinoid tumors are found in the GI tract, with the appendix being the most common site. Nonintestinal sites include the lungs, pancreas, biliary tract, thymus, and ovary. Ileal carcinoids are the most likely to metastasize, even when small, in contrast to appendiceal carcinoids, which rarely metastasize.

RISK FACTORS

Several distinctive characteristics of the small intestine may explain its relative sparing from malignancy. Benzopyrene hydroxylase, an enzyme that converts benzopyrene to a less carcinogenic compound, is found in large amounts in the mucosa of the small intestine. In contrast, anaerobic bacteria, which convert bile salts into potential carcinogens, are generally lacking in the small intestine. Unlike the stomach or colon, the small intestine is protected from the tumorigenic effects of an acidic environment and from the irritating effects of solid GI contents. In addition, the rapid transit of liquid succus entericus through the small bowel is thought to reduce its tumorigenicity by minimizing the contact time between potential enteric carcinogens and the mucosa. Secretory IgA, also found in large quantities in the small intestine, safeguards against oncogenic viruses.

GI dysfunction may predispose the small intestine mucosa to tumorigenesis. Stasis secondary to partial obstruction or blind

Table 10-1.   Sites of origin of carcinoid tumors

Tumor Site	Percentage of Cases
Stomach	2.8
Duodenum	2.9
Jejunoileum	25.5
Appendix	36.2
Colon	6.0
Rectum	16.4
Bronchus	9.9
Ovary	0.5
Miscellaneous	0.2
Unknown primary	3.3

loop syndrome leads to bacterial overgrowth and has been impli-cated in the development of small intestine malignancies.

CLINICAL PRESENTATION

Small-Bowel Malignancy

GI symptoms develop in 75% of patients with malignant lesions of the small bowel, compared with only 50% of patients with be-nign tumors. Sixty-five percent will present with intermittent abdominal pain that is dull and crampy and radiates to the back, 50% with anorexia and weight loss, and 25% with signs and symptoms of bowel obstruction. Only 10% of patients with small-bowel malignancies will develop bowel perforation, most commonly those with lymphomas or sarcomas. A palpable ab-dominal mass is present in 25% of patients. Jaundice may be present in patients with common bile duct obstruction from am-pullary cancer. Episodic jaundice associated with guaiac-positive stool suggests an ampullary malignancy.

The nonspecificity of symptoms, when present, frequently re-sults in a 6- to 8-month delay in diagnosis. The correct diagnosis is established preoperatively in only 50% of cases. Late detec-tion and inaccurate diagnosis contribute not only to the advanced stage of disease at the time of surgery, but also to a 50% rate of metastasis at presentation and thus to the overall poor prognosis for patients with malignant tumors of the small intestine.

Carcinoid Tumors

The presentation of carcinoids varies, depending not only on their physical characteristics and site of origin but also on whether they are producing substances that are hormonally active. In general, most carcinoids are small, indolent tumors that remain asymptomatic and undetected while the patient is alive. Carci-noid tumors are categorized either pathologically by microscopic features or according to their embryologic site of origin. The em-bryologic classification of carcinoids is more commonly used and is outlined in Table 10-2.

This classification system subdivides carcinoids into those of the foregut (stomach, pancreas, and lungs), midgut (small bowel and appendix), or hindgut (colon and rectum).

Table 10-2. Characteristics of carcinoid tumors by embryologic site of origin

Characteristics	Foregut	Midgut	Hindgut
Location	Bronchus	Jejunum	Colon
	Stomach	Ileum	Rectum
	Pancreas	Appendix	
Histology	Trabecular	Nodular, solid nest of cells	Trabecular
Secretion			
Tumor 5-HT	Low	High	None
Urinary 5-HIAA	High	High	Normal
Carcinoid syndrome	Yes	Yes	No
Other endocrine secretions	Frequent	Frequent	No

5-HIAA, 5-hydroxyindoleacetic acid; 5-HT, 5-hydroxytryptamin or serotonin.

Foregut carcinoids are more commonly associated with an atypical presentation due to secretion of peptide hormone products other than serotonin, such as gastrin, adrenocorticotropic hormone, or growth hormone. Pulmonary carcinoids are usually perihilar and patients present with recurrent pneumonia, cough, hemoptysis, or chest pain. Ectopic secretion of corticotropin or growth hormone-releasing factor from these tumors can produce Cushing's syndrome or acromegaly, respectively. Gastric carcinoids are associated with chronic atrophic gastritis type A (CAG-A) in 75% of cases, predominantly women, of which half have pernicious anemia. These tumors usually are identified on endoscopic evaluation for anemia or abdominal pain and are located in the body or fundus of the stomach. Another 5% to 10% of gastric carcinoids are associated with Zollinger-Ellison syndrome in patients with multiple endocrine neoplasia type I. The remaining 15% to 25% of gastric carcinoids are sporadic and found more frequently in men. Sporadic foregut carcinoids are associated with an atypical carcinoid syndrome, which is thought to be histamine-mediated and exhibited mainly as intense erythematous flushing, itching, conjunctival suffusion, facial edema, and occasional urticaria.

Midgut carcinoids produce symptoms of hormone excess only when bulky or metastatic. The vast majority of appendiceal carcinoids are found incidentally, but fewer than 10% cause symptoms since 75% of the tumors are located in the distal one third of the appendix. Patients with small-bowel carcinoids usually present with symptoms similar to those described for other small-bowel tumors. Not uncommonly, as a small-bowel carcinoid progresses, it induces fibrosis of the mesentery, which may by itself cause intestinal obstruction as well as lead to varying degrees of mesenteric ischemia. Most patients with small-bowel carcinoids present with metastases to lymph nodes or to the liver.

Hindgut carcinoids tend to be clinically silent tumors until they are advanced; two thirds are found in the right colon with the average tumor diameter at presentation being 5 cm. They rarely produce serotonin even in the presence of metastatic disease.

Patients with hindgut tumors most commonly present with bleeding but occasionally also have abdominal pain.

The hormonal manifestations of carcinoid tumors (carcinoid syndrome) are seen in only 10% of patients and occur when the secretory products of these tumors gain direct access to the systemic circulation and avoid metabolism in the liver. This clinical syndrome occurs in the following situations: (a) when hepatic metastases are present; (b) when retroperitoneal disease is extensive, with venous drainage directly into the paravertebral veins; and (c) when the primary carcinoid tumor is outside the GI tract, as with bronchial, ovarian, or testicular tumors. Ninety percent of cases of carcinoid syndrome are seen in patients with midgut tumors.

The main symptoms of carcinoid syndrome are watery diarrhea, flushing, sweating, wheezing, dyspnea, abdominal pain, hypotension, or right heart failure due to tricuspid regurgitation or pulmonic stenosis caused by endocardial fibrosis. The flush is often dramatic and is an intense purplish color on the upper body and arms. Facial edema is often present. Repeated attacks can lead to the development of telangiectasias and permanent skin discoloration. The flush can be precipitated by consuming alcohol, blue cheese, chocolate, or red wine, and by exercise. The mediators of these symptoms are shown in Table 10-3.

A life-threatening form of carcinoid syndrome called *carcinoid crisis* is usually precipitated by a specific event such as anesthesia, surgery, or chemotherapy. The manifestations include an intense flush, diarrhea, tachycardia, hypertension or hypotension, bronchospasm, and alteration of mental status. The symptoms are usually refractory to fluid resuscitation and administration of vasopressors.

Table 10-3. Clinical symptoms of carcinoid syndrome and tumor products suspected of causing them

Symptom	Tumor Product
Flushing	Bradykinin
	Hydroxytryptophan
	Prostaglandins
Telangiectasia	VIP
	Serotonin
	Prostaglandins
	Bradykinin
Bronchospasm	Bradykinin
	Histamine
	Prostaglandins
Endocardial fibrosis	Serotonin
Glucose intolerance	Serotonin
Arthropathy	Serotonin
Hypotension	Serotonin

VIP, vasoactive intestinal polypeptide.

DIAGNOSTIC WORKUP

Small-Bowel Malignancies

A high index of suspicion is essential to the early diagnosis and treatment of small-intestine malignancies. The patient presenting with nonspecific abdominal symptoms should undergo a complete history, physical examination, and screening for occult fecal blood. Laboratory workup should include a complete blood cell count, measurement of serum electrolyte levels, and liver function tests. Further laboratory testing, including measurement of urinary 5-hydroxyindoleacetic acid (5-HIAA), should be directed by clinical suspicion.

Retrospective reviews report that 50% to 60% of small-intestine neoplasms are detected by using conventional radiographic techniques, including upper GI series with small bowel follow-through (UGI/SBFT) and enteroclysis. Hypotonic duodenography, using anticholinergic agents or glucagon to reduce duodenal peristalsis, may enhance diagnostic yield to as high as 86% for more proximally located duodenal malignancies. Upper GI endoscopy, when performed to the ligament of Treitz, was diagnostic in eight of nine patients with duodenal malignancies reviewed by Ouriel and Adams (2000). Traditionally, computerized tomography (CT) was not thought to be helpful in diagnosing small-bowel neoplasms. However, several recent reviews have shown that CT was able to detect abnormalities in 97% of patients with small-bowel tumors. Angiography demonstrates a tumor blush in specific subtypes of small-bowel malignancies, most notably carcinoid and leiomyosarcoma, but is rarely indicated in the initial diagnostic workup.

Enteroscopy should be considered when all previous diagnostic studies are negative. Lewis et al. (1991) reviewed the experience at Mt. Sinai Medical Center in New York with two endoscopic techniques—push enteroscopy and small-bowel enteroscopy—in 258 patients with obscure GI bleeding. Push enteroscopy uses a pediatric colonoscope that is passed orally and then pushed distally through the small intestine, facilitating intubation of the jejunum 60 cm distal to the ligament of Treitz. This technique established a diagnosis in 50% of patients examined. Small-bowel enteroscopy, which uses a 120-degree, forward-viewing, 2,560-mm, balloon-tipped endoscope that is carried distally by peristalsis, permitted intubation of the terminal ileum in 77% of cases within 8 hours.

Most retrospective studies report only moderate success in diagnosing small-bowel neoplasms preoperatively, with large series reporting a correct preoperative diagnosis in only 50% of cases, the remainder diagnosed at laparotomy. Exploratory laparotomy remains the most sensitive diagnostic modality in evaluating a patient in whom small-bowel neoplasm is suspected and should be considered in the diagnostic evaluation of a patient with occult GI bleeding, unexplained weight loss, or vague abdominal pain. Because most tumors present as large, bulky lesions with lymph node metastasis, laparoscopy is potentially useful for establishing the diagnosis of malignancy when the workup is otherwise negative and for obtaining adequate tissue samples if a diagnosis of lymphoma is suspected. Early detection and treatment remain the most significant variables in improving outcome from small-bowel malignancy, necessitating thoughtful and expedient diagnostic workup of patients presenting with vague abdominal symptoms.

Carcinoids

The diagnosis of carcinoid tumor is made using a combination of biochemical tests and imaging studies. Overall, approximately 50% of patients with carcinoids have elevated urinary levels of 5-HIAA, irrespective of whether they have symptoms of carcinoid syndrome. One study reported 100% specificity and 70% sensitivity of urinary 5-HIAA for the presence of carcinoid syndrome and 5-HIAA levels seem to correlate with tumor burden. When urinary 5-HIAA levels are nondiagnostic, a more extensive workup should be undertaken, consisting of measurement of urinary 5-hydroxytryptamine (5-HT, serotonin) and 5-hydroxytryptophan (5-HPT), plasma 5-HPT, platelet 5-HT, and serum levels of other secretory products such as chromogranin A, neuron-specific enolase (NSE), substance P, and neuropeptide K. More recently, chromogranin A and NSE levels in serum have been used for the diagnosis of carcinoids. In well-differentiated tumors, the sensitivity of serum chromogranin A is between 80% and 100% and also reflects tumor load. An overview of serotonin metabolism is shown in Fig. 10-1.

Localization of the tumor also may help confirm the diagnosis. Bronchial carcinoids are best visualized with a chest radiograph or CT scan. Gastric, duodenal, colonic, and rectal carcinoids are usually seen on endoscopy and barium studies. Small intestine carcinoids are initially evaluated as described for other small-bowel malignancies. Abdominal CT scan is useful for

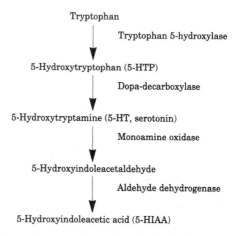

Fig. 10-1.   Biochemical steps in the production of 5-hydroxytryptamine (5-HT, serotonin) and 5-hydroxyindoleacetic acid (5-HIAA).

assessing involvement of the retroperitoneum and presence of liver metastasis. In addition, small-bowel carcinoids have a spoke-wheel appearance on CT due to extensive mesenteric fibrosis, and 70% of cases demonstrate calcifications.

Nuclear medicine scans have also been used in localization. Scans using metaiodobenzylguanidine (MIBG) radiolabeled with iodine 131 (^{131}I) or ^{121}I can identify primary or metastatic carcinoid tumors approximately 50% of the time, when MIBG is taken up by the tumor and stored in its neurosecretory granules. Tyr-3-octreotide, a somatostatin analog, radiolabeled with ^{123}I, has also been used in an attempt to take advantage of the finding that most carcinoids display receptors for somatostatin. Scans using this analog appear useful in localizing 70% to 80% of carcinoids but are not widely available. Eriksson et al. (1998) used positron emission tomography with ^{11}C-labeled 5-HTP and were able to localize carcinoids as small as 0.5 cm.

On occasion, a patient may benefit from angiography or selective venous sampling if other diagnostic maneuvers prove unsuccessful.

STAGING

Only recently has the American Joint Committee on Cancer published a staging system for small-bowel malignancies (Table 10-4).

MALIGNANT NEOPLASMS

The distribution of small-bowel malignancies (reported by Weiss and Yang in a review of nine population-based cancer registries participating in the National Cancer Institute's Surveillance, Epidemiology, and End Results [SEER] Program [1987]) is shown in Table 10-5. Information on tumor biology, modes of lymphatic spread, and patterns of recurrence for small bowel malignancies is limited.

The most common histologic types of malignant tumors of the small intestine are adenocarcinoma (45.3%), carcinoid (29.3%), lymphoma (14.8%), and sarcoma (10.4%). Adenocarcinoma is the most common malignancy in the proximal small intestine, whereas carcinoid is the most common malignancy in the ileum. Sarcoma and lymphoma may develop throughout the small intestine but are more prevalent in the distal small bowel. Mutations of the Ki-*ras* gene are found in 14% to 53% of small intestine adenocarcinomas and are more prevalent in duodenal, rather than jejunal or ileal, adenocarcinomas. In contrast, mutations of the *APC* gene are uncommon in small bowel carcinomas, suggesting that these tumors arise through a different genetic pathway than colorectal carcinomas.

Adenocarcinoma

Pathology

Adenocarcinoma of the small intestine occurs most commonly in the duodenum, with 65% of these neoplasms clustered in the periampullary region. These tumors infiltrate into the muscularis propria and may extend through the serosa and into

Table 10-4.   AJCC staging of small intestine malignancies

Primary tumor (T)

T1   Tumor invades lamina propria or submucosa
T2   Tumor invades muscularis propria
T3   Tumor invades through the muscularis propria into the
        subserosa or into the nonperitonealized perimuscular tissue
        (mesentery or retroperitoneum) with extension ≤ 2 cm
T4   Tumor perforates the visceral peritoneum or directly invades
        other organs or structures (includes other loops of the small
        intestine, mesentery, or retroperitoneum > 2 cm, and
        abdominal wall by way of serosa; for duodenum only,
        invasion of the pancreas)

Regional lymph nodes (N)

N0   No regional lymph node metastasis
N1   Regional lymph node metastasis

Distant metastasis (M)

M0   No distant metastasis
M1   Distant metastasis

Staging

Stage	T	N	M
Stage I	T1-T2	N0	M0
Stage II	T3-T4	N0	M0
Stage III	Any T	N1	M0
Stage IV	Any T	Any N	M1

Adapted from Fleming ID, Cooper JS, Henson DE, et al., eds. *AJCC manual for staging of cancer,* 5th ed. Philadelphia: Lippincott-Raven, 1997.

Table 10-5.   Distribution of primary malignant neoplasms in the small intestine by subsite of cancer and histologic type as percentages of total (*N* = 1,413)

Subsite Specified	Adenocarcinoma	Carcinoid	Lymphoma	Sarcoma
Duodenum	21.9	1.3	0.8	1.8
Jejunum	14.7	2.5	5.1	5.0
Ileum	8.7	25.5	8.9	3.6
Total	45.3	29.3	14.8	10.4

Adapted from NCI SEER Registries 1973–1982. In: Weiss NS, Yang C. Incidence of histologic types of cancer of the small intestine. *J Natl Cancer Inst* 1987;78:653.

adjacent tissues. Ulceration is common, causing occult GI bleeding and chronic anemia. Obstruction may develop from progressive growth of apple core lesions or large intraluminal polypoid masses. It manifests itself as gastric outlet obstruction in cases of duodenal lesions or severe cramping pain in cases of more distally located lesions. Adenocarcinoma of the small bowel follows a pattern of tumor progression similar to that of colon cancer, with similar survival rates when compared stage for stage. Seventy percent to 80% of small-bowel lesions are resectable at the time of diagnosis, with a 5-year survival rate of 20% to 30% reported for patients undergoing resection. Approximately 35% of patients have metastasis to regional lymph nodes at the time of diagnosis, and an additional 20% have distant metastasis. Mural penetration, nodal involvement, distant metastasis, and perineural invasion correlate with a poor prognosis. Large tumor size and poor histologic grade were also associated with decreased survival in a recent study from UCLA, but others have not found the same relationship.

Adenocarcinoma of the small bowel is known to be associated with Crohn's disease, usually occurring in the distal ileum. Risk factors associated with development of a small-bowel cancer in Crohn's disease include duration of disease, male gender, associated fistulous disease, and the presence of surgically excluded bowel loops.

Treatment

Wide excision of the malignancy and surrounding zones of contiguous spread is performed to provide complete tumor clearance for lesions located in the jejunum and ileum. Treatment strategies ranging from pancreaticoduodenectomy to local excision have been proposed for the management of duodenal adenocarcinoma. Pancreaticoduodenectomy has been touted as a superior operation for duodenal adenocarcinoma because of its more radical clearance of the tumor bed and regional lymph nodes. In fact, some authors, including Lai et al. (1988), continue to recommend pancreaticoduodenectomy for all primary duodenal adenocarcinomas. However, segmental resection for adenocarcinoma of the duodenum satisfies the principles of en bloc resection, without the morbidity of a pancreaticoduodenectomy, and should be considered when technically feasible.

Unlike pancreatic cancer, which diffusely infiltrates into the surrounding soft tissues, adenocarcinoma of the duodenum extends into adjacent tissues as a more localized process. Therefore, tumor-free resection margins, critical to a curative extirpation, may be achieved without necessarily resecting a generous portion of the surrounding soft tissues and adjacent organs; however, the tumor-free status of resection margins must be confirmed on frozen-section evaluation of the resected specimen.

In a comparison of pancreaticoduodenectomy to segmental resection for management of duodenal adenocarcinoma at The University of Texas M.D. Anderson Cancer Center, Barnes et al. (1994) found no significant difference in survival rates but did find a difference in 5-year local control rates—76% for pancreaticoduodenectomy and 49% for segmental resection. Several other reviews, including those of Lowell et al. (1992), Joestling et al.

(1981), and van Ooijen and Kalsbeek (1988), which compared survival following pancreaticoduodenectomy or segmental resection for lesions in the third and fourth portions of the duodenum, have demonstrated no significant difference in 5-year survival. In these studies, a more limited resection, with less associated morbidity and mortality, provided a survival benefit equal to that of a more extensive resection.

At M.D. Anderson Cancer Center, a Whipple pancreaticoduodenectomy is performed for lesions involving the proximal duodenum to the right of the superior mesenteric artery (SMA). A segmental resection is performed for duodenal lesions to the left of the SMA. Local excision is considered for small lesions on the antimesenteric wall of the second portion of the duodenum. Two studies have found a higher rate of postoperative complications from Whipple procedures in patients with periampullary malignancies than in those with pancreatic adenocarcinoma, although this did not result in a higher rate of perioperative mortality. A higher pancreatic anastomotic leak rate was present in the group with duodenal carcinoma, presumably because the pancreas in these patients was normal and thus more difficult to sew.

Experimental Therapy

Electron beam intraoperative radiation therapy and external beam radiation therapy have been administered at M.D. Anderson in a limited number of cases of microscopic involvement of resection margins or unresectable disease. However, adenocarcinoma of the small intestine is generally considered to be radiation resistant. Chemotherapy, based on 5-fluorouracil (5-FU) and nitrosoureas, has been recommended in both the adjuvant setting and in cases of unresectable disease, yet most retrospective studies have failed to demonstrate a significant response to chemotherapy. Because most centers have only limited experience treating adenocarcinoma of the small intestine, the efficacy of chemotherapy needs further study, and patients should continue to be enrolled in prospective randomized trials.

Carcinoid

Pathology

Carcinoids are known mainly for their ability to secrete serotonin and are the most common endocrine tumors of the GI system. They arise from enterochromaffin cells, which are located predominantly in the GI tract and mainstem bronchi. In addition to serotonin, these tumors can secrete a number of biologically active substances (Table 10-6), including amines, tachykinins, peptides, and prostaglandins.

Carcinoid tumors occur most frequently in the appendix (40%), small intestine (27%), rectum (15%), and bronchus (11%). Small-bowel carcinoids occur most commonly in the terminal 60 cm of the ileum as tan, yellow, or gray-brown intramural or submucosal nodules. The presence of multiple synchronous nodules in 30% of patients mandates careful inspection of the entire small intestine in these patients.

Primary carcinoid tumors are indolent, slow-growing lesions that become symptomatic late in the course of the disease.

Table 10-6. Biologically active substances that can be secreted by carcinoid tumors

Amines
    5-HT
    5-HIAA
    5-HTP
    Histamine
    Dopamine
Tachykinins
    Kallikrein
    Substance P
    Neuropeptide K
Others
    Prostaglandins
    Pancreatic polypeptide
    Chromogranins
    Neurotensin
    hCGa
    hCGb

5-HT, 5-hydroxytryptamine; 5-HIAA, 5-hydroxyindoleacetic acid; 5-HTP, 5-hydroxytryptophan; hCG, human chorionic gonadotropin.

Rarely ulcerative, these tumors infiltrate the muscularis propria and may extend through the serosa to involve the mesentery or retroperitoneum and to produce a characteristically intense desmoplastic reaction.

Metastatic disease, present in 90% of symptomatic patients, correlates not only with the depth of invasion but also with the size of the primary lesion. For carcinoids less than 1 cm, the risk of metastasis is 2% for appendiceal, 15% to 18% for small bowel, and 20% for rectal primaries. If carcinoid tumors are greater than 2 cm, 33% of appendiceal, 86% to 95% of small bowel, and almost all rectal primaries have metastasized.

Distant sites of metastases include the liver and, to a lesser degree, the lungs and bone. There is no widely accepted histologic classification of carcinoids that accurately predicts metastatic behavior. Morphologic criteria such as mitotic activity, cytologic atypia, and tumor necrosis have been evaluated; however, these features can be affected by ischemia secondary to mesenteric sclerosis in GI carcinoids. An analysis of GI carcinoids by Moyana et al. (2000) revealed that positive immunohistochemical staining for MIB-1 (a marker of proliferation) and p53 was associated with metastatic behavior. In addition, high levels of the nuclear antigen Ki-67 appears to correlate with decreased survival in patients with carcinoid tumors.

Treatment of Localized Disease

Surgical extirpation is the definitive treatment for localized primary carcinoid tumors. The extent of resection is determined by the size of the primary lesion and is based on the likelihood of mesenteric lymph node involvement. The incidence of metastasis depends on the location of the tumor, its depth of invasion, and its size.

Appendiceal carcinoids smaller than 1 cm rarely metastasize and are adequately treated by appendectomy alone unless the base of the appendix is involved, in which case a partial cecectomy may be necessary. Because the incidence of metastasis increases with primary tumor size, treatment of appendiceal carcinoids between 1 and 2 cm is more controversial. In general, most authors recommend appendectomy alone for lesions smaller than 1.5 cm and right hemicolectomy for lesions larger than 1.5 cm or for any lesion with invasion of the mesoappendix, blood vessels, or regional lymph nodes.

In contrast to appendiceal carcinoids, carcinoids of the small bowel are more likely to metastasize even when smaller than 1 cm. As a result, most surgeons recommend a wide en bloc resection that includes the adjacent mesentery and lymph nodes. Such a resection may be difficult at times if the mesentery is fibrotic and foreshortened. Although some surgeons advocate local excision for small midgut carcinoids, up to 70% of these tumors metastasize to the lymph nodes. Therefore a wide resection not only may cure many of these patients but also should provide better local disease control than local excision. Furthermore, a careful and thorough examination of the entire length of bowel is important because 20% to 40% of small-bowel carcinoids are multicentric. Because of the slow-growing nature of these tumors, wide excision is advocated even when distant metastases are present. In addition, approximately 40% of patients with midgut carcinoids have a second GI malignancy. Therefore the entire bowel and colon should be evaluated before any planned surgical intervention.

Rectal carcinoids less than 1 cm, which comprise two thirds of all rectal carcinoids, are adequately treated by wide local excision alone. Tumors between 1 and 2 cm should be locally resected by a wide, local, full-thickness excision with abdominoperineal resection or low anterior resection recommended for tumors that invade the muscularis propria. The treatment of patients with rectal carcinoids greater than 2 cm remains controversial. Even though major cancer operations were once recommended for rectal carcinoids greater than 2 cm, it is now appreciated that the risk of distant metastasis is so high that radical surgery should not be considered if the tumor can be removed by wide local excision. Every attempt should be made for sphincter preservation in patients with carcinoids of the rectum of greater than 2 cm because of the high likelihood of distant relapse and the marginal benefit obtained from radical local therapy.

Long-term prognosis after surgical treatment of patients with GI carcinoids was evaluated in a study from the Mayo Clinic. With median follow-up of 18 years, survival was significantly associated with embryologic origin of the tumor and patient age. Increased survival was found in those patients with midgut carcinoids, compared to those with foregut tumors, as well as in patients younger than 62 years. Overall survival rates at 5 and 10 years were 69% and 53%, respectively.

Treatment of Advanced Disease

The role of surgery for unresectable and metastatic disease is not clearly defined, but it appears that surgery may benefit patients. When metastatic disease is present, it is necessary to establish whether the patient has symptoms of carcinoid syndrome and whether curative resection is possible. If the patient has no contraindications to surgery, then an attempt at complete extirpation should be made because it may lead to prolonged disease-free survival as well as symptomatic relief. Patients with metastatic carcinoid should all begin receiving octreotide therapy preoperatively to prevent a carcinoid crisis (discussed below). Surgical resection of liver metastases has resulted in long-term relief of symptoms. Eighty-two percent of patients with midgut carcinoids metastatic to liver who underwent resection demonstrated partial or complete relief of symptoms with a mean duration of 5.3 years. Patients in whom liver metastases from carcinoid tumor are suspected should undergo an abdominal CT scan. The study should be done before and after intravenous (IV) contrast material to better visualize carcinoid liver metastases, which are usually hypervascular and can be difficult to distinguish from normal liver after injection of IV contrast material.

Patients with mildly symptomatic carcinoid syndrome can be treated medically. Diarrhea can usually be controlled with loperamide, diphenoxylate, or the serotonin receptor antagonist cyproheptadine. Flushing can frequently be controlled with either adrenergic blocking agents (e.g., clonidine or phenoxybenzamine) or a combination of type 1 and 2 histamine receptor antagonists. Albuterol (a beta-adrenergic blocking agent) and aminophylline are effective in relieving bronchospasm and wheezing.

For patients whose symptoms cannot be controlled with these conservative measures or in whom a carcinoid crisis develops, the somatostatin analog octreotide has shown tremendous promise. A trial from the Mayo Clinic found that flushing and diarrhea could be controlled in the vast majority of patients with as little as 150 μg of octreotide administered subcutaneously three times per day. The duration of the responses was on the average more than 1 year. Interestingly, a number of studies have now shown that octreotide is also able to slow tumor growth significantly in more than 50% of patients and to cause tumor regression for variable periods in another 10% to 20% of individuals. Lanreotide, another long-acting somatostatin analog, is available in slow-release formulation. Treatment with lanreotide by injection every 10 to 14 days appears to be as effective as daily octreotide for malignant and nonmalignant endocrine disorders. Furthermore, treatment with a depot formulation of octreotide, 20 mg intramuscularly every 4 weeks, resulted in symptomatic relief and tumor regression in a patient with disseminated carcinoid who had progressed during treatment with lanreotide combined with interferon alfa.

Because such good results can be obtained with octreotide, interferon, or hepatic artery chemoembolization (discussed below), surgical debulking procedures, which used to be recommended for patients with symptomatic carcinoid syndrome and liver metastasis, are rarely required. Patients with unresectable disease, if asymptomatic, should just be monitored. Local complications related to the tumor can be addressed if and when they develop. Our current indications for surgical intervention in unresectable and widely metastatic disease include complications of bulky carcinoid tumors such as obstruction and perforation. In addition, surgical debulking is considered for severe intractable symptoms unresponsive to medical treatment, if a dominant mass or liver metastasis can be identified. For patients who have undergone liver resection for metastatic carcinoids, R2 (vs. R0) resection and pancreatic carcinoids have been associated with poorer prognosis.

Despite the advanced stage of disease at presentation and the limited effectiveness of currently available therapies, the natural history of carcinoids affords affected patients a better prognosis than other malignancies of the small bowel. The 5-year survival rate for localized disease approaches 100% after complete resection. Resection of metastatic disease is associated with a 68% 5-year survival rate, whereas unresectable disease has a 38% 5-year survival rate.

Experimental Therapy

A number of chemotherapeutic agents have been tried in patients with carcinoid tumors. Results of chemotherapy trials with such agents as doxorubicin, dacarbazine, and streptozotocin, either alone or in combination, have been disappointing. Most chemotherapy trials show response rates of less than 30%, with responses lasting only a few months. The role of chemotherapy is still investigational, but for patients with advanced disease that cannot be controlled with standard measures, monitored clinical trials should be recommended.

One biologic agent, interferon, in both the alfa-2a and alfa-2b forms, has shown promising results in diminishing urinary levels of 5-HIAA as well as symptoms of carcinoid syndrome. Most patients in most studies had either a partial regression or stabilization of their disease for a prolonged period. Unfortunately, objective responses with reduction of tumor size occurred in only approximately 15% of patients.

In some centers, hepatic artery occlusion or embolization has been used with some success to diminish the size of liver metastases and decrease levels of biologically active mediators of carcinoid syndrome. However, duration of response is usually short, with median duration ranging from 7 months for hepatic artery occlusion alone to 20 months in a study using hepatic artery occlusion followed by systemic chemotherapy. Furthermore, side effects may be substantial. Liver embolization with Gelfoam performed in patients with neuroendocrine tumors resulted in serious complications in 10%, including renal failure, liver necrosis, and bowel ischemia. Another option for management of carcinoid hepatic metastases is radiofrequency ablation (RFA). In one small series RFA was used as salvage therapy in patients with hepatic metastases that were not amenable to surgical resection and unresponsive to embolization. Although only three patients were treated, all three demonstrated decreases in both the size of the lesions and severity of symptoms. Because RFA can be performed percutaneously or laparoscopically, this may be a useful treatment alternative for patients with disseminated carcinoid tumors.

Although external beam radiation has not proven effective in treating carcinoid tumors, targeted radiation in the form of radioactive iodine coupled to either MIBG or octreotide is a therapeutic strategy that may hold some promise for the future.

Sarcoma

Pathology

Sarcomas of the small intestine are typically slow-growing lesions; they occur more frequently in the jejunum and ileum than in the duodenum. Sharing a similar growth pattern with other GI sarcomas, these malignancies invade adjacent tissues, with metastasis occurring predominantly via the hematogenous route to the liver, lungs, and bones. The most common clinical presentations are pain (65%), abdominal mass (50%), and bleeding. More than 75% of tumors exceed 5 cm in diameter at diagnosis, with extramural extension, rather than intramural or intraluminal extension, representing the typical growth pattern. For this reason, obstruction is rarely a manifestation of this disease process.

CT scan of these lesions typically demonstrates a heterogeneous mass with focal areas of necrosis where the tumor has outgrown its nutrient blood supply and formed localized abscesses.

Leiomyosarcoma accounts for 75% of small-intestine sarcomas; fibrosarcoma, liposarcoma, and angiosarcoma are seen less frequently. In summary, sarcoma represents only 10% of small-bowel malignancies, yet the various subtypes encompass a broad range of biologic behavior, the scope of which exceeds this review.

Treatment

Surgical resection is the primary treatment modality for sarcoma of the small bowel. Because sarcoma infrequently metastasizes to regional mesenteric lymph nodes, unlike adenocarcinoma and carcinoid, an extensive mesenteric lymphadenectomy is unnecessary and will not prolong survival. En bloc resection of the lesion with tumor-free margins is recommended for a potentially curative resection; however, at the time of diagnosis, 50% of lesions are unresectable and most exceed 5 cm in diameter. Local resection should be considered in the presence of widely metastatic disease for control of bleeding and relief of obstruction.

Experimental Therapy

Leiomyosarcomas of the small bowel are resistant to chemotherapy and radiation therapy. Combined chemotherapy and radiation therapy should be offered to patients with leiomyosarcomas only as part of an experimental protocol in an attempt to downstage the disease or possibly make an unresectable lesion resectable. Chemotherapy can be used in the treatment of recurrent or metastatic disease, but again, only as part of an experimental protocol. Currently at M.D. Anderson, chemoembolization with cisplatin is used in patients with metastatic disease to the liver. Sarcomas of other histologic subtypes are discussed in Chapter 5.

Gastrointestinal Stromal Tumors

Definition

Stromal tumors of the GI tract (GISTs) are uncommon tumors, comprising approximately 1% of all GI malignant neoplasms in the United States. Considerable controversy has surrounded the pathologic origin, nomenclature, and prognosis of these tumors. Initially thought to arise from smooth muscle, most GISTs were previously classified as leiomyomas or leiomyosarcomas. More recent studies at the ultrastructural level distinguish GISTs as arising from the interstitial cell of Cajal, an intestinal pacemaker cell, which accounts for its variable features including myogenic, neural, both myogenic and neural (mixed) and undifferentiated forms. Immunohistochemical markers for GISTs include CD34, a myeloid stem cell antigen, and particularly, CD117/c-kit. The c-kit protein is a membrane receptor with tyrosine kinase activity that is present in 80% to 100% of GISTs and is not expressed in smooth muscle or neural tumors. Thus, c-kit positivity is a useful marker to differentiate GISTs from true smooth muscle neoplasms.

Clinical Features

Although GISTs may be found throughout the GI tract, they are most frequently located in the stomach (65%–70%), followed by the small intestine (25%–45%), and less frequently in the esophagus, colon, and rectum. Most studies report no difference in gender distribution, and most patients present in the fifth to seventh decade of life. Malignant GISTs more often present with symptoms such as abdominal mass, GI bleed, or abdominal pain than their benign counterparts. Various series report overall 5-year survival rates for patients with GIST to range from 19% to 56%. No accepted staging system exists for GIST, however, several factors have been identified that seem to correlate with clinical behavior. Malignant tumors are associated with size greater than 5 cm, high cellularity, prominent nuclear pleomorphism, necrosis, greater than one to five mitoses per 10/high-power field, and invasion into adjacent structures. Another strong prognostic marker appears to be a missense mutation in the c-*kit* gene on exon 11 that has been recently identified in 57% of malignant GISTs. Patients with tumors exhibiting this mutation had significantly more frequent recurrences and higher mortality rates than those without the mutation.

Treatment

Surgical resection remains the most effective treatment for GIST. Complete resection of gross tumor, including resection of involved adjacent organs, is associated with higher survival rates (42% 5-year survival rate) than incomplete resection (9% 5-year survival rate), but the status of the final microscopic margin does not seem to affect survival or recurrence rates. Because lymph node involvement is uncommon (<10%), extensive lymphadenectomy appears to provide no added survival benefit. Even when complete surgical resection is achieved, the majority of tumors will recur, often involving the liver and peritoneal surface. The majority of patients for whom surgery fails will experience recurrence within 2 years. In a study of 60 patients with recurrent GIST from Memorial Sloan-Kettering Cancer Center, 76% had local recurrence, and most of these also had associated liver metastases. None of these patients had extra-abdominal disease. Surgical resection for recurrent disease was complete in one third of cases, with median survival of 15 months after salvage surgery. Neither complete nor partial resection of recurrent disease resulted in significantly improved survival, although the subgroup of patients with isolated, resectable hepatic metastases showed a trend toward longer survival. At M.D. Anderson, surgical resection of liver metastases is recommended for patients with a long disease-free survival and disease localized to a limited area of the liver.

With the high recurrence rate after surgery, effective adjuvant therapy is obviously needed. Systemic chemotherapy regimens, which often are doxorubicin-based, have had minimal activity against GISTs. Similarly, radiation therapy has had disappointing results, mainly due to toxicity associated with adjacent tissue. Intraoperative radiation treatment may be a useful approach to deliver more effective doses to the tumor bed itself. Other experimental protocols for patients who are not candidates for surgical resection include hepatic arterial chemoembolization for palliation of liver metastases and intraperitoneal chemotherapy for bulky peritoneal disease. A recently U.S. Food and Drug Administration–approved drug for chronic myeloid leukemia (CML), Gleevec (STI-571), may also be an effective novel therapy for patients with GIST. Gleevec selectively inhibits several tyrosine kinases, including the BCR-ABL fusion protein characteristic of CML as well as the c-kit tyrosine kinase found in the majority of GISTs. Phase III randomized trials are currently underway to evaluate the efficacy of Gleevec in treatment of patients with metastatic GIST.

Lymphoma

Pathology

The distribution of lymphoma in the small intestine parallels the distribution of lymphoid follicles in the small intestine, with the lymphoid-rich ileum representing the most common location of small-bowel lymphoma. Lymphoma arises from the lymphoid aggregates in the submucosa; infiltration of the mucosa can result in ulceration and bleeding. The tumor may also extend to the serosa and adjacent tissues, producing a large obstructing mass associated with cramping abdominal pain. Perforation occurs in as many as 25% of patients. Lymphoma may arise as a primary neoplasm or as a component of systemic disease with GI involvement. As with sarcoma, bulky disease is a characteristic of lymphoma, with approximately 70% of tumors larger than 5 cm in diameter.

Primary tumors are staged according to the Kiel classification (see Chapter 16) as low, intermediate, or high grade, with high-grade lesions being diagnosed most frequently. Prognostic factors include tumor grade, extent of tumor penetration, nodal involvement, peritoneal disease, and distant metastasis. The 5-year survival rate ranges from 20% to 33%.

Treatment

Extended surgical resection of the primary lesion and accompanying regional mesenteric lymph nodes is the mainstay of treatment for lymphoma of the small bowel. Because of the extensive submucosal infiltration of lymphoma, frozen section should be performed to microscopically confirm tumor-free margins. Lymph node metastases are frequent, necessitating an en bloc resection of the adjoining mesentery. Resection alone provides adequate therapy for low-grade lymphomas, whereas resection combined with adjuvant chemotherapy is indicated for intermediate- and high-grade lymphomas. The first-line chemotherapy regimen currently used at M.D. Anderson is cyclophosphamide, doxorubicin, vincristine, and prednisone (CHOP).

Experimental Therapy

Chemoradiation has been used at some institutions for nodal metastasis, positive resection margins, and unresectable disease. However, a survival benefit from such treatment regimens has not been demonstrated. The use of radiation therapy alone has been associated with significant tumor necrosis, bleeding, and bowel perforation but may be considered in elderly patients unable to tolerate the toxicity of chemotherapy.

Metastatic Malignancies

Pathology

Metastases are the most common form of malignancy in the small intestine and develop as a result of hematogenous or lymphatic spread from a primary tumor to the mucosa or submucosal lymphatics of the small intestine. The primary tumors that most commonly metastasize to the small bowel include ovarian, colon, lung, and melanoma. Metastatic melanoma is unique in that once localized in the small bowel, the metastatic focus may further disseminate to the small bowel mesentery and draining lymph nodes. In general, however, small-bowel metastases remain localized to the bowel wall, and they may produce small-bowel obstruction or perforation.

Although the typical presentation of metastatic lesions is obstruction or perforation, the more common cause of obstruction and perforation in patients who have previously undergone resection of a GI primary tumor is related to the initial procedure—that is, either recurrence of the primary tumor or adhesions resulting from the initial exploration.

Segmental bowel resection is the primary treatment for small-bowel metastases. Except for melanoma metastases, which may function as a source of further lymphatic dissemination, a regional lymphadenectomy is not performed for metastatic tumors of the small intestine.

Palliation

At the time of diagnosis, most small-bowel malignancies are locally advanced, with significant bulky disease or metastases. When the advanced stage of disease precludes surgical resection, enteric bypass should be performed to prevent obstruction. In the event of bleeding from an unresectable small-bowel malignancy, intraarterial embolization of nutrient arteries may be considered, but the benefits must be weighed against the significant risks of this procedure. Our experience with this technique at M.D. Anderson Cancer Center has been discouraging because of the significant rate of bowel ischemia and perforation associated with embolization of the small-bowel mesentery.

Chemotherapy or chemoradiation may offer effective control of locally advanced unresectable disease, particularly in the case of lymphoma, and should be considered among palliative treatment options.

SURVEILLANCE

Routine follow-up for patients should include a complete history and physical examination, complete blood cell count, serum electrolyte determination, and liver function tests performed at regular intervals. A chest radiograph should be obtained every 6 months for the first 3 years after resection, followed by subsequent yearly examinations. Assessment of locoregional recurrence in patients who have undergone a right hemicolectomy for ileal malignancy or segmental resection for duodenal malignancy should include endoscopy at 6-month intervals. Assessment for recurrence at other sites may include CT scan, UGI/SBFT, angiography, or enteroscopy and must be directed by clinical suspicion based on patient history and physical and laboratory findings.

RECOMMENDED READING

Ajani JA, Carrasco H, Samaan NA, et al. Therapeutic options in patients with advanced islet cell and carcinoid tumors. *Reg Cancer Treat* 1990;3:235.

Arai M, Shimizu S, Imai Y, et al. Mutations of the Ki-*ras*, *p53* and *APC* genes in adenocarcinomas of the human small intestine. *Int J Cancer* 1997;70:390.

Ashley SW, Wells SA. Tumors of the small intestine. *Semin Oncol* 1988;15:116.

Barnes G, Romero L, Hess KR, et al. Primary adenocarcinoma of the duodenum: Management and survival in 67 patients. *Ann Surg Oncol* 1994;1:73.

Bernstein D, Rogers A. Malignancy in Crohn's disease. *Am J Gastroenterol* 1996;91:3.

Bomanji J, Mather S, Moyes J, et al. A scintigraphic comparison of iodine-123 metaiodobenzylguanidine and iodine-labeled somatostatin analog (tyr-3-octreotide) in metastatic carcinoid tumors. *J Nucl Med* 1992;33:1121.

Carrasco CH, Charnsangavej C, Ajani J, et al. The carcinoid syndrome palliation by hepatic artery embolization. *AJR* 1986;147:149.

Cattell RB, Braasch JW. A technique for the exposure of the third and fourth portions of the duodenum. *Surg Gynecol Obstet* 1960;11:379.

Cheek RC, Wilson H. Carcinoid tumors. *Curr Probl Surg* 1970; Nov:4.

Crist DW, Sitzman JV, Cameron JL. Improved hospital morbidity, mortality, and survival after the Whipple procedure. *Ann Surg* 1987;206:358.

Cubilla AL, Fortner J, Fitzgerald PJ. Lymph node involvement in carcinoma of the head of the pancreas area. *Cancer* 1978;41:880.

Dematteo RP, Lewis JJ, Leung D, et al. Two hundred gastrointestinal stromal tumors: recurrence patterns and prognostic factors for survival. *Ann Surg* 2000;231:51.

Donohue JH. Malignant tumors of the small bowel. *Surg Oncol* 1994;3:61.

Eriksson BK, Larsson EG, Skogseid BM, et al. Liver embolizations of patients with malignant neuroendocrine gastrointestinal tumors. *Cancer* 1998;81:2293.

Farouk M, Niotis M, Branum GD, et al. Indications for and the techniques of local resection of tumors of the papilla of Vater. *Arch Surg* 1991;126:650.

Feldman JM. Carcinoid tumors and syndrome. *Sem Oncol* 1987; 14:237.

Godwin JD II. Carcinoid tumors: an analysis of 2837 cases. *Cancer* 1975;36:560.

Graadt van Roggen JF, van Velthuysen MLF, Hogendoorn, PCW. The histopathological differential diagnosis of gastrointestinal stromal tumours. *J Clin Pathol* 2001;54:96.

Hanson MW, Feldman JE, Blinder RA, et al. Carcinoid tumors: Iodine-131 MIBG scintigraphy. *Radiology* 172:699, 1989.

Joestling DR, Beart RW, van Heerden JA, et al. Improving survival in adenocarcinoma of the duodenum. *Am J Surg* 1981;141:228.

Joensuu H, Roberts PJ, Sarlomo-Rikala M, et al. Effect of the tyrosine kinase inhibitor STI571 in a patient with a metastatic gastrointestinal stromal tumor. *N Engl J Med* 2001;344:1052.

Johnson AM, Harman PK, Hanks JB. Primary small bowel malignancies. *Am Surg* 1985;51:31.

Kulke MH, Mayer, RJ. Medical progress: carcinoid tumors. *N Engl J Med* 1999;340:858.

Kvols LK, Moertel CG, O'Connell MJ, et al. Treatment of the malignant carcinoid syndrome: evaluation of a long acting somatostatin analogue. *N Engl J Med* 1986;315:663.

Lai EC, Doty JE, Irving C, et al. Primary adenocarcinoma of the duodenum: analysis of survival. *World J Surg* 1988;12:695.

Lamberts SW, Bakker WH, Reubi JC, et al. Somatostatin-receptor imaging in the localization of endocrine tumors. *N Engl J Med* 1990;323:1246.

Lewis BS, Kornbluth A, Waye JD. Small bowel tumors: yield of enteroscopy. *Gut* 1991;32:763.

Lowell JA, Rossi RL, Munson L, et al. Primary adenocarcinoma of third and fourth portions of duodenum. *Arch Surg* 1992;127:557.

Maglinte DT, O'Connor K, Bessette J, et al. The role of the physician in the late diagnosis of primary malignant tumors of the small intestine. *J Gastroenterol* 1991;86:304.

Makridis C, Rastad J, Oberg K, et al. Progression of metastases and symptom improvement from laparotomy in midgut carcinoid tumors. *World J Surg* 1996;20:900.

Martin RG. Malignant tumors of the small intestine. *Surg Clin North Am* 1986;66:779.

Moertel CG, Hanley JA. Combination chemotherapy trials in metastatic carcinoid tumor and the malignant carcinoid syndrome. *Cancer Clin Trials* 1979;2:327.

Moertel CG, Weiland LH, Nagorney DM, et al. Carcinoid tumor of the appendix: treatment and prognosis. *N Engl J Med* 1987;317: 1699.

Motojima K, Tsukasa T, Kanematsu T, et al. Distinguishing pancreatic cancer from other periampullary carcinomas by analysis of mutations in the Kirsten-ras oncogene. *Ann Surg* 1991;214:657.

Moyana TN, Xiang J, Senthilselvan A, et al. The spectrum of neuroendocrine differentiation among gastrointestinal carcinoids. *Arch Pathol Lab Med* 2000;124:570.

Nave H, Mossinger E, Feist H, et al. Surgery as primary treatment in patients with liver metastases from carcinoid tumors: a retrospective, unicentric study over 13 years. *Surgery* 2001;129:170.

North JH, Pack MS. Malignant tumors of the small intestine: a review of 144 cases. *Am Surgeon* 2000;66:46.

Oberg K. Carcinoid tumors: current concepts in diagnosis and treatment. *Oncologist* 1998;3:339.

Oberg K, Eriksson B. The role of interferons in the management of carcinoid tumors. *Br J Haematol* 1991;79:74.

O'Rourke MG, Lancashire RP, Vattoune JR. Lymphoma of the small intestine. *Aust NZ J Surg* 1986;56:351.

Ouriel K, Adams JT. Adenocarcinoma of the small intestine. *Am J Surg* 1984;147:66.

Patel SR, Benjamin RS. Management of peritoneal and hepatic metastases from gastrointestinal stromal tumors. *Surg Onc* 2000;9:67.

Pidhorecky I, Cheney RT, Kraybill WG, et al. Gastrointestinal stromal tumors: current diagnosis, biologic behavior, and management. *Ann Surg Oncol* 2000;7:705.

Ryder NM, Ko CY, Hines OJ, et al. Primary duodenal adenocarcinoma. *Arch Surg* 2000;135:1070.

Rothmund M, Kisker O. Surgical treatment of carcinoid tumors of the small bowel, appendix, colon and rectum. *Digestion* 1994;55[suppl 3]:86.

Sohn TA, Lillemoe KD, Cameron JL, et al. Adenocarcinoma of the duodenum: factors influencing long-term survival. *J Gastrointest Surg* 1998;2:79.

Stinner B, Kisker L, Zielke A, et al. Surgical management for carcinoid tumors of small bowel, appendix, colon and rectum. *World J Surg* 1996;20:183.

Strodel WE, Talpos G, Eckhauser F, et al. Surgical therapy for small bowel carcinoid tumors. *Arch Surg* 1983;118:391.

Talamini MA, Moesinger RC, Pitt HA, et al. Adenocarcinoma of the ampulla of Vater. A 28-year experience. *Ann Surg* 1997;225:590.

Thompson GB, van Heerden JA, Martin JK Jr, et al. Carcinoid tumors of the gastrointestinal tract: presentation, management, and prognosis. *Surgery* 1985;98:1054.

Van Ooijen B, Kalsbeek HL. Carcinoma of the duodenum. *Surg Gynecol Obstet* 1988;166:343.

Vinik AI, Thompson N, Eckhauser F, et al. Clinical features of carcinoid syndrome and the use of somatostatin analogue in its management. *Acta Oncol* 1989;28:389.

Wallace S, Ajani JA, Charnsangavej C, et al. Carcinoid tumors: imaging procedures and interventional radiology. *World J Surg* 1996;20:147.

Weiss NS, Yang C. Incidence of histologic types of cancer of the small intestine. *J Natl Cancer Inst* 1987;78:653.

Welch JP, Malt RA. Management of carcinoid tumors of the gastrointestinal tract. *Surg Gynecol Obstet* 1977;145:223.

Wessels FJ and Schell SR. Radiofrequency ablation treatment of refractory carcinoid hepatic metastases. *J Surg Res* 2001;95:8.

Willett CG, Warshaw AL, Connery K, et al. Patterns of failure after pancreaticoduodenectomy for ampullary carcinoma. *Surg Gynecol Obstet* 1993;176:33.

Yeo CJ, Cameron JL, Sohn TA, et al. Six hundred fifty consecutive pancreaticoduodenectomies in the 1990s: pathology, complications, and outcomes. *Ann Surg* 1997;226:248.

Younes N, Fulton N, Tanaka R, et al. The presence of K-12 *ras* mutations in duodenal adenocarcinomas and the absence of *ras* mutations in other small bowel adenocarcinomas and carcinoid tumors. *Cancer* 1997;79:1804.

11

Cancer of the Colon, Rectum, and Anus

Dennis L. Rousseau, Jr., Gregory P. Midis, and Barry W. Feig

EPIDEMIOLOGY

Colorectal cancer is the third most common cancer in males and females. In the year 2000, there were an estimated 130,200 cases diagnosed, including 93,800 cases of colon cancer and 36,400 cases of rectal cancer. Between 1992 and 1996, incidence rates declined approximately 2% per year, a decline thought to be due, in part, to improved screening and treatment of polyps before their progression to invasive cancers. However, colorectal cancer still accounts for 11% of cancer deaths. Estimates for the year 2000 show 56,300 deaths: 47,700 from colon cancer, 8,600 from rectal cancer.

In the United States, the cumulative lifetime risk of developing colorectal cancer is about 6%. The risk of colorectal cancer clearly increases with age. Except in the rare setting of several hereditary forms of colorectal cancer, this disease is rare before age 40. After age 50, there is a rapid increase in the rate of disease, and 90% of the cases of colorectal cancer occur in patients older than 50. These facts are responsible for the recommendations to begin screening at age 50.

When diagnosed, 37% of patients have localized disease, 37% have regional disease, 20% have distant metastasis, and 6% are unstaged. The 5-year survival rates for local, regional, and distant disease are 91%, 66%, and 8.5%, respectively. The relative survival rates at 1 and 5 years for colorectal cancer patients is 80% and 61%, respectively. The 10-year survival rate for colorectal cancer is 54%.

Approximately 75% of colorectal cancer cases are sporadic with the remainder of cases occurring in patients considered to be at increased risk. The patients with increased risk include patients with inflammatory bowel disease, familial adenomatous polyposis (FAP), hereditary nonpolyposis colorectal cancer (HNPCC), as well as patients with a strong family history of colorectal cancer. Colorectal cancer cases are nearly equally divided between men and women.

RISK FACTORS

Diet

Many dietary factors have been studied regarding their effect on colorectal cancer. Consumption of red meat and animal fat, as well as the presence of high fecal levels of cholesterol, correlate with and may be causally related to an increased risk of colorectal carcinoma. Folate supplements have been shown to be protective against colorectal cancer. Calcium supplements have been shown to decrease the formation of new adenomas in patients with a history of adenomas. Vitamins with antioxidant properties including beta-carotene, vitamins C and E have been studied, and at present there are no prospective data that demonstrate a protective effect from colorectal cancer with their use. Dietary fiber has also been studied, and no prospective data support its use for protection from the development of colorectal cancer.

Medications

Several medications have demonstrated protective effects for colorectal cancer. Hormone replacement therapy has been shown to significantly decrease mortality from colorectal cancer in women. Aspirin and other nonsteroidal anti-inflammatory drugs have also demonstrated protective effects. Recent studies with sulindac and the selective COX-2 inhibitor celecoxib demonstrated the ability of these agents to cause regression of colon polyps in patients with FAP. Future studies will evaluate these drugs for safety and efficacy as chemoprevention agents for the general population.

Polyps

Most colorectal cancers arise from polyps. Colorectal polyps are classified histologically as either neoplastic (adenomatous) polyps (which may be benign or malignant) or nonneoplastic (including hyperplastic, mucosal, inflammatory, hamartomatous). Adenomatous polyps are found in approximately 33% of the general population by age 50 and in approximately 50% of the general population by age 70. Most lesions are less than 1 cm in size, with 60% of people having a single adenoma and 40% having multiple lesions. Sixty percent of lesions will be located distal to the splenic flexure.

A genetic model for colon carcinogenesis has been developed from the genetic analysis of colorectal adenomas and carcinomas. This model demonstrates a sequence of genetic alterations responsible for the development of colorectal adenomas and their progression to invasive carcinoma. The National Polyp Study showed that colonoscopic removal of adenomatous polyps significantly reduced the risk of developing colorectal cancer.

Polyps coexist with colorectal cancer in 60% of patients and are associated with an increased incidence of synchronous and metachronous colonic neoplasms. Patients with a primary cancer and a solitary associated polyp have a lower incidence of synchronous and metachronous lesions when compared to patients with multiple polyps. The natural history of polyps supports an aggressive approach to their treatment: invasive cancer will develop in 24% of patients with untreated polyps at the site of that polyp within 20 years.

There are three histologic variants of adenomatous polyps. *Tubular adenomas* represent 75% to 87% of polyps and are found with equal frequency throughout all segments of the bowel. Less than 5% of tubular adenomas are malignant. *Tubulovillous adenomas* constitute 8% to 15% of polyps. They are also equally distributed throughout the bowel, and 20% to 25% are malignant. The remaining 5% to 10% of polyps are *villous adenomas,* which are most commonly found in the rectum; 35% to 40% of these polyps are malignant. Besides histologic characteristics, the size of a polyp and the degree of dysplasia has been associated with malignant potential. Malignancy was found in 1.3% of adenomas less than 1 cm, 9.5% between 1 and 2 cm, and 46% greater than 2 cm. Similarly, 5.7% of mild, 18% of moderate, and 34.5% of adenomatous polyps with severe dysplasia were found to have malignant cells upon complete excision of the polyp. Therefore although only 2% to 5% of adenomatous polyps harbor malignancy at the time of diagnosis, the histologic characteristics, size, and degree of dysplasia can help predict which polyps will be malignant.

The terms *carcinoma in situ* (CIS) and *intramucosal carcinoma* are used to describe severely dysplastic adenomas that have not invaded the muscularis mucosae and therefore have no risk of lymph node metastases. Approximately 5% to 7% of adenomatous polyps contain CIS. If a polyp containing CIS is completely excised endoscopically, the patient should be considered cured.

Overall, 8.5% to 17% of polyps harboring invasive carcinoma will metastasize to regional lymph nodes. Four unfavorable pathologic features of malignant colorectal polyps increase the probability that regional lymph nodes will be involved with tumor: (a) poor differentiation, (b) vascular and/or lymphatic invasion, (c) invasion below the submucosa, and (d) positive resection margin. Poorly differentiated lesions (grade 3) are associated with a higher incidence of lymphovascular involvement and recurrent disease when compared with well and moderately differentiated lesions (grades 1 and 2). Approximately 4% to 8% of malignant polyps will be poorly differentiated. Vascular invasion is uncommon; when it occurs, it is associated with recurrent disease or lymphatic invasion in approximately 40% of patients. Lymphatic invasion occurs in 12% of malignant polyps and carries a poor prognosis. Either type of invasion or poor differentiation is an indication for evaluation for surgical resection. Depth of invasion may be the single most important prognostic factor for mesenteric lymph node involvement with invasive cancer arising in a polyp. Haggitt et al. (1985) approached this depth issue by assigning level 0 to 4 values for invasion from the head of the polyp to the submucosa of the bowel wall (between the stalk and the muscularis propria). Because pathologic studies have shown that lymphatic channels do not penetrate above the muscularis mucosa, they determined that level 4 invasion was the only significant prognostic factor in a multivariate analysis of risk factors for invasive carcinoma in a polyp. Although these findings have been confirmed by other studies, there are frequently multiple adverse prognostic factors seen in patients with higher levels of invasion (i.e., levels 3–4), which makes it difficult to assign depth as the most important factor. A negative resection margin has consistently been shown to be associated with a decreased adverse outcome (recurrence, residual carcinoma, lymph node metastases, decreased survival). Twenty-seven percent of patients with positive or indeterminate tumor margins will have adverse outcomes, compared with 18% with negative margins and poor prognostic features and 0.8% with negative margins and no other poor prognostic features. Therefore a negative margin is important but only a component of the risk factor assessment.

Although clinical factors such as age, location, number of polyps, and gender are collectively known to be prognostic factors, only age greater than 60 years has been identified as an independent risk factor for invasion.

Treatment

When adenomatous polyps are found by sigmoidoscopy, we recommend complete colonoscopy with colonoscopic removal of the polyp and colonoscopic surveillance every 3 years until the examination result is normal. Colonoscopic polypectomy is a safe, effective treatment for nearly all pedunculated polyps. A biopsy is performed on those polyps not amenable to safe polypectomy; surgical resection is recommended (usually for large sessile villous lesions). Fungation, ulceration, and distortion of the surrounding bowel wall are indicative of invasion of the bowel wall and are contraindications to polypectomy. The surgical oncologist will become involved in decisions regarding the necessity of surgical resection after polypectomy.

Colectomy is indicated for patients with residual carcinoma and for those at high risk for lymph node metastases despite complete endoscopic polypectomy. The high-risk pathologic features previously described (positive margin or margin <2 mm, poor differentiation, increased depth of invasion [level 4], and vascular/lymphatic invasion) and the resultant increased risk of lymph node metastasis must be weighed against the risk of surgical resection. Therefore an elderly patient with a completely excised pedunculated polyp with negative margins who has medical factors that increase the risk for open surgery may be best served by endoscopic polypectomy alone.

In a review of 17 studies to evaluate the frequency of lymph node metastases or residual carcinoma in low-risk patients with pedunculated polyps, only a 1% incidence was found. In sessile polyps with low-risk features, the incidence was increased to 4.1%. Because the incidence of nodal metastases is higher in sessile polyps with invasive cancer, those patients at low operative risk should be considered for resection even if no high-risk pathologic features are observed. Stalk invasion in pedunculated polyps is not considered an adverse histologic feature, and treatment of polyps with stalk invasion is the same as that of polyps without stalk invasion (based on risk stratification). Polypoid cancers (almost all the polyp is invaded with carcinoma) are treated no differently from other malignant polypoid lesions. The decision for colectomy must depend on the presence and number of high-risk pathologic factors present in the polyp weighed against the patient's operative risks. Large villous adenomas of the rectum may be amenable to transanal local excision. This provides a complete diagnostic evaluation for malignancy, and if excised with negative margins (with other favorable prognostic features) may be the only therapeutic procedure needed.

Hereditary Polyposis Syndromes

Hereditary polyposis represents a constellation of syndromes rather than a single disease entity. All are characterized by multiple intestinal polyps as well as associated extraintestinal manifestations.

Familial adenomatous polyposis is the best characterized of the syndromes; 1% to 2% of patients diagnosed with colon carcinoma will have FAP. The genetic alteration associated with FAP has been determined to be a point mutation in the adenomatous polyposis coli (APC) gene located on the long arm of chromosome 5 in band q21. It is inherited in an autosomal dominant pattern, with 90% penetrance. The incidence of new mutations in FAP patients is high; approximately 25% of all FAP cases are the result of a *de novo* germline mutation. In affected individuals, polyps develop throughout the gastrointestinal (GI) tract but are most common in the colon. Clinical symptoms usually manifest between the ages of 16 and 50. Without prophylactic colectomy, colorectal cancer will develop in nearly all affected individuals by the sixth decade of life. Commercial genetic testing can identify an APC gene mutation in approximately 80% of FAP families because the mutation in these 80% results in a truncation of the APC protein. The remaining 20% of mutations appear to affect transcription regulatory elements, which have not been identified by current testing methods. Once the specific mutation is identified in a family, the test can differentiate affected from unaffected individuals with 100% accuracy, thereby aiding in surveillance and surgical planning.

Gardner's syndrome is also inherited in an autosomal dominant pattern and is a variant of FAP (including mutation of the APC gene). Colonic as well as extracolonic lesions characterize it. The extracolonic lesions can be divided into three groups. The first group involves lesions of the upper GI tract including periampullary lesions, duodenal lesions, and gastric polyps. The second group involves lesions in the ocular, cutaneous, and skeletal systems. Congenital hypertrophy of the retinal pigment epithelium (CHRPE); osteomata of the mandible, jaw, and calvaria; teeth abnormalities; sebaceous and epidermoid cysts; and fibromas are included in this group. The third group involves malignancies outside the GI tract including mesenteric fibrosis (desmoids), hepatoblastoma, thyroid carcinoma, and brain tumors (Turcot syndrome).

Although the hereditary syndromes are rare, the identification of a genetic alteration in patients with familial polyposis has provided a unique opportunity to investigate the molecular events involved in the pathogenesis of colon cancer.

Hereditary Nonpolyposis Syndromes

HNPCC, also classically known as the Lynch I and II syndromes, is a nonpolyposis autosomal dominant disease that occurs five times more frequently than familial polyposis. HNPCC accounts for 1% to 5% of colon cancers. Isolated colonic involvement occurs in the Lynch I syndrome. Colorectal cancer as well as tumors of the endometrium, ovary, stomach, small bowel, hepatobiliary tract, pancreas, ureter, and renal pelvis characterizes the Lynch II syndrome. Penetrance is between 30% and 70%. There is an estimated 85% lifetime risk of colon cancer. Compared with patients with sporadic colon cancer, patients with HNPCC have cancers that are more right-sided (60%–70% occur proximal to the splenic flexure), occur earlier (about 45 years of age), have a lower stage, have better survival, and have an increased rate of metachronous and synchronous tumors (20%).

The genetic mutations causing HNPCC are in DNA mismatch repair (MMR) genes that prevent replication errors (RER), and hence genetic instability. Five of the DNA MMR genes have been linked to HNPCC. These genes are hMSH2, hMLH1, hMSH6, hPMS1, and hPMS2. The first two genes account for the majority of the cases of HNPCC. Mutations in tumor suppressor genes such as p53, DCC, and APC can be associated with HNPCC because RER are produced in these tumor suppressor genes. Genetic testing is carried out to (a) identify risk within a known family by identifying the specific genetic defect and screening subsequent members and (b) investigate sporadic cancers suspicious for HNPCC by first identifying RER mutations in cancers, then screening for the specific genetic defect.

Inflammatory Bowel Disease

Ulcerative colitis carries a risk of colorectal carcinoma that is 30 times greater than that of the general population. The incidence increases steadily with increasing duration of disease. After 30 years, the risk of colorectal cancer increases to 35% in this population. Crohn's disease is also associated with a 10- to 20-fold increased risk of cancer. The risk associated with inflammatory bowel disease underscores the importance of surveillance in this patient population.

Previous Colon Carcinoma

A second primary colon carcinoma is three times more likely to develop in patients with a history of colon cancer than in the general population; metachronous lesions develop in 5% to 8% of these patients.

History of First-Degree Relatives with Bowel Cancer

People with a first-degree relative with colorectal cancer have a 1.8- to 8-fold higher risk of colorectal cancer than the general population. The risk is higher if more than one relative is affected, and higher cancer developed in the relative at a young age (<45).

SCREENING

Screening can be defined as stratification of risk among apparently asymptomatic, average-risk individuals. Those with a positive screen are subjected to surveillance, and those with a positive surveillance test or symptoms are subjected to a diagnostic evaluation. As many as 19% of the general population are at risk of developing adenomatous polyps, and 5% of sporadic polyps may progress to colorectal carcinoma. These data make it likely that screening patients for polyps and early cancers and treatment of these lesions could decrease overall mortality from colorectal carcinoma. Recently, this reduction in mortality has been shown in prospective, randomized trials.

Fecal occult blood testing (FOBT) (using Hemoccult or Hemoquant), endoscopy, and double-contrast barium enemas (DCBE) are the most useful screening tools for colorectal cancer. The sensitivity and specificity of FOBT for the detection of colorectal cancer varies from 30% to 90%, and from 90% to 99%, respectively, and depends on whether the specimens are rehydrated or not (increases sensitivity but decreases specificity, which increases the numbers of colonoscopies). Nevertheless, there is proof from three randomized trials that FOBT detects cancers at an earlier stage than those detected in populations without testing and that there is a reduction in colorectal cancer mortality. Rehydration of specimens is not recommended at this time. There is recent evidence that screening with FOBT, and subsequent colonoscopy, is cost-effective.

Although the introduction of flexible sigmoidoscopy has improved patient comfort and decreased risk compared with rigid sigmoidoscopy, the incidence of cancers proximal to the splenic flexure has increased, especially in women, which decreases the sensitivity of the test. Despite this, flexible sigmoidoscopy and polyp clearance has resulted in a decreased incidence of colorectal cancer, and hence a decreased mortality from this disease.

The value of colonoscopy in screening can be appreciated if one considers that approximately 40% of colon cancers arise proximal to the splenic flexure and that 75% of proximal colon cancers do not have an index lesion within reach of the flexible sigmoidoscope. Most studies using screening colonoscopy in average-risk patients report an average of 30% of neoplastic lesions detected. Cost is an important issue, however, if colonoscopy is considered the ultimate screening tool. Currently, screening colonoscopy is cost-effective if a 10-year interval is used once the colon is cleared of polyps.

DCBE is used less frequently than colonoscopy for screening and can detect colorectal carcinoma and polyps greater than 1 cm with an accuracy equal to that of colonoscopy. It is used in patients who refuse or cannot have full colonoscopy to the cecum, as an adjunct to flexible sigmoidoscopy to evaluate the remainder of the colon, and for difficult-to-visualize turns in the colon. The difficulty with this method is that lesions detected by DCBE require further evaluation, decreasing the cost-effectiveness of the method.

The study of Winawer et al. (1997) from Memorial Sloan-Kettering Cancer Center showed a reduction in mortality (43%) in people who were screened with FOBT and rigid sigmoidoscopy, but this was not statistically significant ($p = 0.053$). Other prospective randomized trials have shown that tumors identified in screened populations tend to be earlier-stage tumors at the time of diagnosis, as compared with tumors found in control groups of unscreened patients. However, a significant reduction in cancer-specific mortality has been demonstrated to date in only one study, the Minnesota Colon Cancer Control Study. Other studies, including three European randomized trials that have shown a significant decrease in the stage of detected cancers compared with the control group, may show a reduction in mortality when the data are more mature. A recent meta-analysis of the randomized trials indicates that hemoccult testing is associated with a 19% reduction in the mortality rate from colorectal carcinoma.

Carcinoembryonic antigen (CEA) has no role in screening for primary lesions. The sensitivity ranges from 30% to 80%, depending on the stage of disease. False-positive results occur in benign disease (lung, liver, and bowel) as well as malignancies of the pancreas, breast, ovary, prostate gland, head and neck, bladder, and kidney. The CEA level is also increased in smokers. Overall, 60% of tumors will be missed by CEA screening alone.

Screening Recommendations

Recently, an expert panel, after reviewing all pertinent data to late 1996, made the following recommendations regarding screening (Winawer et al., 1997) (Table 11-1).

Table 11-1. Screening recommendations

Symptomatic patients
  Diagnostic studies
Average risk, asymptomatic (age ≥50)
  FOBT each year (full colonoscopy or DCBE/flex sig if+)
  Flex sig every 5 yr (full colonoscopy if +, except tubular adenomas <1 cm)
  FOBT + flex sig (as described earlier)
  Alternative: DCBE every 5–10 yr
  Alternative: colonoscopy every 10 yr
Increased risk, asymptomatic (close relatives with colorectal cancer or polyps)
  Same recommendations for average-risk patients, begin at 40 yr of age or 10 yr earlier than the age of the first colorectal cancer case in the family
Increased risk, family history of FAP
  Genetic counseling and possible testing
  Gene carriers or indeterminate cases: flex sig every 12 mo, begin at puberty
  Polyps present: consider timing of colectomy
Increased risk, family history of HNPCC
  Full colonoscopy every 1–2 yr starting between the ages of 20 and 30 or at an age at least 10 yr younger than the youngest family member with colorectal cancer
  Full colonoscopy every year after age 40
Increased risk, history of adenomatous polyps
  1-cm polyp or multiple polyps found, repeat initial examination in 3 yr
  Second examination: normal or single, small, or tubular adenoma, repeat examination in 5 yr
  Second examination: multiple or large polyps, etc; repeat examination per clinician judgment
Increased risk, history of colorectal cancer
  Complete resection, full colonoscopy within 1 yr of surgery
  Second examination: normal, repeat examination in 3 yr
  Third examination: normal, repeat examination in 5 yr

DCBE, double-contrast barium enema; FAP, familial adenomatous polyposis; Flex sig, flexible sigmoidoscopy; FOBT, fecal occult blood testing; HNPCC, hereditary nonpolyposis colorectal cancer.

PATHOLOGY

Histologically, more than 90% of colon cancers are adenocarcinomas. On gross appearance, there are four morphologic variants of adenocarcinoma. Ulcerative adenocarcinoma is the most common configuration seen and is most characteristic of tumors in the descending and sigmoid colon. Exophytic (also known as polypoid or fungating) tumors are most commonly found in the ascending colon, particularly in the cecum. These tumors tend to project into the bowel lumen, and patients often present with a right-sided abdominal mass and anemia. Annular (scirrhous) adenocarcinoma tends to grow circumferentially into the wall of the colon, resulting in the classic apple core lesion seen on barium enema radiologic study. Rarely, a submucosal infiltrative pattern can be observed that is similar to linitis plastica seen with gastric adenocarcinoma.

Other epithelial histologic variants of colon cancer that are occasionally seen include mucinous (colloid) carcinoma, signet-ring cell carcinoma, adenosquamous carcinoma, and undifferentiated carcinoma. Other rare tumors include carcinoids and leiomyosarcomas (to be discussed later in the chapter).

The most commonly used grading system is based on the degree of formation of glandular structures, nuclear pleomorphism, and number of mitoses. Grade 1 tumors have the most developed glandular structures with the fewest mitoses, grade 3 is the least differentiated with a high incidence of mitoses, and grade 2 is intermediate between grades 1 and 3.

STAGING

The Dukes and TNM staging systems for colorectal carcinoma are presented in Tables 11-2 and 11-3. Although most clinicians are familiar with both staging systems, clinical trial and treatment planning should be based on the TNM staging system. The Dukes staging system is important for historical perspective.

Table 11-2. Modified Astler-Coller classification of the Dukes staging system for colorectal cancer

Stage	Description
A	Lesion not penetrating submucosa
B1	Lesion invades but not through the muscularis propria
B2	Lesion through intestinal wall, no adjacent organ involvement
B3	Lesion involves adjacent organs
C1	Lesion B1 invasion depth, regional lymph node metastasis
C2	Lesion B2 invasion depth; regional lymph node metastasis
C3	Lesion B3 invasion depth; regional lymph node metastasis
D	Distant metastatic disease

Table 11-3.   TNM staging classification of colorectal cancer

Primary tumor (T)

T1	Invades submucosa
T2	Invades muscularis propria
T3–T4	
Serosa	
T3	Invades into subserosa, but not through serosa
T4	Invades through serosa into free peritoneal cavity or into contiguous organ
No Serosa	
T3	Invades through muscularis propria
T4	Invades contiguous organs

Regional lymph nodes (N)

N0	No lymph node metastasis
N1	Lymph node metastasis in 1–3 nodes
N2	Lymph node metastasis in 4 or more nodes
N3	Lymph node metastasis in central nodes

Distant metastases (M)

M0	No distant metastasis
M1	Distant metastases present

CLINICAL PRESENTATION

Patients with colorectal cancer present with bleeding, abdominal pain, change in bowel habits, anorexia, weight loss, nausea, vomiting, fatigue, and anemia. Pelvic pain or tenesmus in rectal cancer may be associated with an advanced stage of disease indicating involvement of pelvic nerves. Metastatic disease is suspected in patients with right upper quadrant pain, fevers and sweats, hepatomegaly, ascites, effusions, and supraclavicular adenopathy. Central nervous system and bone metastasis are seen in less than 10% of autopsy cases, and are very rare in the absence of advanced liver or lung disease. The incidence of complete obstruction in newly diagnosed colorectal cancer is 5% to 15%. In a large study from the United Kingdom, 49% of obstructions occurred at the splenic flexure, 23% occurred in the left colon, 23% occurred in the right colon, and 7% occurred in the rectum. Obstruction increases the risk of death from colorectal cancer 1.4-fold and is an independent covariate in multivariate analyses. Perforation occurs in 6% to 8% of colorectal carcinoma cases. Perforation increases the risk of death from cancer 3.4-fold. Using TMN staging and Surveillance, Epidemiology, and End Results (SEER) Program data, 15% of patients present with stage I disease, 30% with stage II, 20% with stage III, and 25% with stage IV. The remainder have unknown staging.

DIAGNOSIS

Colon Cancer

Clinical evaluation of carcinoma of the colon should include colonoscopy and biopsy, air-contrast barium enema if the entire colon could not be visualized by colonoscopy, chest radiograph, complete blood cell count, CEA determination, urinalysis, and liver function tests (LFTs).

The use of abdominopelvic computed tomography (CT) in the preoperative evaluation of patients with colon cancer is controversial. The abdomen and pelvis should be evaluated with CT in patients with large, bulky lesions to detect involvement of contiguous organs, para-aortic lymph nodes, and the liver. Some authors only recommend CT scan when preoperative LFTs are abnormal. Both lactate dehydrogenase and alkaline phosphatase (AP) levels are useful for detecting hepatic involvement. However, abnormal LFTs are present in only approximately 15% of patients with liver metastases. In contrast, the false-positive rate for elevated LFTs is close to 40%. Therefore a significant number of unnecessary CT scans would be performed if all patients with abnormal LFTs underwent CT scan. The preoperative CEA level can also reflect disease extent and prognosis: CEA levels surpassing 10 to 20 ng/mL are associated with increased chances of disease failure for both node-negative and node-positive patients. Some surgeons believe that preoperative evaluation of the liver is important because 15% to 20% of liver metastases will be nonpalpable at the time of surgery. However, 10% to 15% of lesions will be missed by combined preoperative and operative evaluation. Intraoperative ultrasonography has been shown to be the most accurate method of detecting liver metastasis.

Most patients with colon cancer will require an operative procedure even in the presence of liver metastasis; surgery is the best method to prevent the complications of colon tumors, such as obstruction and bleeding. Therefore the only advantages of a preoperative CT scan are in helping to plan possible treatment options for metastatic disease to the liver or to plan operative procedures when contiguous organ involvement is present. At the University of Texas M.D. Anderson Cancer Center, we do not routinely obtain preoperative CT scans in patients with colon tumors. The decision to perform a preoperative CT scan is individualized based on the results of physical examination, LFTs, and CEA level.

The role of routine preoperative urinary tract evaluation is controversial. Patients who are symptomatic or have large, bulky lesions should have a preoperative intravenous pyelogram or CT scan to evaluate the urinary tract. Up to 40% of these patients will have urinary tract abnormalities.

Rectal Cancer

In addition to the history and physical examination, chest radiograph, complete blood cell count, LFTs, electrolytes, and urinalysis, endorectal ultrasound (EU), proctoscopic examination, full colonoscopy, and abdominopelvic CT scan should be performed to accurately stage patients with rectal cancer. Symptomatic patients undergo evaluation of their urinary tract as described earlier for colon cancer.

Accurate preoperative staging tools are critical in rectal cancer because disease stage may influence treatment decisions such as transanal resection or preoperative multimodality therapy. EU is the most accurate tool in determining tumor (T) stage. All layers of the rectal wall can be identified with 67% to 93% accuracy. The

EU characteristics of T1 and T3 tumors make them relatively easy to differentiate. However, the distinction between T2 and T3 tumors is not as well defined, yet it is vital in determining treatment planning. Limitations of EU include operator experience, differentiating lymph nodes from blood vessels and other structures, differentiating T2/T3 tumors, differentiating peritumoral edema from tumor, evaluating a tumor after radiation therapy, and overstaging (10%–15%) or understaging (1%–2%) errors. Stenotic lesions may make EU impossible secondary to the inability to pass the probe. EU evaluation of the depth of bowel wall penetration is superior to that of either CT (52%–83% accuracy) scanning or magnetic resonance imaging (MRI) (59%–95% accuracy). CT and MRI are most valuable for locally advanced tumors because they can delineate the relationship of the tumor to surrounding viscera and pelvic structures. Neither CT nor MRI is more useful for the evaluation of locoregional disease after neoadjuvant chemoradiation treatment because radiation changes can be difficult to accurately differentiate from tumor.

Lymph node staging in rectal cancer has proven more difficult than primary tumor staging, with EU accuracies of 62% to 83%, CT accuracies of 35% to 73%, and MRI accuracies of 39% to 84% reported. Despite descriptions of methods to radiologically predict metastases in lymph nodes, only nodal enlargement can be detected with most current technologies. Fifty percent to 75% of positive lymph nodes in rectal cancer may be normal in size, thereby limiting accurate evaluation. Similarly, lymph nodes may be enlarged from inflammation, giving false-positive results. Accuracy can be increased by combining size and ultrasonographic characteristics. Lymph nodes that are greater than 3 mm and hypoechoic are more likely to contain metastatic deposits. In addition, it is possible to perform fine-needle aspiration of suspicious lymph nodes under EU guidance. EU is invaluable when evaluating patients for preoperative adjuvant therapy, but it cannot accurately assess response to preoperative adjuvant therapy due to the obliteration of tissue planes by edema and fibrosis.

Abdominopelvic CT scanning is important in assessing the presence of distant spread of disease and involvement of adjacent organs. In the management of rectal cancer it is extremely important to accurately assess the local spread of disease, including the potential involvement of the levator muscles and other pelvic structures. Although EU is superior to CT in detecting depth of penetration, CT provides a better assessment of contiguous organ involvement. MRI may provide better delineation of contiguous organ involvement than CT scan (e.g., bladder, blood vessel involvement); however, this advantage has not been definitively established.

The staging of recurrent rectal cancer is complicated by radiation and postoperative changes that are often difficult to distinguish from tumor. At present, EU is not useful in distinguishing scar from recurrent tumor. Similarly, there is poor correlation of post–radiation therapy EU in preoperative regimens to final pathologic findings (postresection), indicating the limited value of EU in assessing tumor in an irradiated milieu. CT is useful to assess extent of disease and adjacent organ involvement if recurrent tumor is obvious. MRI is equally useful and can provide sagittal images that may provide additional information on resectability. In cases where recurrence is unknown but suspected, CT is more useful if a baseline study is available for comparison. Positron emission tomography (PET) has recently been introduced with early reports of increased accuracy in distinguishing postoperative changes from recurrent tumor. Further studies are required before this test can be recommended for use on a routine basis. Currently at M.D. Anderson Cancer Center, we obtain both a CT scan and MR image of the pelvis in cases of isolated recurrent rectal carcinoma because we believe these studies are complementary in their provision of critical staging and resectability information.

MANAGEMENT OF COLON CANCER

The goal of primary surgical treatment of colon carcinoma is to eradicate disease in the colon, the draining nodal basins, and contiguous organs. Careful surgical planning is essential. Patient age, stage of disease, extent of tumor, and presence of synchronous colonic tumors are significant factors in determining the optimal surgical approach. Overall medical condition is also important because most perioperative deaths result from cardiovascular or pulmonary complications.

Anatomy

Thorough knowledge of the arterial, venous, and lymphatic anatomy of the colon and rectum is essential to appropriate surgical management (Fig. 11-1). The ascending and proximal transverse colon are embryologically derived from the midgut and receive their arterial blood supply from the superior mesenteric artery via the ileocolic, right, and middle colic arteries. The distal transverse, descending, and sigmoid colon are hindgut derivatives whose arterial blood supply arises from the inferior mesenteric artery (IMA) through the left colic and sigmoid arteries. The rectum, also a hindgut derivative, receives its blood supply to the upper third from the IMA via the superior hemorrhoidal artery. The middle and lower thirds of the rectum are supplied by the middle and inferior hemorrhoidal arteries, which are branches of the hypogastric artery. Collateral blood supply for the colon is provided through the marginal artery of Drummond. The venous drainage of the colon and rectum parallels the arterial supply, with the majority draining directly into the portal venous system. This provides a direct route for metastatic spread of tumor to the liver. The only minor anatomic variation in the venous drainage compared with the arterial supply is that the inferior mesenteric vein (IMV) joins the splenic vein before emptying into the portal system. The rectum has dual venous drainage; the upper rectum drains into the portal system, and the distal one-third of the rectum drains into the inferior vena cava via the middle and inferior hemorrhoidal veins, providing a direct route for hematogenous spread outside of the abdomen.

The lymphatic drainage of the bowel is more complex than the vascular supply. Lymphatics begin in the bowel wall as a plexus beneath the lamina propria and drain into the submucosal and intramuscular lymphatics. The epicolic lymph nodes drain the

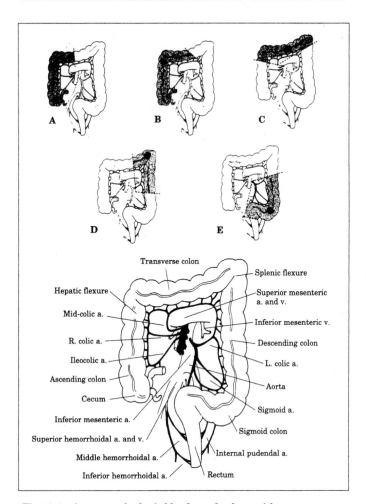

Fig. 11-1. Anatomy of colonic blood supply along with a pictorial description of the various anatomic resections used for colon carcinoma. A: Right hemicolectomy. B: Extended right hemicolectomy. C: Transverse colectomy. D: Left hemicolectomy. E: Low anterior resection. (From Sugarbaker PH, MacDonald J, Gunderson L. Colorectal cancer. In: DeVita VT, Hellman S, Rosenberg SA, eds. *Cancer: principles and practice of oncology,* 3rd ed. Philadelphia: Lippincott, 1984.)

subserosa and are located in the colon wall. This nodal group runs along the inner bowel margin between the intestinal wall and the arterial arcades. These nodes in turn drain into the paracolic nodes, which follow the routes of the marginal arteries. The epicolic and paracolic nodes represent the majority of the colonic lymph nodes and are the most likely sites of regional metastatic disease. The paracolic nodes drain into the intermediate nodes, which follow the main colic vessels. Finally, the intermediate nodes drain into the principal nodes, which begin at the origins of the superior and inferior mesenteric arteries and are contiguous with the paraaortic chain.

The route of lymphatic flow parallels the arterial and venous distribution of the colon. The right colon will drain to the superior mesenteric nodes through the intermediate nodes or to the portal system via the lymphatics of the superior mesenteric vein. The left colon's lymphatic drainage follows the marginal artery to the left colic intermediate nodes and finally to the inferior mesenteric nodes. The lymphatic drainage of the upper third of the rectum follows the IMV, whereas the lower two-thirds drain into the hypogastric nodes, which, in turn, drain into the paraaortic nodes. The lower third of the rectum can also drain along the pudendal vessels to the inguinal nodes.

Surgical Options

At resection, the primary tumor and its lymphatic, venous, and arterial supply are extirpated, as well as any contiguously involved organs. Our current use of intraoperative ultrasound is limited to the evaluation of non-palpable hepatic abnormalities identified on preoperative CT scan. We do not believe that the "no-touch" isolation technique is necessary; we support high ligation of appropriate vessels in colon cancer resections.

The various surgical options, as well as their indications and major morbidities, are briefly discussed next.

Right Hemicolectomy

This operation involves removal of the distal 5 to 8 cm of the ileum, right colon, hepatic flexure, and transverse colon just proximal to the middle colic artery. This procedure is indicated for cecal, ascending colonic, and hepatic flexure lesions. Major morbidities include ureteral injury, duodenal injury, and rarely bile acid deficiency.

Extended Right Hemicolectomy

This procedure includes resection of the transverse colon (including resection of the middle colic artery at its origin) in addition to the structures removed in the right hemicolectomy. Indications for the procedure are hepatic flexure or transverse colon lesions. Morbidities include anastomotic dehiscence and diarrhea in addition to the complications associated with right hemicolectomy.

Transverse Colectomy

This procedure involves the segmental resection of the transverse colon and is indicated for middle transverse colon lesions. The major morbidity is anastomotic dehiscence. At M.D. Anderson this procedure is rarely performed because of the potential difficulty in achieving a tension-free anastomosis with adequate blood supply (as the marginal artery of Drummond is sacrificed). We prefer to perform an extended right hemicolectomy with an ileo-descending colon anastomosis.

Left Hemicolectomy

This resection involves the removal of the transverse colon distal to the right branch of the middle colic artery and the descending colon up to but not including the rectum, plus IMA ligation and division. Indications for the procedure are left colon and splenic flexure lesions. Morbidities include anastomotic dehiscence.

Low Anterior Resection

This procedure includes removal of the distal descending colon, the sigmoid colon, the upper two-thirds of the rectum, and ligation of IMA (and IMV) at its origin. The procedure is indicated for sigmoid and proximal rectal lesions. Morbidities include anastomotic dehiscence and bowel ischemia (secondary to inadequate flow through the marginal artery of Drummond).

Subtotal Colectomy

This resection involves the removal of the entire colon to the rectum with an ileorectal anastomosis. This procedure is indicated for multiple synchronous colonic tumors, patients with a second primary colon cancer, and distal transverse colon lesions in patients with a clotted IMA. Morbidities include diarrhea, perineal excoriation, and anastomotic dehiscence.

The surgical treatment of the familial polyposis syndromes depends on the age of the patient and the polyp density in the rectum. Surgical options include proctocolectomy with Brooke ileostomy, proctocolectomy with continent ileostomy, total abdominal colectomy with ileorectal anastomosis, or proctocolectomy with mucosectomy and ileal pouch–anal canal anastomosis. The first two operations are rarely performed in the FAP population today. Total abdominal colectomy and ileorectal anastomosis have a low complication rate, provide good functional results, and are a viable option for younger patients and those with few polyps in the rectum. These patients must be observed with 6-month proctoscopic examinations to remove polyps and detect signs of cancer. If rectal polyps become too numerous, a trial of sulindac or conversion to an ileoanal pouch is warranted. The risk of cancer in the retained rectal stump increases to approximately 8% at 50 years of age and 29% at 60 years of age.

Proctocolectomy with ileal pouch–anal canal anastomosis has the advantage of removing all of the large intestine mucosa at risk for cancer while preserving transanal defecation. Complication rates are low when this procedure is done in large centers. Morbidity from the procedure includes incontinence, multiple loose stools, impotence, retrograde ejaculation, dyspareunia, and pouchitis. Approximately 7% of patients have to be converted to a permanent ileostomy due to complications after the procedure.

Laparoscopic Resection for Colorectal Carcinoma

Recent studies have confirmed that laparoscopy for colorectal carcinoma resection is technically feasible, is safe, and yields an equivalent number of resected lymph nodes compared to open colectomy. It may reduce hospital stay, be less morbid, and decrease convalescence, although this has yet to be proven in a randomized prospective trial. Despite reports of equivalent lymphadenectomies being performed laparoscopically, only prospective randomized studies with long-term follow-up will determine whether this translates into equivalent local and distant recurrence rates, and disease-specific survival. Laparoscopy clearly has a role in performing diverting ostomies in colorectal and anal carcinoma, in palliative resections in patients with metastatic disease, and in the resection of large polyps. Several single and multi-institutional prospective randomized trials are under way to answer the critical questions regarding laparoscopic versus open resection for colorectal carcinoma, including the issue of port-site recurrences and oncologic outcome. Multiple nonrandomized studies have shown that laparoscopic colon resection can be performed with similar oncologic results when compared to historical controls. Until the results of the prospective randomized trials are disseminated, patients should only be offered laparoscopic resection with curative intent in the context of one of these trials.

Obstructing Colorectal Cancers

Obstructing colorectal cancers are usually treated in two stages: resection and Hartmann's procedure, followed by colostomy takedown and reanastomosis. An alternative is a one-stage procedure with either subtotal colectomy and primary anastomosis or a segmental resection and intraoperative colonic lavage for carefully selected patients. (Contraindications include multiple primary cancers, advanced peritonitis, hemodynamic instability, poor general health, steroid therapy or immunosuppressed state.) In the SCOTIA prospective randomized trial using these two treatment modalities in 91 patients with malignant left-sided colonic obstruction, the morbidity and mortality rates were similar. Laser fulguration and endoscopic stenting of obstructive lesions can be used for palliation to allow for bowel preparation and subsequent single-step resection. Obstructing right-sided cancers can be effectively treated with resection and anastomosis in one stage.

Survival

Nodal involvement is the primary determinant of 5-year survival. In node-negative disease, the 5-year survival rate is 90% for patients with T1 and T2 lesions and 80% for those with T3 lesions. For node-positive cancers, the 5-year survival ranges from 69% (one positive node) to 27% with six or more positive nodes. Other factors that are proven prognostic indicators include grade, bowel perforation, and obstruction. Patients who present with unresectable metastatic disease have an overall 8% 5-year survival rate.

Adjuvant Therapy

Most patients with colon cancer present with disease that appears localized and can be completely resected with surgery. However, almost 33% of patients undergoing curative resection will relapse with recurrent disease secondary to unresected occult microscopic metastasis. Adjuvant therapy is administered to treat and hopefully eradicate this residual micrometastatic disease. 5-Fluorouracil (5-FU) is the most effective single agent for colon carcinoma, with response rates of 15% to 30% when it is used alone as treatment for patients with advanced disease.

History

With the identification of the anticancer activity of 5-FU in patients with colorectal cancers, there have been numerous studies of 5-FU in combination therapies. Adjuvant trials using 5-FU and semustine (MeCCNU; Veterans Administration Surgical Oncology Group, VASOG no. 5) failed to demonstrate an overall survival benefit from adjuvant therapy with this combination. However, subset analysis of patients with one to four positive lymph nodes did reveal a significant improvement in 5-year survival in patients receiving surgery and 5-FU/semustine versus surgery alone (51%–31%, respectively). A second large trial was the National Surgical Adjuvant Breast and Bowel Project (NSABP) C-01 protocol, which compared surgery alone to surgery followed by MOF chemotherapy (MeCCNU, vincristine, and 5-FU). With over 1,100 patients randomized, the study demonstrated an 8% improvement in 5-year survival in the adjuvant therapy arm. While these initial results were positive, they were not sufficient to recommend adjuvant therapy for colorectal cancer. They did, however, stimulate further studies combining 5-FU with other agents.

5-Fluorouracil/Levamisole

The first major success of adjuvant therapy for colon cancer was demonstrated in trials of 5-FU in combination with levamisole, an antihelminthic agent with immunostimulatory properties. The use of levamisole in the adjuvant setting was based on initial studies in patients with advanced stages of colon cancer that showed this agent had some activity when used as single-agent therapy. Later studies showed that 5-FU/levamisole was more effective than levamisole alone. A pilot prospective randomized study comparing 5-FU/levamisole, levamisole, and surgery alone was conducted by the North Central Cancer Treatment Group (NCCTG). This study demonstrated improved 5-year disease free survival with levamisole and 5-FU/levamisole as compared to surgery alone. The improvement in the levamisole only arm was less significant than that of the 5-FU/levamisole arm when examining overall 5-year survival. This initial study led to the National Cancer Institute Intergroup Trial (NCI-INT) protocol 035, a larger study comparing the same treatment arms. In this study, patients with stage III disease were shown to have a 41% reduction in the risk of recurrence when treated with

5-FU/levamisole. These patients also demonstrated a 33% improvement in overall 5-year survival. Interestingly, the levamisole-only arm failed to show any improvement in disease-free and overall 5-year survival rates compared to the surgery-only arm. Additionally, the data suggested an improvement in disease-free and overall survival for patients with stage II colon carcinoma; however, statistical significance was not reached for this group of patients. Based on these results, the National Institutes of Health Consensus Conference in 1990 recommended that all patients with stage III colon carcinoma receive adjuvant chemotherapy with 5-FU and levamisole. Adjuvant chemotherapy for patients with stage II colon carcinoma remained of unproved benefit.

5-Fluorouracil/Leucovorin

The addition of leucovorin (LV) to 5-FU has been shown to increase antitumor activity in both in vitro and in vivo models. LV works by stabilizing the 5-FU thymidylate synthase complex, thus prolonging the inhibition of thymidylate synthase and increasing tumor cytotoxicity. Initial efficacy of this combination was demonstrated in the NCI-INT protocol 089, which demonstrated a 30% improvement in 5-year survival when compared to surgery alone. An Italian study also demonstrated both improved disease-free and overall survival using the 5-FU/LV combination. More recent studies have compared 5-FU/LV to previously tested combinations. The NSABP C-03 trial compared 5-FU/LV to MOF chemotherapy (MOF was used in NSABP C-01). This study was reported early because 5-FU/LV was significantly superior to MOF in terms of overall survival and it was much less toxic than MOF (1% severe hematologic toxicity vs. 16% for MOF). NSABP C-04 compared 5-FU/LV to 5-FU/levamisole and 5-FU/LV/levamisole. Duration of therapy for this trial was 1 year. The results showed that the 5-FU/LV combination was slightly superior to 5-FU/levamisole, with disease-free survival of 64% versus 60% and overall survival of 74% versus 69%, respectively ($p = 0.05$). The 5-FU/LV/levamisole combination did not improve outcome, but had marked increased toxicity. Finally, NSABP C-05 compared 5-FU/LV with 5-FU/LV and interferon (IFN). No difference in disease-free and overall survival was demonstrated with the addition of IFN.

Duration of Therapy

Most of the adjuvant trials used 1 year of treatment for the adjuvant treatment arms. Optimal treatment duration was examined in two trials: the NCI-INT protocol 089 and an NCCTG trial. These studies examined 12 month and 6 month treatment courses for 5-FU/LV and 5-FU/levamisole. Reduction of treatment from 12 to 6 months for 5-FU/levamisole resulted in an 8% increase in mortality. No increase in mortality was noted comparing 12-month and 6-month treatment with 5-FU/LV. Overall, 6 months of 5-FU/LV was shown to be equivalent to 1 year of 5-FU/levamisole. For 5-FU/LV, maximal benefit of adjuvant therapy for the patient is achieved with 6 months of therapy.

Adjuvant Therapy for Stage II Disease

While adjuvant therapy has been proven to benefit patients with stage III disease, the issue of benefit for patients with stage II disease remains controversial. While many of the adjuvant trials included patients with stage II disease, subgroup analysis shows trends toward benefit without reaching statistical significance. This issue was addressed in a recent study that examined the relative efficacy of adjuvant chemotherapy by stage in the four NSABP trials C-01 to C-04. This analysis concluded that adjuvant chemotherapy in stage II patients provided a relative improvement in overall 5-year survival that was comparable to that of stage III patients (30% relative improvement). The absolute improvement in overall survival was 5%, which was statistically significant. However, routine use of adjuvant chemotherapy for stage II patients is still not common practice. Currently, work is in progress to determine molecular and genetic prognostic markers that will be useful in selecting those stage II patients who would benefit most from routine use of adjuvant therapy.

New Adjuvant Agents Under Investigation

New agents that have demonstrated efficacy in the treatment of metastatic disease are now being tested in an adjuvant setting. The first group of agents is oral fluoropyrimidines. UFT, a combination of oral uracil and the 5-FU prodrug tegafur, is currently under investigation in the NSABP C-06 trial. Other oral agents under study include emiluracil, an agent which makes small oral doses of 5-FU clinically effective, and capecitabine, a drug with rapid GI absorption that undergoes a three-step enzymatic conversion to 5-FU in tumor tissue. Irinotecan (CPT-11), a topoisomerase I inhibitor, has been shown to improve survival in patients with metastatic colon cancer when used in combination with 5-FU and LV. The role of irinotecan in the adjuvant setting remains under investigation. A recent U.S. intergroup trial was stopped early due to an increased number of deaths in the group receiving irinotecan. Further investigation involving different infusion schedules of CPT-11 will be required to determine the safety and efficacy of irinotecan. Oxaliplatin, a new platinum derivative with activity against colorectal cancer, will be examined in the NSABP C-07 trial. Finally, tumor-specific monoclonal antibodies are being evaluated. The murine monoclonal antibody Mab 17-1A has shown efficacy in the adjuvant setting and is currently under study in randomized trials.

Treatment of Locally Advanced Colon Cancer

Colon cancers that are adherent to adjacent structures have a 36% to 53% chance of local failure after complete resection. Approximately 10% of carcinomas present in this fashion. Strategies designed to reduce local recurrence would benefit these patients.

Surgical Strategy

Resection of colorectal cancer that has invaded adjacent structures involves en bloc resection of all involved structures; failure to do so results in significantly increased local recurrence and decreased survival. Of importance, all adhesions between the carcinoma and adjacent structures should be assumed to be malignant and not taken down because 33% to 84% are malignant when examined histologically. The affected organ should have resection limited to the involved area with a rim of normal tissue. A patient who has a margin-negative multivisceral resection has the same survival as a patient with no adjacent organ involvement on a stage-matched basis.

Adjuvant Therapy

Retrospective series have shown subsets of patients who have benefited from postoperative radiation therapy with or without 5-FU–based chemotherapy. Unfortunately, there are no consistent criteria to use in assessing increased risk of local failure. The value of adjuvant radiation therapy after complete resection of high-risk colon cancer is currently being evaluated in a randomized prospective fashion (NCCTG 91-46-52). In this trial, patients with B3 or C3 (modified Astler-Coller) tumors are randomized to receive postoperative 5-FU/levamisole or 5-FU/levamisole and radiation therapy. Patients with subtotally resected cancers fare worse than those with positive microscopic disease, as one would expect. It has been found that radiation therapy is more effective in microscopic than in macroscopic disease, and that it is more effective when combined with 5-FU. In a recent retrospective Mayo Clinic study of 103 mostly stage B3 and C3 (modified Astler-Coller) patients, in which 49% had no residual disease, 17% had microscopic residual disease, and 34% had gross residual disease, the local failure rate was 10% for patients with no residual disease, 54% for those with microscopic residual disease, and 79% for those with gross residual disease. If there is any question regarding the ability to achieve a margin negative resection, surgical clips should be used to outline the area of the tumor bed. If the margin is positive on final pathologic studies, radiation should be administered with concomitant 5-FU–based chemotherapy.

MANAGEMENT OF RECTAL CANCER

There are four goals in the successful management of rectal cancer: (a) cure, (b) local control (negative margin resection of tumor, and resection of all draining lymph nodes), (c) restoration of intestinal continuity, and (d) preservation of the anorectal sphincter, sexual function, and urinary function. Because of the anatomic constraints of the bony pelvis, it may be difficult to achieve adequate sphincter, sexual, and urinary function without compromising cure and local control.

Local control is clearly related to the adequacy of the surgical procedure. Although local control is critical for increasing the chances of cure, many patient- and tumor-related factors are associated with overall outcome. Data suggest that there is a significant surgeon-related and center-related variability in patient outcome after treatment for rectal cancer. The Stockholm Rectal Cancer Study Group found that "specialists" and centers with higher volumes of rectal cancer cases had lower local failure rates and increased survival rates. It is not unusual to see local recurrence rates ranging from 3.7% to 43% in various series for curative surgical resection, with or without adjuvant therapy. Obviously, other factors are involved, such as methods of adjuvant therapy, patient selection, and disease factors. These varying results have hindered an accurate assessment of the vital components of an adequate oncologic operation and prevented an accurate assessment of the value of adjuvant chemoradiation in rectal cancer. Consequently, there are some who believe that with an adequate oncologic procedure by an experienced surgeon, only large T3 and T4 (fixed) lesions need adjuvant chemoradiation treatment. Treating all other T3 patients and those with N1-N2 disease merely attempts to make up for "bad surgery." Others contend that the significant decrease in local recurrence and possibly some improvement in survival associated with adjuvant radiation or chemoradiation justify its application in all patients with tumors that are T3 or greater, or those with node-positive disease. Nevertheless, surgical technique is critical to the success of the treatment of rectal cancer.

When planning surgical treatment of a rectal cancer, the rectum can be divided into three regions in relation to the anal verge. The upper rectum is defined as 11 to 12 cm from the anal verge. Tumors greater than 12 cm behave more like colonic cancers and are therefore generally considered to be distal sigmoid or "rectosigmoid" cancers. Tumors 6 to 10 cm from the anal verge are defined as middle rectal cancers, and tumors from 0 to 5 cm are defined as low rectal cancers. Note that low rectal cancers can be associated with the internal and external sphincters, anal canal, or levator muscles, or can be above the pelvic floor.

Surgical Aspects
In addition to understanding the anatomic site of the tumor, it is important to understand the principles influencing the extent of radical extirpative surgery regardless of the type of resection planned.

Resection Margin
Optimal treatment of all malignancies requires an adequate margin of resection. Histologic examination of the bowel wall distal to the gross rectal tumor reveals that only 2.5% of patients will have submucosal spread of disease greater than 2.5 cm. In addition, patients with distal submucosal disease spread greater than 0.8 cm have a poor prognosis and will probably not benefit from more radical surgery. At M.D. Anderson we try to obtain a distal resection margin of at least 2 cm. Although irrigation of the rectal stump is performed routinely at other institutions, we do not use this technique in rectal cancer surgery.

Lymphadenectomy
An adequate lymphadenectomy should be performed for accurate staging and local control. Spread from the primary tumor occurs in a lateral and upward direction, with distal spread occurring in less than 5% of patients. In a large series no distal spread was seen with T1 and T2 lesions. With T3 and T4 lesions, the most distal spread into the mesorectum was 4 cm for upper rectal lesions and 3 cm for lower rectal lesions. Total mesorectal

excision (TME) provides an adequate lymphadenectomy for rectal cancer. The technique involves sharp excision and extirpation of the mesorectum by dissecting outside of the investing fascia of the mesorectum. TME optimizes the oncologic operation by not only removing draining lymph nodes, but also maximizing lateral resection margins around the tumor. Although no randomized prospective trial has compared TME with conventional mesorectal excision, some institutions have shown a significant decrease in the local recurrence rate compared with historical controls using conventional surgery (to the range of 6.3%–7.3%). The major morbidity associated with TME is an increased rate of anastomotic leak, thought to be due to devascularization of the rectal stump. Leak rates of 11% to 16% have been reported for TME as compared to 8% for non-TME resections done by the same group of surgeons.

The TME dissection can be facilitated by ligation of the IMA (and IMV) at or near its origin ("high ligation"). The data on whether high ligation also results in a decreased local recurrence remain equivocal. Data do suggest that negative lateral (radial) margins are major determinants of survival that may be more important than longitudinal resection margins. Lateral margin clearance can be maximized by sharp dissection outside the mesorectum on the endopelvic fascia. The bony pelvis, which inherently limits the maximal extent of lateral dissection, may serve as the best explanation of why distal rectal cancers have a higher local recurrence rate than their more proximal counterparts when comparing patients with tumors of similar stage. It is controversial whether the entire mesorectum must be excised for all rectal cancers or whether the mesorectum can be sharply divided at the distal resection margin. At M.D. Anderson Cancer Center (MDACC), we excise the mesorectum to the distal resection margin, which would include nearly the entire mesorectum for lower and the lower half of middle rectal cancers, while preserving a portion of the mesorectum for the upper and upper half of middle rectal cancers. We think that this does not compromise an adequate oncologic operation and may lessen the complication rate (anastomotic leak from devascularization of the rectal stump). It is important to remember that although a 2-cm distal mucosal margin is adequate, local control of rectal cancer requires maximal extirpation of the mesorectal and lateral pararectal tissues. A proven benefit of sharp mesorectal excision in a defined anatomic plane is the ability to perform an adequate cancer operation with preservation of the pelvic autonomic nerves. No benefit in survival or local disease control has been attainable with the use of more extended lymphadenectomy (iliac/periaortic nodes, pelvic sidewall, etc.), and the complication rates are higher with these more extensive surgical procedures.

Surgical Approaches to Rectal Cancer

Surgical approaches to the rectum include transabdominal procedures (abdominoperineal resection [APR], low anterior resection [LAR], coloanal anastomosis [CAA]), transanal approaches, and transsacral approaches (York-Mason, Kraske). These latter two approaches will be discussed in detail in the section on local treatment of rectal cancer. APR, an operation devised by Ernest Miles in the 1930s, was the only previous treatment for all rectal cancers. With the advent of better preoperative staging, improved adjuvant and neoadjuvant therapy, and a better understanding of this disease, the use of APR has decreased significantly. APR is now reserved for patients with primary sphincter dysfunction and incontinence, patients with direct tumor invasion into the sphincter complex, patients with large or poorly differentiated lesions in the lower third of the rectum that do not have adequate tumor clearance for sphincter-preservation surgery (located 0–3 cm from the anal verge), and patients with large rectal tumors invading adjacent pelvic organs.

Sphincter-Preservation Procedures

Besides local excision, sphincter-preservation procedures include LAR and proctectomy/CAA either alone or combined with neoadjuvant radiation and chemoradiation. Another option includes the addition of a colonic reservoir for improved function. These procedures can only be performed if the oncologic result is not compromised and the functional results are acceptable. It was demonstrated as early as 20 years ago that there is no difference in local recurrence rate or survival in patients with mid-rectal cancers who undergo LAR rather than APR. The technical feasibility of LAR in this setting was increased with the advent of circular stapling devices and the knowledge that distal margins of resection of 2 cm were adequate. Survival was found to depend on the distance of the tumor from the anal verge, the presence of positive lymph nodes, and the lateral extent of dissection. Therefore many studies comparing the two procedures included high-risk low rectal cancers treated by APR, and higher, lower-risk rectal cancers treated with LAR. More recently, a retrospective study (Rullier et al., 1997) in 106 patients with low to middle rectal cancers treated by APR or LAR showed no difference in local recurrence or survival, confirming earlier results with middle and upper rectal cancers. An alternative to LAR is proctectomy with CAA. Originally, this was used for technically difficult LAR procedures in mid-rectal cancers. It is used now for low middle rectal cancers and very select low rectal cancers, with the stapled or hand-sewn anastomosis between the dentate line and the anorectal ring. Most surgeons use temporary fecal diversion when this procedure is performed. The use of proctectomy and CAA for low rectal cancers is usually in the context of preoperative radiation or chemoradiation protocols. Using either LAR or proctectomy with CAA (and adjuvant therapy), local recurrence rates of 3% to 6.5% have been reported by MDACC and Memorial Hospital. Functional results have been good, with 60% to 86% patients attaining continence by 1 year, 10% to 15% requiring laxative use, and some with mild soiling at night. Preoperative chemoradiation does not seem to have a negative impact on these functional results. Obviously, the lower the anastomosis (i.e., coloanal), the greater the bowel dysfunction.

Data, mostly retrospective, show that the oncologic results of proctectomy with CAA are similar to those of anterior proctectomy with TME with and without sphincter preservation: a local recurrence rate of 7% to 22% and a 5-year survival rate of 69% to 73%.

Colonic J Pouch

Although continence can be maintained in patients with a CAA, there is a degree of incontinence in some patients, and others require antidiarrheal agents. This is probably due to lack of compliance in the neorectum. This led to the introduction of the colonic J pouch for low rectal cancers that showed better results in terms of stool frequency, urgency, nocturnal movements, and continence than straight coloanal anastomoses. There is some reduction in functional advantage of the pouch at 1 year, particularly regarding difficulty in pouch evacuation (20% of patients). Prospective randomized studies carried out to 3 years show superior functional advantage of the colonic J pouch to straight reconstructions. As in anterior resection, the functional outcome of patients with CAA (with or without a J pouch) may take 1 to 3 years to stabilize and is related to the level of the anastomosis (lower anastomoses tend to have poorer function). The pouch is usually constructed with a 6-cm efferent limb. Unfortunately, many patients with low rectal cancers do not have enough remaining colonic length to construct a J pouch. Studies have shown that postoperative radiation therapy does not adversely affect pouch function.

Proximal Diversion

Proximal diversion after sphincter preservation is indicated in the following circumstances: (a) anastomosis less than 5 cm above the anal verge, (b) patients who have received preoperative radiation therapy, (c) patients on corticosteroids, (d) when the integrity of the anastomosis is in question, and (e) any case of intraoperative hemodynamic instability.

Local Approaches to Rectal Cancer

Local treatment alone as definitive therapy of rectal cancer was first applied to patients with severe coexisting medical conditions unable to tolerate radical surgery. Currently, conservative, sphincter-saving local approaches are being more widely considered. Early studies of local excision demonstrate up to a 97% local control rate and 80% disease-free survival for properly selected individuals. Local treatment is best applied to rectal cancers within 10 cm of the anal verge, tumors less than 3 cm in diameter involving less than one fourth of the circumference of the rectal wall, exophytic tumors, tumors staged less than T2 by EU, highly mobile tumors, and tumors of low histologic grade. The decision to use local excision alone or to employ adjuvant therapy after local excision is based on the pathologic characteristics of the primary cancer (with negative margins) and the potential micrometastases in draining lymph nodes. T1 lesions have positive lymph nodes in 5% to 10% of cases, whereas the rate for T2 and T3 lesions is 10% to 20% and 30% to 70%, respectively. T2 tumors treated with local resection alone can have local recurrence rates of 15% to 44%. Most authors recommend adjuvant chemoradiation after local excision of T2 or greater lesions, and select T1 lesions with poor prognostic features. A phase II cooperative group study of 110 T1 to T2 low to middle rectal cancers was performed where T1 cancers received no further therapy, whereas all T2 cancers received postoperative chemoradiation treatment. At a median follow-up of 48 months, four of 59 patients with T1 lesions and ten of 51 patients with T2 lesions recurred. Of the T1 lesions, two recurred locally, one recurred with metastatic disease, and one recurred with both local and metastatic disease. Of the T2 recurrences, five were local, three were metastatic only, and two were both local and metastatic recurrences. Overall and disease-free survival rates were 85% and 78%, respectively, at 48 months. This study is evidence that local treatment for highly selected patients with selective use of adjuvant therapy can provide adequate cancer control without undergoing complex operative procedures with their attendant morbidity and mortality (Table 11-4).

Local therapy of distal rectal cancers can be accomplished by transanal excision, posterior proctectomy, fulguration, or endocavitary irradiation.

Transanal excision is the most straightforward approach to removing distal rectal cancers. The deep plane of the dissection is the perirectal fat. Tumors should be excised with an adequate circumferential margin.

Posterior proctotomy (Kraske procedure) can be used for tumors in the middle and upper rectum and is more suitable for larger, low rectal lesions. In this procedure, a perineal incision is made just above the anus, the coccyx is removed, and the fascia is

Table 11-4. Recommended surgical treatment strategy for rectal cancer

Location	T-stage	Resection	Mesorectal Excision to
Upper rectum	T1	TEM or Kraske	—
	≥T2	LAR[a]	Distal resection margin
Middle rectum	T1	TAE, Kraske,	—
	T2	LAR	Distal resection margin or entire
	≥T3	CXRT/LAR	Distal resection margin or entire
Low rectum	T1	TAE	—
	T2	Proctectomy/ CAA,[b] (±J pouch), APR	Entire
	≥T3	CXRT/proctectomy/ CAA[b] (±J pouch), APR	Entire

APR, abdominoperineal resection; CAA, coloanal anastomosis; CXRT, preoperative chemoradiation; LAR, low anterior resection; TAE, transanal excision; TEM, transanal endoscopic microsurgery.
[a]LAR distal resection margin >2 cm.
[b]CAA hand-sewn; protective ileostomy.

divided. The rectum can then be mobilized for a sleeve resection, or a proctotomy is performed for excision of the tumor. The disadvantages of this procedure are fistula formation and the potential to seed the posterior wound with malignant cells.

Fulguration uses either standard electrocautery or laser to ablate the tumor. *Endocavitary radiation* is a high-dose, low-voltage irradiation technique that applies contact radiation to a small rectal cancer through a special proctoscope. Fulguration and endocavitary radiation have the disadvantage of not providing an intact specimen for histologic analysis.

Transanal endoscopic microsurgery (TEM) provides accessibility to tumors of the middle and upper rectum that would otherwise require a laparotomy or transsacral approach, with improved visibility and instrumentation. Almost any adenoma 15 to 20 cm from the anal verge is amenable to this approach. The procedure requires special training and equipment, which is expensive and therefore has limited its acceptance in the United States. This procedure is not recommended for tumors within 5 cm of the anal verge. These tumors are optimally treated with a standard transanal approach. Patient selection is important and it is recommended that patients have preoperative EU to select superficial lesions. Patients with deeper lesions and metastatic disease or comorbid conditions that would preclude laparotomy are also candidates. Although local procedures have become more commonly used, few randomized prospective trials have evaluated oncologic and functional outcomes compared with anterior resection or APR. Winde et al. (1996) prospectively randomized 50 patients with T1 adenocarcinoma of the rectum to either anterior resection or TEM. Similar local recurrence and survival rates, as well as decreased morbidity rates for local excision, were found in the two study arms, confirming the advantages of local excision.

At MDACC, transanal excision is used for low rectal cancers, whereas a Kraske procedure is used for higher rectal lesions. Optimal local excision includes at least a 1-cm resection margin circumferentially, a full-thickness excision, and an excision that is not fragmented or piecemeal. An inadequate local excision mandates an alternate resection strategy, not merely the addition of adjuvant therapy. If preoperative T stage is increased after pathologic evaluation following local excision, the appropriate standard resection is recommended. T1 tumors are treated with local therapy alone unless any of the following poor prognostic features are identified: tumor greater than 4 cm, poorly differentiated histologic type, lymphatic or vascular invasion, or clinical or radiologic evidence of enlarged lymph nodes. Those T1 tumors with poor prognostic features and tumors T2 and greater are treated with adjuvant radiation therapy with or without concomitant chemotherapy. T3 cancers are treated with local excision alone only if the patient refuses standard resection. Adjuvant chemoradiation treatment is strongly recommended postoperatively.

Treatment for Locally Advanced Rectal Cancer

Occasionally, patients will present with involvement of adjacent structures (bladder, vagina, ureters, seminal vesicles, sacrum, etc.). These patients with stage T4, N1 to N3, M0 disease clearly benefit from multimodality therapy, including preoperative or postoperative chemoradiation treatment, intraoperative radiation therapy (IORT), or brachytherapy. The goal of surgical therapy is resection of the primary tumor, with en bloc resection of adjacent involved structures to obtain negative margins. The confines of the pelvis and the proximity to nerves and blood vessels that cannot be resected decrease the resectability rate of rectal tumors compared with locally advanced colon cancer. Increased resectability rates and margin-negative resections have been demonstrated for locally advanced rectal cancers after preoperative chemoradiation treatment. Furthermore, in patients requiring pelvic exenteration for locally advanced rectal cancer, the addition of preoperative radiation therapy decreases the locoregional recurrence rates. At the Mayo Clinic, the addition of IORT to standard external beam radiation therapy with 5-FU in patients with locally advanced rectal cancer has shown significantly improved local disease control and possibly some improvement in survival (Gunderson et al., 1997). Preoperative chemoradiation has also been shown to improve rates of sphincter preservation in patients who were initially thought to need APR for curative resection. The best chance of cure in patients with locally advanced disease appears to involve preoperative chemoradiation treatment, maximal surgical resection, and IORT; randomized, controlled trials are needed to confirm these findings.

In the situation of unresectable locally advanced disease, significant rates of resectability have been reported after preoperative radiation therapy. Moreover, patients who are resected with negative margins have improved survival over those resected with close or positive margins.

At MDACC, preoperative chemoradiation is standard treatment for locally advanced rectal cancer. An evaluation of 40 patients (29 with locally advanced disease; 11 with recurrence) requiring pelvic exenteration for local disease control with negative margins demonstrated that chemoradiation may significantly improve survival and that chemoradiation response and S-phase fraction were important determinants of survival (Meterissian et al., 1997). Patients with low-risk factors had a 65% 5-year survival, whereas high-risk patients had only a 20% survival.

Survival after Surgical Therapy

Seventy-five percent to 90% of node-negative rectal cancers are cured by radical surgical resection. Only one-third of patients with regional lymph node metastases will survive 5 years. As mentioned previously, 25% of patients who fail will fail in the pelvis alone. However, local failure will occur in up to 75% of patients who die of the disease.

The survival rate after local therapy varies from 70% to 86%, with recurrence rates of 10% to 50%. The overall local recurrence rate is 30%, and increasing recurrence rates are seen with increasing stage of disease and decreasing distance from the anal verge. Many of these patients can be salvaged with radical surgery after a local recurrence. When analyzing the results of local therapy, it must be remembered that this represents a carefully selected group of patients.

Complications of Surgical and Adjuvant Therapy for Rectal Cancer

Complications of surgical and adjuvant therapy for rectal cancer include all the complications associated with major abdominal surgery (bleeding, infection, adjacent organ injury, ureteral injury, and obstruction), with the addition of some complications that are unique to pelvic surgery. Specifically, anastomotic leak occurs in 5% to 10% of cases overall, with increasing rates seen in lower anastomoses, those associated with immunocompromised states, and those associated with preoperative radiation therapy. The incidence of anastomotic leak is decreased with a defunctioning stoma. At MDACC, a defunctioning loop ileostomy is used in all anastomoses below the peritoneal reflection in patients who have received preoperative radiotherapy and in patients with CAA. Autonomic nerve preservation is part of all pelvic dissections unless tumor involvement necessitates the sacrifice of these structures. With careful dissection during TME, 75% to 85% of patients have a return to preoperative sexual and urinary function. Other complications include stoma dysfunction, perineal wound complications, hemorrhage from presacral vessels, and anastomotic stricture. The mortality rate from surgical resection varies from 2% to 6%.

The complications associated with chemoradiation treatment include radiation enteritis and dermatitis, hematologic toxicity, stomatitis (mostly with continuous 5-FU infusions), and venous access infections. The frequency and intensity of these complications depend on multiple factors, including radiation therapy total dosing, fractionation, field technique, and whether the radiation therapy is given preoperatively or postoperatively. There are no good predictors of which patients will have these complications and to what degree they will have them.

Adjuvant Therapy of Rectal Cancer

The two main components of adjuvant therapy for rectal cancer are radiation therapy to the pelvis and 5-FU–based chemotherapy. The goal of chemotherapy is to increase tumor radiation sensitivity and to decrease the chance of distant failure. The goal of radiation therapy is to increase local control, and in the preoperative setting to increase margin-negative resection rates and sphincter preservation. It must be emphasized that successful multimodality treatment of rectal cancer requires close collaboration between radiation therapists, medical oncologists, and surgeons.

Postoperative Radiation

Three randomized trials have been performed comparing surgery alone with surgery plus postoperative radiation therapy for T3 or N1 to N2 rectal cancer. The only trial to show a decrease in local recurrence rate was the NSABP R-01 trial. Local recurrence was decreased from 25% in the surgical arm to 16% in the postoperative radiation therapy arm ($p = 0.06$). Several nonrandomized trials have shown a decrease in local recurrence rates to the 6% to 8% level; the differences between these trials may reflect radiotherapy dosing and patient selection. These trials showed that postoperative radiation therapy could reduce local recurrence, but total radiation therapy dose and technique were important to achieve this effect. Higher radiation doses are proportional to higher local control rates. Despite the performance of several large prospective trials, survival, local pelvic control, and extrapelvic recurrence rates have not been improved consistently by radiation doses of 45 to 50 Gy. This prompted the addition of chemotherapy to radiation therapy in the postoperative period (see below).

Preoperative Radiation Therapy (± Chemotherapy)

Several theoretical advantages to the use of preoperative radiation therapy have led to its use in recent trials:

1. A reduction in the size of the tumor increases the potential for sphincter preservation.
2. There is a decreased risk of local failure and distant metastasis from cells shed at operation.
3. There is a decreased risk of late radiation enteritis because the small bowel can more readily be excluded from the radiation field in a preoperative setting.
4. Some tumors considered unresectable may become resectable with therapy.
5. Tumor cells are well oxygenated when treated preoperatively because there has been no surgical manipulation of the blood supply to the tumor. Well-oxygenated cells are thought to have increased radiation sensitivity, and therefore tumor cell killing may be increased.
6. There is no delay of therapy as in some cases of postoperative therapy due to operative morbidity.
7. Systemic therapy is initiated earlier than in postoperative therapy.
8. Preoperative radiotherapy may be more dose efficient than postoperative radiation therapy secondary to the tumor cells being better oxygenated.

Until now there have been ten randomized trials evaluating the role of preoperative radiation therapy in resectable rectal cancer. Although five report significant decreases in local recurrence, only one study identifies a significant survival advantage for the total patient group (Swedish Rectal Cancer Trial, 1997). In this trial, 25 Gy was delivered in five fractions (1 week), followed by curative resection to one group, whereas the control group received curative surgery only. The local recurrence rate and 9-year disease-specific survival were 11% and 74%, respectively, versus 27% and 65% for the control group. In the United States, preoperative radiation therapy trials have usually included chemotherapy in a more protracted course. Although there has not been a significant increase in survival, there have been reports of increased sphincter preservation rates, decreased local recurrence, and acceptable toxicities. Many nonrandomized studies demonstrate local recurrence rates of 8% to 15% for T1 to T3 disease in either long- or short-course 40- to 50-Gy total dose radiation therapy without chemotherapy. Three-fourths of patients initially declared to need APR have been found in some trials to be able to receive sphincter preservation, with 75% to 80% of these patients having good to excellent sphincter function postoperatively. Factors shown to be predictive of tumor downstaging have included higher total radiation dose, tumor differentiation, and a longer interval before surgery.

Given the increased success of combined chemotherapy and radiation therapy compared with radiation therapy alone in the postoperative setting as well as the increased morbidity from short-course preoperative radiotherapy, recent trials have included combined modality therapy over a protracted preoperative period. Several nonrandomized trials, including an MDACC trial (described later), have shown that preoperative 5-FU–based chemoradiation regimens for resectable T2 to T3 rectal cancer results in a 4% to 5% local failure rate, and up to a 93% 5-year survival rate, with tolerable toxicities. An important advance in this area has been the appreciation that infusional 5-FU versus bolus treatment may enhance the radiation therapy effect while reducing combined treatment-induced toxicity. It has also been shown that the pathologic response rate can be correlated with the local control rate; this has not been definitely proven for disease-free and overall survival.

The addition of leucovorin to 5-FU in the preoperative period has recently been evaluated at Memorial Sloan-Kettering Cancer Center in 32 patients (Grann et al., 1997). There was an 85% sphincter preservation rate in those patients initially thought to need an APR, with no local failure (median follow-up 22 months), a 60% 3-year disease-free survival rate, and a 9% complete pathologic response rate. Pending trials (NSABP R-03 and INT 0147) compare preop to postop 5-FU with leucovorin chemoradiation therapy and should allow answers to which treatment modality is optimal. Functional data are also being collected to address this often-overlooked aspect of adjuvant therapy in rectal cancer.

Intraoperative Radiation Therapy

IORT is used for both recurrent and locally advanced rectal cancer. Its advantages include increased local control in high-risk cancers, accurate treatment of focal areas at risk, ability to adjust the depth of the radiation beam, and ability to shield sensitive structures. Even preoperative chemoradiation in high-risk tumors can result in high local recurrence rates. IORT allows treatment of areas with close or microscopically positive margins in this situation. At the Massachusetts General Hospital, IORT is used for focal areas of tumor adherence, close or positive margins, and areas of gross residual disease. IORT dosing depends on the clinical situation: 10 to 13 Gy is given for close margins (<5 mm), 15 Gy is given for microscopically positive margins, and 17 to 20 Gy is used for areas of gross residual disease. In a recent 2-year analysis of IORT in the RTOG study of locally advanced disease, the local control rate was 77%, with a 2-year survival of 88% and a complication rate of 16%. For facilities able to deliver this type of therapy, there is a clear advantage in local control in select patients with advanced and recurrent disease. At MDACC, IORT (10–20 Gy) is used selectively in patients with locally advanced or recurrent disease where there is a close or positive margin as demonstrated by frozen section. Another option is brachytherapy, particularly in areas where the IORT beam cannot be focused due to anatomic constraints of the pelvis.

Postoperative Radiation Therapy and Chemotherapy

The addition of chemotherapy to radiation therapy has been used to enhance the radiation-responsiveness of tumors and impact on distant disease. Several studies have shown not only a reduction in local recurrence, but increases in survival. Two large studies of postoperative chemotherapy and radiation therapy conducted by the Gastrointestinal Tumor Study Group (GITSG) and NCCTG have provided evidence that combination therapy may affect local control and distant failure. In the GITSG trial there was a decrease in pelvic failure for the group treated by surgery and postoperative chemoradiation therapy (11% vs. 24% for surgery alone). In addition, a statistically significant survival advantage was found at 7 years using the combination of resection, radiation, and chemotherapy. The NCCTG trial did not have a surgery-alone control. However, there was a significant decrease in pelvic recurrence (14% vs. 25%) and a significant decrease in cancer-related deaths for the group treated by resection, radiation, and chemotherapy compared with the group treated with resection and radiation therapy.

The findings from these studies prompted the publication of a clinical advisory by the NCI Consensus Conference in 1990 recommending adjuvant treatment for patients with Duke's B2 and C rectal carcinoma (T3–T4, N0; T3–T4, N1–N3) consisting of six cycles of fluorouracil-based chemotherapy and concurrent radiation therapy to the pelvis. This regimen has remained the standard by which all current adjuvant rectal cancer protocols are compared. In the United States, postoperative chemoradiation is by far the most common mode of delivering adjuvant therapy. This is usually given as a continuous infusion of 5-FU and approximately 55 Gy of irradiation delivered to the pelvis in 1.8 to 2.0 Gy fractions (6-week treatment). Although the trend in Europe is treatment with radiation therapy and no chemotherapy, the addition of chemotherapy in the United States has been shown to decrease the rate of distant metastases, something not attainable with radiation therapy alone. In addition, there has consistently been a 10% to 15% survival advantage when radiation therapy is compared to radiation therapy with chemotherapy. The Intergroup 0114 trial has recently demonstrated that there is no statistically significant advantage to the addition of levamisole in the postoperative period to 5-FU and pelvic radiation; the results for modulation with leucovorin are unclear at this point.

M.D. Anderson Experience

Our preferred management of T3 to T4, or any T, N1 or greater rectal cancer is to use preoperative radiation therapy with a protracted intravenous infusion of 5-FU. We deliver 45 Gy of preoperative radiation therapy with standard fractionation 1.8 Gy/fraction (Gy/fxn). A continuous infusion of 5-FU at a dose of 300 mg m^{-2} day^{-1} is given 5 days per week. Surgery is performed 6 to 8 weeks after completion of therapy. In patients with

T3 disease, 61% had either a complete response or microscopic residual disease. Sixty-six percent of patients could have sphincter-preserving procedures, with a local control rate of 96%, and a negative-margin resection rate of 99%. Grade 3 to 4 toxicity was seen in only 3% to 4% of patients, and the 3-year survival was 88%. In patients with fixed T3 to T4 tumors, the same regimen was used with the addition of IORT boost for positive or close margins. The local control rate was 97% with an 82% 5-year survival. The use of this regimen for recurrences will be presented in that section.

Future Trends in Multimodality Treatment

Although some institutions will advocate TME alone for most rectal cancers, surgeons globally are now looking to identify those patients who will benefit most from adjuvant therapy, what therapy should be used (chemotherapy and radiation therapy dosing), and what setting (preoperative or postoperative) is best. Ongoing studies are investigating whether there is an advantage to continuous or bolus 5-FU and whether 5-FU should be combined with leucovorin or levamisole. Lower radiation doses (e.g., 25 Gy) are being used in shorter preoperative courses to see if a lower preoperative dose confers the same advantage of decreased local recurrence. Some centers are exploring the use of IORT and brachytherapy as adjuncts to neoadjuvant chemoradiation treatments to increase the local disease control in select patients who are at high risk for local recurrence. Various molecular markers are being evaluated in fresh or archival specimens to aid in identifying patients who will benefit from treatment.

RECURRENT AND METASTATIC DISEASE

More than 50% of patients who undergo curative surgery for colorectal cancer have tumor recurrences. Of the patients who have recurrences, 85% do so during the first 2.5 years after surgery. The remaining 15% experience recurrence during the subsequent 2.5 years. Recurrence develops in less than 5% of patients who are disease-free at 5 years. The risk of recurrence is higher with stage II or III disease. Other recurrence risk modifiers include race, presentation, grade of tumor, aneuploidy, and adjacent organ invasion. Many molecular markers are currently being evaluated for their usefulness in predicting recurrence risk. Recurrences may be local, regional, or distant. Distant disease recurrence, the most common presentation, occurs either alone or concomitantly with locoregional recurrence. Local recurrence develops in 20% to 30% of patients who undergo initial curative resections for rectal cancer, and in 50% to 80% of these patients, the local recurrence is the only site of disease. For all recurrence sites, complete resection results in a 25% to 30% cure rate. Recurrence isolated to the anastomosis (intramural) is rare and usually indicates inadequate surgical resection. Liver involvement occurs in approximately 50% of patients with colon cancer, whereas lung, bone, and brain involvement occurs in 10%, 5%, and less than 5%, respectively. Symptomatic recurrences present with a constellation of symptoms ranging from the vague and nonspecific to the clinically overt.

CEA is invaluable for postoperative monitoring. It is most useful in patients in whom levels are increased preoperatively and return to normal following surgery. Levels should be determined preoperatively, 6 weeks postoperatively, and then according to the schedule described in the surveillance section. The absolute level and rate of increase in CEA and the patient's clinical status are important in determining prognosis and treatment. Postoperative CEA levels that do not normalize within 4 to 6 weeks suggest incomplete resection or recurrent disease, although false-positive results do occur. CEA levels that normalize postoperatively and then start to increase are indicative of recurrence. This may represent occult or clinically obvious disease. A rapidly increasing CEA level suggests liver or lung involvement, whereas a slow, gradual rise is associated with locoregional disease. Despite the reliability of an increased CEA level in predicting tumor recurrence, 20% to 30% of patients with locoregionally recurrent tumors have a normal CEA level. Poorly differentiated tumors may not make CEA, which is one explanation for such false-negative results. In contrast, CEA is increased in 80% to 90% of patients with hepatic recurrences. A prospective randomized trial of the value of CEA in follow-up was undertaken in 311 patients (McCall et al., 1994). The survival data have not matured, but some valuable information is available. The study followed asymptomatic patients with increased CEA levels until symptoms developed; then a full workup was initiated. The purpose was to define the "natural history" of an elevated CEA. The sensitivity, specificity, and positive predictive values of an increased CEA level were 58%, 93%, and 79%, respectively. The median lead time of the increased CEA to detection by other means was 6 months, a result found in other studies. Seven percent of patients who had an increased CEA failed to have recurrent disease on workup. This and other newer studies call into question the cost-effectiveness and value of CEA monitoring. At MDACC, we routinely monitor CEA values because of the potential to detect liver metastases in a subgroup of patients who may benefit from early recurrence detection.

Treatment of the asymptomatic patient with an increased CEA level can be challenging. An increased level should be confirmed by a repeat CEA determination approximately 1 month later. A thorough clinical investigation that includes LFTs; CT scan of the abdomen, pelvis, and chest; colonoscopy; and, if clinically indicated, bone scan or CT of the brain should be performed. If the CEA level is increasing and the radiologic workup is negative, attention should be directed to a radiolabeled monoclonal antibody study or a PET scan.

Radiolabeled monoclonal antibodies (MoAbs) directed against tumor-specific antigens and CEA have been approved for imaging the extent and location of extrahepatic metastases. This modality is particularly useful in the evaluation of recurrent disease where postsurgical or postradiation changes are not easily differentiated from tumor on CT or MRI. One agent OncoScint CR/OV (Cytogen Corp., Princeton, NJ) is an indium-111–labeled MoAb B72.3 that targets the tumor-associated glycoprotein TAG-72, which is reactive with approximately 83% of colorectal tumors. An anti-CEA preparation that is technetium labeled is also available

(CEA-Scan). These agents were found to be superior to CT in evaluating extrahepatic and pelvic disease, whereas CT was better for detecting metastatic disease to the liver. Most studies of labeled MoAbs show a sensitivity range of 70% to 86%, with a higher specificity, and positive predictive values greater than 90%. These studies are most useful for the detection of recurrent disease in a patient with an increasing CEA level and negative radiologic workup, or to rule out metastatic disease in a patient with locoregional recurrence who may be suitable for surgical therapy (i.e., hepatic resection/cryotherapy, pelvic exenteration, etc.). Side effects occur in less than 4% of patients, and antimurine antibody formation is more problematic and may limit the ability to rescan patients (dose related). In the future, the use of antibody fragments or peptides may resolve the problem of murine antibodies and shorten imaging times.

PET imaging relies on the increased metabolic uptake of glucose (fluorine-labeled analog of 2-deoxyglucose or FDG) in tumors compared with normal tissues. Its value may lie in distinguishing postsurgical and postradiation changes from tumor, in measuring tumor response to chemotherapy or radiation therapy, or in evaluating the source of an increased CEA level in the patient with a negative radiologic workup. Initial studies have been promising, however, further prospective studies are required to determine the sensitivity and specificity of PET scan in patients with colorectal cancer. Limitations of this technology include expense and limited access to PET scanners in the United States.

If the metastatic evaluation is negative in the face of an increased CEA level, a second-look laparotomy should be performed. Approximately 60% to 90% of patients with asymptomatically increased CEA levels will have recurrent disease at laparotomy; 12% to 60% of these patients will have resectable disease at the time of laparotomy; and 30% to 40% will survive 5 years following resection of the recurrence. Early detection of asymptomatic disease results in a higher resectability rate than when resection is performed for symptomatic disease (60% vs. 27%). The liver is the most common site of recurrence, followed by adjacent organs, the anastomotic site, and the mesentery. Resectability rates correspond to the level of CEA elevation, with CEA levels less than 11 ng/mL being associated with higher resectability rates.

In recent years, radioimmuno-guided surgery (RIGS) has been used to detect recurrences intraoperatively. This technique is useful in directing the surgeon to disease sites that would otherwise be left behind. In addition, it is especially useful in patients with resectable liver lesions who have extranodal disease that is otherwise not detectable. ^{125}I-labeled monoclonal antibodies directed against CEA are injected 6 weeks before the second-look surgery. The antibodies localize to the tumor sites and can be detected intraoperatively by a handheld gamma probe. Tumor is accurately detected in 81% of patients. Sixteen percent of patients will have tumor that is detected by RIGS alone. Despite this novel modality for detecting and treating disease in the asymptomatic patient, no study has demonstrated a survival advantage with this technique.

Treatment

The appropriate treatment of resectable recurrent disease depends on the location of disease. If two disease sites are detected that are completely resectable, the procedure is undertaken in select patients. Otherwise, individual treatment modalities are used as needed for palliation of pelvic symptoms. As in locally advanced disease, potentially resectable recurrent disease is treated in a multimodality fashion using preoperative chemotherapy (with our without radiation), surgery, IORT, if available, and brachytherapy. For recurrence involving the sacrum, en bloc sacral resection can sometimes result in 4-year survival rates of 30%. Contraindications to sacral resection include pelvic sidewall involvement, sciatic notch involvement, higher than S2 involvement, encasement of iliac vessels, and extrapelvic disease. A review of pelvic recurrence at Memorial Sloan-Kettering Cancer Center revealed that there were no predictors either in the initial tumor or in the recurrent tumor to indicate survival. Complete resection of the recurrence, however, improved survival. Symptoms of recurrent disease could be adequately palliated with surgery. At MDACC, potentially resectable pelvic recurrences are treated with preoperative chemoradiation, followed by surgery and the use of IORT and brachytherapy as needed for close or positive margins. Using this approach in 43 patients, the overall resection rate was 77%, with an 88% margin-negative resection rate, a 64% local control rate, and a 58% 5-year survival. Although the usual surgical procedure for resectable recurrent rectal cancer is APR, select cases can be treated with sphincter preservation.

Chemotherapy for recurrent and metastatic disease has undergone recent changes. Standard therapy was the combination of 5-FU/LV. Recent studies have demonstrated that the addition of irinotecan (CPT-11) to 5-FU/LV resulted in significantly longer progression-free survival and overall survival as well as a higher rate of confirmed response. Oxaliplatin also appears to confer additional progression-free survival benefit when added to 5-FU/LV therapy. Oral agents including UFT (uracil with 5-FU prodrug tegafur), emiluracil, and capecitabine have also shown promise in the treatment of metastatic disease.

Liver

Approximately 70% of patients who die of colon cancer have hepatic involvement. The liver is the site of metastatic or recurrent disease in 50% of patients and is the primary determinant of patient survival. Colorectal hepatic metastases are discussed in detail in Chapter 12.

Lung

Pulmonary metastases occur in 10% to 20% of patients with colorectal cancer. They are most commonly seen in the setting of a large hepatic tumor burden or extensive metastatic disease. Isolated pulmonary metastases occur most commonly with distal rectal lesions, as the venous drainage of the distal rectum bypasses the portal system and allows metastasis to travel directly to the lungs.

The finding of a solitary lesion on a chest radiograph should prompt evaluation with thoracic CT scanning and, for a centrally located lesion, bronchoscopy with biopsy. Peripheral lesions may be amenable to CT-guided needle biopsy or video-assisted thoracoscopic surgery. Fifty percent of patients with solitary pulmonary nodules will have primary lung tumors rather than colorectal metastases.

Patients with locally controlled primary tumors, no evidence of metastases elsewhere, good pulmonary reserve, and good medical condition are candidates for resection. Patients with solitary metastases experience the best survival, but patients with as many as three lesions (unilateral or bilateral) can experience up to a 40% 5-year survival. The optimum surgical approach is a median sternotomy to allow for bilateral pulmonary exploration, because contrast-enhanced CT scan has up to a 25% false-negative and false-positive rate for the detection of metastases. As in liver resection for metastatic disease, the optimum surgery involves the minimal procedure to obtain negative margins (i.e., wedge resection vs. pneumonectomy).

The overall 5-year survival rate following resection of pulmonary metastases ranges from 20% to 40%. In newer series involving only colorectal cancer metastases, the rate is closer to 40% to 43% 5-year survival. Age, sex, location of the primary disease, disease-free interval, or involvement of hilar or mediastinal lymph nodes does not seem to influence survival. The number of metastases in most series is inversely correlated with 5-year survival. Recurrence confined to the lung after resection is an indication by some for repeat resection.

Bone and Brain

Metastatic disease to the brain is uncommon and usually occurs after established lung involvement. Symptomatic solitary lesions can be treated by palliative craniotomy and resection. In a very small subpopulation of patients, cranial disease may be the only site of involvement, and excision in this setting may increase survival. Bone metastases are quite uncommon and are best managed with radiation therapy.

Ovary

Because 1% to 7% of women who undergo potentially curative resections subsequently develop ovarian metastases, it has been suggested that prophylactic oophorectomy may benefit these patients. Unfortunately, it has never been proven that removal of ovarian micrometastatic disease, or the potential for metastases at this site, improves survival. In most cases ovarian metastases develop in the presence of widespread disease, and it would not be expected that prophylactic oophorectomy would alter survival. In the postmenopausal patient with isolated unilateral or bilateral metastatic disease to the ovaries, a bilateral oophorectomy is performed. In the premenopausal patient with unilateral involvement, a unilateral oophorectomy is performed. Prophylactic oophorectomy is not performed routinely at the MDACC when resecting potentially curable colorectal carcinoma.

Pelvis

Local recurrence in the pelvis is a major problem after treatment for rectal cancer. These patients are infrequently saved by additional surgery. Radiation affords good palliation; however, if the patient has previously received adjuvant radiotherapy, external beam radiation therapy may no longer be an option. Radical surgical procedures, including pelvic exenteration and sacrectomy, may benefit a select group of patients whose disease can be completely extirpated by these procedures. IORT and brachytherapy may be useful adjuvants in the setting of radical surgery for recurrent disease.

SURVEILLANCE

Patients with a history of colon carcinoma require close surveillance. The data to support this, however, are lacking. In a Danish prospective randomized study in 597 colorectal cancer patients, patients had either close follow-up (every 6 months for the first 3 years) or yearly for 3 years (including examination/stool heme test, colonoscopy, laboratory testing [except CEA], and chest radiograph). The frequency of recurrent cancer was the same in both groups, but it was diagnosed earlier in the close follow-up group. The close follow-up group had more resections for curative intent (local and distant), but there was no cancer-specific survival difference. Other studies, mostly retrospective, show similar findings. However, a recent meta-analysis (Rosen et al., 1998) of randomized and comparative cohort studies was able to demonstrate that intensive follow-up resulted in a significantly higher curative re-resection rate as well as an improved 5-year survival for those patients with recurrence.

History and physical examination, hemoccult stool testing, and laboratory tests (complete blood cell count, CEA determination, LFTs) are performed at MDACC every 3 months for the first 3 years after surgery, every 6 months during years 4 and 5, and yearly thereafter. Colonoscopy should be performed after 1 year, and then at 3 years if normal. A baseline CT scan of the abdomen and pelvis is obtained 3 to 4 months after resection of rectal carcinoma. Because of the 47% false-positive rate, the utility of routine CT scanning in surveillance is controversial. However, in the presence of symptoms or abnormal laboratory tests, CT should be performed. A chest radiograph is obtained every 6 months for the first 2 years and yearly thereafter. It has traditionally been proposed that patients should be monitored closely for local recurrence during the first 2 years postoperatively (time at which most local recurrences appear). Recent data show that the addition of adjuvant radiation therapy may extend this period of vulnerability such that 50% of local recurrences may occur more than 2 years from surgery.

UNCOMMON COLORECTAL TUMORS

Lymphoma

Lymphoma is an uncommon tumor that occurs in 0.4% of patients with intestinal lymphoma presenting anywhere between the second and eighth decades. Almost all are non-Hodgkin's lymphomas. Twenty-five percent of patients may present with fever, occult blood loss, anemia, a palpable mass, or an acute abdomen. The diagnosis is often made intraoperatively. A history of abdominal pain, fever, and weight loss in a patient who is younger than the expected age for a colorectal tumor should raise the suspicion of intestinal lymphoma.

Abdominal CT and endoscopy with biopsy are the most useful diagnostic tests because lesions are often missed on barium enema examination. A thickened bowel, adjacent organ extension, or nodal enlargement may be seen. If the lesion is intraluminal, endoscopic biopsy will facilitate the diagnosis. Most of these lesions are intermediate- to high-grade B-cell lymphomas. If a diagnosis is made preoperatively in an otherwise asymptomatic patient, bone marrow biopsy should be performed. A primary lesion is defined as a lesion with no associated organ or lymphatic involvement, negative chest CT, and a negative peripheral blood smear and bone marrow.

Surgery is performed in the clinical setting of obstruction, bleeding, perforation, or an uncertain diagnosis. Surgery is also performed, although not consistently, for complete resection of a primary lesion. A thorough exploration is performed and all suspicious nodes or organs are biopsied to assess the stage of disease. The primary intestinal lesion should be resected with negative margins whenever possible. The bowel mesentery should be resected with the tumor so that regional nodes can be assessed pathologically. Intestinal continuity should be restored whenever possible. If a large tumor is found to be unresectable and is not obstructing the bowel, a bypass can be performed. Surgical clips should be placed to facilitate identification of the tumor by the radiation oncologist.

Intestinal lymphoma requires a combined-modality approach using surgery and chemotherapy with or without radiation. For rectal lymphoma, complete resection is followed by radiation treatments to the pelvis. Chemoradiation is used if the resection was incomplete. The overall survival for stages I and II disease is approximately 80%. This decreases to 35% with advanced disease.

Leiomyosarcoma

Leiomyosarcomas comprise less than 1% of colonic tumors. The peak incidence occurs in the sixth decade. Most of these tumors present as large intramural masses. They may invade the mesenteric and pericolic fat, prostate gland, vagina, and ischiorectal fossa.

Patients can present with pain, bleeding, obstruction, nausea, vomiting, anemia, tenesmus, or hematuria. Ulceration is present in 30% to 50% of patients. A thorough clinical evaluation should be conducted to exclude metastatic disease. Excision with wide surgical margins is the treatment of choice. Colonic tumors are excised with adjacent mesentery. Wide nodal excision is not indicated in the absence of clinically evident disease. Small tumors of the rectum and anal canal can be removed transrectally or endoscopically. A recent report from Memorial Sloan-Kettering Cancer Center showed promising results for rectal and anal leiomyosarcomas using transanal resection with brachytherapy.

As with other sarcomas, prognosis depends on tumor size, grade, and presence or absence of adjacent organ involvement. The 5-year survival rate with tumors less than 5 cm is 71%, compared with 25% in tumors greater than 5 cm. Survival decreases to 28% at 5 years with adjacent organ involvement. Grade is the most important prognostic factor. Survival with low-grade tumors is 62%, whereas that with high-grade tumors is only 12%. The liver and peritoneum are the most common sites of recurrence, followed by lymph nodes. Prognosis is poor in recurrent disease. Neither radiation therapy nor chemotherapy is of proven benefit in the management of this disease.

Carcinoid

Carcinoids are neuroendocrine tumors derived from Kulchitsky's cells, which are uncommonly found in the colon and rectum. They constitute 11% to 50% of all alimentary tract carcinoids. They are usually discovered incidentally unless they are large. Size and depth of invasion are the best predictors of clinical behavior. Tumors in this location almost never produce the carcinoid syndrome. Although large tumors may present with bleeding, obstruction, or constipation, tumors less than 2 cm are frequently asymptomatic. Diagnosis is made by endoscopic biopsy. In general, tumors less than 1 cm rarely metastasize, whereas those greater than 2 cm usually metastasize; in the 1- to 2-cm range, 10% to 20% will metastasize. This makes treatment decisions for tumors in the 1- to 2-cm range problematic. Small lesions (<1 cm) are commonly well differentiated and can be adequately treated with endoscopic excision. Tumors greater than 1 cm have associated lymphatic and distant metastases in 90% and 60% of cases, respectively. Lesions less than 2 cm can be treated with local excision. It is recommended that larger lesions, those that demonstrate invasion through the muscle wall, or inadequate resection margins be treated with standard resection techniques using either an anterior approach or APR. However, a recent retrospective review from this institution on 44 rectal carcinoids revealed that extensive surgery offered no survival advantage over local excision. At MDACC, we locally excise tumors less than 2 cm and resect those greater than 2 cm if sphincter preservation is possible. The experience with radiation therapy and chemotherapy in rectal carcinoids is not extensive enough to make recommendations regarding its use.

Squamous Carcinoma of the Anus

Epidemiology and Etiology

Anal cancers constitute 1% to 2% of all anorectal cancers. Anal cancer occurs most frequently during the sixth decade of life, except in the male homosexual population where the mean age at diagnosis is 39 years of age. Groups reported to be at increased risk of anal cancer include northern Brazilian females, homosexual males regardless of human immunodeficiency virus (HIV) status, women practicing receptive anal sex, and organ transplant patients.

Anal cancers are divided into two groups that differ in epidemiology, histologic type, and prognosis. Anal canal cancers (tumors proximal to the anal verge) comprise 67% of anal cancers. These cancers are three to four times more common in women than in men. Anal margin cancers (tumors distal to the anal verge) are more common in males. There are significantly more cases of anal margin cancers in homosexual males.

Anal cancer is associated with poor personal hygiene, chronic anal irritation, infection, cigarette smoking, and immune suppression. Other risk factors for the development of anal cancer include genital condyloma acuminatum, a history of gonorrhea in men, herpes simplex virus type I seropositivity, and a history of *Chlamydia trachomatis* infection. The presence of human papillomavirus (HPV) infection, especially serotypes 6, 11, 16, and 18, has been strongly linked to anal squamous carcinoma. Up to 54% of HIV-positive patients have HPV DNA in their anal canal, which may account for the increased incidence of anal cancers seen in this group.

Pathologic Characteristics

More than 80% of malignant anal lesions are histologically squamous cell carcinomas. With the exception of melanoma (see later), small cell carcinoma, and anal adenocarcinoma, all other histologic subtypes behave similarly and are treated according to their anatomic location. Basaloid carcinoma (basal cell carcinoma with a massive squamous component), mucoepidermoid carcinoma (originating in anal crypt glands), and cloacogenic carcinoma are all variants of squamous carcinoma. Malignant anal tumors may be preceded by or coexist with premalignant dysplasia or anal intraepithelial neoplasia.

The prognosis of anal margin cancers is favorable. The rate of local recurrence is higher than the rate of distant metastases, which are rare. When they do occur, metastases most commonly are found in the superficial inguinal lymph nodes (approximately 15% of cases). It is unusual for anal margin cancers to metastasize to mesenteric or internal iliac nodes.

Anal canal cancers are associated with aggressive local growth and if untreated will extend to the rectal mucosa and submucosa, subcutaneous perianal tissue and perianal skin, ischiorectal fat, local skeletal muscle, perineum, genitalia, lower urinary system, and even the pelvic peritoneum and the broad ligament. Historically, mesenteric lymph node metastases have been detected in 30% to 50% of surgical specimens. More than 50% of patients present with locally advanced disease. The most common sites of distant metastases are the liver, lung, and abdominal cavity. However, most cancer-related deaths are due to uncontrolled pelvic or perineal disease.

Diagnosis

The initial symptoms of anal cancer include bleeding, pain, and local fullness. These symptoms are similar to those caused by the common benign anal diseases, which accompany anal cancer in more than 50% of cases. A detailed history, including previous anal pathosis and sexual habits, should precede a meticulous physical examination. Physical examination should attempt to identify the lesion, its size and anatomic boundaries, and any

associated scarring or condylomata. It is also important to determine the resting and voluntary anal sphincter tone. Occasionally, an examination under general anesthesia may be necessary to complete the local evaluation. Pelvic and abdominal
CT scans and a chest radiograph are important in assessing extent of local disease and distant spread. Proctosigmoidoscopy is
essential to assess the proximal extent of disease and to obtain
tissue for biopsy. Endorectal ultrasound is the method of choice
for determining depth of tumor invasion as well as for detection of
early recurrence. Palpable inguinal lymph nodes should be evaluated by fine-needle aspiration.

Staging

The current American Joint Committee on Cancer (AJCC) staging system for anal margin and anal canal cancers is depicted in
Tables 11-5 and 11-6.

Treatment

ANAL MARGIN CANCER. Squamous cell carcinoma of the anal margin is defined currently by the AJCC as a lesion originating in an
area between the anal margin and 5 cm in any direction onto
the perianal skin. Note that the data supporting the treatment
of these uncommon, heterogeneous lesions derive from small,
single-institution, mostly retrospective studies. Moreover, many
of these studies include lesions of the lower anal canal (dentate
to anal verge) that were included previously in older definitions
of the anal margin. The rationale for any modality of therapy
derives from the proportional increase in chance of metastases
with increasing tumor size; in tumors less than 2 cm, lymph node
metastases are rarely found. For lesions between 2 and 5 cm,
and those greater than 5 cm, the rates are 24% and 25% to 67%,
respectively.

Small (<5 cm), superficial (T1–T2) anal margin cancers that do
not invade the sphincter complex can be treated by a negative-
margin wide local excision alone, with a 5-year survival rate
greater than 80%. Wide local excision may include parts of the
superficial internal and external anal sphincters without compromising anal continence. Radiation as primary treatment for
these smaller cancers can produce similar survival rates, with
local control in 80% of patients with 5-year survival rates in the
78% to 90% range. Complication rates are slightly higher with radiation therapy. Patients with local recurrence are treated with
further excision or APR, with excellent salvage rates.

Larger T2, T3 to T4, or T1 to T2, N-positive lesions are best
treated with multimodality therapy, as in anal canal cancers,
given the higher local recurrence rate. Prophylactic inguinal node
radiation is given to patients with T3 to T4 N0 lesions, and higher
doses of radiation are given to patients with positive inguinal
nodes. Lymph node dissection is reserved for those patients with
residual or recurrent disease. It is not known if the treatment of
inguinal disease translates into improved survival. Patients with
T3 to T4 and poor sphincter function are given APR. For all patients, the 5-year disease-specific survival is 71% to 88%, and the
local control rate after initial therapy is 70% to 100%.

Table 11-5. AJCC staging of anal canal cancer

Primary tumor (T)

TX	Primary tumor cannot be assessed
T0	No evidence of primary tumor
Tis	Carcinoma *in situ*
T1	Tumor ≤2 cm in greatest dimension
T2	Tumor >2 cm but not >5 cm in greatest dimension
T3	Tumor >5 cm in greatest dimension
T4	Tumor of any size invades adjacent organ(s)

Lymph nodes (N)

NX	Regional lymph nodes cannot be assessed
N0	No regional lymph node metastasis
N1	Metastasis in perirectal lymph node(s)
N2	Metastasis in unilateral internal iliac and/or inguinal lymph node(s)
	Metastasis in perirectal and inguinal lymph nodes and/or bilateral internal iliac and/or inguinal lymph nodes

Distant metastasis (M)

MX	Presence of distant metastasis cannot be assessed
M0	No distant metastasis
M1	Distant metastasis

Stage grouping

0	Tis	N0	M0
I	T1	N0	M0
II	T2	N0	M0
	T3	N0	M0
IIIA	T1	N1	M0
	T2	N1	M0
	T3	N1	M0
	T4	N0	M0
IIIB	T4	N1	M0
	Any T	N2	M0
	Any T	N3	M0
IV	Any T	Any N	M1

ANAL CANAL CANCER. Until the 1980s, APR with permanent colostomy was the recommended treatment for all anal canal cancers. This treatment, however, was attended by low survival rates as a result of distant failure. Radiation therapy in the range of 50 to 60 Gy was also used as definitive treatment of these cancers, with recurrence and survival rates similar to those seen using APR. The pioneering chemoradiation protocol developed by Nigro et al. (1983), which has since been confirmed and modified by others, has radically changed the approach to this disease. Currently, surgery is reserved for (a) T1 and small T2 lesions, which may be locally excised; (b) salvage treatment for patients with persistent disease (within 6 months of chemoradiation) or recurrent disease (after 6 months); (c) severely symptomatic patients (perineal sepsis, intractable urinary or fecal fistulae, intolerable

Table 11-6. AJCC staging of anal margin cancer

Primary tumor (T)

TX	Primary tumor cannot be assessed
T0	No evidence of primary tumor
Tis	Carcinoma *in situ*
T1	Tumor ≤2 cm in greatest dimension
T2	Tumor >2 cm but not >5 cm in greatest dimension
T3	Tumor >5 cm in greatest dimension
T4	Tumor invades deep extradermal structures (i.e., cartilage, skeletal muscle or bone)

Lymph nodes (N)

NX	Regional lymph nodes cannot be assessed
N0	No regional lymph node metastasis
N1	Regional lymph node metastasis

Distant metastasis (M)

MX	Presence of distant metastasis cannot be assessed
M0	No distant metastasis
M1	Distant metastasis

Stage grouping

0	Tis	N0	M0
I	T1	N0	M0
II	T2	N0	M0
	T3	N0	M0
III	T4	N0	M0
	Any T	N1	M0
IV	Any T	Any N	M1

incontinence); (d) inguinal lymph node dissection for persistent inguinal disease, recurrent inguinal disease (treated first with radiation therapy unless associated with local recurrence), or primary disease in the inguinal basin where the disease is bulky or fungating; and (e) temporary fecal diversion in patients with nearly obstructing lesions.

Since the initial work of Nigro et al. (1983), studies have been performed to dissect out the vital components and doses of the chemoradiation treatments to optimize treatment. There is evidence that (a) higher doses of radiation produce better local control rates using a constant mitomycin-C dose (Rich 1997); (b) 5-FU and mitomycin-C with radiation therapy produces better local control rates than radiation therapy alone; (c) 5-FU, mitomycin-C with radiation therapy produces better local control rates than 5-FU with radiation therapy; and (d) cisplatin with 5-FU and radiation therapy produces local control and survival rates similar to 5-FU, mitomycin-C mitomycin, and radiation therapy, possibly with less toxicity.

The current regimen for primary treatment of anal canal cancer and large anal margin cancers is chemoradiation therapy (Table 11-7). This has recently been changed from a 5-FU, mitomycin, radiation therapy protocol (45–55 Gy, with boosts up to 60 Gy) because of improved response rates, decreased toxicity,

Table 11-7. Treatment protocol for anal canal cancer

Days 1–4	5-FU, 750–1,000 mg/m^2 over 24-hr continuous IV infusion
Day 1	Mitomycin C, 10–15 mg/m^2, IV bolus (alternatively, bleomycin, 15 units once a week, or cisplatin, 4 mg m^{-2} d^{-1} with 5-FU dose reduced to 250–300 mg/m^2)
Days 1–35	Radiation therapy 5 d/wk for total dose of 45–55 Gy. Boosts of up to 60 Gy may be given to the anus and/or inguinal basins
Days 29–32	5-FU, 750–1,000 mg/m^2 over 24-hr continuous IV infusion

5-Fu, 5-fluorouracil; IV, intravenous.

and similar survival data. Complete responses with this treatment can be expected in up to 90% of patients, with 5-year survival rates approaching 85%. Patients with acquired immunodeficiency syndrome and anal cancer are poor candidates for high dose radiation therapy and the use of mitomycin. Current research is being directed at different chemotherapy regimes with lower dose radiation for this group.

Controversial issues involving the surgical oncologist include when to perform a biopsy after completion of the chemoradiation protocol and what therapy to initiate. It has been shown that a persistent mass after therapy will demonstrate cancer on biopsy in 18% to 34% cases. Moreover, the longer the time after completion of treatment, the higher the chances a mass will be a cancer on biopsy. There are reports of positive biopsy specimen results 6 to 8 weeks after therapy (persistent disease), which will revert to negative biopsy results in patients who have refused surgery. This implies that there may be a delayed radiation effect for up to several months after treatment. At MDACC we do not routinely obtain a biopsy specimen of the treated tumor site; instead we wait for clinical evidence of locally recurrent disease in follow-up visits.

Patients with local recurrence or persistent disease are almost all salvaged with APR. However, cisplatin-based chemotherapy with additional radiation therapy has been used successfully to salvage up to one third of patients with locally recurrent disease. These findings may allow a nonsurgical option, or a combined modality approach to recurrent or persistent disease.

Surveillance

Patients should be followed for detection of local and systemic failures as well as treatment complications. Local inspection, digital examination, anoscopy, and biopsy of any suspicious area are recommended every 3 months after chemoradiation treatment for 2 years, and twice a year thereafter. Early detection of local recurrence may enable less extensive salvage surgical procedures. Distant failures of epidermoid cancer are responsive to radiation therapy, and up to 30% of patients respond to second-line chemotherapy. Therefore chest radiography, LFTs, and pelvic CT are recommended every 6 to 12 months for 2 to 3 years after initial therapy. Patients with anal margin cancers should have careful, close follow-up, given the indolent nature of these tumors and the benefits of further local therapy.

Paget's and Bowen's Disease

Although not cancers, the uncommon lesions of Paget's and Bowen's disease are precancerous. Paget's disease is an intraepithelial adenocarcinoma that occurs mostly in elderly women. The lesion (a well-demarcated, eczematoid plaque) is usually characteristic; however, morphologic variations can occur, making the diagnosis difficult by inspection alone. The diagnosis is made histologically by the presence of large, vacuolated Paget's cells, which stain periodic acid-Schiff (PAS) positive (from high mucin content). There is some evidence for the association of perianal Paget's disease with other invasive carcinomas, but this relationship is not as strong as that seen with Paget's of the breast. Invasion can develop in these lesions, and the prognosis is poor in those cases.

Bowen's disease is an intraepithelial squamous cell carcinoma that develops in mostly middle-aged women. The lesion is raised, irregular, scaly, plaque-like, with eczematoid features. Histologically, large atypical haloed cells (Bowenoid cells) are seen that stain PAS negative. As in Paget's disease, there is an association in some studies with invasive carcinomas, suggesting the need for colonoscopy or barium enema examination.

The treatment for these lesions is not completely uniform, given their rarity. However, most small series report excellent long-term results with complete excision (minimal clear margins). Local recurrence is common, but reexcision provides excellent local control. Because the lesion can microscopically extend beyond the visible boundary, perianal mapping is suggested to outline all involved areas and to help plan the local excision (four quadrant biopsies at anal margin, anal verge, and dentate line). Because of the increased incidence of these lesions in immunocompromised patients, particularly HIV patients, other treatments have been used successfully, including 5-FU topical cream. This treatment is also useful in patients with widespread perianal disease where excision would be too morbid.

Anorectal Mucosal Melanoma

Epidemiology

Primary melanoma of the anus or rectum is a rare tumor, accounting for 0.4% to 1.6% of all melanomas and less than 1.0% of all tumors of the anorectum. The overall prognosis for patients with anorectal melanoma is dismal. The reported 5-year survival rate is only 6% to 17%, and the median survival time is only 19 to 25 months.

Pathologic Characteristics

Melanomas arising from the true rectum are less common than those developing at the squamocolumnar junction in the anal canal. Nodal metastases in the pelvis are more commonly associated with rectal tumors, whereas inguinal node disease is more likely to result from anal lesions. Most patients present with a clinically localized but advanced polypoid or nodular primary tumor. Prognosis is related to tumor thickness, as with cutaneous melanomas.

Diagnosis

Patients most commonly present with rectal bleeding. Some patients will complain of a painful rectal mass. Occasionally, melanoma will be an incidental pathologic finding after hemorrhoidectomy. Physical examination should include evaluation of the rectal mass as well as palpation of the inguinal nodes. A chest radiograph and LFTs should be performed to determine whether distant metastases are present. Abdominal and pelvic CT scans are helpful in determining the extent of local and regional disease.

Treatment

Although most patients will die of their disease regardless of therapy, there may be a group with disease confined to the primary site (smaller lesions) or mesenteric nodes that may benefit from more aggressive local therapy (APR). It has been found that, unlike epidermoid carcinoma of the anal canal, melanoma may preferentially spread to mesenteric rather than to inguinal lymph nodes. This argues in favor of APR rather than local excision because there is no better way to select patients for less aggressive, potentially curative surgery. On the other hand, sphincter-saving approaches have been advocated because, despite higher local recurrence rates, the overall outcome of these patients is the same. Certainly, APR is the treatment of choice for large, bulky tumors and recurrent disease. Therapeutic inguinal node dissection is indicated for palpable nodal disease. Because of the high incidence of local recurrence and inguinal nodal disease, regardless of treatment used, postoperative adjuvant irradiation of the tumor bed and nodal basins may be warranted.

RECOMMENDED READING

Arbman G, Nilsson E, Hallbrook O, et al. Local recurrence following total mesorectal excision for cancer. *Br J Surg* 1996;83:375.

Ballhausen WG. Genetic testing for familial adenomatous polyposis. *Ann NY Acad Sci* 2000;910:36.

Blend MJ, Abdel-Nabi H. New methods for the staging of colorectal cancer using noninvasive techniques. *Semin Surg Oncol* 1996;12:253.

Boland CR. Molecular genetics of hereditary nonpolyposis colorectal cancer. *Ann NY Acad Sci* 2000;910:50.

Boland CR, Sinicrope FA, Brenner DE, et al. Colorectal cancer prevention and treatment. *Gastroenterology* 2000;118:S115.

Brady MS, Kavolius JP, Quan SHQ. Anorectal melanoma: a 64-year experience at Memorial Sloan-Kettering Cancer Center. *Dis Colon Rectum* 1995;38:146.

Burt RW. Screening of patients with a positive family history of colorectal cancer. *Gastrointest Endosc Clin North Am* 1997;7:65.

Cawthorn SJ, Parums DV, Gibbs NM, et al. Extent of mesorectal spread and involvement of lateral resection margin as prognostic factors after surgery for rectal cancer. *Lancet* 1990;335:1055.

Cohen AM, Minsky BD, Friedman MA. Rectal cancer. In: DeVita VT, Hellman S, Rosenberg SA, eds. *Cancer: principles and practice of oncology*, 5th ed. Philadelphia: Lippincott, 1997.

Cohen AM, Minsky BD, Schilsky RL. Colon cancer. In: DeVita VT, Hellman S, Rosenberg SA, eds. *Cancer: principles and practice of oncology*, 5th ed. Philadelphia: Lippincott, 1997.

Cohen AM. Radical surgery for rectal cancer: why we fail and rationale for current clinical trials of adjuvant therapy. *Surg Onc Clin North Am* 2000;9:741.

Cranley JP. Proper management of the patient with a malignant colorectal polyp. *Gastrointest Endosc Clin North Am* 1993;3:661.

De Gramont A, Figer A, Seymour M, et al. Leucovorin and fluorouracil with or without oxaliplatin as first-line treatment in advanced colorectal cancer. *J Clin Oncol* 2000;18:2938.

Enker WE. Sphincter-preserving operations for rectal cancer. *Oncology* 1996;10:1673.

Enker WE, Paty PB, Minsky BD, et al. Restorative or preservative operations in the treatment of rectal cancer. *Surg Oncol Clin North Am* 1992;1:57.

Farouk R, Nelson H, Gunderson LL. Aggressive multimodality treatment for locally advanced irresectable rectal cancer. *Br J Surg* 1997;84:741.

Fisher B, Wolmark N, Rockette H, et al. Postoperative adjuvant chemotherapy or radiation therapy for rectal cancer: results from the NSABP Protocol R-01. *J Natl Cancer Inst* 1988;90:21.

Fleshman JW, Myerson RJ. Adjuvant radiation therapy for adenocarcinoma of the rectum. *Surg Clin North Am* 1997;77:15.

Franklin ME, Rosenthal D, Medina DA, et al. Prospective comparison of open vs. laparoscopic colon surgery for carcinoma. *Dis Colon Rectum* 1996;39:S35–S46.

Fuchs CS, Mayer RJ. Adjuvant chemotherapy for colon and rectal cancer. *Semin Oncol* 1995;22:472.

Galanis E, Alberts SR, O'Connell MJ. New adjuvant therapy for colon cancer. *Surg Oncol Clin North Am* 1988;9:813.

Gerard A, Buyse M, Nordlinger B. Preoperative radiotherapy as adjuvant treatment in rectal cancer: final results of a randomized study of the European Organization for Research and Treatment of Cancer (EORTC). *Ann Surg* 1988;208:606.

Gastrointestinal Tumor Study Group. Prolongation of the disease free interval in surgically treated rectal carcinoma. *N Engl J Med* 1985;312:1465.

Grann A, Minsky BD, Cohen AM, et al. Preliminary results of preoperative 5-fluorouracil, low dose leucovorin, and concurrent radiation therapy for clinically resectable T3 rectal cancer. *Dis Colon Rectum* 1997;40:515.

Grann A, Paty PB, Guillem JG, et al. Sphincter preservation of leiomyosarcoma of the rectum and anus with local excision and brachytherapy. *Dis Colon Rectum* 1999;42:1296.

Guleserian KJ, Bland KI. Current protocols and outcomes for colonic cancer. *Surg Oncol Clin North Am* 2000;9:725.

Gunderson LL, Nelson H, Martenson JA, et al. Locally advanced primary colorectal cancer: intraoperative electron and external beam irradiation < 5-FU. *Int J Radiol Oncol Biol Phys* 1997;37:601.

Haggitt RC, Glotzbach RE, Soffer EE, et al. Prognostic factors in colorectal carcinomas arising in adenomas: implications for lesions removed by endoscopic polypectomy. *Gastroenterology* 1985;89: 328.

Heriot AG, Grundy A, Kumar D. Preoperative staging of rectal carcinoma. *Br J Surg* 1999;86:17.

Hida J, Yasutomi M, Maruyama T, et al. Lymph node metastases detected in the mesorectum distal to carcinoma of the rectum by the clearing method: justification of total mesorectal excision. *J Am Coll Surg* 1997;184:584.

Janne PA, Mayer RJ. Primary care: chemoprevention of colorectal cancer. *N Engl J Med* 2000;342:1960.

Jessup JM, Bothe A, Stone MD, et al. Preservation of sphincter function in rectal carcinoma by a multimodality treatment approach. *Surg Oncol Clin North Am* 1992;1:137.

Jones DJ, James RD. Anal cancer. *BMJ* 1992;305:169.

Kafka NJ, Coller JA. Endoscopic management of malignant colorectal polyps. *Surg Oncol Clin North Am* 1996;5:633.

Kjeldsen BJ, Kronberg O, Fenger C, et al. A prospective randomized study of follow-up after radical surgery for colorectal cancer. *Br J Surg* 1997;84:666.

Koura A, Giacco G, Curley S, et al. Carcinoid tumors of the rectum. *Cancer* 1997;79:1294.

Lavery IC, Lopez-Kostner F, Pelley RJ, et al. Treatment of colon and rectal cancer. *Surg Clin North Am* 2000;80:535.

Lowy AM, Rich TA, Skibber JM, et al. Preoperative infusional chemoradiation, selective intraoperative radiation, and resection for locally advanced pelvic recurrence of colorectal adenocarcinoma. *Ann Surg* 1996;223:177.

Lynch HT, De la Chapelle A. Genetic susceptibility to non-polyposis colorectal cancer. *J Med Genet* 1999;36:801.

Mamounas E, Weiand S, Wolmark HD, et al. Comparative efficacy of adjuvant chemotherapy in patients with Duke's B versus Duke's C colon cancer: results from four National Surgical Adjuvant Breast and Bowel Project adjuvant studies (C-01, C-02, C-03, and C-04). *J Clin Oncol* 1999;17:1349.

Markowitz AJ, Winawer SJ. Management of colorectal polyps. *CA Cancer J Clin* 1997;47:93.

McCall JL, Black RB, Rich CA, et al. The value of serum carcinoembryonic antigen in predicting recurrent disease following curative resection of colorectal cancer. *Dis Colon Rectum* 1994;37: 875.

McCormack PM, Burt ME, Bains MS, et al. Lung resection for colorectal metastases: 10-year results. *Arch Surg* 1992;127:1403.

Mendenhall WM, Zlotecki RA, Vauthey J-N, et al. Squamous cell carcinoma of the anal margin. *Oncology* 1996;10:1843.

Meterissian SH, Skibber JM, Giacco GG, et al. Pelvic exenteration for locally advanced rectal carcinoma: factors predicting improved survival. *Surgery* 1997;121:479.

Milsom JW. Pathogenesis of colorectal cancer. *Surg Clin North Am* 1993;73:6.

Minsky BD. Multidisciplinary management of resectable rectal cancer. *Oncology* 1996;10:1701.

Moertel CG, Fleming TR, MacDonald JS, et al. Levamisole and fluorouracil for adjuvant therapy of resected colon carcinoma. *N Engl J Med* 1990;322:352.

Moertel CG, MacDonald JS. Fluorouracil plus levamisole as effective adjuvant therapy after resection of stage III colon carcinoma: a final report. *Ann Intern Med* 1995;122:321.

Nelson RL, ed. Anal and perianal cancer. *Semin Colon Rectal Surg* 1995;6:131.

Nigro ND, Sydel HG, Considine B, et al. Combined preoperative radiation and chemotherapy for squamous cell carcinoma of the anal canal. *Cancer* 1983;51:1286.

NIH Consensus Conference. Adjuvant therapy for patients with colon and rectal cancer. *JAMA* 1990;264:1444.

Nivatvongs S, Rojanasakul A, Reiman HM, et al. The risk of lymph node metastases in colorectal polyps with invasive adenocarcinoma. *Dis Colon Rectum* 1991;34:323.

Ota DM, Skibber R, Rich TA. M.D. Anderson Cancer Center experience with local excision and multimodality therapy for rectal cancer. *Surg Oncol Clin North Am* 1992;1:147.

Papillon J, Gerard JP. Role of radiotherapy in anal preservation for cancer of the lower third of the rectum. *Int J Radiat Oncol Biol Phys* 1990;19:1219.

Petros JG, Lopez MJ. Pelvic exenteration for carcinoma of the colon and rectum. *Surg Oncol Clin North Am* 1994;3:257.

Philipshen SJ, Heilweil M, Quan SHQ, et al. Patterns of pelvic recurrence following definitive resections of rectal cancer. *Cancer* 1983;53:1354.

Phillips RKS. Familial adenomatous polyposis: the surgical treatment of the colorectum. *Semin Colon Rectal Surg* 1995;6:33.

Quirke P, Durdey P, Dixon MF, et al. Local recurrence of rectal adenocarcinoma due to inadequate surgical resection. *Lancet* 1986; 11:996.

Ranshoff DF, Lang CA. Screening for colorectal cancer with the fecal occult blood test: a background paper. *Ann Intern Med* 1997;126: 811.

Rich TA. Infusional chemoradiation for operable rectal cancer: post-, pre-, or nonoperative management? *Oncology* 1997;11:295.

Rich TA, Skibber JM, Ajani JM, et al. Preoperative infusional chemoradiation therapy for stage T3 rectal cancer. *Int J Radiat Oncol Biol Phys* 1995;32:1025.

Rosen M, Chan L, Beart RWJ, et al. Follow-up of colorectal cancer: a meta-analysis. *Dis Colon Rectum* 1998;41:1116.

Rowe VL, Frost DB, Huang S. Extended resection for locally advanced colorectal carcinoma. *Ann Surg Oncol* 1997;4:131.

Rullier E, Laurent C, Charles J, et al. Local recurrence of low rectal cancer after abdominoperineal and anterior resection. *Br J Surg* 1997;84:525.

Saclarides TJ, Bhattacharyya AK, Britton-Kuzel C, et al. Predicting lymph node metastases in rectal cancer. *Dis Colon Rectum* 1994; 37:52.

Saltz LB, Cox JV, Blanke C, et al. Irinotecan plus fluorouracil and leucovorin for metastatic colorectal cancer. *N Engl J Med* 2000; 343:905.

Schild SE, Gunderson LL, Haddock MG, et al. The treatment of locally advanced colon cancer. *Int J Radiat Oncol Biol Phys* 1997;37:51.

SCOTIA Study Group. Single-stage treatment for malignant left-sided colonic obstruction: a prospective randomized clinical trial comparing subtotal colectomy with segmental resection following intraoperative irrigation. *Br J Surg* 1995;82:1622.

Scott N, Jackson P, Al-Jaberi T, et al. Total mesorectal excision and local recurrence: a study of tumor spread in the mesorectum distal to rectal cancer. *Br J Surg* 1995;82:1031.

Smith LE, Ko ST, Saclarides T, et al. Transanal endoscopic microsurgery-USA Registry results. *Dis Colon Rectum* 1995;38: P33.

Soreide O, Norstein J. Local recurrence after operative treatment of rectal carcinoma: a strategy for change. *J Am Coll Surg* 1997; 184:84.

Steele GD, Herndon JE, Burgess AM, et al. Sphincter sparing treatment for distal rectal adenocarcinoma: a phase II intergroup study. *Proc ASCO* 1997;16:256.

Stockholm Colorectal Cancer Study Group. Randomized study on preoperative radiotherapy in rectal carcinoma. *Ann Surg Oncol* 1996;3:423.

Swedish Rectal Cancer Trial. Improved survival with preoperative radiotherapy in resectable rectal cancer. *N Engl J Med* 1997;336: 980.

Tempero M, Brand R, Holdeman K, et al. New imaging techniques in colorectal cancer. *Semin Oncol* 1995;22:448.

Tepper JE, O'Connell MJ, Petroni GR, et al. Adjuvant postoperative fluorouracil-modulated chemotherapy combined with pelvic radiation therapy for rectal cancer: initial results of Intergroup 0114. *J Clin Oncol* 1997;15:2030.

Wanebo HJ, Koness RJ, Vezeridis MP, et al. Pelvic resection of recurrent rectal cancer. *Ann Surg* 1994;220:586.

Weinstein GD, Rich TA, Shumate CR, et al. Preoperative infusional chemoradiation and surgery with or without an electron beam intraoperative boost for advanced primary rectal cancer. *Int J Radiat Oncol Biol Phys* 1995;32:197.

Winawer SJ, Fletcher RH, Miller L, et al. Colorectal cancer screening: clinical guidelines and rationale. *Gastroenterology* 1997;112: 594.

Winde G, Nottberg H, Keller R, et al. Surgical cure for early rectal carcinomas (T1). Transanal endoscopic microsurgery vs. anterior resection. *Dis Colon Rectum* 1996;39:969.

Wolmark N, Rockette H, Fisher B, et al. The benefit of leucovorin modulated fluorouracil as postoperative adjuvant therapy for primary colon cancer: results from National Surgical Adjuvant Breast and Bowel Project Protocol C-03. *J Clin Oncol* 1993;11:1879.

Hepatobiliary Cancers

Syed A. Ahmad, Eddie K. Abdalla, Francis R.
Spitz, Michael Bouvet, and Alan M. Yahanda

SURGICAL ANATOMY OF THE LIVER

A basic knowledge of the anatomy of the liver is essential to the management of hepatic or biliary tract neoplasms. On the most elementary level, the liver can be divided into two parts (Fig. 12-1), or classic lobes. Cantlie described the functional anatomy of the liver in 1898 and more accurately divides the liver into two lobes by an imaginary line drawn between the gallbladder bed and the vena cava (Cantlie's line). The left lobe is further divided by the falciform ligament into the medial segment (the portion between the falciform ligament and Cantlie's line) and the lateral segment (the portion to the left of the falciform ligament). The right lobe is divided into anterior and posterior segments.

Most surgeons further conceptualize the segmental anatomy of the liver in the manner described by Couinaud. Each of the eight segments of the liver is defined by its distinct and separate arterial and portal vascular supply, as well as its biliary drainage (portal pedicle). Furthermore, the three main hepatic veins divide the liver into four sectors (Fig. 12-2). For example, the left hepatic vein divides segments 2 and 3 from segment 4. The middle hepatic vein divides segment 4 from segments 5 and 8, and the right hepatic vein divides segments 5 and 8 from segments 6 and 7. This sectoral anatomy forms the foundation on which modern hepatic surgery is performed. Finally, the portal pedicles are surrounded by Glisson's sheath, and this distinguishes this structure from hepatic veins when intraoperative ultrasonography is performed.

Liver resections can be classified as a trisegmentectomy (removal of the right lobe and the medial segment of the left lobe, or removal of the left lobe and either the anterior or posterior segment of the right lobe), a lobectomy (removal of the entire left or right lobe), a segmentectomy (removal of an anatomic segment of the liver, based on Couinaud's segmental anatomy), and a subsegmental or nonanatomic resection (see Fig. 12-1). An additional type of resection is a total hepatectomy, which can be done only in the setting of liver transplantation.

Anatomic variations of the hepatic artery are frequent. At The University of Texas M.D. Anderson Cancer Center, hepatic arterial variants are divided into ten types (Table 12-1). By far the most common types are I, II, and III, which constitute approximately 76% of all cases.

PRIMARY HEPATOCELLULAR CARCINOMA

Epidemiology

Primary hepatocellular carcinoma (HCC) is relatively rare in the United States, with an annual incidence of less than five cases

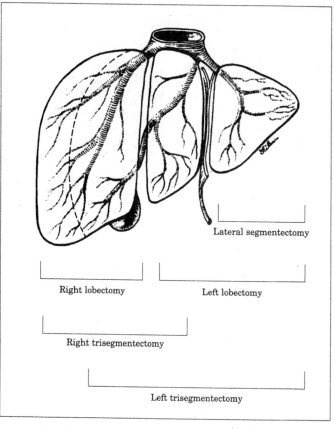

Lateral segmentectomy

Right lobectomy

Left lobectomy

Right trisegmentectomy

Left trisegmentectomy

Fig. 12-1. Liver anatomy with the description of common anatomic hepatic resections. (From Iwatsuki S, Sheahan DG, Starzl TE. The changing face of hepatic resection. *Curr Probl Surg* 1989;26:291.)

per 100,000. It is ranked as the 22nd most common type of cancer in the country. Globally, however, HCC is among the most common of solid human malignancies. It is one of the ten most common cancers in the world and is one of the most lethal malignancies, with a mortality index of 0.94. Chronic hepatitis B virus (HBV) and C virus (HCV) infections have been implicated as important etiologic factors in the development of HCC (2–5). A literature review reveals that among all patients diagnosed with HCC, the range of coexistent chronic HBV or HCV infection is 13% to 73% and 11% to 88%, respectively. The highest rates are found in countries in Southeast Asia including China, Korea, and Taiwan. In these countries, the incidence of HCC is greater than 20 per 100,000. The lowest rates are found in North America and Europe.

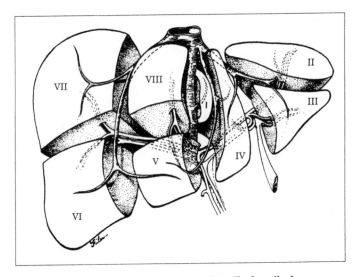

Fig. 12-2. Segmental liver anatomy as originally described by Couinaud. Each of the eight segments is based on its separate and distinct blood supply and biliary drainage. (From Iwatsuki S, Sheahan DG, Starzl TE. The changing face of hepatic resection. *Curr Probl Surg* 1989;26:291.)

Table 12-1. Hepatic arterial variations

Type I	RHA, MHA, and LHA arise from the CA (55%)
Type II	RHA and MHA arise from the CA, replaced LHA from the LGA (10%)
Type III	MHA and LHA arise from the CA, replaced RHA from the SMA (11%)
Type IV	MHA arises from the CA, replaced RHA from the SMA and replaced LHA from the LGA (1%)
Type V	RHA, MHA, LHA arise from the CA, accessory LHA from the LGA (1%)
Type VI	RHA, MHA, LHA arise from the CA, accessory RHA from the SMA (7%)
Type VII	RHA, MHA, LHA are from the CA, accessory LHA from the LGA, and accessory RHA from the SMA (1%)
Type VIII	Replaced RHA and an accessory LHA; or replaced LHA and an accessory RHA (2%)
Type IX	Absent celiac HA. Entire hepatic trunk arises from the SMA (4.5%)
Type X	Absent celiac HA. Entire hepatic trunk arises from the LGA (0.5%)
Type X	Double celiac HA (no common HA) (variant)

CA, celiac artery; HA, hepatic artery; LGA, left gastric artery; LHA, left hepatic artery; MHA, middle hepatic artery; RHA, right hepatic artery; SMA, superior mesenteric artry.

A number of other risk factors also have been implicated in HCC. Alcohol-related cirrhosis is probably the leading cause of HCC in the United States, Canada, and Western Europe. Dietary intake of aflatoxins is elevated in several countries with a high incidence of HCC. HCC also has been reported in association with several metabolic disorders, such as hemochromatosis, Wilson's disease, hereditary tyrosinemia, type I glycogen storage disease, familial polyposis coli, alpha-1 antitrypsin deficiency, and Budd-Chiari syndrome. Chemicals such as nitrites, hydrocarbons, and polychlorinated biphenyls also have been implicated as hepatic carcinogens. The resultant cirrhosis or chronic hepatocellular injury may be the common etiologic factor.

HCC is more likely to develop in men than in women. In high-incidence areas, the male-to-female ratio is approximately 8:1, and in low-incidence areas, the ratio is 4:1. HCC develops early in life in the high-incidence areas, whereas it occurs predominantly in the elderly in low-incidence areas. More important than the actual age of the patient, however, is the chronicity of the hepatitis viral infection or the cirrhosis.

Pathology

The majority of primary malignancies of the liver are HCC (85%–90%), with cholangiocarcinoma, angiosarcoma, and hepatoblastoma being much less common.

The histologic variations of HCC are of little importance in determining the treatment and prognosis of a patient. However, two exceptions should be noted. First, fibrolamellar carcinoma, is found in younger patients without cirrhosis, and is believed to carry a better prognosis. Second, adenomatous hyperplasia is a premalignant lesion that develops within a regenerating nodule in a cirrhotic liver. Therefore complete resection of adenomatous hyperplasia is curative.

HCC frequently spreads by local extension to the diaphragm and adjacent organs and into the portal and hepatic veins. Metastatic spread occurs most often to regional lymph nodes (periportal), lungs, bone, adrenal glands, and brain.

Clinical Presentation

Most patients with HCC have a history of HBV or HCV infection, alcoholic liver disease, or cirrhosis. The incidence of HCC increases with age in all populations. HCC usually presents at a late stage, often with upper abdominal pain or discomfort, a palpable right upper quadrant mass, weight loss, ascites, or other sequelae of portal hypertension. Jaundice is relatively uncommon. Physical examination may reveal firm, nodular hepatomegaly, a hepatic rub, or an arterial bruit in the right upper quadrant. The triad of abdominal pain, weight loss and an abdominal mass is the most common clinical presentation. In fewer than 5% of cases, patients present with tumor rupture. Numerous paraneoplastic complications have been described, including hypoglycemia, hypercalcemia, erythrocytosis, and hypertrophic pulmonary osteoarthropathy.

Diagnosis

HCC usually is diagnosed at a late stage, unless found accidentally during other investigations. Certain laboratory and radiologic findings should raise one's suspicion for HCC. Alpha-fetoprotein (AFP) is increased in 50% to 90% of all patients with HCC, with levels greater than 400 ng/mL usually found in those with large tumors or rapidly growing tumors. In healthy adults, serum AFP levels normally are less than 20 ng/mL. A patient with a small HCC may have minimal or even no elevation of AFP. Transient increases in AFP also may be seen with inflammatory hepatic disease or cirrhosis. Serum AFP measurements are used to monitor patients for tumor recurrence because levels should fall to normal after curative resection. Studies also have shown a correlation between AFP elevation, tumor stage, and patient prognosis.

Radiologic confirmation of a mass in the liver can be made by either ultrasound (US) or computed tomography (CT). US, which is as sensitive and specific as CT for detecting small lesions (<3 cm in diameter), has the advantage of being relatively inexpensive. As a result, US has been used extensively as a screening tool in regions with a high incidence of HCC. Although US has these advantages, the sensitivity and specificity of transabdominal US are low, with an overall false-negative rate of more than 50%. In addition, lesions at the dome of the liver adjacent to the lung base may be difficult to image. Intraoperative US, however, is considered the gold standard for the detection of liver lesions.

Conventional CT can detect larger lesions in the liver and assess the presence of extrahepatic disease. At M.D. Anderson Cancer Center, the imaging modality of choice is one of the newer generation helical CT scanners, which have the advantage of speed and can image the abdomen at various phases of contrast enhancement. Three phases of enhancement have been observed: after an injection of a bolus of contrast material, an early vascular or arterial phase, a portal phase, and a delayed phase can be seen. The early arterial phase is used to image hypervascular tumors, such as HCC or metastatic neuroendocrine tumors. The portal-dominant phase is used to detect hypovascular tumors, such as metastatic adenocarcinoma or cholangiocarcinoma. Sensitivity can be improved by using CT angiography, in which a contrast agent is injected into the hepatic artery during the study. The blood supply to HCC is derived almost entirely from the hepatic artery; thus, the tumor will appear as a hyperdense area on the scan. The accuracy of the study depends on the uniform distribution of the contrast agent to both lobes of the liver. Unfortunately, this is not always possible in a diseased, cirrhotic liver or with variant hepatic arterial anatomy. At M.D. Anderson, this test is performed only when there is a concern about the hepatic arterial anatomy, such as when the placement of a hepatic infusion pump is planned.

CT with arterial portography (CTAP) has proved to be the best method to study mass lesions in the liver. In CTAP, a contrast agent is injected into the superior mesenteric artery or the splenic artery before the scan. Delayed images are then taken when contrast material has entered the portal venous system. Because it is not well perfused by the portal system, HCC is seen as a low-density area against the surrounding liver parenchyma. The sensitivity of CTAP in identifying liver lesions is reported to be as high as 97%.

More recently, magnetic resonance imaging (MRI) with magnetic resonance angiography has demonstrated reliable sensitivity, and the technique provides good information concerning the anatomic relationship of the tumor and major vessels. MRI has an advantage over CT in that it does not rely on the use of contrast agents for detecting lesions.

Lipiodol has been used in Asia and Europe to aid in evaluating small HCCs. Lipiodol, an oily derivative of the poppy seed combined with iodine contrast medium, is retained by HCC cells. It is injected into the hepatic artery, and a CT scan is performed 1 to 2 weeks later. Lesions as small as a few millimeters can be detected with this technique.

The histologic diagnosis of HCC can be obtained by percutaneous needle biopsy or by fine-needle aspiration of the mass, usually under US guidance. However, the risk of hemorrhage following this procedure is not insignificant, because most HCCs are hypervascular, and patients may have ascites or some degree of coagulopathy. Tumor seeding of the biopsy track, a rare event, has been reported. Therefore a preoperative liver biopsy is unnecessary unless the workup has demonstrated that the lesion is unresectable and tissue is needed to plan appropriate alternative therapy.

The evaluation of the patient is completed with a chest radiograph to exclude pulmonary metastases. Further studies, such as a CT scan of the brain or a bone scan, are not indicated in the absence of clinical indications of metastases to these areas.

Staging

The current American Joint Committee on Cancer (AJCC) staging system for HCC is shown in Table 12-2.

Evaluation of Operative Risk

Before contemplating major surgery, let alone hepatic resection, in a patient with a diseased liver, one must determine whether the patient has adequate liver function to tolerate surgery and anesthesia. In addition, one must try to predict whether the remaining liver will have adequate hepatic function after tumor resection. This assessment has been plagued by the lack of specific tests to determine hepatic function and hepatic reserve. Traditionally, the Child-Pugh classification or its modifications have been applied to liver resection in the same manner in which they were used originally in portosystemic shunt surgery. The parameters measured in this classification scheme give a rough estimation of the gross synthetic and detoxification capacity of the liver. Numerous studies have validated this system as a predictor of survival in cirrhotic patients. Several other tests have been devised, to better evaluate liver function, including the urea-nitrogen synthesis rate, galactose elimination capacity, indocyanine green (ICG) clearance, and Bromsulphalein and aminopyrine breath tests.

Table 12-2. AJCC staging system for primary liver cancer

Primary tumor (T)

TX	Primary tumor cannot be assessed
T0	No evidence of tumor
T1	Solitary tumor ≤2 cm without vascular invasion
T2	Solitary tumor ≤2 cm with vascular invasion; or multiple tumors ≤2 cm, limited to one lobe without vascular invasion; or solitary tumor >2 cm without vascular invasion
T3	Solitary tumor >2 cm with vascular invasion; or multiple tumors ≤2 cm, limited to one lobe with vascular invasion; or multiple tumors, any >2 cm, limited to one lobe, with or without vascular invasion
T4	Multiple tumors in more than one lobe; or tumor involving a major branch of the portal or hepatic vein(s)

Regional lymph nodes (N)

NX	Regional lymph nodes cannot be assessed
N0	No regional lymph node metastasis
N1	Regional lymph node metastasis

Distant metastasis (M)

MX	Presence of distant metastasis cannot be assessed
M0	No distant metastasis
M1	Distant metastasis

Stage grouping

Stage I	T1	N0	M0
Stage II	T2	N0	M0
Stage IIIA	T3	N0	M0
Stage IIIB	T1–3	N1	M0
Stage IVA	T4	Any N	M0
Stage IVB	Any T	Any N	M1

Adapted from *AJCC Manual for Staging of Cancer*, 5th ed. Philadelphia: Lippincott-Raven, 1998.

At M.D. Anderson, portal vein embolization (PVE) is performed preoperatively in selected patients before extensive liver resections when the potential exists for postoperative complications as a result of inadequate volume of remaining liver. The rationale for this technique is to induce hypertrophy of the future liver remnant (FLR). FLR is calculated based on CT volumetric analysis as well as a standardized formula incorporating age, sex and body surface area. PVE is performed if the anticipated liver remnant volume is 25% or less of the total liver volume, and for patients with compromised liver function when the liver remnant volume is 40% or less.

In experienced hands, liver resection is safe, with a 1% to 5% mortality. Most perioperative deaths are due to liver failure, hemorrhage, and sepsis. The most common complications after liver surgery include perihepatic abscess, wound infection, bile leak, and pneumonia.

The preoperative evaluation of liver function at M.D. Anderson is based primarily on the Child-Pugh classification scheme. The age of the patient is taken into consideration. Coexisting medical problems, such as ischemic heart disease and chronic obstructive pulmonary disease, are investigated, as these are known to be poor prognostic factors. We do not use any other tests, such as the aminopyrine breath test or ICG clearance, in the preoperative workup of liver function.

Surgical Therapy

The definitive treatment for resectable HCC remains surgery. Unfortunately, of the patients presenting with HCC, only 10% to 30% will be eligible for surgery, and of those patients who undergo exploration, only 50% to 70% will have a resection with curative intent. The criteria that render a tumor unresectable include (a) the presence of extrahepatic disease, (b) evidence of severe hepatic dysfunction, (c) extensive tumor that would leave too little liver remaining following extirpation, and (d) tumor involvement of the portal vein or vena cava. The latter criterion has become more of a relative contraindication because many surgeons are now resecting portions of involved portal vein and hepatic artery.

The operative approach to the patient with a potentially resectable HCC should begin with a thorough surgical exploration of the abdomen, searching for any evidence of extrahepatic disease. In particular, care is taken to evaluate the periportal lymph nodes, as well as the nodes in the hepatoduodenal ligament. The liver is then completely mobilized to allow full examination of the organ. Intraoperative US should be used to define both the size of the tumor and its relationship to the major vascular and biliary structures. Intraoperative US has been shown to alter the surgical management plan in 18% of patients.

Once the tumor has been determined to be resectable, the decision must be made as to how much liver to remove. This will depend, in part, on the size of the mass, the number of nodules, the tumor's proximity to vascular structures, and the severity of the liver disease. Most surgeons believe a 1-cm margin of uninvolved tissue around a tumor is adequate. Larger HCCs, especially those in cirrhotic livers, should have the widest margin possible that will leave a sufficient amount of remnant tissue. In such cases, it may be necessary to compromise on the 1-cm tumor-free margin. A segmentectomy is usually practical only for small tumors. Several series have demonstrated that for HCCs smaller than 3 cm, the best operation is a segmentectomy. More radical surgeries for these lesions are accompanied by higher operative morbidity and mortality without any reduction in the recurrence rate or improvement in survival. On the other hand, lesser operations, such as wedge resections, should be discouraged, because they are associated with high rates of recurrence. The extent of the resection is often limited by the concomitant presence of cirrhosis and impaired liver function. In these cases, nonanatomic or subsegmental resections are useful to preserve as much liver as possible.

Recurrence rates following hepatic resection range from 30% to 70% in the literature. The site of recurrence usually is intrahepatic. Tumor size, number, and positive margin of resection are by far the most significant factors predicting tumor recurrence. Other risk factors include capsular or vascular invasion by tumor cells, high histologic grade, absence of a pseudocapsule, presence of cirrhosis, and tumor located deep in the liver. Positive HBV or HCV serology also seems to increase the risk of tumor recurrence. We recently reviewed the records of 77 patients who underwent margin-negative resections for HCC. With a median follow-up of 30 months, a significantly decreased local disease-free survival (LDFS) was seen in HBV-positive (5-year LDFS, 26%) and HCV-positive (5-year LDFS, 38%) patients compared to those with negative serology (LDFS, 79%). A trend toward a decreased overall survival was noted in patients with positive hepatitis serology compared to patients with negative serology (37% vs. 79%).

Survival data vary, depending on the patient population. In western countries where HCC is less frequently associated with HBV infection or cirrhosis, 2- and 3-year survival rates are 23% to 51%. In countries where patients have a history of hepatitis and cirrhosis, 5-year survival is 10% to 39%.

In a series by Yamanaka et al. (1997), in selected patients with no vascular invasion, solitary lesions, tumor diameter less than 5 cm and a negative margin of resection of more than 1 cm, the 5-year survival rate following resection was as high as 78%.

The role of orthotopic liver transplantation (OLT) in the treatment of HCC is not completely defined. In theory, total hepatectomy seems advantageous because it would remove the entire diseased organ, thereby reducing recurrences and improving survival. In the larger series reported in the literature, the survival rates for patients undergoing OLT for HCC range from 15% to 35% at 5 years and are no better, or are even worse, than those reported for subtotal resection. Likewise, the tumor recurrence rates with OLT are similar to those for subtotal hepatic resection. The risk factors that predict cancer recurrence following OLT are similar to those that predict a high risk of recurrence after partial hepatectomy. These include vascular invasion, tumor size greater than 5 cm, multiple hepatic tumors, lymph node metastases, and advanced stage of disease. However, OLT may confer improved survival in several subpopulations. The Pittsburgh group found that when HCC was associated with cirrhosis, OLT provided a significant survival advantage over subtotal resection at each tumor stage. This survival advantage was absent in the noncirrhotic patients. More recent studies have demonstrated that if OLT is restricted to patients with solitary HCC less than 5 cm or to patients with less than three tumor nodules each less than 3 cm, recurrence is low and 4-year survival rates are 75%. The Pittsburgh group reported 20 patients who underwent preoperative, intraoperative, and post-OLT systemic doxorubicin infusion, resulting in an overall survival of 59% and a disease-free survival of 54% at 3 years.

Cryosurgery has been advocated as an alternative to resection for HCC. With this technique, liquid nitrogen is circulated through a vacuum-insulated metal probe placed in the tumor.

Placement of the probe and treatment are monitored by intraoperative US. Each freezing takes 15 to 20 minutes, and multiple areas may be treated, particularly with larger tumors. This technique generally has been reserved for patients with unresectable tumors, although it can be used in combination with a resection. Cryosurgery has the advantage of treating the tumor and a small area of surrounding liver parenchyma; a disadvantage is that it necessitates both an anesthetic and a laparotomy. Serious complications that can occur with cryosurgery include intraoperative hemorrhage from the cryoprobe tract, bile duct fistula, and renal failure related to myoglobinuria. In a study of 107 patients treated with cryosurgical therapy, Zhou et al. (1993) found 5- and 10-year survival rates of 22% and 8.2%, respectively. For a subset of 32 patients with HCC less than 5 cm in diameter, the 5- and 10-year survival rates were 49% and 17%, respectively.

Management of previously resected HCC that recurs in the liver is difficult. Further liver resection usually is not possible without subjecting the patient to certain postoperative liver failure. Most patients should be treated with surgical therapies that do not require resection, such as cryosurgery, or with nonoperative therapies, such as percutaneous ethanol injection (PEI) or chemoembolization. As mentioned, OLT can be considered in highly selected cases.

PEI has been used with some success in patients with cirrhosis who are ineligible for surgery. Absolute alcohol induces cellular dehydration, necrosis, and vascular thrombosis, causing tumor cell death. PEI is contraindicated in patients with gross ascites, coagulopathy, and obstructive jaundice. With this technique, US is used to direct the placement of a needle into the tumor. Eight to 10 mL of 95% ethanol is injected through the needle.

These treatments are repeated once or twice a week on an outpatient basis. Several studies have documented survival rates following this treatment that are similar to, or even better than, those obtained with hepatic resection. The largest reported series is by Livraghi et al. (1992), who treated 207 cirrhotic HCC patients with PEI. These patients were deemed to have unresectable tumors or to be at too high a surgical risk, or they had refused surgery. Most of the patients were Child's class A (66%) and had lesions less than 5 cm in diameter. The 3-year survival rates for patients with single and multiple lesions were 63% and 31%, respectively. Currently, patients with HCC less than 3 cm and with fewer than three lesions are candidates for PEI. Liver recurrence after PEI is high, in the range of 50% at 2 years.

Radiofrequency ablation (RFA) has recently been used to treat primary liver tumors. A combined report of 110 patients from the University of Texas M.D. Anderson Cancer Center and the G. Pascale National Cancer Institute in Naples, Italy has been published recently. The HCC tumor size treated with RFA in this patient population ranged from 1 to 7 cm in greatest dimension. As the size of the tumor increased, the number of deployments of the multiple array needle electrode and the total time of applying RF energy increased. Primary liver tumors tend to be highly vascular, so a vascular heat sink phenomenon may contribute to the extended ablation times.

All 110 patients with HCC in this recent study were observed for a minimum of 12 months after RFA; the median follow-up was 19 months. Percutaneous or intraoperative RFA was performed in 76 (69%) and 34 patients (31%), respectively. A total of 149 discrete HCC tumor nodules were treated with RFA. Median diameter of tumors treated percutaneously (2.8 cm) was smaller than lesions treated during laparotomy (4.6 cm) (P <0.01). Local tumor recurrence at the RFA site developed in four patients (3.6%), all with tumors greater than 4.0 cm in diameter; in all four patients, recurrent HCC subsequently developed in other areas of the liver. New liver tumors or extrahepatic metastases developed in 50 patients (45.5%), but 56 patients (50.9%) have no evidence of recurrence. Clearly, a longer follow-up period is required to establish long-term disease-free and overall survival rates.

Chemotherapy

Systemic chemotherapy has little activity against HCC. Single-agent chemotherapy provides response rates of 15% to 20%, and the responses usually are short lasting. Combination chemotherapy does not seem to improve these results. The most active agent appears to be doxorubicin, with an overall response rate pooled from several trials of 19%.

A variety of regional treatments have been studied in an effort to improve the poor results obtained with systemic chemotherapy. Intraarterial infusion of chemotherapeutic agents is advantageous for several reasons. Because the blood supply to HCC is derived from the hepatic arteries, intraarterial infusion allows high concentrations of cytotoxic drugs to be delivered directly to the tumor. In addition, because these agents are metabolized in the liver, their systemic levels can be minimized.

Numerous studies have evaluated the effects of intraarterial infusion of single and multiple chemotherapeutic agents. Although intraarterial therapy appears to be associated with some survival benefit, few prospective trials have compared it with standard intravenous (IV) systemic chemotherapy. Intraarterial doxorubicin, alone or in combination with other agents, has produced the best response rates. Recently, transarterial chemotherapy and lipiodolization of hydrophilic drugs, such as epirubicin, have been tested. Improved response rates and a trend toward improved survival have been noted.

Hepatic artery ligation or occlusion has been used as a palliative treatment for unresectable HCC. It can offer significant symptomatic relief in some patients. This palliation, however, usually is transient, because collateral vessels quickly revascularize the liver.

Transcatheter arterial embolization (TAE) is basically a combination of both intraarterial infusion chemotherapy and hepatic artery occlusion. Chemotherapeutic agents are either infused into the liver before embolization or impregnated in the gelatin sponges used for the embolization. Lipiodol also has been used in conjunction with TAE. When it is combined with cytotoxic drugs or radionuclides and injected into the hepatic artery,

Lipiodol will remain selectively in HCC tissue for an extended period, delivering locally concentrated therapy. The treatment protocols that have produced the highest survival rates are TAE with gelatin sponges containing the chemotherapeutic agent or TAE with gelatin sponges and Lipiodol mixed with the chemotherapeutic agent. There was a slight survival difference in favor of those treated by the former regimen, with 2-year survival rates of 55% and 43%, respectively. However, prospective randomized trials have failed to demonstrate an advantage for chemoembolization over embolization.

More recently, immunotherapy, chemo-immunotherapy, and hormonal therapy have been used to manage unresectable HCC. Improved response rates have been obtained with interferon alfa when compared to systemic doxorubicin. A combination of cisplatin, doxorubicin, 5-fluorouracil (5-FU), and interferon alfa resulted in a partial response rate of 26%. Finally, data on the anti-estrogen drug tamoxifen remain unclear. Several randomized trials have shown improved response rates and survival with tamoxifen when compared to placebo in patients with unresectable HCC. Other randomized trials, however, have found no difference.

Radiation Therapy

External beam radiation therapy has limited usefulness in the treatment of HCC. The dose that can be safely delivered to the liver is approximately 30 Gy; higher doses cause radiation hepatitis. Radiation therapy can, however, provide palliative, symptomatic relief among patients with HCC. Alternatively, locally concentrated doses of radiation can be delivered with intraarterial infusion of Lipiodol or with antiferritin antibodies that are coupled with radioactive iodine.

Multimodality Therapy

Combinations of surgical and nonsurgical therapies are currently the state of the art in the treatment of HCC. Some tumors that previously were considered unresectable now can be rendered resectable with intraarterial chemotherapy and radiation therapy. A variety of chemotherapeutic agents have been studied in the neoadjuvant setting, including doxorubicin, 5-FU, mitomycin C, and cisplatin. Furthermore, tumor recurrence may be prevented by the administration of adjuvant intraarterial chemotherapy after surgical resection, ethanol injection, or cryosurgery.

METASTASIS TO THE LIVER

Virtually every malignant tumor has been known to metastasize to and proliferate in the liver. Most of these metastases are from gastrointestinal primary tumors, especially from the colon and rectum. In collected series of resected noncolorectal metastases to the liver, 5-year survivors are uncommon. However, in series of highly selective groups of patients with noncolorectal metastases, 5-year survival rates of 40% have been reported. These patient series represent a small percentage of patients with noncolorectal metastasis, and presently no well-defined criteria have been established for selecting patients for surgical resection. The exceptions to this appear to be metastases from neuroendocrine tumors, Wilms' tumor, and, to a lesser extent, renal cell carcinoma. With neuroendocrine tumors, even a subtotal resection of gross disease can provide significant palliation by decreasing the volume of hormone-secreting tumor. Given that the vast majority of liver metastases that are considered for resection are from colorectal primary tumors, the remainder of this discussion is concerned with their management.

Epidemiology and Etiology

Based on data from the American Cancer Society, colorectal cancer represents the third most common type of cancer for both men and women, with an estimated incidence of 130,000 new cases per year in the United States. Approximately 85% of these patients will have malignancies that are amenable to surgical cure but half of these resected cancers will recur within 5 years. Only 20% of these recurrences will be solely or predominantly in the liver, and fewer still will be amenable to surgical resection. It has been estimated that less than 5,000 patients a year are potential candidates for resection of their liver metastases.

Metastatic disease is discovered in the liver at the time of the initial presentation for the primary lesion (synchronous lesions) in approximately 25% of patients. The remainder will have their metastatic disease found some time following resection of the primary (metachronous) lesions. Metachronous lesions are associated with a stage III primary tumor in approximately 60% of cases, and the disease-free interval is usually less than 2 years.

Clinical Presentation

Symptoms or clinical signs suggesting metastatic disease in the liver usually are late occurrences. Consequently, findings such as ascites, jaundice, right upper quadrant pain, and increases in liver function values are associated with a poor prognosis.

Diagnosis

In the vast majority of patients, metastases to the liver are found through routine postoperative carcinoembryonic antigen (CEA) screening or radiologic imaging following resection of their colorectal primary tumor. Any patient with an increasing CEA level should undergo a thorough diagnostic evaluation, including a chest radiograph and a contrast-enhanced CT scan of the abdomen and pelvis. A slowly increasing CEA usually indicates local or regional recurrence, whereas a rapidly increasing CEA suggests hepatic metastases. Overall, 75% to 90% of patients with hepatic colorectal metastases have an increased CEA. In addition, the colon should be examined by either a barium enema examination or, preferably, colonoscopy to exclude a metachronous colon or rectal primary tumor as the source of the increasing CEA.

Determining Resectability

In cases in which the initial evaluation suggests that the metastatic disease is isolated to the liver, one must determine whether the patient is a candidate for surgical resection. Patients should be studied further with triple-phase helical CT scans or with

CTAP to better depict small lesions that might have been missed by standard CT. The rationale for CTAP in this setting is the same as that for primary tumors of the liver: metastatic lesions derive the majority of their blood supply from the hepatic artery, not the portal vein. At the time of CTAP, visceral angiography is performed to exclude tumor encasement of major blood vessels and the presence of any hepatic arterial anomalies.

MRI has been used more often. In the T1-weighted images, metastases are low intensity, and angiographic or three-dimensional reconstructive images can demonstrate the relationship of the tumor to major blood vessels.

Many investigators have attempted to identify the group of patients who will benefit from hepatic resection. The only true contraindication to resection of hepatic colorectal metastases is the presence of extrahepatic disease and the inability to achieve complete resection. The number of metastases and the presence of bilobar disease, although found to influence the prognosis in some studies, have not been found to consistently impact survival and therefore are no longer considered contraindications to resection. In one series among 12 long-term survivors in whom four or more metastases were removed, nine remained disease-free at 5 to 14 years after surgery. Other relative contraindications to hepatic resection include tumor size greater than 10 cm (5-year survival <14%) and presence of coexisting serious medical problems. In a recent report by Fong et al. (1997) patient age greater than 70 was not associated with a worse prognosis (5-year survival <36%). Although positive margins appear to nearly universally affect survival, long-term survival for patients with less than 1 cm margin is possible; however, the overall survival rate is reduced by inadequate margins. Overall 5- and 10-year survivals are 37% and 21%, respectively, with 1- to 9-mm margin versus 43% and 28%, respectively with 10 mm or greater margin. An anticipated close resection margin (1–9 mm) does not constitute a contraindication to resection. The presence of extrahepatic metastases traditionally has been considered another contraindication to hepatic resection. Hughes et al. (1988), however, found that patients with extrahepatic metastases resected simultaneously with the hepatic resection did not have statistically significant reduced overall survival. The disease-free survival, nonetheless, was significantly shorter.

In patients whose liver metastases are deemed resectable by preoperative evaluation, histologic identification of the mass before exploration is not necessary. Percutaneous biopsy of lesions under US or CT guidance may be necessary, however, before initiation of alternative therapies in patients for whom surgical resection is not indicated.

Evaluation of Operative Risk

Patients undergoing surgery for metastases to the liver differ from those with HCC in that cirrhosis usually is not present. This does not relieve the surgeon of the responsibility of determining the preoperative condition of the liver parenchyma and the expected adequacy of hepatic reserve following tumor resection. The preoperative evaluation of liver function is the same as that outlined for patients with HCC. A preoperative CT scan of the abdomen and pelvis and a chest radiograph should be obtained in all surgical candidates. In addition, all patients require full colonoscopy to rule out local recurrence or metachronous colorectal cancer.

Surgical Therapy

Once the metastases are deemed to be potentially resectable, the patient should undergo a thorough exploratory laparotomy. Particular attention should be paid to the presence of any extrahepatic disease and enlarged portal and celiac lymph nodes. The colon should be examined for any local recurrences of the primary tumor. The liver is examined first by visual inspection and palpation and then by intraoperative US. This study will help define the relationship of the tumor(s) to the portal veins, hepatic veins, and vena cava. In addition, it can identify small lesions that were not palpable or demonstrable on preoperative imaging studies. Suspicious areas can be sampled by fine-needle aspiration under US guidance. Complete exploration combined with intraoperative US reveals that nearly half of all patients have unresectable disease. In a prospective trial conducted by the Gastrointestinal Tumor Study Group (GITSG), 42% of patients who underwent surgical exploration were found to have unresectable tumors, and only 46% underwent curative resection. More than two-thirds of the patients had tumors deemed unresectable as a result of anatomic constraints, such as the proximity of the tumor to major blood vessels or the presence of bilobar disease.

The type of resection performed will depend on the size, number, and location of the lesions. In all cases, the resection must achieve at least a 1-cm tumor-free margin. Thinner margins invariably are associated with local recurrences and shorter survival times. Solitary lesions smaller than 4 cm usually can be extirpated with either a nonanatomic resection or a segmentectomy. Larger lesions should be approached with an anatomic lobectomy, if at all possible. This strategy is supported by Yamamoto's studies on the pattern of intrahepatic spread in 89 patients with metastatic colorectal cancer. Nine patients had gross extension to Glisson's sheath, eight had bile duct invasion, and one had neural invasion. The distance from the edge of the tumor to the tip of the extension ranged from 4 mm to 23 mm.

The presence of bilobar metastases is not necessarily a contraindication to resection. Patients with multiple unilobular metastases have no survival advantage or prolongation of disease-free survival compared with patients with a comparable number of bilobar metastases. What dictates resectability is the amount of normal, functioning liver parenchyma that will remain after the lesions are removed. Small lesions are best treated with multiple segmentectomies; these can be performed safely in up to three isolated segments. Larger bilobar lesions or those involving more than three segments should be removed with a trisegmentectomy if their locations and the patient's hepatic reserve allow such a major procedure.

In experienced hands, liver resection is safe, with a 1% to 5% mortality. The most common cause of death is perioperative hemorrhage or liver failure. Postoperative complications occur in 12% to 43% of all patients. The most common sources of morbidity are hepatic failure, bile leak (biloma or biliary fistula), intraabdominal hemorrhage, and subphrenic or intraabdominal abscess. In most reported series of hepatic resection for colorectal metastases, the 5-year survival rate ranges from 25% to 40%, with a median survival of 33 to 42 months.

Despite surgical removal of all gross tumor, most patients will have a tumor recurrence after hepatic resection. In the two large series compiled by Hughes et al. (1986) and by Fong et al. (1997), the recurrence rates were 70% and 51%, respectively. Results from the GITSG study were better, with a reported recurrence rate of 49%. The patterns of recurrence have been described in detail by Hughes et al. (1986). Of 607 patients treated with hepatic resection, 316 had initial recurrences at one site. The liver (47%) and lung (23%) were the most common sites of initial recurrence. Analysis of late recurrences showed a similar distribution, with involvement of the liver in 43% of patients and the lungs in 31%. Late recurrent disease arose in the liver alone in only 16% of patients. Fong et al. (1997) have reported the liver as the first site of recurrence in 41% of their patients. As a result, patients who have recurrences after hepatic resection for liver metastases are seldom candidates for further resective surgery. Nevertheless, several authors have reported results of hepatic surgical resections for recurrent colorectal metastasis, with median survivals ranging from 23 to 39 months.

Synchronous liver metastases, in general, should not be resected at the same operation as the primary tumor. The exception would be a solitary, small, peripherally located lesion in a healthy, hemodynamically stable patient that could be adequately excised with a wedge resection. Lesions that are larger or that will require a major hepatic resection are best approached during a second operation after further evaluation and staging. A delay of weeks to months between surgeries has not been shown to have a negative impact on survival. Obviously, at the time of the initial operation, a thorough exploration should be conducted to rule out the presence of extrahepatic metastases. The liver also should be examined by intraoperative US, if available.

Cryosurgical ablation, as described in the previous section, has been applied to colorectal cancer liver metastases. Several studies have shown the efficacy and safety of hepatic cryosurgery, with mortality rates reported between 0% and 4%. Seifert et al. (1999) analyzed 85 patients who were not candidates for resection and who underwent cryoablation of colorectal liver metastases over a 7-year period. At a median follow-up of 22 months, local recurrence at the cryosite was observed in 33% of patients, liver recurrence in 65%, and extrahepatic recurrence in 56%. Multivariate analysis indicated that metastases larger than 3 cm was the only independent factor associated with local recurrence. In a separate analysis of 116 patients, Seifert et al. (1998) found the following factors to be independently associated with a favorable outcome: low presurgical serum CEA, metastases smaller than 3 cm, complete cryoablation, and good-to-moderate differentiation of the primary tumor. In this series, 37% of patients were alive at a follow-up of 23 months. Median survival was 26 months, with a five-year survival of 13%. Ravikumar et al. (1991) reported 32 patients who underwent cryosurgery, including 24 patients with colorectal metastases. The median follow-up was 24 months and the 5-year actuarial disease-free survival and overall survival were 24% and 62%, respectively. There were no operative mortalities. Bleeding from the probe sites was controlled with packing of thrombogenic materials. Transient increases in temperature, liver function enzyme levels, and white blood cell count were seen, but these returned to normal in the postoperative period.

Cryotherapy also has been used in conjunction with surgery when the resection margin is involved or suboptimal (<1 cm). Seifert et al. (1999) reported cryotherapy of the resection edge in 44 patients after liver resection for colorectal liver metastases with an involved or inadequate resection margin. At a median follow-up of 19 months, 16 patients were alive and disease free, and recurrences that involved the liver developed in 19 patients, but only five were at the resection edge (9%).

RFA is the newest technique for local ablation of tumors not amenable to resection. An RFA needle is placed within the substance of a tumor under radiographic guidance (i.e. CT, US). As the array is deployed, thermal energy is generated. The cell membranes are destroyed and the intracellular proteins degenerate when the temperature exceeds 45° C to 50° C. Curley et al. (1999) recently reported a series of 123 patients with primary or metastatic hepatic malignancies, who were treated with RFA. Of these, 61 were hepatic colorectal metastases. No treatment-related deaths occurred, and the complication rate was 2.4%. With a median follow-up of 15 months, only 1.8% of tumors had recurred at the RFA site. Unfortunately, 28% of patients experienced recurrences at distant sites.

At M.D. Anderson, we are continuing to investigate these forms of therapies for patients who are not candidates for surgical resection. Our present eligibility criteria include:

1. Age greater than 18 years;
2. Biopsy-proven metastatic disease, or suspicious lesion on CT scan;
3. Intraoperative US that demonstrates unresectable lesions;
4. No extrahepatic disease; and
5. Ability to ablate all disease with either RFA or RFA in combination with surgical resection.

Patients with prothrombin times greater than 14 seconds, bilirubin greater than 2 mg/dL, white blood cell count below 2,000, or platelet count below 100,000 are excluded.

Chemotherapy

Systemic chemotherapy has been applied in the adjuvant or neoadjuvant setting for patients undergoing liver resection. Several nonrandomized trials have analyzed this issue. Unfortunately, no randomized trials have compared systemic chemotherapy to surgery alone. The majority of these studies have been retrospective, with median survival ranging from 30 months to more than 60 months. Using historical controls, no significant difference in survival is evident between patients treated with resection alone and resection with adjuvant chemotherapy.

Chemotherapy for unresectable metastatic colorectal cancer consists of 5-FU–based regimens. The current standard is a combination of 5-FU and leucovorin (LV). Response rates have ranged from 12% to 40% with median survival of 10 to 17 months. Two new drugs that have shown promise are irinotecan (CPT-11) and oxaliplatin. Overall response rates for these drugs are 23% to 40%. In summary, systemic chemotherapy does not offer any potential for cure of metastatic colorectal cancer. Second-line regimens may provide some response in patients who fail 5-FU–based therapy but are associated with minimal improvement in survival.

Patients with unresectable metastatic disease confined to the liver, without evidence of extrahepatic disease, may be considered for regional chemotherapy, administered via a hepatic arterial infusion (HAI) pump. Although 5-FU is the favored drug in systemic chemotherapy, its first-pass clearance by the liver is low. Consequently, the relative increase in hepatic exposure to the drug by HAI is estimated to be only five- to tenfold. A related pyrimidine antagonist, floxuridine (fluorodeoxyuridine [FUDR]), has a much higher extraction on the first pass through the liver. The estimated increase in the liver's exposure to this drug when delivered by HAI is 100- to 400-fold, making it an ideal drug for this purpose. The following tenets support the use of HAI: (a) metastases larger than 3 mm derive their blood supply from the hepatic artery; (b) prolonged exposure to continuous infusion allows for increased response rates with pyrimidine derivatives (5-FU and FUDR); (c) FUDR is 15-fold higher in hepatic metastases after hepatic artery infusion as opposed to systemic infusion; and (d) FUDR by HAI has minimal systemic toxicity.

The possibility of extrahepatic or nodal metastases must be excluded before implantation of the HAI pump. In addition, a good-quality arteriogram is necessary for proper positioning of the catheter. Once the decision has been made to proceed with pump placement, a cholecystectomy should first be performed to prevent the development of chemical cholecystitis, a well-documented complication of HAI. In the presence of normal hepatic arterial anatomy, the infusion catheter is placed into the gastroduodenal artery (GDA), in a retrograde direction, with its tip just at the take-off of this artery from the common hepatic artery. The right gastric artery and any accessory arteries distal to the GDA should be ligated to prevent inadvertent perfusion of extrahepatic tissues. The pump usually is positioned in a subcutaneous pocket in the right lower quadrant of the abdomen, with the catheter tunneled through the anterior abdominal wall. When the catheter is in place, a fluorescein dye study should be performed. A Wood's lamp is used to confirm that no extrahepatic perfusion is present. In the postoperative period and before the initiation of chemotherapy, a radionuclide pump study is performed to reconfirm proper functioning of the catheter.

Variant hepatic arterial anatomy must be recognized and defined clearly on a preoperative arteriogram. When present, accessory lobar vessels are ligated to prevent inhomogeneous perfusion of drug to that lobe. Replaced hepatic arteries are managed in several ways. Two catheters can be placed, one to infuse the main hepatic artery and the other to supply the replaced vessel. One or two infusion pumps may be required. The method used at M.D. Anderson is to ligate the replaced vessel and use a single catheter

Table 12-3. Major randomized trials comparing hepatic arterial infusion and IV chemotherapy for unresectable liver metastases from colorectal cancer

Study	No. of Patients	HAI Response Agent (%)	IV Response Agent (%)
MSKCC	162	FUDR (50)	FUDR (20)
NCI	64	FUDR (62)	FUDR (17)
NCOG	115	FUDR (42)	FUDR (10)
Mayo	69	FUDR (48)	5-FU (21)
France	163	FUDR (43)	5-FU (9)

France, multicenter French cooperative study (Rougier P, et al. *J Clin Oncol* 1992;10:1112); 5-FU, 5-fluorouracil; FUDR, floxuridine; HAI, hepatic arterial infusion; Mayo, Mayo Clinic (Martin JK, et al. *Arch Surg* 1990;125:1022); MSKCC, Memorial Sloan-Kettering Cancer Center (Kemeny N, et al. *Ann Intern Med* 1987;107:459); NCI, National Cancer Institute (Chang AE, et al. *Ann Surg* 1987;206:685); NCOG, Northern California Oncology Group (Hohn DC, et al. *J Clin Oncol* 1989;7:1646).

to infuse the main hepatic artery. The lobe with the ligated accessory artery will rapidly develop collateral flow from the other lobe, allowing it to be perfused with the drug.

Interest in HAI increased after the development of the totally implantable Infusaid pump. This device allows both continuous and bolus injection of drug into the hepatic artery. Initial studies using this delivery system for the infusion of FUDR demonstrated remarkable response rates, some as high as 83%. Since then, five major randomized trials have compared the efficacy of HAI to that of standard IV chemotherapy (Table 12-3) for unresectable colorectal metastases. All studies showed significantly better response rates for patients receiving HAI chemotherapy (43%–62%) when compared to response rates with systemic chemotherapy (10%–21%). Because of differences in study design and length of follow-up, survival data are not as easily compared. All studies showed a tendency for longer survival in patients treated with HAI; however, only the National Cancer Institutes trial demonstrated a statistically significant improvement in survival. In this study, the 2-year survival rates for HAI and systemic regimens were 44% and 13%, respectively.

Table 12-4 lists randomized trials using HAI as adjuvant chemotherapy following liver resection. In prospective randomized studies (Wagman et al., 1990; Lorenz et al., 1998), adding HAI chemotherapy to surgery resulted in no survival advantage. However, patient accrual was insufficient in both studies, and the study by Lorenz et al. lacked FUDR, which has a higher hepatic extraction rate than 5-FU. Recently, Kemeny et al. (1999) published a single-center randomized study comparing patients receiving FUDR and dexamethasone via an implantable pump and systemic 5-FU and LV to patients receiving systemic 5-FU and LV alone after liver resection. Kemeny et al. found a significant difference in 2-year survival (86% vs. 72%, $P = 0.03$) and hepatic disease-free survival (90% vs. 60%, $P < 0.001$) when

Table 12-4. Major randomized trials using hepatic arterial infusion chemotherapy for resectable liver metastases from colorectal cancer

Trial	No. of Patients	Chemotherapy	Route	Survival	P
Wagman, 1990	6[a]	None	—	Median: 28 mo	NS
	5[a]	FUDR	HAC	Median: 37 mo	
Lorenz, 1998	111	None	—	Median: 41 mo	NS
	108	5-FU and LV	HAC	Median: 35 Mo	
Kemeny, 1999	82	5-FU and LV	Systemic	72% at 2 yr	
	74	FUDR, DM and 5-FU, LV	HAC Systemic	86% at 2 yr[a]	0.03

DM, dexamethasone; 5-FU, 5-fluorouracil; FUDR, floxuridine; HAC, hepatic arterial chemotherapy; HAI, hepatic arterial infusion; LV, leucovorin.
[a]Patients with solitary resectable metastases.

comparing arterial infusion chemotherapy to systemic chemotherapy, respectively. This has been the only published randomized trial comparing HAI chemotherapy to systemic 5-FU and LV after liver resection; however, further data accrual and follow-up are necessary before any conclusions can be made.

The efficacy of HAI therapy can be further evaluated by the patterns of responses and failures. In a Memorial Sloan-Kettering Cancer Center study, 82% of patients in the systemic group experienced disease progression in the liver, compared with 37% in the HAI group. On the other hand, extrahepatic disease developed in 56% of patients who received HAI, compared with 37% of patients who received systemic chemotherapy. These data demonstrate, once again, that regional control of the disease alone may not be adequate, because most people treated with HAI ultimately die of extrahepatic disease.

This problem has been the impetus for several studies aimed at reducing the rate of extrahepatic failure in patients receiving HAI. One approach has been to infuse IV chemotherapy concomitantly with HAI infusion. Safi et al. (1989) compared patients treated with intrahepatic FUDR with those treated with both intrahepatic and IV FUDR. Both groups had comparable response rates and survival durations; however, the rates of extrahepatic failure differed between the two treatment groups. Extrahepatic metastases developed in 61% of patients in the HAI group compared to 33% of patients in the HAI/IV group. Another approach used at M.D. Anderson is alternating administration of FUDR and 5-FU via the HAI pump. The use of 5-FU not only reduces the toxicity to the liver but also, because of the lower first-pass clearance of that drug by the liver, allows significant systemic levels to be attained. This treatment has resulted in a 50% response rate and a prolongation of survival, compared with intrahepatic FUDR alone.

Presently, the most active regimen for HAI chemotherapy is a combination of FUDR, 5-FU, LV, and dexamethasone. Response rates of up to 80% have been reported with this regimen.

Although HAI significantly decreases the systemic toxicity of chemotherapy, it is by no means a benign procedure. The locally concentrated dose of drug is associated with a number of complications, including chemical hepatitis, biliary sclerosis, gastritis, and gastric or duodenal ulcer disease. Careful monitoring of liver function during chemotherapy and prompt reduction of the dose can avert permanent hepatic damage if evidence of chemical hepatitis is noted.

CANCER OF THE EXTRAHEPATIC BILE DUCT

Epidemiology and Etiology

Cancer of the extrahepatic bile duct (cholangiocarcinoma) is extremely rare, comprising 2% of all cancers. In most reported series, the male-to-female incidence ratio is equal and patients are in their seventh decade. There is no significant geographic variation in the prevalence of the tumor.

The etiology of cholangiocarcinoma is unknown. Several diseases are associated with an increased risk of such tumors: sclerosing cholangitis, ulcerative colitis, and choledochal cysts. No convincing evidence links gallstones or infection with Clonorchis sinensis, in which the risk of cholangiocarcinoma also is increased. The common cancer-causing factor in all these conditions is unclear, although chronic inflammation of the bile duct probably plays a role.

Pathologic Characteristics

Histologically, cholangiocarcinoma can be classified as papillary, nodular, or sclerosing adenocarcinomas. The papillary variety has a better prognosis than do the other two types. Papillary tumors usually are well differentiated and can present with multiple lesions within the duct. The worst prognosis is associated with the sclerosing type, which is usually poorly differentiated. The sclerosing types are located around the hilum, whereas nodular and papillary types are located distally.

Most cholangiocarcinomas are located in the proximal portion of the duct. A tumor arising at the confluence of the right and left hepatic ducts is termed a Klatskin's tumor, following the description of 13 such lesions by Klatskin in 1965.

Cholangiocarcinomas are slow growing and most often spread by local extension or metastasis to regional lymph nodes. Hematogenous spread is rare. Lesions of the proximal and middle thirds of the extrahepatic bile duct can compress, constrict, or invade the underlying portal vein or hepatic artery. In addition, proximal tumors can invade the liver parenchyma. Hilar cholangiocarcinomas will involve the parenchyma of the caudate lobe in as many as 36% of patients. Distant metastases from cholangiocarcinomas are rare.

A number of pathologic findings are important in predicting the outcome of patients with cholangiocarcinoma. These factors include infiltration to the serosa of the bile duct, lymph node metastases, vascular invasion, and perineural invasion.

Clinical Presentation

The most common presenting symptom in patients with cholangiocarcinoma is obstructive jaundice. Rarely, a very proximal tumor may block a segmental or lobar bile duct without the occurrence of clinical jaundice. Other symptoms that may occur are pruritus, weight loss, fatigue, vague abdominal pain, and nausea. A patient may present with cholangitis and sepsis resulting from contamination of the obstructed bile. Except for the jaundice, the physical findings in a patient with bile duct cancer are nonspecific. In cases of middle or distal duct obstruction, a distended gallbladder may be palpable.

Diagnosis

When extrahepatic bile duct obstruction is suspected, the first radiologic test that should be performed is US, which can provide information about the level and nature of an obstructing lesion. CT is as sensitive as US in demonstrating bile duct dilation. Because of its higher cost, however, CT should not be used routinely as the initial diagnostic test. If US demonstrates extrahepatic bile duct dilation that is not a result of common bile duct stones, a CT scan should be obtained. CT has the advantage of depicting the actual tumor mass more often than US can. In addition, CT is better able to demonstrate the relationship of the tumor to surrounding structures and to evaluate the remainder of the abdomen for metastatic spread.

The actual location of the tumor and, more importantly, its proximal extent must be defined before planning any surgical intervention. This goal can be accomplished in one of two ways: percutaneous transhepatic cholangiography (PTC) or endoscopic retrograde cholangiopancreatography (ERCP). If the point of obstruction is thought to be proximal, PTC is the preferred method for depicting the biliary tract. For suspected distal bile duct lesions, ERCP is superior, because it allows imaging of both the bile duct and the pancreatic duct. MRI cholangiopancreatography is a noninvasive study recently shown to facilitate diagnosis of pancreaticobiliary neoplasia and depict the anatomy.

The workup for a suspected cholangiocarcinoma is completed with visceral angiography and portography. As mentioned previously, these tumors have a tendency to involve the portal vein and the hepatic artery by local invasion. Evidence of encasement of these vascular structures suggests that the lesion is unresectable. This criterion has become more a relative contraindication, because many surgeons are now resecting portions of involved portal vein and hepatic artery.

Obtaining tissue to confirm the diagnosis of bile duct cancer is essential if non-surgical or protocol-based therapy is being considered. Fine-needle aspiration, which can be done under US or CT guidance, has a sensitivity of 77%. Cytologic evaluation of bile is positive in 47% of patients with a malignancy. In most instances, the decision to operate is based on the preoperative radiologic examinations, not histologic confirmation.

Table 12-5.   Differential diagnosis for focal bile duct obstruction

Malignant lesions

Primary cholangiocarcinoma
Mucoepidermoid carcinoma
   Direct invasion
   Hepatoma
   Gallbladder carcinoma
   Pancreatic carcinoma
   Retroperitoneal sarcoma
Metastasis to hilar or periportal lymph nodes
Lymphoid tumors (Hodgkin's and non-Hodgkin's lymphoma)

Benign lesions

Choledocholithiasis
Sclerosing cholangitis
Iatrogenic bile duct stricture
Mirizzi's syndrome
Idiopathic focal stenosis
Tuberculosis
Clonorchis or *Ascaris* infestation

The differential diagnosis for focal stenosis or obstruction of the bile duct is given in Table 12-5. Although the list is extensive, choledocholithiasis and cholangiocarcinoma are the most common causes.

Staging

The current AJCC staging system for cholangiocarcinoma is shown in Table 12-6.

Surgical Therapy

The definitive therapy for all extrahepatic bile duct carcinomas is surgical resection; however, only a fraction of these lesions will ultimately be resectable. Overall resectability rates range from 10% to 85%, depending on the series. Lesions of the lower third of the bile duct have the best rates of resectability, followed by those of the middle third. Proximal cholangiocarcinomas are technically difficult to approach, resulting in the lowest rate of resectability among bile duct tumors. Standard criteria that render a tumor unresectable are (a) lymph node involvement outside the hepatic pedicle, (b) distant metastases, (c) bilateral tumor extension into secondary hepatic ducts, (d) bilateral extension of tumor into hepatic parenchyma, and (e) a combination of unilateral vascular involvement and contralateral ductal spread. As stated earlier, many surgeons would resect involved portal vein, therefore making vascular involvement a relative contraindication.

The need for preoperative biliary drainage has been debated at length in the literature. Earlier reports noted that preoperative hyperbilirubinemia was a poor prognostic indicator and that normalization of the bilirubin level before surgery was associated

Table 12-6. AJCC staging system for cancer of the extrahepatic bile duct

Primary tumor

TX	Primary tumor cannot be assessed
T0	No evidence of tumor
Tis	Carcinoma in situ
T1	Tumor invades subepithelial connective tissue or fibromuscular layer
	T1a Tumor invades subepithelial connective tissue
	T1b Tumor invades fibromuscular layer
T2	Tumor invades perifibromuscular connective tissue
T3	Tumor invades adjacent structures: liver, pancreas, duodenum, gallbladder, colon, stomach

Regional lymph nodes

NX	Regional lymph nodes cannot be assessed
N0	No regional lymph node metastasis
N1	Metastasis in cystic duct, pericholedochal and/or hilar lymph nodes (i.e., in the hepatoduodenal ligament)
N2	Metastasis in peripancreatic (head only), periduodenal, periportal, celiac, and/or superior mesenteric and/or posterior pancreaticoduodenal lymph nodes

Distant metastasis

MX	Presence of distant metastasis cannot be assessed
M0	No distant metastasis
M1	Distant metastasis

Stage grouping

Stage 0	Tis	N0	M0
Stage I	T1	N0	M0
Stage II	T2	N0	M0
Stage III	T1–T2	N1–N2	M0
Stage IVA	T3	Any N	M0
Stage IVB	Any T	Any N	M1

Adapted from *AJCC Manual for Staging of Cancer*, 5th ed. Philadelphia: Lippincott-Raven, 1998.

with reduced morbidity and mortality. Three prospective randomized trials have examined the role of preoperative percutaneous biliary drainage. No reduction in morbidity or mortality was evident in these studies. Nevertheless, Cameron advocates routine preoperative placement of biliary drainage catheters to facilitate identification and dissection of the bile duct during surgery and to aid the intraoperative placement of larger, softer Silastic transhepatic stents. At M.D. Anderson, we believe routine biliary drainage has no effect on perioperative complication rates and is indicated only in patients with sepsis and cholangitis.

Resectable lesions of the lower third of the bile duct are best treated with a pancreaticoduodenectomy. The proximal bile duct should be resected to the point that the surgical margin is negative for tumor. Occasionally, this may require removal of most of the extrahepatic biliary tract with a high hepaticojejunostomy.

The operative approach for a pancreaticoduodenectomy at M.D. Anderson is outlined in Chapter 13.

Lesions of the middle third of the bile duct are in proximity to the hepatic artery and the portal vein and have a tendency to invade these structures. If such a tumor has been deemed resectable, it is best treated by local excision and regional lymph node dissection. All efforts should be made to achieve a microscopically negative margin. Care must be taken not to disrupt the soft tissues containing the blood supply to the remaining proximal bile duct, to which the hepatoenteric anastomosis will be performed; otherwise, a postoperative bile duct stricture may result. Biliary drainage is reestablished using a Roux-en-Y hepaticojejunostomy.

The surgical management of proximal cholangiocarcinomas is challenging and remains controversial. Numerous reports have suggested that radical excision of the duct and any involved liver improves survival and quality of life. However, some surgeons believe the morbidity and mortality associated with major hepatic resection for this tumor are too high to justify its use. Part of the controversy involves the necessity of resecting the caudate lobe (segment I) en bloc with the bile duct. Proponents of this approach state that pathologic examination of resected specimens demonstrates direct invasion of tumor into the liver parenchyma or the bile ducts of the caudate lobe in as many as 35% of patients. In addition, the caudate lobe is often the site of tumor recurrence following bile duct resection. Therefore several surgeons have recommended routine caudate lobectomy with bile duct excision. Other surgeons believe the caudate lobe should be removed only if it is invaded by the tumor, citing equivalent survival data for those who had caudate lobectomy and those with similar lesions who did not. The difficulty and potential benefits of obtaining a negative margin have been demonstrated in a recent report by Burke et al. (1998). In this series, 69 patients with hilar cholangiocarcinoma were evaluated for possible resection. Thirty patients underwent resection, 26 of which were R0 resections. The median survival for all patients was 40 months. Patients with positive margins had a median survival of 22 months, and patients with negative margins had a median survival of more than 60 months. The 5-year survival for the latter group was 56%.

A final area of controversy is the use of total hepatectomy and OLT for tumors with bilateral extension into secondary intrahepatic biliary ducts. Thus far, there is no convincing evidence that liver transplantation is of benefit to these patients.

At M.D. Anderson, the surgical approach to proximal bile duct tumors depends on their location relative to the confluence of the right and left bile ducts and on their proximal extension. Lesions in this region are classified according to the scheme described by Bismuth and Corlette (1975) (Fig. 12-3). Type I and II lesions are treated by local excision and local lymph node dissection. We do not perform routine caudate lobe resections for type II tumors unless they have invaded into the lobe. Type IIIa and IIIb lesions undergo local excision and either right or left hepatic lobectomy, respectively. Type IV lesions are not considered resectable. We do not advocate the use of OLT in patients with such advanced disease.

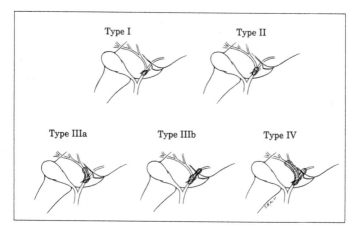

Type I
Type II
Type IIIa
Type IIIb
Type IV

Fig. 12-3. **Classification of extrahepatic bile duct tumors according to the location of the obstructing lesion (Bismuth classification).**

Despite aggressive surgical management, most patients with bile duct carcinoma will succumb to their tumors. Previous survival rates after resection of distal bile duct tumors were believed to be greater than those after resection of hilar cholangiocarcinoma. However, this assumption was founded in older literature that did not take into account the status of margin-negative resections. Reported 5-year survival rates for hilar cholangiocarcinoma range from 22% to 56%, and 5-year survival rates for distal bile duct tumors range from 16% to 40%.

The optimal palliation for patients with unresectable tumors is unclear. If the tumor has been deemed unresectable before exploration, the bile duct can be intubated either percutaneously or endoscopically. The use of metallic in-dwelling stents, which are more durable than traditional stents, has made this option more appealing. If the tumor has been found to be unresectable at exploration, the duct can be intubated with either transhepatic Silastic stents or a T tube after dilation of the lesion. When technically feasible, operative biliary bypass, with or without concomitant tumor resection, provides the best survival and quality of life for patients with unresectable tumors. Unresectable lesions at the bile duct confluence, especially Bismuth type III and IV lesions, can be particularly difficult to palliate. A left intrahepatic cholangioenteric anastomosis has been used with success in these situations. In this technique, the left hepatic duct branch is located between segments III and IV and is drained into a Roux-en-Y limb of jejunum.

Chemotherapy

No chemotherapeutic agents are clearly effective in the treatment of cholangiocarcinoma. Single-agent trials using 5-FU have demonstrated response rates less than 15%. Other agents, such as doxorubicin, mitomycin C, and cisplatin, used alone or in combination with 5-FU, have been no more successful.

Radiation Therapy

Several studies have investigated the role of adjuvant radiation therapy after bile duct resection. Two separate studies from Johns Hopkins found no benefit to adjuvant radiation therapy. Kamada et al (1996), however, have shown radiation to be beneficial in patients with histologically positive margins. At M.D. Anderson, postoperative chemoradiation is given to patients with resected bile duct cancers. Patients receive a continuous-infusion of 5-FU concomitantly with 54 Gy of radiation to the tumor bed. Although patient numbers are small and follow-up duration is short, initial results suggest a prolongation of survival in treated patients when compared with untreated, historical controls. Radiation therapy also has been found to be effective in the palliation of unresectable bile duct cancers. Doses of 40 to 60 Gy have resulted in a median survival rate of 12 months, as well as symptomatic improvement.

Multimodality Therapy

At the M.D. Anderson Cancer Center, we currently are investigating the role of preoperative chemoradiation in patients with proximal cholangiocarcinomas in an effort to improve local control and potentially improve resectability rates. The results of this approach are not yet available.

PERIAMPULLARY CARCINOMA

Pathology

Adenocarcinoma accounts for 95% of malignancies of the periampullary area and may develop from four different tissues of origin at this site: head of pancreas, ampulla of Vater, distal bile duct, and periampullary duodenum. Although the modes of presentation and treatment are similar, the prognosis for each of these malignancies is different. The 5-year survival rate for adenocarcinoma of the head of the pancreas is reported to be 18%; of the ampulla, 36%; of the distal bile duct, 34%; and of the periampullary duodenum, 33%. Determination of the tissue of origin is therefore critical, because it affects management decisions regarding potential for cure and extent of resection necessary to obtain tumor-free resection margins. The current AJCC staging system for ampullary tumors is shown in Table 12-7.

Determination of the tissue of origin may be made from fine-needle aspiration biopsy or endoscopic biopsy and is based on mucin production and the degree of cellular differentiation. Anatomic information based on thin-section CT and ERCP may also contribute to the determination of the tissue of origin. Detection of a mutation in the Kirsten (Ki)-ras proto-oncogene, which occurs in 75% to 90% of pancreatic adenocarcinomas, may be helpful in differentiating these neoplasms from other periampullary tumors.

Locoregional spread of periampullary adenocarcinoma results from lymphatic invasion and direct tumor extension to adjacent soft tissues. In a prospective study of regional lymph node metastases in patients undergoing pancreaticoduodenectomy for

Table 12-7.   AJCC staging system for cancer of the ampulla of Vater

Primary tumor

TX	Primary tumor cannot be assessed
T0	No evidence of primary tumor
Tis	Carcinoma in situ
T1	Tumor limited to the ampulla of Vater or sphincter of Oddi
T2	Tumor invades duodenal wall
T3	Tumor invades ≤ 2 cm into the pancreas
T4	Tumor invades >2 cm into pancreas and/or into other adjacent organs

Regional lymph nodes

NX	Regional lymph nodes cannot be assessed
N0	No regional lymph node metastasis
N1	Regional lymph node metastasis

Distant metastasis

MX	Presence of distant metastasis cannot be assessed
M0	No distant metastasis
M1	Distant metastasis

Stage grouping

Stage 0	Tis	N0	M0
Stage I	T1	N0	M0
Stage II	T2	N0	M0
	T3	N0	M0
Stage III	T1	N1	M0
	T2	N1	M0
	T3	N1	M0
Stage IV	T4	Any N	M0
	Any T	Any N	M1

Adapted from *AJCC Manual for Staging of Cancer,* 5th ed. Philadelphia: Lippincott-Raven, 1998.

periampullary adenocarcinoma, Cubilla et al. (1978) found significant variability in both the frequency of lymph node metastases and the pattern of lymph node involvement, depending on the tissue of origin. Ampullary lesions metastasized to regional lymph nodes in only 33% of cases, typically involving only a single lymph node in the posterior pancreaticoduodenal group. Duodenal adenocarcinomas had an intermediate risk of nodal metastasis with metastases to several lymph nodes in different subgroups of the paraduodenal area. Pancreatic adenocarcinoma, with its propensity to invade the rich lymphatic network of the pancreas and its ability to directly invade adjacent tissues, had the highest frequency of lymph node involvement (88%); metastases typically involved multiple lymph nodes, multiple subgroups, and distant sites.

Treatment

The standard Whipple pancreaticoduodenectomy is thought to provide adequate tumor clearance in the case of nonpancreatic periampullary carcinoma because disease spread is usually localized. Although biopsy-proved paraduodenal lymphadenopathy is thought by most surgeons to preclude curative resection in patients with pancreatic adenocarcinoma, one may appropriately consider en bloc resection in patients with duodenal, ampullary, or distal bile duct tumors in the presence of regional lymph node metastasis if the disease is confined to the field of resection. A detailed description of operative technique is provided in Chapter 13.

The effectiveness of locoregional control of periampullary adenocarcinoma by surgery alone and the potential benefits of adjuvant chemoradiation continue to be examined. In a retrospective review of 41 patients with periampullary carcinoma, Willett et al. (1993) identified patients with low-risk pathologic features (tumor limited to ampulla or duodenum, well- or moderately well-differentiated histologic characteristics, negative resection margins, and uninvolved lymph nodes) who had significantly better 5-year actuarial local control and survival rates–100% and 80%, respectively. In contrast, patients with high-risk pathologic features (tumor invasion of pancreas, poorly differentiated histologic characteristics, positive resection margins, and involved lymph nodes) had 5-year actuarial local control and survival rates of 50% and 38%, respectively. Based on these findings, the authors have proposed a course of preoperative chemoradiation to improve local disease control and survival rates in patients with locally advanced, poorly differentiated tumors.

GALLBLADDER CANCER

Epidemiology and Etiology

Although carcinoma of the gallbladder is a rare tumor, it is actually the most common malignancy of the biliary system and the fifth most common cancer of the gastrointestinal tract. The tumor has been reported in almost all age groups but is most often found in patients in their seventh and eighth decades. There is a striking difference in the incidence of the tumor between the sexes; females are affected three to four times as often as males. Evaluation of the Surveillance, Epidemiology, and End Results database reveals an incidence of 1.2 cases per 100,000 population per year in the United States.

The exact etiology of carcinoma of the gallbladder is not known; however, there are several entities with which it is frequently associated. Cholelithiasis is found in 75% to 92% of gallbladder carcinoma cases. Furthermore, gallbladder carcinoma can be found in 1% to 2% of all cholecystectomy specimens, a rate that is several times higher than that reported in autopsy studies. Chronic cholecystitis, especially cases in which the gallbladder is calcified (porcelain gallbladder), also has been associated with an increased risk of cancer, with an incidence as high as 61%. Other factors linked to gallbladder carcinoma include inflammatory bowel disease, advanced age, female sex, and familial predisposition. There is no association between gallbladder carcinoma and hepatitis B or C virus infection.

Pathologic Characteristics

Adenocarcinoma of the gallbladder is a slow-growing tumor that arises from the fundus in 60% of cases. Grossly, the gallbladder is firm and the walls are thickened. The tumor has a tendency to invade surrounding structures, including the liver, bile duct, and duodenum. The papillary adenocarcinoma subtype characteristically grows intraluminally and spreads intraductally. It is a less aggressive tumor that, consequently, carries a better prognosis when compared to other histologic subtypes.

Gallbladder cancer can spread by hematogenous or lymphatic routes and can directly invade the liver. It has the ability to seed the peritoneal cavity after spillage and cause tumor implantation in biopsy tracts or abdominal wounds. Lymph node metastases are found in 50% to 75% of gallbladder carcinoma cases. The cystic duct node, at the confluence of the cystic and hepatic ducts, is the initial focus of regional lymphatic spread. Invasion of the liver, either by direct extension or via draining veins that empty into segments IV and V, is seen in more than 50% of patients and usually occurs early. Distant hematogenous spread is rare and is usually seen only in the later stages of the disease. The most common site of distant extra-abdominal spread is the lung.

Clinical Presentation

In most series, the most common presenting complaint is abdominal pain. Nausea, vomiting, weight loss, and jaundice are other common symptoms. Most patients have had symptoms for 3 months or less before presentation. On physical examination, patients may have right upper quadrant pain with hepatomegaly or a palpable, distended gallbladder. In advanced cases, patients may have jaundice, cachexia, and ascites. The tumor markers CEA and CA19-9 may be increased in patients with gallbladder cancer.

Diagnosis

Unfortunately, no laboratory or radiologic tests are routinely accurate in the diagnosis of gallbladder carcinoma. That inconsistency, along with the paucity of clinical signs and symptoms, has made the tumor's preoperative diagnosis difficult. In fact, a correct preoperative diagnosis of gallbladder cancer is made in fewer than 10% of cases in most series. In the Roswell Park experience, none of the 71 cases were diagnosed correctly preoperatively. The most common preoperative diagnoses are acute and chronic cholecystitis and malignancies of the bile duct or pancreas.

In the rare event when a diagnosis of gallbladder carcinoma is suspected preoperatively, US or CT may demonstrate a mass with local hepatic extension or suspicious portal adenopathy. Angiography may demonstrate encasement of the cystic or hepatic arteries or the portal vein. Vascularity around the gallbladder may be increased. Cholangiography is valuable in jaundiced patients because it allows the location and extent of biliary obstruction to be determined.

Numerous staging systems have been described for gallbladder cancer. The original staging system, as described by Nevin,

**Table 12-8. Nevin's staging system
for gallbladder carcinoma**

Stage I	Intramucosal involvement only
Stage II	Involvement of the mucosa and muscularis
Stage III	Transmural involvement of gallbladder wall
Stage IV	Metastases to the cystic duct lymph nodes
Stage V	Involvement of the liver by direct extension or metastasis, or metastases to any other organ

is based on the depth of invasion and the spread of tumor (Table 12-8). The standard AJCC staging scheme is shown for comparison in Table 12-9. However, neither of these classification systems is entirely accurate, because a recent Memorial-Sloan Kettering Cancer Center review indicated that patients with nodal metastases had worse prognoses when compared to patients with direct liver invasion greater than 2 cm. The bulk of the literature on gallbladder cancer is based on the Nevin staging system, although the AJCC staging system is used most commonly today.

Surgical Therapy

The surgical treatment for gallbladder carcinoma is dictated by the stage of the tumor. In fact, in developing his staging system, Nevin found that survival was inversely correlated with the depth of invasion and the extent of spread. Most patients with gallbladder carcinoma present with advanced disease (AJCC stage IV). Approximately 10% to 30% of patients present with disease that can be resected for cure.

Standard criteria that make a tumor unresectable include (a) distant hematogenous or lymphatic metastases, (b) peritoneal implants, or (c) invasion of tumor into major vascular structures such as the celiac or superior mesenteric arteries, vena cava, or aorta. Tumors involving the hepatic artery or portal vein have been extirpated with an en bloc vascular resection and reconstruction, but such an extensive procedure would not be considered standard therapy and should be performed only at very specialized centers. Because of the dismal prognosis for patients with AJCC stage IV cancers, many surgeons advocate palliative procedures rather than resection.

The optimal treatment for patients with AJCC stage II and III tumors is an extended cholecystectomy. The components of this procedure are a cholecystectomy, regional lymph node dissection in the hepatoduodenal ligament, and a wedge resection of the gallbladder bed (including at least a 3-cm margin of normal parenchyma). The rationale for this operation is that the incidence of lymph node spread in T1b and T2 tumors is 16% and 56%, respectively. The incidence of lymph node positivity for T3 tumors is 75%. Several series have shown a 5-year survival rate of 29% with this operative approach, compared to a 0% 5-year survival rate for patients undergoing simple cholecystectomy.

AJCC stage I carcinoma of the gallbladder can be treated adequately with cholecystectomy alone, with 5-year survival rates

Table 12-9. AJCC staging system for cancer of the gallbladder

Primary tumor

TX	Primary tumor cannot be assessed
T0	No evidence of primary tumor
Tis	Carcinoma in situ
T1	Tumor invades lamina propria or muscle layer
	T1a Tumor invades lamina propria
	T1b Tumor invades muscle layer
T2	Tumor invades perimuscular connective tissue; no extension beyond serosa or into liver
T3	Tumor perforates serosa (visceral peritoneum) or directly invades on adjacent organ, or both (extension ≤2 cm into liver)
T4	Tumor extends >2 cm into liver and/or into two or more adjacent organs (stomach, duodenum, colon, pancreas, omentum, extrahepatic bile ducts, any involvement of liver)

Regional lymph nodes

NX	Regional lymph nodes cannot be assessed
N0	No regional lymph node metastasis
N1	Metastasis in cystic duct, pericholedochal and/or hilar lymph nodes (i.e., in the hepatoduodenal ligament)
N2	Metastasis in peripancreatic (head only), periduodenal, periportal, celiac, and/or superior mesenteric lymph nodes

Distant metastasis

MX	Presence of distant metastasis cannot be assessed
M0	No distant metastasis
M1	Distant metastasis

Stage grouping

Stage 0	Tis	N0	M0
Stage I	T1	N0	M0
Stage II	T2	N0	M0
Stage III	T1–T2	N1	M0
	T3	N0–N1	M0
Stage IVA	T4	N0–N1	M0
Stage IVB	Any T	N2	M0
	Any T	Any N	M1

Adapted from *AJCC Manual for Staging of Cancer,* 5th ed. Philadelphia: Lippincott-Raven, 1998.

as high as 100% in several series. Hepatic resection and lymphadenectomy are not justified for patients with stage I disease.

Nonoperative Therapy

The use of single and multiple chemotherapeutic agents, either as primary therapy or as adjuvant therapy, has been disappointing. The response rate to 5-FU regimens in patients with locally advanced cancer is approximately 12%; 5-FU combined with doxorubicin has produced response rates of 30% to 40%.

HAI chemotherapy produces response rates of 50% to 60% in patients with unresectable disease. These responses are short lived, however, and most patients die of progressive disease within 12 months.

Radiation therapy has shown some promise in the postoperative adjuvant setting, although most series are small. Intraoperative radiation therapy also has been used with some success. External beam radiation of 45 Gy can produce tumor reduction in 20% to 70% of cases and relieve jaundice in up to 80% of patients. At M.D. Anderson, patients with gallbladder cancer are treated postoperatively with a combination of continuous-infusion chemotherapy and external beam radiation in an approach similar to that used among patients with cholangiocarcinoma.

RECOMMENDED READING

Ahmad SA, Bilimoria MM, Wang X, et al. Hepatitis B or C virus serology as a prognostic factor in patients with hepatocellular carcinoma. *J Gastroint Surg* 2001;5:468–476.

Abdalla EK, Hicks ME, Vauthey JN. Portal vein embolization: rationale, technique and future prospects. *Br J Surg* 2000;88:165–175.

Bartlett DL, Fong Y, Fortner JG, et al. Long-term results after resection for gallbladder cancer. Implications for staging and management. *Ann Surg* 1996;224(5):639.

Bismuth H, Corlette MB. Intrahepatic cholangioenteric anastomosis in carcinoma of the hilus of the liver. *Surg Gynecol Obstet* 1975;140:170.

Bismuth H, Nakache R, Diamond T. Management strategies in resection for hilar cholangiocarcinoma. *Ann Surg* 992;1215:31.

Blumgart LH, Kelley CJ. Hepaticojejunostomy in benign and malignant high bile duct stricture: approaches to the left hepatic ducts. *Br J Surg* 1984;71:257.

Bruix J, Castells A, Bosch J, et al. Surgical resection of hepatocellular carcinoma in cirrhotic patients: prognostic value of preoperative portal pressure. *Gastroenterology* 996;1111(4):1018.

Burke EC, Jarnagin WR, Hochwald SN, et al. Hilar cholangiocarcinoma: patterns of spread, the importance of hepatic resection for curative operation, and a presurgical clinical staging system. *Am Surg* 1998;228:385–394.

Cady B, Stone MD, McDermott WV, et al. Technical and biological factors in disease-free survival after hepatic resection for colorectal cancer metastases. *Arch Surg* 1992;127:561.

Cameron JL, Broe P, Zuidema GD. Proximal bile duct tumors: surgical management with silastic transhepatic biliary stents. *Ann Surg* 1982;196:412.

Cameron JL, Pitt HA, Zinner MJ, et al. Management of proximal cholangiocarcinomas by surgical resection and radiotherapy. *Am J Surg* 1990;159:91.

Cubilla AL, Fortner J, Fitzgerald PJ. Lymph node involvement in carcinoma of the head of the pancreas area. *Cancer* 1978;41:880.

Curley SA, Izzo F, Delrio P, et al. Radiofrequency ablation of unresectable primary and metastatic hepatic malignancies. Results in 123 patients. *Ann Surg* 1999;230: 1–8.

Curley SA, Izzo F, Ellis LM, et al. Radiofrequency ablation of hepatocellular cancer in 110 patients with cirrhosis. *Ann Surg* 2000;232:381–391.

Di Bisceglie AM, Rustgi VK, Hoofnagle JH, et al. Hepatocellular carcinoma. *Ann Intern Med* 1988;108:390.

Feldman D, Kulling D, Kay C, et al. Magnetic resonance cholangiopancreatography (MRCP): a novel approach to the evaluation of pancreaticobiliary neoplasms. Abstract 55. Presented at the 50th Annual Cancer Symposium of the Society of Surgical Oncology, 1997.

Fong Y, Cohen AM, Fortner JG, et al. Liver resection for colorectal metastases. *J Clin Oncol* 1997;15(3):938.

Fong Y, Kemeny N, Paty P, et al. Treatment of colorectal cancer: hepatic metastasis. *Semin Surg Oncol* 1996;12(4):219.

Gagner M, Rossi RL. Radical operations for carcinoma of the gallbladder: recent status in North America. *World J Surg* 1991;15:344.

Groupe d'Etude et de Traitement du Carcinome Hepatocellulaire. A comparison of lipiodol chemoembolization and conservative treatment for unresectable hepatocellular carcinoma. *N Engl J Med* 1995;332(19):1256.

Hohn DC, Stagg RJ, Friedman MA, et al. A randomized trial of continuous intravenous versus hepatic intraarterial floxuridine in patients with colorectal cancer metastatic to the liver: the Northern California Oncology Group Trial. *J Clin Oncol* 1989;7:1646.

Hughes KS, et al. Resection of the liver for colorectal carcinoma metastases: a multi-institutional study of indications for resection. *Surgery* 1988;103:278.

Hughes KS, Simon R, Songhorabodi S, et al. Resection of the liver for colorectal carcinoma metastases: a multi-institutional study of patterns of recurrence. *Surgery* 1986;100:278.

Iwatsuki S, Sheahan DG, Starzl TE. The changing face of hepatic resection. *Curr Probl Surg* 1989;26:283.

Iwatsuki S, Starzl TE, Sheahan DG, et al. Hepatic resection versus transplantation for hepatocellular carcinoma. *Ann Surg* 1991;214:221.

Kamada T, Saito H, Takemura A, et al. The role of radiotherapy in the management of extrahepatic bile duct cancer: an analysis of 145 patients. *Int J Radiat Oncol Biol Phys* 1996;34(4):767–774.

Kanematsu T, Matsumata T, Shirabe K, et al. A comparative study of hepatic resection and transcatheter arterial embolization for the treatment of primary hepatocellular carcinoma. *Cancer* 1993;71:2181.

Karl RC, Morse SS, Halpert RD, et al. Preoperative evaluation of patients for liver resection: appropriate CT imaging. *Ann Surg* 1993;217:226.

Kawai S, Okamura J, Ogawa M, et al. Prospective and randomized clinical trial for the treatment of hepatocellular carcinoma: a comparison of Lipiodol-transcatheter arterial embolization with and without adriamycin (first cooperative study). The Cooperative Study Group for Liver Cancer Treatment of Japan. *Cancer Chemother Pharmacol* 1992;31(suppl):S1.

Kemeny N, Daly J, Reichman B, et al. Intrahepatic or systemic infusion of fluorodeoxyuridine in patients with liver metastases from colorectal carcinoma: a randomized trial. *Ann Intern Med* 1987;107:459.

Kemeny N, Huang Y, Cohen AM, et al. Hepatic arterial infusion of chemotherapy after resection of hepatic metastases from colorectal cancer. *N Engl J Med* 1999;341:2039–2048.

Klatskin G. Adenocarcinoma of the hepatic duct at its bifurcation within the portahepatis: an unusual tumor with distinctive clinical and pathological features. *Am J Med* 1965;38:241.

Klempnauer J, Ridder GJ, Von Wasielewski R, et al. Resectional surgery of hilar cholangiocarcinoma: a multivariate analysis of prognostic factors. *J Clin Oncol* 1997;15:947.

Langer JC, Langer B, Taylor BR, et al. Carcinoma of the extrahepatic bile ducts: results of an aggressive surgical approach. *Surgery* 1985;98:752.

Livraghi T, Bolondi L, Lazzaroni S, et al. Percutaneous ethanol injection in the treatment of hepatocellular carcinoma in cirrhosis: a study of 207 patients. *Cancer* 1992;69:925.

Llovet JM, Bruix J, Fuster J, et al. Liver transplantation for hepatocellular carcinoma. Results of a restrictive policy. *Hepatology* 1996;24:350A.

Lorenz M, Muller HH, Schramm H, et al. Randomized trial of surgery versus surgery followed by adjuvant hepatic arterial infusion with 5-fluorouracil and folinic acid for liver metastases of colorectal cancer. *Ann Surg* 1998;228(6):756–762.

MacIntosh EL, Minuk GY. Hepatic resection in patients with cirrhosis and hepatocellular carcinoma. *Surg Gynecol Obstet* 1992;174:245.

Mazzaferro V, Regalia E, Doci R, et al. Liver transplantation for the treatment of small hepatocellular carcinomas in patients with cirrhosis. *N Engl J Med* 1996;334(11):693.

McPherson DAD, Benjamin IS, Hodgson HJF, et al. Preoperative percutaneous transhepatic biliary drainage: the results of a controlled trial. *Br J Surg* 1984;71:371.

Morrow CE, et al. Primary gallbladder carcinoma: significance of serosal lesions and results of aggressive surgical treatment and adjuvant chemotherapy. *Surgery* 1983;94:709.

Nagorney DM, van Heerden JA, Ilstrup DM, et al. Primary hepatic malignancy: surgical management and determinants of survival. *Surgery* 1989;106:740.

Nevin JE, Moran TJ, Kay S, et al. Carcinoma of the gallbladder: staging, treatment and prognosis. *Cancer* 1976;37:141.

Ogura Y, Mizumoto R, Tabaya M, et al. Surgical treatment of carcinoma of the hepatic duct confluence: analysis of 55 resected carcinomas. *World J Surg* 1993;17:85.

Order SE, Stillwagon GB, Klein JL, et al. Iodine-131 antiferritin, a new treatment modality in hepatoma: a radiation therapy oncology group study. *J Clin Oncol* 1985;3:1573.

Pitt HA, Somes AS, Lois JF, et al. Does preoperative percutaneous biliary drainage reduce operative risk or increase hospital cost? *Ann Surg* 1985;201:545.

Ravikumar TS, Kane R, Cady B, et al. A 5-year study of cryosurgery in the treatment of liver tumors. *Arch Surg* 1991;126:1520.

Rich TA. Adjuvant therapy for primary biliary and pancreatic cancer. In: Niederhuber JE, ed. *Current therapy in oncology* St. Louis: Mosby-Year Book, 1993.

Rivera JA, Rattner DW, Fernandez-del Castillo C, et al. Surgical approaches to benign and malignant tumors of the ampulla of Vater. *Surg Oncol Clin North Am* 1996;5(3):689.

Rougier P, Laplanche A, Huguier R, et al. Hepatic arterial infusion of floxuridine in patients with liver metastases from colorectal carcinoma: long-term results of a prospective randomized trial. *J Clin Oncol* 1992;10:1112.

Safi F, Bittner R, Rosher R, et al. Regional chemotherapy for hepatic metastases of colorectal carcinoma (continuous intraarterial versus continuous intraarterial/intravenous therapy): results of a controlled clinical trial. *Cancer* 1989;64:379.

Saltz LB, Ahmad SA, Vauthey JN. Colorectal cancer: management of advanced disease. In: Kelsen DP, Daly JM, Kern SE, et al. *Gastrointestinal oncology: principles and practice* Philadelphia: Lippincott Williams & Wilkins, 2002:825–852.

Scheele J, Stangl R, Altendorf-Hofmann A, et al. Resection of colorectal liver metastases. *World J Surg* 1995;19:59–71.

Seifert JK, Morris DL. Indicators of recurrence following cryotherapy for hepatic metastases from colorectal cancer. *Br J Surg* 1999;86: 234–240.

Seifert JK, Morris DL. Prognostic factors after cryotherapy for hepatic metastases from colorectal cancer. *Ann Surg* 1998;228:201– 208.

Shirai Y, Yoshida K, Tsukada K, et al. Inapparent carcinoma of the gallbladder: an appraisal of a radical second operation after simple cholecystectomy. *Ann Surg* 1992;215:326.

Silk YN, Douglass HO, Nava HR, et al. Carcinoma of the gallbladder: the Roswell Park experience. *Ann Surg* 1989;210:751.

Sitzmann JV, Abrams R. Improved survival for hepatocellular cancer with combination surgery and multimodality treatment. *Ann Surg* 1993;217:149.

Sitzmann JV, Coleman JA, Pitt HA, et al. Preoperative assessment of malignant hepatic tumors. *Am J Surg* 1990;159:137.

Stagg RJ, Venook AP, Chase JL, et al. Alternating hepatic intraarterial floxuridine and fluorouracil: a less toxic regimen for treatment of liver metastases from colorectal cancer. *J Natl Cancer Inst* 1991;83:423.

Stain SC, Baer HU, Denison AR, et al. Current management of hilar cholangiocarcinoma. *Surg Gynecol Obstet* 1992;175:579.

Steele G Jr, Bleday R, Mayer RJ, et al. A prospective evaluation of hepatic resection for colorectal carcinoma metastases to the liver: Gastrointestinal Tumor Study Group protocol 6584. *J Clin Oncol* 1991;9:1105.

Steele G Jr, Ravikumar TS. Resection of hepatic metastases from colorectal cancer: biologic perspectives. *Ann Surg* 1989;210:127.

Suenaga M, Nakao A, Harada A, et al. Hepatic resection for hepatocellular carcinoma. *World J Surg* 1992;16:97.

Tuttle TM, Curley SA, Roh MS. Repeat hepatic resection as effective treatment of recurrent colorectal liver metastases. *Ann Surg Oncol* 1997;4(2):125.

Wagman LD, Kemeny MM, Leong L, et al. A prospective, randomized evaluation of the treatment of colorectal cancer metastatic to the liver. *J Clin Oncol* 1990;8:1885.

Wanebo HJ, Castle WN, Fechner RE. Is carcinoma of the gallbladder a curable lesion? *Ann Surg* 1982;195:624.

Willett CG, Warshaw AL, Convery K, et al. Patterns of failure after pancreaticoduodenectomy for ampullary carcinoma. *Surg Gynecol Obstet* 1993;176:33.

Yamanaka N, Tanaka T, Tanaka W, et al. Correlation of hepatitis virus serologic status with clinicopathologic features in patients undergoing hepatectomy for hepatocellular carcinoma. *Cancer* 1997;79:1509–1515.

Yamamoto J, Sugihara K, Kosuge T, et al. Pathologic support for limited hepatectomy in the treatment of liver metastases from colorectal cancer. *Ann Surg* 1995;221:74–78.

Yu YQ, Xu DB, Zhou XD, et al. Experience with liver resection after hepatic arterial chemoembolization for hepatocellular carcinoma. *Cancer* 1993;71:62.

Zhou X, Yu Y, Tang Z, et al. An 18-year study of cryosurgery in the treatment of primary liver cancer. *Asian J Surg* 1992;15:43.

Zhou XD, Tang ZY, Yu YQ, et al. The role of cryosurgery in the treatment of hepatic cancer: a report of 113 cases. *J Cancer Res Clin Oncol* 1993;120:100.

Pancreatic Adenocarcinoma

Ana M. Grau, Francis R. Spitz, Michael Bouvet,
George M. Fuhrman, and David H. Berger

EPIDEMIOLOGY

Pancreatic cancer is the eighth most common malignancy and the fifth leading cause of adult cancer death in the United States. Only 1% to 4% of all patients diagnosed with pancreatic cancer can expect to survive 5 years. In the year 2000, 28,300 new cases of adenocarcinoma of the pancreas were diagnosed in the United States, and 28,200 patients died of this aggressive malignancy. Thus, incidence rates are virtually identical to mortality rates. The incidence of pancreatic cancer in the United States steadily increased for several decades but has leveled off over the past 20 years as a result of a steady decline in the rate for white men. In contrast, rates for white women, black men, and black women have not decreased and may have increased slightly, bringing the male-to-female ratio to 1.3:1.0. The risk of developing pancreatic cancer increases sharply after age 50 years, and most patients are between 65 and 80 years old at diagnosis.

The etiology of pancreatic adenocarcinoma is uncertain. Epidemiologic studies reported that cigarette smoking increases the risk of developing pancreatic cancer threefold. The risk of pancreatic cancer increases as the amount and duration of smoking increase. Coffee, alcohol, organic solvents, and petroleum products have been linked epidemiologically to pancreatic cancer. However, the data are conflicting, and none of these agents are conclusively causal. Diabetes mellitus has been implicated as both an early manifestation of pancreatic carcinoma and a predisposing factor. Recent studies have shown that pancreatic cancer occurs more frequently in patients with long-standing diabetes. Reports have validated the epidemiologic association between chronic pancreatitis and pancreatic cancer, but the magnitude of the risk of pancreatic cancer attributable to pancreatitis remains controversial. Approximately 5% to 8% of pancreatic cancer cases have been associated with a familial predisposition. Because high-risk groups of patients have not been well defined, screening presently has only a very limited role.

CLINICAL PRESENTATION

The presenting signs and symptoms of patients with pancreatic cancer are shown in Table 13-1. The most common presenting symptoms are weight loss, pain, and jaundice. Pain is initially of low intensity, is visceral in origin, and is poorly localized to the upper abdomen. This pain may mimic peptic ulcer disease. Severe pain localized to the lower thoracic or upper lumbar area is more characteristic of advanced disease due to invasion of the celiac and superior mesenteric plexus.

Anorexia and weight loss are common in pancreatic cancer patients. Weight loss results from malabsorption and decreased

Table 13-1. Presenting signs and symptoms of patients with carcinoma of the head of the pancreas

Sign or Symptom	Percentage of Patients
Weight loss	90
Pain	75
Malnutrition	75
Jaundice	70
Anorexia	60
Pruritus	40
Courvoisier's sign	33
Diabetes mellitus	15
Ascites	5
Gastric outlet obstruction	5

caloric intake. The sudden onset of diabetes mellitus in non-obese adults older than 40 years warrants evaluation for pancreatic cancer.

Painless jaundice as the sole presenting symptom is more frequently seen with ampullary or distal bile duct tumors but can be present with adenocarcinoma of the head or uncinate process of the pancreas. Small tumors of the pancreatic head may obstruct the intrapancreatic portion of the bile duct and cause the patient to seek medical attention when the tumor is still localized and potentially resectable. In the absence of extrahepatic biliary obstruction, few patients present with potentially resectable disease. Courvoisier's sign, a palpable gallbladder at presentation, is seen in less than one-third of patients.

NATURAL HISTORY

Pancreatic cancer spreads early to regional lymph nodes, and microscopic involvement of the liver is frequently present at diagnosis. Patients who undergo surgical resection for localized adenocarcinoma of the pancreatic head have a median survival of 13–20 months. Survival and local control are improved with either preoperative or postoperative chemoradiation. With improved locoregional control, the liver has become the most frequent site of recurrence for these patients. Patients with locally advanced disease and patients with metastatic disease have median survivals of 6–10 and 3–6 months, respectively. Therefore, improvements in systemic or regional therapy directed to the liver and the development of screening strategies for earlier diagnosis will be necessary to change the natural history of this disease.

PREOPERATIVE EVALUATION

An algorithm for the current diagnostic and therapeutic management of pancreatic adenocarcinoma at the M.D. Anderson Cancer Center is presented in Fig. 13-1. When pancreatic cancer

$\longrightarrow$

Fig. 13-1. Algorithm for the management of pancreatic carcinoma. EUS-FNA, endoscopic ultrasound guided fine needle aspiration biopsy; ERCP, endoscopic retrograde cholangiopancreatography.

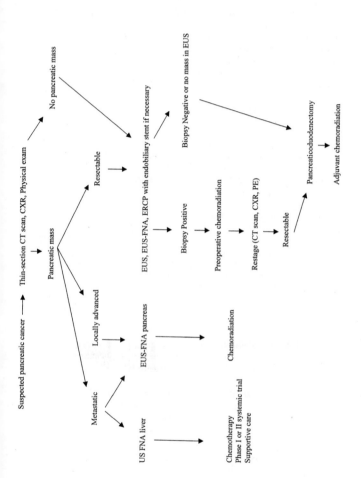

is suspected, radiologic confirmation should be attempted. Several large reviews of pancreatic cancer noted delays of more than 2 months from the onset of symptoms to diagnosis in most patients. Ultrasound should be the initial diagnostic test in the jaundiced patient to confirm extrahepatic biliary ductal dilatation and to assess the pancreatic head and liver.

Thin-section computed tomography (CT) scanning through the pancreas with an intravenous bolus injection of contrast remains the test of choice to evaluate the extent of disease and to assess tumor resectability. Local tumor resectability is most accurately assessed before surgery. Laparotomy should be therapeutic, not diagnostic. At M.D. Anderson, we use objective and reproducible radiologic criteria to operate only on patients with potentially resectable disease. Resectability is defined as the absence of extrapancreatic disease; the absence of direct tumor extension to the superior mesenteric artery (SMA) and celiac axis, as defined by the presence of a fat plane between the low-density tumor and these arterial structures; and a patent superior mesenteric-portal vein confluence. The accuracy of this form of radiographic staging is supported by previous work at M.D. Anderson and validated by a high resectability rate (94 of 118, 80%) and low rate of microscopic retroperitoneal margin positivity (17%). The accuracy of CT in predicting unresectability and the inaccuracy of intraoperative assessment of resectability are both well established. The use of standardized, objective radiologic criteria for preoperative tumor staging allows physicians to develop detailed treatment plans for their patients, avoid unnecessary laparotomy in patients with locally advanced or metastatic disease, and improve rates of resectability at laparotomy. Therefore, we recommend a system for clinical (radiologic) staging illustrated in Table 13-2. The current American Joint Committee on Cancer Staging (AJCC) staging for pancreatic cancer is listed in Table 13-3. The AJCC staging system provides only one system

Table 13-2.   Clinical/radiologic staging of pancreatic cancer

Stage	Clinical/Radiologic Criteria
I	Resectable (T1–2, selected T4[a], NX, M0) No encasement of the celiac axis or SMA Patent SMPV confluence No extrapancreatic disease
II	Locally advanced (T4, NX–1, M0) Arterial encasement (celiac axis or SMA) or venous occlusion (SMV or portal vein) No extrapancreatic disease
III	Metastatic (T1–4, NX–1, M1) (liver, peritoneum, lungs)

SMA, superior mesenteric artery; SMV, superior mesenteric vein; SMPV, superior mesenteric-portal vein.
[a]Resectable T4 tumors include those with isolated involvement of the SMPV, and without encasement of the celiax axis or SMA.

Table 13-3. AJCC staging of pancreatic cancer

Primary tumor (T)

Tis	Carcinoma in situ
T1	Tumor limited to the pancreas ≤ 2 cm in greatest dimension
T2	Tumor limited to the pancreas > 2 cm in greatest dimension
T3	Tumor extends directly into any of the following: duodenum, bile duct, peripancreatic tissues
T4	Tumor extends directly into any one of the following: stomach, spleen, colon, adjacent large vessels

Regional lymph nodes (N)

N0	No regional lymph node metastasis
N1	Regional lymph node metastasis

Distant metastasis

M0	No distant metastasis
M1	Distant metastasis

Stage grouping

Stage I	T1–T2	N0	M0
Stage II	T3	N0	M0
Stage III	T1–T3	N1	M0
Stage IVA	T4	Any N	M0
Stage IVB	Any T	Any N	M1

for both clinical (radiographic) and pathologic staging. Pathologic staging can be applied only to patients who undergo pancreatectomy; in all other patients, only clinical staging, based on radiographic examinations, can be performed. Without surgery the histologic status of the regional lymph nodes cannot be determined. In addition, treatment and prognosis are based on whether the tumor is potentially resectable, locally advanced, or metastatic, definitions that may not directly correlate with TNM status. For example, both potentially resectable and locally advanced tumors may be categorized as T4; isolated involvement of the superior mesenteric vein (SMV) would be considered T4 disease but does not preclude resection in the absence of arterial encasement.

Endoscopic ultrasound with fine-needle aspiration biopsy (EUS-FNA) has emerged as a helpful diagnostic tool and has proven to be safe and accurate. Pretreatment confirmation of malignancy is mandatory in patients with locally advanced or metastatic disease prior to chemotherapy or external beam radiation therapy (EBRT) and before initiation of neoadjuvant therapy in patients with resectable pancreatic cancer. In our experience, EUS-FNA has a specificity and positive predictive value of 100% while sensitivity and negative predictive values are 90% and 38%, respectively. In addition to patients with large tumors, EUS-FNA is successful in most patients with small, resectable tumors, allowing for the delivery of protocol-based neoadjuvant therapy. Negative results with EUS-FNA should not be interpreted as definitive proof that a malignancy does not exist.

Although pretreatment pancreatic fine-needle aspiration (FNA) biopsy is frequently performed, physicians should be cautioned about the use of intraoperative pancreatic biopsy. In patients with resectable disease, there is no indication for routine intraoperative pancreatic biopsy and the use of preoperative EUS-FNA should be limited to those patients receiving preoperative chemoradiation for whom cytologic confirmation of malignancy is needed. Unlike FNA, surgical manipulation and intraoperative large-needle biopsy during surgery increases the risk of peritoneal dissemination of tumor cells. Having undergone a previous laparotomy with tumor biopsy prior to definitive pancreaticoduodenectomy is the only factor associated with an increased risk of locoregional tumor recurrence. Further, intraoperative pancreatic biopsy has been associated with significant complications such as pancreatitis, pancreatic fistula, and hemorrhage.

Endoscopic retrograde cholangiopancreatography (ERCP) is used to differentiate choledocholithiasis and chronic pancreatitis from malignant obstruction of the distal common bile duct when a mass is not seen by CT. To prevent cholangitis in patients who undergo diagnostic ERCP because of extrahepatic biliary obstruction, endoscopic stents are routinely placed. Endoscopic stents are also placed in patients with elevated bilirubin levels who are enrolled in preoperative chemoradiation protocols. We are currently performing EUS-FNA and ERCP under monitored anesthesia as one procedure.

Angiography has been used to demonstrate encasement of the celiac or mesenteric vessels; however, this information is more accurately obtained by thin-section contrast-enhanced CT. Currently, the only indication for routine angiography in the work-up of these patients is to exclude the possibility of aberrant arterial anatomy. This information prevents iatrogenic arterial injury of a replaced right hepatic artery. Because a replaced right hepatic artery can be identified at laparotomy, we utilize angiography in the evaluation of patients who were operated on prior to referral in whom dissection is often more difficult.

Laparoscopy has been advocated for the diagnosis of extrapancreatic disease in patients with radiologic evidence of localized disease. Recent investigations suggest that extrapancreatic disease not visible by CT is uncommon, being found in only 4% to 15% of patients with pancreatic tumors considered resectable following high-quality CT. Laparoscopy before laparotomy (during a single anesthesia induction) is a reasonable approach in patients with biopsy-proven or suspected potentially resectable pancreatic cancer in whom a decision has been made to proceed with pancreaticoduodenectomy. However, data are not available to support the cost-effectiveness of routinely using laparoscopy as a staging procedure under a separate anesthesia induction prior to treatment planning.

PATHOLOGY

Approximately 90% of pancreatic exocrine tumors arise from the pancreatic ductules, and 80% of these tumors are adenocarcinomas. Pancreatic adenocarcinomas arise in the head of the gland in 60% to 70% of cases. The rest of the tumors are located in the body or tail, or diffusely throughout the pancreas.

In gross histologic examination, pancreatic adenocarcinoma is firm and white with poorly defined margins. An associated surrounding area of pancreatitis is often present and can make pathologic diagnosis difficult. An intense desmoplastic reaction is identifiable on both gross and microscopic examination. Histologic identification of mucin production is helpful in diagnosing an adenocarcinoma. Perineural invasion can be identified in most specimens. The degree of differentiation reported on microscopic examination is based on the degree of formation of tubular glandular structures.

SURGICAL TREATMENT

Surgical resection of carcinoma of the pancreatic head remains the only potentially curative treatment modality. Five surgical techniques are used to resect pancreatic cancer: (a) the standard pancreaticoduodenectomy, modified from Whipple's initial description in 1935; (b) pylorus-preserving pancreaticoduodenectomy; (c) total pancreatectomy; (d) regional pancreatectomy; and (e) the M.D. Anderson extended resection. Thorough abdominal exploration should precede resection. There is no role for resection of adenocarcinoma in the presence of metastatic disease. Exploration should include intraoperative inspection and palpation of the liver, peritoneal surfaces, para-aortic lymphatics, and root of the mesentery to define the tumor's extent.

The surgical resection is divided into the following six clearly defined steps (Fig. 13-2).

1. A Cattell-Braasch maneuver is performed by mobilizing the right colon and incising the visceral peritoneum to the ligament of Treitz. When complete, this maneuver allows cephalad retraction of the right colon and small bowel, exposing the third and fourth portions of the duodenum. Mobilization of the retroperitoneal attachments of the mesentery is of particular importance in patients who require venous resection and reconstruction. The omental bursa is entered by taking the greater omentum from the transverse colon. The middle

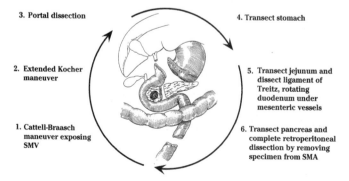

3. Portal dissection

4. Transect stomach

2. Extended Kocher maneuver

5. Transect jejunum and dissect ligament of Treitz, rotating duodenum under mesenteric vessels

1. Cattell-Braasch maneuver exposing SMV

6. Transect pancreas and complete retroperitoneal dissection by removing specimen from SMA

Fig. 13-2. Six surgical steps of pancreaticoduodenectomy (clockwise resection). (From Tyler DS, Evans DB. Reoperative pancreaticoduodenectomy. *Ann Surg* **1994;219:214.)**

colic vein is identified, ligated, and divided before its junction with the SMV. Routine division of the middle colic vein allows greater exposure of the infrapancreatic SMV and prevents iatrogenic traction injury during dissection of the middle colic vein-SMV junction.

2. The Kocher maneuver is begun at the junction of the ureter and right gonadal vein. The right gonadal vein is ligated and divided, and all fibro-fatty and lymphatic tissue overlying the medial aspect of the right kidney and inferior vena cava is removed with the tumor specimen. The gonadal vein is again ligated at its entrance into the inferior vena cava. The Kocher maneuver is continued to the left lateral edge of the aorta, with careful identification of the left renal vein.

3. The portal dissection is initiated exposing the common hepatic artery proximal and distal to the gastroduodenal artery. The gastroduodenal artery is then ligated and divided. Two large lymph nodes are commonly encountered during portal dissection: one along the inferior border of the common hepatic artery, and one behind the portal vein seen after transection of the common bile duct. Removal of these lymph nodes (en bloc with the specimen) is necessary to mobilize the hepatic artery and portal vein. However, they rarely contain metastatic disease. Lymph node metastases from pancreatic cancer are commonly small and are almost always found by the pathologist rather than the surgeon. The gallbladder is dissected out of the liver bed and the common hepatic duct transected just cephalad to its junction with the cystic duct. The anterior wall of the portal vein is easily exposed following division of the common hepatic duct and medial retraction of the common hepatic artery. This connective tissue anterior to the portal vein is divided in a caudal direction to the junction of the portal vein and the neck of the pancreas. A constant venous tributary, the posterior pancreatic duodenal vein, can be located at the supralateral aspect of the portal vein. Bleeding caused by traction injury to the venous tributary may be difficult to control at the time of the operation. The portal dissection is made more difficult in the presence of anomalous hepatic artery circulation. Rarely, the hepatic artery (distal to the origin of the gastroduodenal artery) courses posterior to the portal vein. More commonly, an accessory or replaced right hepatic artery arises from the proximal SMA and lies posterior and lateral to the portal vein. The common hepatic artery may arise from the SMA (type IX hepatic arterial anatomy). Fatal hepatic necrosis can result if this is unrecognized and the vessel is sacrificed. Identification of aberrant arterial anatomy is generally not difficult except in reoperative portal dissections

4. The stomach is transected at the level of the third or fourth transverse vein on the lesser curvature and at the confluence of the gastroepiploic veins on the greater curvature. The omentum is divided at the level of the greater curvature transection.

5. The jejunum is transected approximately 10 cm distal to the ligament of Treitz, and its mesentery is sequentially ligated

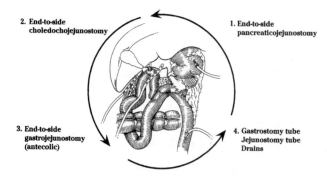

Fig. 13-3. Four surgical steps of counterclockwise reconstruction following standard pancreaticoduodenectomy. (From Tyler DS, Evans DB. Reoperative pancreaticoduodenectomy. *Ann Surg* 1994;219:214.)

and divided. The duodenal mesentery is similarly divided to the level of the aorta; the duodenum and jejunum are then reflected beneath the mesenteric vessels.

6. After traction sutures are placed on the superior and inferior borders of the pancreas, the pancreas is transected with an electrocautery at the level of the portal vein. If there is evidence of tumor adherence to the portal vein or SMV, the pancreas can be divided at a more distal location in preparation for segmental venous resection. The specimen is separated from the SMV by ligating and dividing the small venous tributaries to the uncinate process and the pancreatic head. Complete removal of the uncinate process combined with medial retraction of the superior mesenteric-portal vein confluence facilitates exposure of the SMA, which is then dissected to its origin at the aorta. Total exposure of the SMA avoids iatrogenic injury and ensures direct ligation of the inferior pancreaticoduodenal artery.

Reconstruction proceeds in the counterclockwise direction, and again in a stepwise and orderly fashion (Fig. 13-3).

1. The pancreatic remnant is mobilized from the retroperitoneum and splenic vein for a distance of 2 to 3 cm. Failure to adequately mobilize the pancreatic remnant results in poor suture placement at the pancreaticojejunal anastomosis. The transected jejunum is brought through a small incision in the transverse mesocolon to the right or left of the middle colic vessels. A two-layer, end-to-side, duct-to-mucosa pancreaticojejunostomy is performed over a small Silastic stent. Following completion of the posterior row of 3-0 seromuscular sutures, a small, full-thickness opening in the bowel is made. The anastomosis between the pancreatic duct and small-bowel mucosa is completed with 4-0 or 5-0 monofilament sutures. Each stitch incorporates a generous bite of

pancreatic duct and a full-thickness bite of jejunum. The posterior knots are tied on the inside, and the lateral and anterior knots are tied on the outside. Prior to the anterior sutures being tied, the stent is placed across the anastomosis so that it extends into the pancreatic duct and into the small bowel for a distance of approximately 2 to 3 cm. The anastomosis is completed with a placement of an anterior row of 3-0 seromuscular sutures. When the pancreatic duct is not dilated and/or the pancreatic substance is soft (not fibrotic), a two-layer anastomosis that invaginates the cut end of the pancreas into the jejunum is recommended. The outer posterior row of 3-0 sutures is placed as outlined earlier. The bowel is then opened for its full length to the transverse diameter of the pancreatic remnant. Using a running, double-armed, 4-0 non-absorbable monofilament suture, the pancreatic remnant is sewn to the jejunum. The anastomosis is completed with placement of an anterior row of 3-0 seromuscular sutures.

2. A single-layer biliary anastomosis is performed using interrupted, 4-0 absorbable monofilament sutures. It is important to align the jejunum with the bile duct to avoid tension on the pancreatic and biliary anastomosis. A stent is rarely used in the construction of the hepaticojejunostomy.

3. An anti-colic, end-to-side gastrojejunostomy is constructed in two layers. Starting from the greater curvature, 6 to 8 cm of gastric staple line is removed. A posterior row of silk sutures is followed by a running, monofilament, full-thickness inner layer; the anterior row of silk sutures completes the anastomosis. The distance between the biliary and gastric anastomosis should allow the jejunum to assume its anti-colic position (for the gastrojejunostomy) without tension. There is no harm in making a long (25 to 35 cm) afferent limb.

4. Gastrojejunostomy and feeding jejunostomy tubes are placed using the Witzel technique, and then closed suction drains are placed.

Traverso and Longmire introduced the concept of pyloruspreserving pancreaticoduodenectomy in 1978 in an attempt to eliminate the postgastrectomy syndromes seen after antrectomy. This operation technically differs from a standard Whipple procedure only in the preservation of the blood supply to the proximal duodenum. This can be accomplished by carefully preserving the right gastroepiploic arcade after ligation of the right gastroepiploic artery and vein close to their origin. The right gastric artery can be spared in some cases to provide additional blood supply to the duodenum. The most significant morbidity of pylorus preservation is transient gastric stasis. Operative time and blood loss are slightly reduced compared with those of classic pancreaticoduodenectomy. Pylorus preservation should not be performed in patients with bulky tumors or tumors involving the first and second portion of the duodenum.

Some authors have advocated routine total pancreatectomy as definitive therapy for adenocarcinoma of the head of the pancreas. They cite the possible multicentric nature of pancreatic cancer and the avoidance of a pancreatic anastomosis as justification for this approach. However, the incidence of pathologic documentation of multicentricity of pancreatic adenocarcinoma is less than 10% and does not justify the additional operative morbidity and lifelong insulin dependence that results from total pancreatectomy. The significant operative morbidity and mortality from pancreaticoduodenectomy is historically attributed to pancreaticojejunal anastomotic leak. However, anastomotic complications are rare at institutions experienced with this operation. Also, more effective management of pancreatic anastomotic leakage with hyperalimentation, percutaneous drainage, and somatostatin analog has reduced the magnitude of this problem. Total pancreatectomy is only indicated if there is tumor at the pancreatic margin on serial frozen sections or if the pancreas is not suitable for an anastomosis.

Regional pancreatectomy includes extensive retroperitoneal and hepatoduodenal lymph node dissection and sleeve resection of the SMV-portal venous confluence. Superior mesenteric and hepatic arterial resections have also been included by proponents of this more radical approach. The potential oncologic advantages of regional pancreatectomy are offset by its increased morbidity and mortality.

Venous resection should be considered when the lesion has been deemed resectable, the pancreatic neck is divided, and, while dissecting the uncinate process from the SMV, the tumor is found to be adherent to the posterior-lateral portion of the vein. Vein resection is preferable to shaving the tumor from the portal-superior mesenteric venous confluence. In addition, venous resection for any tumor involving the SMV-portal venous confluence should be performed as long as the vein has been demonstrated to be patent by preoperative CT. An interposition internal jugular vein graft is our preferred method of reconstruction. Unlike other recent reports, data from our institution suggest that resection of the SMV at pancreaticoduodenectomy can be performed safely, is not associated with retroperitoneal margin positivity (when high-quality preoperative imaging is performed), and does not negatively influence patient survival.

Intraoperative decision-making in the surgical treatment of pancreatic cancer can challenge the most experienced surgeon. The morbidity and mortality associated with pancreaticoduodenectomy are greater than those seen with many other procedures and should be performed only by experienced surgeons. This conclusion is supported by Lieberman et al. (1995), who reported the experience with pancreaticoduodenectomy in New York State from 1984 to 1991. More than 75% of patients who underwent pancreaticoduodenectomy had their operations performed at hospitals that reported less than seven of these operations per year. For patients who received their surgical care at those hospitals, mean perioperative hospital stay was greater than 1 month, and the risk-adjusted perioperative mortality was 12% to 19%. Patients and their families must be informed preoperatively of the required complex postoperative care and potential complications of pancreaticoduodenectomy. This is most critical when there is no preoperative histologic confirmation of the diagnosis. Neoplasms of the pancreatic head can obstruct the pancreatic duct, resulting in pancreatitis, which makes definitive histologic diagnosis difficult. An intraoperative transduodenal biopsy specimen that reveals inflammation does not exclude the possibility of malignancy. Because of this, many experienced pancreatic surgeons do not routinely perform intraoperative biopsies if malignancy is suspected. In our institution we do not routinely perform intraoperative biopsies in patients with radiographic (CT or ERCP) studies consistent with malignancy. Occasionally, a surgeon suspects that a malignancy exists but cannot establish radiologic or histologic confirmation. Every large series of pancreatic resections includes a few patients resected for benign disease. The potential morbidity of an unnecessary pancreatic resection is preferred to leaving a potentially curable lesion in situ. Repeated biopsies to obtain histologic confirmation of malignancy are inadvisable because of the risk of pancreatic fistula, pancreatitis, and hemorrhage. Patients should be aware of the potential need to perform a resection without histologic confirmation of malignancy.

RESULTS OF SURGERY

Aggressive surgical resection of pancreatic head tumors has come under intense scrutiny, although presently, pancreaticoduodenectomy remains the only procedure capable of curing adenocarcinoma of the pancreatic head. Postoperative morbidity rates that were greater than 50% in the late 1960s, are now less than 25% in the most recently reported series. Postoperative mortality rates have also decreased, from a high of more than 20% to as low as 3% in the most recent reviews.

The presence of fever after postoperative day 3 or 4 should prompt careful evaluation. Potential sources of fever include those common to all abdominal surgeries as well as intraabdominal abscess as a result of pancreaticojejunostomy leak. Gastric and biliary anastomoses rarely leak. The study of choice is CT scan of the abdomen with CT-guided drainage of any localized fluid collection. Pancreaticojejunostomy anastomotic leaks generally close when adequately drained. The use of octreotide in this setting should be individualized. Postoperative gastrointestinal or drain tract bleeding should prompt immediate angiography to evaluate for arterial-enteric fistula. The most common cause is pancreaticojejunostomy leak followed by a herald bleed due to blowout of the ligated gastroduodenal artery stump. This is a rare complication and should be managed by embolization at the time of diagnostic angiography.

Despite the improvement in morbidity and mortality, there has been little change in long-term patient survival. The 5-year survival rate following curative pancreaticoduodenectomy for carcinoma of the pancreatic head remains less than 25%, with a median survival of 20 to 25 months.

Body and tail tumors are often considered to have a poorer prognosis than lesions of the pancreatic head because the former frequently go undetected until they are locally advanced or metastatic. At our institution, these lesions account for only 2% of the pancreatectomies performed. However, a Mayo Clinic report suggested that the few patients with body or tail lesions amenable to resection for cure have long-term survival rates similar to those patients who have undergone complete resection of the more common carcinoma of the pancreatic head.

ADJUVANT THERAPY

Because the 5-year survival rate of patients with resected pancreatic cancer is poor, it is imperative to examine the potential benefit of adjuvant therapy for this disease. Autopsy series have indicated that 85% of patients will experience recurrences in the field of resection. Furthermore, approximately 70% of patients will develop metastasis to the liver. Therefore, adjuvant therapy must address the possibility of distant disease (chemotherapy) as well as the possibility of locoregional recurrence (radiation therapy). The initial studies examining adjuvant therapy of pancreatic cancer were based on results from studies on patients with advanced disease.

Most widely used chemotherapeutic agents have limited activity against pancreatic cancer. 5-Fluorouracil (5-FU) is the only active agent, and its effect is marginal. Most studies report an overall response of 15% to 28% in patients with advanced disease. Studies of 5-FU have also demonstrated the ability of this agent to act as a radiation sensitizer. Gemcitabine, a deoxycytidine analogue capable of inhibiting DNA replication and repair, has demonstrated activity against pancreatic cancer. In a randomized trial of patients with advanced disease, patients treated with gemcitabine experienced a modest but statistically significant improved response rate and median survival and an improved quality of life compared with patients treated with 5-FU.

Combined 5-FU and radiation therapy have been reported to significantly increase survival in patients with locally advanced disease. In a study by the GITSG, patients with unresectable pancreatic cancer were randomized to receive high-dose, postoperative radiation therapy (60 Gy) alone, high-dose postoperative radiation therapy (60 Gy) plus concomitant 5-FU, or standard-dose postoperative radiation therapy (40 Gy) and 5-FU. Patients receiving 5-FU and radiation therapy experienced a significant survival advantage compared with patients who received radiation therapy alone. The higher dose of radiation therapy did not confer an additional survival advantage.

The combination of postoperative EBRT and concomitant 5-FU as adjuvant therapy after resection was also investigated by the GITSG. Patients were randomized to receive surgery alone or surgery followed by radiation therapy (40 Gy delivered in two 20-Gy courses) and 5-FU (500 mg/m^2 by IV bolus delivered daily for the initial 3 days of each radiation therapy course and then weekly for 2 years). Median survival was 20 months in the group that received adjuvant therapy; this was significantly longer than the 11-month median survival seen in patients treated with surgery alone.

Unlike surgery for adenocarcinoma of the esophagus, stomach, or colorectum, pancreaticoduodenectomy requires complete reconstruction of the upper gastrointestinal tract, including reanastomosis of the pancreas, bile duct, and stomach. The magnitude of the operation and its associated morbidity may result in a lengthy recovery, preventing the timely delivery of postoperative therapy.

In most large series, approximately 25% of patients who undergo pancreaticoduodenectomy do not receive postoperative chemoradiation because of prolonged recovery.

The risk of delaying adjuvant therapy, combined with small preliminary experiences of successful pancreatic resection following EBRT, prompted many institutions to initiate studies of chemoradiation before pancreaticoduodenectomy for patients with potentially resectable or locally advanced adenocarcinoma of the pancreas. The preoperative use of chemoradiation is supported by the following considerations:

1. Radiation therapy is more effective on well-oxygenated tumors that have not been devascularized by surgery.
2. Peritoneal spread of tumor cells as a result of surgery may be prevented by preoperative chemoradiation.
3. The high frequency of positive-margin resections recently reported supports the concern that the retroperitoneal margin of excision, even when negative, may be only a few millimeters. Surgery alone may therefore be inadequate for local tumor control.
4. Patients with disseminated disease evident on restaging studies after chemoradiation will not be subjected to laparotomy and therefore will be spared the associated morbidity and risk of treatment-related mortality. Repeat staging CT after chemoradiation reveals liver metastases in approximately 25% of patients. It is probable that the liver metastases were already present subclinically at diagnosis and if these patients had undergone pancreaticoduodenectomy then, they would have had a major surgical procedure only to have liver metastases found soon after surgery.
5. Because radiation therapy and chemotherapy are given first, long postoperative recovery will have no effect on the delivery of all components of the multimodality treatment, a frequent problem in postoperative adjuvant therapy studies.

The standard-fractionation preoperative chemoradiation regimen at M.D. Anderson was delivered over 5.5 weeks to a total dose of 50.4 Gy (1.8 Gy/fraction) concurrently with continuous-infusion 5-FU at a dosage of 300 mg/m^2/day, 5 days per week, through a central venous catheter. To avoid the gastrointestinal toxicity seen with this standard 5.5-week program, a rapid-fractionation program of chemoradiation was designed. Rapid-fractionation chemoradiation is delivered over 2 weeks to a total dose of 30 Gy (3 Gy/fraction) for 5 days per week. 5-FU is given concurrently by continuous infusion at a dosage of 300 mg/m^2/day, 5 days per week. This program is based on the principle that the total radiation dose required to obtain a given biologic effect decreases as the dose per fraction increases. Restaging with chest radiography and abdominal CT is performed 4 weeks after chemoradiation. Patients with localized disease on restaging undergo pancreaticoduodenectomy with electron-beam intraoperative radiation therapy (EB-IORT). In our recently published series, patients with radiographically resectable localized adenocarcinoma of the pancreatic head were entered onto this preoperative protocol. Thirty-five patients received this treatment, 27 had surgery, and 20 (74%) underwent successful pancreaticoduodenectomy.

Local tumor control and patient survival were equal to the results reported with standard-fractionation (5.5-week) chemoradiation: locoregional recurrence developed in only two (10%) of the 20 patients who underwent resection, and the median survival time for all 20 patients was 25 months. This protocol had minimal toxicity, maximized the proportion of patients who received all components of therapy, was significantly shorter than standard therapy, and avoided pancreaticoduodenectomy on patients with metastatic disease on restaging.

The role of preoperative rapid-fractionation EBRT and concomitant gemcitabine for patients with resectable adenocarcinoma of the pancreatic head is currently being evaluated. A dose of 400 mg/m^2 of gemcitabine is administered weekly for 7 weeks. A total radiation dose of 30 Gy in 10 fractions over 2 weeks (Monday to Friday) is given beginning 4 days after the first dose of gemcitabine. Pancreaticoduodenectomy is performed 4 weeks after completion of therapy if restaging CT demonstrates resectable disease. So far, 69 patients have been entered in this study and 65 have completed preoperative therapy. Fifty patients have had surgery and 42 had resection. No treatment-related mortality has been observed. Table 13-4 summarizes the most recent published reports of adjuvant and neoadjuvant therapy for pancreatic cancer.

One potential barrier to neoadjuvant therapy for pancreatic cancer is the need for stent placement for biliary decompression. At M.D. Anderson, the rates of biliary stent–related complications and mortality were evaluated in 300 patients undergoing preoperative chemoradiation therapy, 207 of whom received stents. On multivariate analysis, stent placement was associated only

Table 13-4. Recent chemo-radiation therapy studies of patients with resectable pancreatic cancer

Author (year)	No. of Patients	EBRT (Gy)	Chemotherapy	Median Survival (mo)
Postoperative				
Kalser (1985)	21	40	5-FU	20
Surgery alone	22	—	—	11
GITSG (1987)	30	40	5-FU	18
Yeo (1997)	120	40–57.6	5-FU	19.5
Surgery alone	53	—	—	13.5
Klinkenbijl (1999)	60	40	5-FU	17.1
Surgery alone	54	—	—	12.6
Preoperative				
Breslin (2000)	132	30–50.4	5-FU, paclitaxel or gemcitabine	21

EBRT, external beam radiation therapy; 5-FU, 5-fluorouracil; GITSG, Gastrointestinal Tumor Study Group.

with an increased rate of wound infection after pancreaticoduodenectomy. Stents did not result in prohibitive morbidity during preoperative chemoradiation therapy.

Investigators from our institution studied a regimen of preoperative EBRT (50.4 Gy in 28 fractions or 30 Gy in 10 fractions) and concomitant protracted-infusion 5-FU (300 mg/m^2/day) followed by pancreaticoduodenectomy and EB-IORT (10–20 Gy) to the resection bed. EB-IORT was delivered with minimal morbidity after preoperative chemoradiation and pancreaticoduodenectomy. The median survival duration in our most recent report was 25 months. Disease recurred in 70% of the patients at a median follow-up of 37 months; 86% of the recurrences were distant, and only 14% were locoregional. The results of these studies indicated that EB-IORT can be safely combined with pancreaticoduodenectomy and current chemoradiation regimens. Although EB-IORT appears to improve local control, marked improvements in survival have not been demonstrated. At present, the use of EB-IORT should be limited to investigational protocols. EB-IORT for locally advanced unresectable tumors has been reported to reduce symptoms from advanced disease and to prolong survival. A National Cancer Institute–controlled prospective trial of adjuvant radiation therapy for pancreatic cancer examined the benefit of EB-IORT (20 Gy) in addition to EBRT (50 Gy) after resection. Although EB-IORT did not have an impact on overall survival in this small study, patients who received EB-IORT experienced prolonged disease-free survival and improved local control.

SURVEILLANCE

Patients should be seen at 3 to 4 months after potentially curative resection of pancreatic adenocarcinoma or earlier if symptoms develop. Follow-up visits should include a thorough history, chest radiograph, and abdominal CT.

There have been numerous attempts to identify a tumor marker for pancreatic cancer. The most frequently measured antigens are carcinoembryonic antigen, CA 19-9, and pancreatic-oncofetal antigen. Some encouraging results have been reported with use of CA 19-9 to predict recurrence following resection of pancreatic adenocarcinoma.

Postoperatively, all patients receive some form of enteral nutritional supplementation via a jejunostomy tube for at least 6 weeks. Nutritional status, including serum albumin level, dietary history, and general body habitus, should be carefully assessed at each clinic visit. Patients must also be evaluated for signs of malabsorption resulting from pancreatic enzyme insufficiency. This is readily treatable with pancreatic enzyme replacement.

PALLIATION

Patients with unresectable or recurrent pancreatic cancer frequently require palliative treatment for biliary obstruction, gastric outlet obstruction, and pain. Historically, palliation for these patients was undertaken at laparotomy after a tumor was deemed unresectable. Operative biliary bypass, gastric bypass, and splanchnicectomy are effective methods of palliation.

However, with current improved diagnostic techniques, unresectability should be determined before laparotomy. Biliary diversion can then be achieved either endoscopically or percutaneously. Gastric outlet obstruction occurs in only 10% to 15% of patients and is often a preterminal event and so does not mandate surgical correction. CT-guided alcohol splanchnicectomy is an effective option for the palliation of pain in the occasional patient unresponsive to narcotics. Therefore, the surgeon can avoid laparotomy in most patients who have a limited life expectancy.

BILIARY OBSTRUCTION

Jaundice is a common presenting symptom in patients who have carcinoma of the head of the pancreas. Prolonged biliary obstruction leads to coagulopathy, hepatic dysfunction, malabsorption, and altered bile salt metabolism. Patients often complain of severe, disabling pruritus. Relief of biliary obstruction significantly palliates these problems and improves overall patient well-being. It is helpful to group patients with pancreatic cancer into four separate categories when considering operative versus nonoperative biliary decompression:

1. Patients in poor health who would not tolerate laparotomy and are clearly best served by nonoperative palliative measures.
2. Patients with concomitant gastric outlet obstruction who require laparotomy for palliation of that symptom and for whom the benefit of avoiding the complications of a stent or transhepatic drain warrants the limited additional morbidity of a surgical biliary bypass.
3. Patients undergoing operation for resection but who are found to have unsuspected unresectable disease; these patients are also best served by an operative biliary bypass.
4. Patients who have unresectable pancreatic cancer on diagnostic evaluation and are an acceptable medical risk for laparotomy; these patients are candidates for operative or nonoperative management, depending on the judgment of the surgeon and the expertise of the available endoscopist or invasive radiologist. (At M.D. Anderson, these patients are treated successfully with nonoperative palliative measures.)

Surgical biliary diversion can be accomplished by either choledochoenteric or cholecystenteric bypass. Constructing a Roux limb requires an additional anastomosis and longer operative time than making a simple loop of small bowel for biliary bypass. Roux reconstruction is necessary when an unresectable tumor prevents a loop from reaching the right upper quadrant without tension. Most authorities advocate either loop choledochojejunostomy or cholecystojejunostomy for surgical palliation of malignant biliary obstruction. Cholecystojejunostomy has the advantage of being simple to perform; however, there is the possibility of recurrent biliary obstruction after this procedure. The advantage of choledochojejunostomy is that it provides a more proximal biliary anastomosis and therefore obstruction by progressive extension of the tumor is less likely. The high operative mortality and short median survival associated with each procedure are due to the aggressive nature of the malignancy rather than to the technique used. The choice of surgical option ultimately depends on local tumor considerations and the surgeon's experience.

Nonoperative palliative biliary decompression can be accomplished endoscopically or percutaneously. Experienced endoscopists report a success rate of greater than 90%. In randomized studies comparing endoscopic biliary decompression with conventional surgical bypass, the procedures have resulted in identical survival times and relief of jaundice. Total hospital stay is also similar for the two procedures because of the need for occasional readmissions to change stents after endoscopic decompression. Percutaneous transhepatic biliary drainage has provided successful palliation in 80% to 90% of patients. External catheters are being replaced by newer indwelling endoprostheses, which are associated with a lower rate of infectious complications. Although endoscopic biliary decompression is the preferred method of nonoperative palliation, the choice of technique depends on the expertise available.

We use a selective approach to biliary decompression. Outpatient endoscopic stenting is performed in all patients who are not candidates for pancreaticoduodenectomy. In patients with a life expectancy of 3 to 5 months (i.e., those with poor performance status or liver or peritoneal metastases), an 11.5-F polyethylene stent is placed. In patients with a life expectancy of 6 to 12 months (i.e., those with locally advanced, nonmetastatic disease), a self-expanding metal stent is preferred. However, patients in whom early stent occlusion or migration develops or who by clinical criteria appear to do poorly with endoscopic biliary decompression are quickly referred for operative biliary bypass. A multidisciplinary approach to these patients is critical—the medical oncologist, gastroenterologist, and surgeon must communicate and avoid overly dogmatic approaches to palliative care.

GASTRIC OUTLET OBSTRUCTION

Patients with pancreatic cancer rarely present with duodenal obstruction. Furthermore, less than 15% of patients will require operative correction of gastric outlet obstruction before death. Clearly, patients with unresectable disease and gastric outlet obstruction require a gastrojejunostomy for palliation. There is controversy about whether all patients undergoing palliative laparotomy should undergo prophylactic gastroenterostomy. Complications resulting from longer surgery and additional anastomosis are minimal. However, the incidence of subsequent duodenal obstruction in asymptomatic patients who undergo only biliary bypass is low. In addition, gastric outlet obstruction often occurs shortly before death and does not require treatment. In general, we do not perform prophylactic surgery in patients with pancreatic cancer.

If a patient is found to have unresectable disease during surgery for planned pancreaticoduodenectomy, gastrojejunostomy is considered when clinical symptoms or anatomic findings suggest impending obstruction. However, in patients with locally advanced or limited metastatic disease with good performance status, prospective randomized data would support the creation of a gastrojejunostomy.

Table 13-5. Differentiation of inflammatory pseudocysts from cystic neoplasms of the pancreas

Patient History, CT and FNA Findings	Mucinous Neoplasm (adenoma or carcinoma)	Serous Cystadenoma	Inflammatory Pseudocyst
History of pancreatitis, alcohol abuse, complicated biliary disease	No	No	Yes
CT	Small number ($\leq$ 6) of large cysts (> 2 cm)	Many small cysts	No loculations
Cyst fluid analysis/cytology	Positive for mucin; malignant (if carcinoma)	No mucin; positive for glycogen	Negative
Cyst fluid CEA (ng/mL)	Usually > 500; highly variable	< 5	> 50% elevated, but usually < 400
Cyst fluid amylase (U/mL)	50% > 2,000; variable	< 5,000	> 5,000

CEA, carcinoembryonic antigen; CT, Computed tomography; FNA, fine needle aspiration.

CYSTIC NEOPLASMS

Cystic neoplasms of the pancreas account for approximately 1% of all pancreatic cancers and 10% of all pancreatic cystic lesions. These tumors are typically large, are located in the distal pancreas, and affect women three times more frequently than men. The diagnosis of a cystic neoplasm must be considered in patients with radiographic evidence of a pancreatic cyst and no prior symptoms or history of pancreatitis.

Cystic neoplasms with a cuboidal epithelial lining (serous cystadenoma) have no malignant potential. When a columnar epithelial lining is present in the cyst wall, the lesion is frankly malignant (mucinous cystadenocarcinoma) or premalignant (mucinous cystic neoplasm).

It is often impossible to distinguish malignant from benign cystic neoplasms preoperatively or intraoperatively, because the epithelial lining is often incomplete. Therefore, all cystic neoplasms should be resected for potential cure. Patients with malignant cystic neoplasms who undergo complete resection have a 40% to 60% 5-year survival rate. Table 13-5. offers clinical and laboratory tools to help differentiate inflammatory pseudocysts from neoplastic cystic lesions of the pancreas.

RECOMMENDED READING

Bold RJ, Charnsangavej C, Clearly KR, et al. Major vascular resection as part of pancreaticoduodenectomy for cancer: radiologic, intraoperative, and pathologic analysis. *J Gastrointestinal Surg* 1999;3(3):233.

Breslin TM, Hess KR, Harbison DB, et al. Neoadjuvant chemoradiotherapy for adenocarcinoma of the pancreas: treatment variables and survival duration. *Ann Surg Oncol* 2000;8(2):123.

Burris HA, Moore MJ, Andersen J, et al. Improvements in survival and clinical benefit with gemcitabine as first-line therapy for patients with advanced pancreas cancer: a randomized trial. *J Clin Oncol* 1997;15(6):2403.

Crist DW, Sitzman JV, Cameron JL. Improved hospital morbidity, mortality, and survival after the Whipple procedure. *Ann Surg* 1987;206:358.

Dalton RR, Sarr MG, van Heerden JA. Carcinoma of the body and tail of the pancreas: is curative resection justified? *Surgery* 1992;111:489.

Evans DB, Abbruzzese JL, Cleary KR, et al. Rapid-fractionation preoperative chemoradiation for malignant periampullary neoplasms. *J R Coll Surg Edinb* 1995;40:319.

Evans DB, Abbruzzese JL, Willeett CG. Cancer of the pancreas. In: DeVita Jr VT, Hellman S, Rosenberg SA, eds. *Cancer: principles and practice of oncology,* 6th ed. Philadelphia: Lippincott, 2000.

Fortner JG. Regional pancreatectomy for cancer of the pancreas, ampulla, and other related sites. *Ann Surg* 1984;199:418.

Foo ML, Gunderson LL, Nagorney DM, et al. Patterns of failure in grossly resected pancreatic ductal adenocarcinoma treated with adjuvant irradiation +5 fluorouracil. *Int J Radiat Oncol Biol Phys* 1993;26:483.

Fuhrman GM, Charnsangavej C, Abbruzzese JL, et al. Thin-section contrast-enhanced computed tomography accurately predicts the resectability of malignant pancreatic neoplasms. *Am J Surg* 1994; 167:104.

Fuhrman GM, Leach SD, Staley CA, et al. Rationale for en bloc vein resection in the treatment of pancreatic adenocarcinoma adherent to the superior mesenteric-portal venous confluence. *Ann Surg* 1996;223:154.

Gastrointestinal Tumor Study Group. Further evidence of effective adjuvant combined radiation and chemotherapy following curative resection of pancreatic cancer. *Cancer* 1987;59:2006.

Geer RJ, Brennan MF. Prognostic indicators for survival after resection of pancreatic adenocarcinoma. *Am J Surg* 1993;165:68.

Itani KM, Coleman RE, Akwari OE, et al. Pylorus-preserving pancreaticoduodenectomy: a clinical and physiologic appraisal. *Ann Surg* 1986;204:655.

Leach SD, Rose JA, Lowy AM, et al. Significance of peritoneal cytology in patients with potentially resectable adenocarcinoma of the pancreatic head. *Surgery* 1995;118:472.

Lieberman MD, Kilburn H, Lindsey M, et al. Relation of perioperative deaths to hospital volume among patients undergoing pancreatic resection for malignancy. *Ann Surg* 1995;222:638.

Moertel CG, Frytak S, Hahn RG, et al. Therapy of locally unresectable pancreatic carcinoma: a randomized comparison of high dose (6000 rads) radiation alone, moderate dose radiation and 5-fluorouracil. *Cancer* 1981;48:1705.

Pisters PWT, Abbruzzese JL, Janjan NA, et al. Rapid-fractionation preoperative chemoradiation, pancreaticoduodenectomy, and intraoperative radiation therapy for resectable pancreatic adenocarcinoma. *J Clin Oncol* 1998;16:3843.

Pisters PWT, Hudec WA, Lee JE, et al. Preoperative chemoradiation for patients with pancreatic cancer: toxicity of endobiliary stents. *J Clin Oncol* 2000;18:860.

Rumstadt B, Schwab M, Schuster K, et al. The role of laparoscopy in the preoperative staging of pancreatic carcinoma. *J Gastrointestinal Surg* 1997;1(3):245.

Shepherd HA, Royle G, Ross APR. Endoscopic biliary endoprothesis in the palliation of malignant obstruction of the distal common bile duct: a randomized trial. *Br J Surg* 1988;75:1166.

Sindelar WF, Kinsella TJ. Randomized trial of intraoperative radiotherapy in resected carcinoma of the pancreas. *Radiat Oncol Biol Physiol* 1986;12:148.

Spitz FR, Abbruzzese JL, Lee JE, et al. Preoperative and postoperative chemoradiation strategies in patients treated with pancreaticoduodenectomy for adenocarcinoma of the pancreas. *J Clin Oncol* 1997;15:928.

Warshaw AL, Compton CC, Lewandrowski K, et al. Cystic tumors of the pancreas. *Ann Surg* 1990;212:432.

Yeo CJ, Cameron JL, Lillemoe KD, et al. Pancreaticoduodenectomy for cancer of the head of the pancreas: 201 patients. *Ann Surg* 1995;221:721.

Yeo CJ, Abrams RA, Grochow LB, et al. Pancreaticoduodenectomy for pancreatic adenocarcinoma: postoperative adjuvant chemoradiation improves survival. A prospective, single-institution experience. *Ann Surg* 1997;225(3):621.

Pancreatic Endocrine Tumors and Multiple Endocrine Neoplasia

Jeffrey T. Lenert, Richard J. Bold, Jeffrey J. Sussman, and Douglas S. Tyler

PANCREATIC ENDOCRINE TUMORS

Pancreatic endocrine tumors are relatively rare, with approximately five clinically recognized cases occurring per one million people annually. However, some series of carefully performed, unselected autopsies have demonstrated an incidence as high as 0.5% to 1.5%. Many of these tumors are functional and patients present with symptoms attributable to excess hormone production and secretion. The tumors tend to arise in the islet cells of the pancreas but can also be located in the small bowel, especially the duodenum, and in other intraabdominal sites. Although the islet cells have long been thought to be of neural crest origin because of metabolic characteristics shared with other cells of neuroectodermal origin, specifically the amine precursor uptake and decarboxylation (APUD) cells, more recent studies suggest they may be of endodermal origin (e.g., pancreatic ductal epithelium).

Islet cell tumors are usually divided into functioning and nonfunctioning tumors. More than 75% of the islet cell tumors diagnosed clinically are functioning and frequently produce, and often secrete, more than one hormone. The tumors are categorized by the major hormone producing the clinical syndrome. The hormones may include gastrin, insulin, glucagon, somatostatin, neurotensin, pancreatic polypeptide (PP), vasoactive intestinal polypeptide (VIP), growth hormone-releasing factor (GRF), and adrenocorticotropic hormone (ACTH). The tumors are considered entopic, or orthoendocrine, if they produce hormones or peptides usually found within the pancreas (e.g., insulinomas, glucagonomas, somatostatinomas, and PPomas) or ectopic (paraendocrine) if the hormones or peptides are not native to the normal pancreas (e.g., gastrinomas, VIPomas, GRFomas, neurotensinomas, and ACTHoma). An overview of the characteristics of pancreatic endocrine tumors is shown in Table 14-1.

The diagnosis of pancreatic endocrine tumors is usually made by the recognition of the clinical syndrome caused by excess hormone secretion. The specific hormone excess also allows assessment of a patient's response to therapy and provides a mechanism for observing the long-term status of the disease. However, PPomas and nonfunctioning islet cell tumors do not secrete clinically apparent hormones and hence are diagnosed as a result of mass-effect symptoms or as an incidental finding on computed tomography (CT) scans of the abdomen for unrelated reasons. Unlike in patients with functioning neuroendocrine tumors, response to treatment and long-term follow-up of patients with

Table 14-1. Characteristics of pancreatic endocrine neoplasms

Tumor Name	Hormone Secreted	Pancreatic Cell Type	Clinical Syndrome	Malignant (%)	Association with MEN 1 (%)
Gastrinoma	Gastrin	D or D variant	Peptic ulcers, diarrhea, GERD	60–90	25–30%
Insulinoma	Insulin	β	Hypoglycemia, neurologic symptoms, adrenergic excess symptoms	5–15	10%
VIPoma	Vasoactive intestinal peptide	H	Watery diarrhea, achlorhydria, hypokalemia	60–80	Rare
Glucagonoma	Glucagon	α_2	Hyperglycemia dermatitis (necrolytic migratory erythema) cachexia, thrombophlebitis	60–70	Rare
Ppoma	Pancreatic polypeptide	PP	None	>60	Occasional
Somatostatinoma	Somatostatin	δ or α	Hyperglycemia Steatorrhea Gallstones	90	Never
GRFoma	Growth hormone-releasing factor		—	—	—
ACTHoma	Adrenocorticotropic hormone		—	—	—
PTHrp-oma	Parathyroid hormone-related protein		—	—	—
Nonfunctioning	None		None	>60	Frequent

GERD, gastroesophageal reflux disease; MEN 1, multiple endocrine neoplasia type 1.

Table 14-2. Anatomic distribution of pancreatic endocrine tumors within the pancreas (head, body, and tail) as well as the extrapancreatic tissue, including the duodenum

Tumor	Head (%)	Body (%)	Tail (%)	Extrapancreatic/ duodenal (%)
Gastrinoma	30	12	14	44[a]
Insulinoma	25	41	33	1
Glucagonoma	23	37	40	0
PP-secreting tumor	52	14	14	20
Somatostatinoma	62	4	12	22

Adapted from Howard TJ, Stabile BE, Zinner MJ, et al. Anatomic distribution of pancreatic endocrine tumors. *Am J Surg* 1990;159:258.
[a]More recent series show that two-thirds are extrapancreatic.

nonfunctioning tumors is not aided by measurement of hormones specific to the tumor in question; however, more general tumor markers can be used. Functioning and nonfunctioning pancreatic neuroendocrine tumors secrete several tumor markers, including chromogranins, PP, and subunits of human chorionic gonadotropin. Chromogranin A (CgA) in particular may be a useful marker to supplement specific markers in functioning tumors and may be useful by itself or with other general markers when tumors are nonfunctioning. Histologic diagnosis of the islet cell tumor can be obtained with CT-guided fine-needle aspiration, although this is often not required, given the syndrome of pancreatic hormonal excess and a localizing study. (See Table 14-2 for the distribution of these tumors within the pancreas.)

In general, pancreatic endocrine tumors are more indolent than ductal adenocarcinoma and carry a better prognosis; even patients with hepatic metastasis may have a mean survival time of 5 years.

Gastrinoma: Zollinger-Ellison Syndrome

In 1955, Zollinger and Ellison described a syndrome characterized by the triad of severe, atypical peptic ulceration; gastric hypersecretion and hyperacidity; and a non-insulin–producing islet cell tumor of the pancreas. They theorized that a humoral factor arising from the tumor was responsible for the syndrome. Several years later, the hormone gastrin was discovered and found to be the underlying cause of the peptic hyperacidity, and the term Zollinger-Ellison syndrome (ZES) was applied to the clinical complex.

Epidemiology

At least 0.1% of patients with duodenal ulcer disease and approximately 2% of patients with recurrent ulcers after appropriate medical therapy are found to have a gastrinoma, making it the most common functioning malignant pancreatic endocrine tumor. Approximately 75% of gastrinomas occur sporadically; the remaining 25% are associated with the multiple endocrine neoplasia type 1 syndrome (MEN 1). The mean age at onset of symptoms is 50 years, and approximately 60% of those diagnosed with ZES are men. Gastrinomas that occur as part of MEN 1 are more often benign, multicentric, and extrapancreatic and occur at an earlier age than sporadic gastrinomas. In more than half of the patients with MEN 1 syndrome, the pancreatic tumors are gastrinomas.

Clinical Presentation

High levels of gastrin stimulate the parietal cells within the stomach to secrete excess acid in an unregulated state. This leads to severe ulcer diathesis and injury to the small bowel mucosa well past the ligament of Treitz, resulting in varying degrees of malabsorption. Profuse watery diarrhea occurs in up to 50% of patients because of the combination of acid hypersecretion and small bowel mucosal injury. In addition to secreting gastrin, the majority of gastrinomas secrete at least one other peptide hormone, such as insulin, PP, glucagon, or even ACTH.

The clinical manifestations of gastrinomas are almost invariably due to hypergastrinemia. Ninety percent of patients have endoscopically documented ulcerations of the upper gastrointestinal (GI) tract. Most of these ulcers are accompanied by abdominal pain, which is the most frequent single symptom. Bleeding occurs in 30% to 50% of patients and perforation in 5% to 10%. Secretory diarrhea is the only clinical manifestation of the syndrome in 20% of patients, although diarrhea and pain in combination is more frequent than either symptom alone. Symptoms of gastroesophageal reflux disease are also being recognized more often in association with ZES. The syndrome is often initially misdiagnosed due to the frequency of typical peptic ulcer disease (PUD) and a broad differential diagnosis. The mean duration of symptoms before diagnosis is often several years. Clinical situations in which ZES should be suspected and the differential diagnoses are listed in Tables 14-3 and 14-4.

Table 14-3. Clinical situations warranting further evaluation for gastrinoma

Recurrent peptic ulcers after appropriate medical or surgical therapy
Failure of peptic ulcer to heal on appropriate medical therapy, including treatment for *H. pylori* if present
Multiple UGI ulcers or ulcers in atypical locations
Family history of peptic ulcer disease
Peptic ulcer or GERD with diarrhea
Persistent diarrhea without clear etiology
Peptic ulcer in the absence of *H. pylori*
Personal or family history of MEN 1 tumors or endocrinopathies
Prominent gastric rugae with PUD
PUD resulting in complication (bleeding, perforation, obstruction)

GERD, gastroesophageal reflux disease; MEN 1, multiple endocrine neoplasia type 1; PUD, peptic ulcer disease; UGI, upper gastrointestinal.

**Table 14-4. Differential diagnosis of hypergastrinemia
and gastric hypersecretion**

H. pylori infection
Gastric outlet obstruction
Antral G-cell hyperfunction/hyperplasia
Chronic renal failure
Retained gastric antrum syndrome
Short bowel syndrome
Zollinger-Ellison syndrome

Adapted from Jensen RT. Zollinger-Ellison syndrome. In: Doherty GM, Skögseid B, eds. *Surgical endocrinology.* Philadelphia: Lippincott Williams & Wilkins, 2001.

Biochemical Diagnosis

The diagnosis of gastrinoma requires confirmation with laboratory studies. A fasting serum gastrin measurement should be the first test obtained and is increased in greater than 90% of patients with gastrinoma (normal is 100–200 pg/mL). A level greater than 1,000 pg/mL is usually diagnostic of a gastrinoma and is seen in approximately 30% of patients. Most patients with gastrinomas have more moderate elevation of fasting gastrin levels (in the 200–1,000 pg/mL range). In addition to hypergastrinemia, gastric acid hypersecretion is required for the diagnosis of gastrinoma because hypergastrinemia is a normal physiologic response to achlorhydria or hypochlorhydria. Documentation of a gastric pH less than 2.5 rules out this physiologic response as the cause of hypergastrinemia. One third of patients with gastrinoma will have serum gastrin levels greater than 1,000 pg/mL and a gastric pH less than 2.5, which confirms the diagnosis. In the remaining two thirds, measurement of gastric acid output is required. Typically, patients with gastrinomas have a basal acid output of more than 15 mEq/hour or greater than 5 mEq/hour if they have had a previous ulcer operation aimed at reducing gastric acid secretion. A basal acid output/maximal acid output ratio greater than 0.6 also helps support the diagnosis of gastrinoma.

Provocative testing using the secretin stimulation test helps confirm the diagnosis in patients with more moderate hypergastrinemia (200–1000 pg/mL) and gastric acid hypersecretion. After an overnight fast, the patient is given 2 units of secretin per kilogram of body weight intravenously. Serum gastrin levels are measured at 15 and 2 minutes before secretin injection and 0, 2, 5, 10, and 20 minutes following injection. A paradoxical increase in the serum concentration of gastrin by more than 200 pg/mL over baseline levels is diagnostic of gastrinoma. Patients with either antral G-cell hyperplasia or hypertrophy do not respond to secretin injection, although they do have postprandial gastrin elevation.

Tumor Localization

Tumor localization has become increasingly important in recent years with the demonstration that resection of gastrinomas is associated with an excellent prognosis and is frequently curative. Historically, numerous tests have been used to localize gastrinomas preoperatively, often without a well-designed strategy. This approach has used any, and frequently many, of the following modalities: CT scans, magnetic resonance imaging (MRI), transabdominal ultrasound, selective visceral angiography, selective venous sampling of portal venous tributaries, intraarterial secretin with hepatic venous sampling for gastrin, and conventional upper endoscopy. Two newer diagnostic methods—somatostatin receptor scintigraphy (SRS) and endoscopic ultrasonography (EUS)—are now complementing, and often replacing, the more traditional localization techniques. SRS, which takes advantage of the presence of high-affinity somatostatin receptors on the majority of pancreatic endocrine tumors, has been shown to have a sensitivity and specificity as high as 90% and 80%, respectively, equal to or greater than those for all other conventional localizing techniques combined (CT, MRI, US, angiography). The one relative weakness of SRS is in detecting small duodenal gastrinomas: it has been reported to miss up to one third of such lesions ultimately identified surgically. Because more than half of all lesions in recent surgical series have been duodenal gastrinomas, EUS has shown promise in complementing the information gained by SRS. Endoscopic ultrasound can localize up to half of duodenal lesions as well as most pancreatic gastrinomas. The combination of SRS and EUS should allow preoperative localization of most extrahepatic gastrinomas. When both of these studies are negative, an intraarterial secretin injection with hepatic venous sampling for gastrin is recommended by some because of its high sensitivity (approximately 89%) and ability to detect lesions independent of size, a drawback with SRS and EUS. CT and MRI can be used to address specific questions, if necessary (e.g., extent of liver metastases).

The introduction of SRS and EUS has clearly improved preoperative localization; still, up to one third of patients at experienced institutions will undergo exploration when preoperative imaging is negative. Although somewhat controversial, surgical exploration is warranted in patients with sporadic gastrinoma without diffuse liver metastases, even without successful preoperative localization. This scenario underscores the need for a careful operative strategy to ensure identification of the lesions to be resected.

Because most gastrinomas are found in the gastrinoma triangle (an anatomic area bounded by the junction of the body and neck of the pancreas medially, the junction of the second and third portion of the duodenum inferiorly, and the junction of the cystic duct and common bile duct superiorly), the operative focus is on this region. However, one must remember that primary gastrinomas can be found in numerous sites, including the lymph nodes, stomach, jejunum, mesentery, liver, ovary, and kidney. The combined use of an extensive Kocher maneuver for bimanual palpation of the pancreatic head and intraoperative ultrasonography detects virtually all intrapancreatic lesions. Detection of duodenal lesions requires more effort. Intraoperative endoscopy with duodenal transillumination will increase the duodenal gastrinoma detection rate above that of palpation and intraoperative ultrasound, but the key—some would advocate mandatory—maneuver is duodenotomy with careful palpation of the duodenal wall. The use of these intraoperative techniques has resulted in the ability to identify nearly all gastrinomas (including fairly small tumors, <5 mm) and essentially eliminated the nonproductive laparotomy. A final intraoperative technique using the gamma probe and radiolabeled octreotide to detect microscopic and otherwise undetected abdominal neuroendocrine tumors is currently being evaluated.

Treatment

Once the diagnosis of gastrinoma is suspected, the first step is to control the gastric acid hypersecretion and its end-organ effects. After initiation of appropriate medical therapy, definitive diagnosis and evaluation may proceed. Total gastrectomy warrants only a historical note and is rarely indicated because effective medical treatment is now readily available. Historically, total gastrectomy served as the only modality to eliminate the potentially lethal sequelae of gastric hypersecretion. H_2-blockers initially control acid secretion in most patients with gastrinomas, but over time most of these individuals require increasing dosages. In addition, up to 65% of patients, depending on the series, will fail to respond to this form of medical therapy. On the other hand, omeprazole, a gastric proton pump inhibitor, is associated with a considerably lower failure rate (0%–7.5%) and a more convenient dosing schedule. Omeprazole, or one of the newer proton pump inhibitors (e.g., lansoprazole, pantoprazole), is currently the drug of first choice. Long-term use may lead to drug-induced achlorhydria or hypochlorhydria with resultant vitamin B12 deficiency. Similarly, the question of increased incidence of gastric carcinoids—particularly in patients with MEN 1—has yet to be resolved satisfactorily. The somatostatin analogue, octreotide acetate, or the longer-acting lantreotide, may also be useful for symptomatic relief by decreasing the release of gastrin and other peptide hormones from gastrinomas and directly inhibiting gastric parietal cells.

In a patient with a sporadic gastrinoma, surgical exploration with attempted curative resection should follow localization studies regardless of whether the tumor is identified preoperatively. Because as many as 10% to 40% of tumors may not be localized before surgery, a standardized approach to exploration should be undertaken. The exploration should be done through a bilateral subcostal incision and the abdomen completely explored for evidence of metastasis, especially the regional lymph nodes and the liver, because up to 50% of gastrinomas are malignant with demonstrable disease at exploration. A complete mobilization of the pancreas is essential to allow inspection and palpation of the gland. Any suspicious lymph node or mass should be evaluated by frozen-section examination, as it is unclear whether surgical resection in the presence of metastasis prolongs survival or alleviates medical management of gastric hypersecretion. Some groups do recommend aggressive debulking of all tumor deposits if they are unresectable because survival may be improved and medical management of the acid disease may be better controlled. Intraoperative ultrasound may help identify intrapancreatic lesions, while intraoperative endoscopy with transillumination of the duodenal wall may help to identify duodenal gastrinomas.

If no tumor is identified, a longitudinal duodenotomy should be made in the second portion of the duodenum. Careful bimanual examination of the bowel wall, along with its eversion, helps identify duodenal gastrinomas, which are frequently located submucosally with decreasing frequency from the proximal to the distal duodenum. When the tumor is small (<2 cm), duodenal gastrinomas can be resected with a small margin of normal tissue, whereas pancreatic gastrinomas should be enucleated, if possible, particularly in the head of the pancreas. Larger tumors often require pancreatic resection, either distal pancreatectomy or pancreaticoduodenectomy, particularly with tumors that are clearly invasive or abut critical ductal or vascular structures.

Despite extensive preoperative localizing studies and careful surgical exploration, the tumor of some patients cannot be identified even at laparotomy. "Blind" pancreatic head resection is controversial, especially given the dichotomous nature of gastrinoma whereby 75% of tumors pursue a fairly nonaggressive course. Patients with ZES in whom no tumor is found have an excellent prognosis, with 5- and 10-year survival rates of more than 94% and 87%, respectively. If gastric hypersecretion remains problematic despite maximal medical management, consideration may be given to performing a highly selective vagotomy. Total gastrectomy should be considered in patients who have had previous life-threatening complications from their ulcer disease despite appropriate medical management.

Medical management of ZES in patients with MEN 1 can be more difficult because of decreased sensitivity to antisecretory drugs, especially H_2-blockers. Parathyroidectomy and control of hypercalcemia can increase the potency of both proton pump inhibitors and H_2-blockers. The role of surgery in patients with ZES and MEN 1 is controversial. Resection of gastrinomas in patients with MEN 1 rarely results in normal serum gastrin levels, suggesting that the probability of curing these patients with surgery is extremely low. However, patients with MEN 1 tend to experience the less aggressive disease process and have a considerably long survival time even without complete surgical resection. As a result, many authorities have recommended that patients with MEN 1 and gastrinomas do not undergo exploration. Other groups think that resection of localized, larger (>2.5–3 cm) tumors may help reduce the risk of distant metastatic disease and presumably alter the natural history of the disease; therefore, they recommend that patients with MEN 1 undergo exploration. More extensive resections are generally discouraged because of the more favorable natural history, in addition to the problematic presence of multiple, synchronous, nonfunctioning pancreatic endocrine tumors, the prognostic effect of which is unclear.

Metastatic Disease

Now that medical treatment of gastric acid hypersecretion in ZES is so effective, patients rarely die from complications related to PUD. As a result, they live longer, only to die from metastatic disease. Given the propensity of malignant gastrinomas to metastasize to the liver, it is not surprising that patients ultimately die of liver failure. When feasible (approximately 15% of the time), cytoreductive hepatic resection can play a significant role in palliation of metastatic gastrinoma, often improving symptoms and extending life expectancy. When debulking procedures are not practical, nonsurgical therapy is often targeted directly at the liver in the form of peripheral hepatic artery embolization or chemoembolization and, in very selected cases, hepatic transplantation. Hepatic artery embolization with or without chemotherapeutic or radiotherapeutic agents takes advantage of the hypervascular morphology of pancreatic endocrine tumors derived preferentially from the hepatic artery. The nature of systemic therapy is to treat the entire body at risk for metastases and any currently manifest lesions. Systemic strategies include traditional chemotherapy, interferon-alpha, and somatostatin analogues used with and without radioisotopes (e.g., ^{90}yttrium). The larger series of gastrinoma patients report a 50% to 90% incidence of metastatic disease. Chemotherapy rarely results in cure, although some regimens have reasonable rates of response. The most promising regimen appears to be a combination of streptozocin and 5-fluorouracil, with or without doxorubicin; this combination gives response rates of 50% to 70%. Importantly, although many gastrinomas may not decrease demonstrably in volume, patients may have a symptomatically significant biochemical response. The somatostatin analogues appear effective in controlling symptoms of gastrinomas but show a disappointing objective tumor response rate of 10% to 20%. Interferon alfa has also been studied alone and in combination with chemotherapy and somatostatin therapy. It also may result in biochemical response, with fewer patients realizing a reduction in tumor volume. Generally, traditional chemotherapy is considered first line nonsurgical therapy.

When to initiate therapy for metastatic disease remains a controversial topic. Metastatic gastrinoma appears to follow at least three distinct clinical courses. In patients with rapidly progressing symptomatic disease, there would be little disagreement regarding the need to initiate potentially toxic therapy. However, in patients with slowly progressing, or even stable disease with easily controlled symptoms, the decision becomes less clear. Ultimately, the decision must be individualized to maximize the quality of the patient's remaining life.

Insulinoma

Epidemiology

In most series, insulinomas are the most common islet cell tumors of the pancreas, with a reported incidence estimated between less than one and four cases per 1 million people per year. These tumors occur slightly more often in women than in men. The average patient's age at presentation is between 40 and 50 years. These tumors are almost always benign and overwhelmingly small (<2 cm), solitary lesions within the pancreas unless associated with MEN 1, when they tend to occur in a multicentric fashion.

Clinical Presentation

The original diagnostic criteria for an insulinoma are known as Whipple's triad and were proposed by Whipple, who initially

Table 14-5. Symptoms associated with an insulinoma and their respective frequency

Symptoms	Frequency (%)
Neuroglycopenic symptoms	
Visual disturbances	59
Confusion	51
Altered consciousness	38
Weakness	32
Seizures	23
Symptoms related to hypoglycemic catecholamine release	
Sweating	43
Tremulousness	23
Tachycardia	23

described the syndrome. This triad consists of symptoms of hypoglycemia at fasting, documentation of blood glucose levels less than 50 mg/dL, and relief of symptoms following administration of glucose. However, Whipple's triad has proven not to be very specific, underscoring the importance of clinical suspicion and careful, systematic evaluation. The clinical symptoms of insulinomas are due to the hypoglycemia induced by excess insulin secretion and are commonly characterized as either neuroglycopenic or autonomic adrenergic. No truly hypoglycemic disorder presents with exclusively excess adrenergic symptoms. Many patients learn to recognize their specific symptom onset and thus avoid them by frequent meals or snacks. This is reflected in the often long duration of symptoms before diagnosis, frequently measured in months if not years. A list of the common symptoms and their frequency is shown in Table 14-5. Hunger, nausea, weight gain, and vomiting are also reported occasionally.

Biochemical Diagnosis

The measurement of normal serum glucose concentration documented during characteristic symptoms eliminates the diagnosis of insulinoma. The most reliable method of diagnosing an insulinoma is the provocative 72-hour supervised fast. Blood glucose and insulin levels are measured every 4 to 6 hours during the fast until serum glucose levels decrease below 60 mg/dL, at which time the frequency is increased to every 1 to 2 hours. Eighty percent of patients with insulinoma become symptomatic within 24 hours of starting the fast, and almost all are symptomatic if the fast is continued for 72 hours. The presence of hypoglycemia with concurrent elevation of serum insulin concentrations higher than 6 μU/mL (lack of appropriate suppression) and an insulin to glucose ratio of more than 0.3 confirm the diagnosis. One large series found, however, that 19% of patients with excised insulinomas had insulin:glucose ratios less than 0.3, pointing out the potential diagnostic weakness of the ratio. Measurement of the beta cell products C-peptide and proinsulin is important because both are usually increased in patients with insulinoma. In fact, the half-life of C-peptide is roughly twice that of insulin; therefore measurable C-peptide in a hypoglycemic patient is indicative of an endogenous insulin source. Patients who surreptitiously administer insulin to themselves usually have low levels of C-peptide and proinsulin, because commercial insulin does not contain the insulin precursor or its cleavage fragments. Patients taking oral hypoglycemic agents have normal or elevated levels of C-peptide and proinsulin, so differentiation from an insulinoma is made by measurement of plasma levels of sulfonylureas. Occasionally, ancillary tests such as the C-peptide suppression test and the tolbutamide test may provide evidence to support the diagnosis of insulinoma in equivocal cases.

Tumor Localization

Most insulinomas are small (<2 cm in diameter), and only approximately 10% of insulinomas are multicentric. There are no histologic criteria of malignancy for insulinomas; therefore, the diagnosis of a malignant tumor is based on the demonstration of metastatic disease, which is noted in 10% of cases. As with gastrinomas, all of the different modalities noted have also been used in an attempt to preoperatively localize insulinomas. Historical experience has demonstrated that, as with gastrinomas, no single technique is consistently reliable in localizing insulinomas short of exploration. Dynamic CT scanning is often the first localizing study performed, because it can detect approximately two thirds of the primary tumors and most metastatic lesions. When no tumor is seen with the CT scan, visceral angiography with digital subtraction techniques is successful in visualizing lesions approximately 60% to 90% of the time, although over the past decade the sensitivity of this study has fallen considerably in several reports. Selective portal venous sampling is reserved mainly for patients whose tumors cannot be visualized with CT or angiography. Portal venous sampling is able to define the general area of the tumor in 90% of patients overall and in approximately 75% of patients in whom other localizing tests are negative. The perfect study does not exist and thus the decision of which technique(s) will be used should revolve around institutional expertise and expected yield, the risk to the patient, and the cost of the total evaluation relative to its expected yield. In some experienced hands, preoperative localization is limited to transabdominal ultrasound.

Newer modalities are encouraging but continue to undergo definitive evaluation. Endoscopic ultrasound has shown promise, as it has with intrapancreatic gastrinomas, although its success becomes more limited when evaluating more distal pancreatic lesions. Lesions in the head of the pancreas can be visualized up to 95% of the time, while those in the body and tail were visualized in 78% and 60%, respectively, in one series. Unfortunately, insulinomas often (30%–90% of cases) do not possess appropriate somatostatin receptors, limiting the benefit of SRS in insulinomas as compared with other pancreatic endocrine tumors. Regardless of preoperative imaging, intraoperative ultrasound has been uniformly helpful in locating lesions not identified before exploration or by manual palpation alone and for ruling out or identifying multiple tumors.

Treatment

At exploration, reddish-purple or white tumors may be visible on the surface of the gland; however, the pancreas must be completely mobilized as described previously for intrapancreatic gastrinomas. Small insulinomas located away from the main pancreatic duct can be enucleated. Small lesions in proximity to the main pancreatic duct can also be enucleated, and such a procedure is aided by intraoperative ultrasound guidance to avoid injury to the duct. Distal pancreatectomy is recommended for small lesions near the pancreatic duct to minimize the risk of a pancreatic fistula. Large lesions in the head of the pancreas may require pancreaticoduodenectomy, whereas those in the body and tail can be treated with a distal pancreatectomy. Resection is also preferred when signs of malignancy are present (e.g., hard tumors, puckering of adjacent tissue, infiltration, or tumors causing distal ductal obstruction). Intraoperative ultrasound can help identify tumors that could not be localized preoperatively using standard imaging techniques. Insulinomas are identified approximately 95% of the time at initial exploration. As with gastrinomas, blind resection of the pancreas is not recommended when no tumor is identified. Given the fairly uniform distribution of insulinomas throughout the pancreas, the logic behind "blind" resection is unclear, although there are those that would consider a "regionalizing" transhepatic portal venous sampling study adequate localization, particularly after an initial failed exploration and inadequate control of symptoms by appropriate medical therapy. If no tumor is identified at exploration, then pancreatic biopsy to rule out beta cell hyperplasia and adult nesidioblastosis is advisable. Beta cell hyperplasia or adult nesidioblastosis can generally be successfully treated by subtotal pancreatectomy.

Metastatic Disease

Patients with successful resection of insulinomas can expect an otherwise normal life expectancy. However, in those patients whose tumors are not found at exploration, are unsuitable for operative exploration, or have metastatic disease, symptoms can often be managed pharmacologically with diazoxide, verapamil, phenytoin, propranolol, or octreotide. Nonetheless, patients with metastatic disease should be considered for resection of the primary tumor and accessible metastatic lesions. Median disease-free survival is approximately 5 years in patients with malignant insulinoma who undergo curative resection. Approximately 65% of patients with malignant tumors will have recurrences at a mean of about 2.8 years. Although the chances for cure after resection are low in patients with malignant insulinoma, 10-year survival rates are 29%. Tumor debulking may improve control of hypoglycemic symptoms, but is recommended only if greater than 90% of disease can be resected.

Palliation can be achieved with medical therapy as well as surgery. Diazoxide can control the endocrine symptoms of insulinomas in 50% to 70% of patients by inhibiting the release of insulin from islet cells directly and by enhancing glycogenolysis indirectly. Octreotide controls symptoms in 40% to 60% of patients; however, its effect may be unpredictable in individual patients with tumors having atypical beta granules or none at all. Of the chemotherapeutic agents used for patients with metastatic disease, streptozocin, 5-fluorouracil, and doxorubicin have shown the best response rates.

Vasoactive Intestinal Polypeptidoma

Epidemiology

Although not a normal product of pancreatic islet cells, VIP can be secreted by islet cell tumors. The syndrome of excessive VIP secretion is associated with watery diarrhea, hypokalemia, and either hypochlorhydria or achlorhydria. First described in association with islet cell tumors in 1958, the syndrome has many names, including Verner-Morrison syndrome, pancreatic cholera, and WDHA (watery diarrhea, hypokalemia, and achlorhydria). Subsequently, it has been realized that 80% to 90% of so-called VIPomas are located in the pancreas, most often the body and tail (75%). Extrapancreatic tumors are often located in the chest and retroperitoneum (lung, esophagus, adrenal medulla [as ganglioblastomas, neuroblastomas, and ganglioneuromas] and along the autonomic nervous system). Ten percent of cases are due to islet cell hyperplasia. To date, approximately 200 well-documented cases of VIPoma have been described, and in most cases the tumor is malignant. An interesting bimodal distribution is noted, with younger patients (<10 years old) having less aggressive and extrapancreatic tumors.

Clinical Presentation / Tumor Localization

Patients usually present with excessive secretory diarrhea, often greater than 3 L/day that is aggravated by oral food intake and persists despite fasting. The patients become hypokalemic secondary to fecal potassium loss and acidotic from loss of fecal bicarbonate. The presence of a VIPoma is confirmed by demonstrating an increased fasting serum VIP level (>200 pg/mL) in the setting of secretory diarrhea with the presence of a mass. There are no provocative or inhibitory confirmatory studies. Pancreatic VIPomas are usually solitary, are greater than 3 cm in diameter, and most often are located in the tail of the pancreas. Diarrhea is such a nonspecific symptom that the evaluation should focus on eliminating more common causes (i.e., infectious, inflammatory, mechanical, even gastrinoma) before proceeding to serum VIP levels or localization studies. Typically, preoperative localization is easily achieved by abdominal and chest CT scans or by SRS. Mesenteric arteriography and hepatic portal venous sampling (HPVS) may be useful if the tumor location is still in question.

Treatment

Surgical excision remains the only effective method of cure. Preoperative preparation should include adequate rehydration and correction of electrolyte imbalances. The first-line therapy for control of the diarrhea is the use of long-acting somatostatin analogues. However, administration of steroids, nonsteroidal anti-inflammatory drugs, or phenothiazines may also be helpful. At exploration, most tumors are located in the distal pancreas and are amenable to a complete resection by a distal pancreatectomy. A careful evaluation of both adrenal glands is mandatory if no tumor is found in the pancreas. Approximately 50% of the time, metastatic disease is found outside the pancreas at exploration. If curative resection is not possible, surgical debulking is often indicated to help palliate symptoms.

Long-term survival is relatively poor at approximately 15%. Streptozocin and interferon are currently the most active chemotherapeutic agents for advanced disease, and these are generally believed to be more effective against VIPomas than against other pancreatic endocrine tumors. Octreotide and other somatostatin analogues are useful for symptomatic relief from diarrhea in patients with metastatic disease and have been shown by some investigators to have some effect on tumor growth.

Glucagonoma

Glucagonomas arise from the A cells in the pancreatic islets of Langerhans. The syndrome caused by this tumor is due to excess secretion of glucagon. In contrast to other pancreatic endocrine tumors, glucagonomas are frequently fairly large at diagnosis (>5 cm) and are rarely found outside the pancreas. Approximately 70% of these tumors are malignant.

Clinical Presentation / Diagnosis

The most common and usually initial symptom in patients with glucagonoma is mild glucose intolerance (occurring in >90% of patients) that rarely requires insulin administration. The most striking and characteristic feature is a severe dermatitis called necrolytic migratory erythema, seen in approximately 70% of patients. The skin rash is most often located on the lower abdomen, perineum, perioral area, or feet. Other symptoms include a catabolic state, hypoaminoacidemia, stomatitis, anemia (normochromic/normocytic), weight loss, glossitis, depression, and venous thrombosis.

The diagnosis is confirmed by documenting the presence of an increased fasting serum glucagon level; levels greater than 1,000 pg/mL (normal, 0–150 pg/mL) are virtually diagnostic. Other conditions may cause hyperglucagonemia (e.g., hepatic insufficiency, severe stress, bacteremia, and starvation), but serum glucagon levels rarely exceed 500 pg/mL. In addition, the diagnosis can be confirmed by the characteristic findings on biopsy of the skin rash.

Tumor Localization

CT scanning is the first localization study. Most tumors are large at the time of diagnosis, ranging from 5 to 10 cm, and occur most often in the body and tail of the pancreas. As with the other pancreatic endocrine tumors, SRS localizes glucagonomas very reliably. Given the large size of these lesions, additional localization studies are rarely needed, although angiography and portal venous sampling may be required for glucagonomas that are difficult to identify.

Treatment

Surgical exploration should be undertaken in any patient whose tumor is thought to be resectable. Preoperative preparation of patients to reverse catabolism should include the use of somatostatin analogues and replenishment of amino acids—helping to ameliorate the catabolic state and often leading to resolution of the associated dermatitis. Sixty-eight percent of patients will have metastatic disease diagnosed by preoperative studies or at the time of exploration. Patients who are symptomatic due to metastatic disease frequently benefit from surgical resection. Patients with widely metastatic disease in whom surgical debulking is impossible can often benefit from medical therapy. Octreotide has been successful in controlling the diabetes and dermatitis in 60% to 90% of patients. Dacarbazine and streptozocin have been successfully used to treat some unresectable or recurrent glucagonomas. Although glucagonomas are rarely cured, long-term survival of up to 50% at 5 years is reported due to the frequent resectability and slow-growing nature of the lesions.

Somatostatinoma

Somatostatinomas arise from the D cells of the islets of Langerhans and are among the rarest endocrine neoplasms, with an estimated yearly incidence of one in 40 million. Generally mild hyperglycemia, cholelithiasis, steatorrhea, and diarrhea mark the somatostatinoma syndrome associated with these tumors. This "classic" syndrome is seen in patients with pancreatic tumors, while it is typically absent in those with duodenal somatostatinomas. Although duodenal tumors are not often associated with the classic somatostatinoma syndrome, they have been noted retrospectively to be often associated with neurofibromatosis. This has resulted in the proposal of a new MEN syndrome and should cause the clinician to be aware of the possibility of concurrent pheochromocytoma.

Early detection is difficult because symptoms are frequently mild and nonspecific. Diagnosis is often serendipitous during cholecystectomy, exploratory laparotomy, or radiologic or endoscopic evaluation of nonspecific abdominal symptoms. Confirmation of diagnostic suspicion can be achieved by demonstration of serum somatostatin levels 50-fold higher than normal. Provocative testing is not routinely available, although tolbutamide has been reported to cause an increase in serum levels in patients with somatostatinomas and not in controls. Most of these lesions are large and solitary and located in the head of the pancreas, and they are easily localized by CT scan or ultrasound (duodenal lesions are usually smaller but can be confirmed by esophagogastroduodenoscopy or radiography). Up to 90% of the lesions are malignant, and metastatic disease is found in most cases. In the absence of distant metastatic disease, resection is the treatment of choice; debulking, when possible, can offer symptomatic relief. Patients undergoing surgery for attempted resection should also have a cholecystectomy performed because of the high incidence of cholelithiasis. Medical therapy has proven disappointing, with 13% 5-year survival and only 48% 1-year survival reported.

Miscellaneous Functioning Tumors

Many islet cell tumors previously thought to be nonfunctioning have been found to secrete PP. Because this substance can now be measured, these tumors are referred to as *PPomas*. (Interestingly, 28%–70% of all functioning pancreatic endocrine tumors also secrete PP, the most likely being VIPomas and least likely insulinomas.) When an increased level of PP (>300 pmol/L) is detected in conjunction with a pancreatic mass, the diagnosis of PPoma is made by excluding the possibility of other functioning islet cell tumors. The excess secretion of PP is not associated with any clearly defined clinical syndrome; thus these tumors are usually large at diagnosis, presenting with symptoms related to local growth. Nonspecific symptoms such as diarrhea and weight loss may be present, however, possibly due to the inhibitory nature of PP on pancreatic secretion and gallbladder contraction. Surgical excision is the treatment of choice for resectable tumors, which can usually be easily localized by CT scan. PPomas are usually located in the head of the pancreas and are almost always malignant, though often slow-growing. Sixty percent are metastatic at the time of diagnosis. As with other pancreatic endocrine tumors, streptozocin is the chemotherapy of choice; however, because of the absence of hormonally related symptoms, no specific role for somatostatin analogues has been identified. The 5-year overall survival rate is 44%.

Growth hormone–releasing factor (GRF) is another hormone that has recently been identified as a tumor product. Referred to as GRFomas, tumors that secrete GRF are located in the pancreas 30% of the time, the lung 55% of the time, and the intestine 15% of the time. Approximately 30% of these lesions are malignant. Patients usually present with acromegaly, but these tumors also may secrete other products. In addition to GRFomas, 40% of patients have ZES, and 40% have Cushing's syndrome. Although octreotide can significantly suppress the levels of circulating growth hormone in this syndrome, surgical excision, if possible, is the treatment of choice.

Other uncommon islet cell tumors include those that secrete neurotensin, ACTH, or a parathyroid hormone–like peptide.

Carcinoid

The classic carcinoid tumor of the pancreas is extremely rare, although anecdotal cases have been reported. Pancreatic carcinoids are grouped with foregut carcinoids, and patients with these tumors may have normal serum levels of serotonin (may be increased or tumor stain for 5-hydroxytryptamine) but commonly have elevated urinary levels of 5-hydroxyindolacetic acid. Furthermore, the typical carcinoid syndrome is more common than in other foregut carcinoids. Pancreatic carcinoids generally are larger than midgut, hindgut, or other foregut carcinoids and therefore patients often present with mass-effect symptoms such as epigastric pain, weight loss, or jaundice from common bile duct compression. Localization has traditionally been by CT scan because most of these tumors are several centimeters in diameter at the time of diagnosis, although octreotide scanning has shown promise as a method to diagnose the disease and follow these patients after resection. Generally, carcinoid tumors grow slowly and invade adjacent organs late in the course of the disease, making resection possible in most patients. Unfortunately, at least 70% of patients have distant metastases at the time of diagnosis, minimizing the likelihood of long-term survival. However, in the absence of distant metastases, complete resection of the primary tumor offers an excellent possibility of long-term survival.

Nonfunctioning Tumors

Recent series report that 35% to 50% of pancreatic islet tumors are nonfunctioning, that is, they do not secrete detectable levels of functional hormones. Instead of a well-defined clinical syndrome, the presentation of these tumors is similar to that of pancreatic ductal adenocarcinoma. Since many nonfunctioning pancreatic tumors stain for one or many known hormones or precursor hormones, several hypotheses have been proposed to account for the lack of manifest symptoms. First, the hormones secreted in excess may not produce signs or symptoms. Second, a clinically active hormone may be secreted in clinically irrelevant amounts. Finally, the secreted hormone product may actually be either a precursor hormone or one that has yet to be identified. Common symptoms include abdominal pain, weight loss, and jaundice. Most of these tumors are found in the head of the pancreas, and most are malignant.

Diagnosis can be made by CT-guided fine-needle aspiration as well as by the characteristic hypervascular appearance on arteriography. However, conventional CT scans may have features characteristic of pancreatic islet cell tumors in contrast to adenocarcinoma of the pancreas. These features include a high degree of enhancement, cystic degeneration, and calcification. Additionally, endocrine tumors are less likely to encase vascular structures or obstruct the pancreatic duct. Following localization studies, operative exploration for attempted curative resection is often indicated.

The prognosis for patients with nonfunctioning islet cell tumors is significantly better than that for patients with pancreatic ductal adenocarcinoma, with the overall median survival rate in the former group reported at over 3 years. In patients with localized and completely resected disease, however, median overall survival is as long as 7 years. Even when localized disease is unresectable, the prognosis can remain fairly good, with a median survival of over 5 years. Chemotherapy with streptozocin and 5-fluorouracil has shown some favorable results and should be considered early in the course of the disease because median survival for unresectable metastatic disease is less than 2 years.

MULTIPLE ENDOCRINE NEOPLASIA

There are currently three well-defined MEN syndromes (MEN 1, MEN 2A, and MEN 2B), characterized by a familial predisposition to the development of tumors (often multiple) in various endocrine glands. Recognition of the individual components of each syndrome may be synchronous but more often is over a long period of follow-up. Typically, not all of the clinical manifestations of the "classic" syndromes are expressed. A descriptive overview

Table 14-6. Features of multiple endocrine neoplasia syndromes and the associated tumors (approximate incidence of tumor with each syndrome)

	MEN 1	MEN 2A	MEN 2B
Acronym	Werner's syndrome	Sipple's syndrome	None
Genetic mutation	Chromosome 11q13	RET proto-oncogene chromosome 10q11.2	RET proto-oncogene chromosome 10q11.2
Tumors	Parathyroid (90%)	MTC (100%)	MTC (100%)
	Pancreas (80%)	Pheo (20%–50%)	Pheo (20%–50%)
	Pituitary adenoma (55%)	Parathyroid (20%–35%)	Neuromas (~100%)
	Adrenal adenomas (30%)	Cutaneous lichen amyloidosis	Skeletal deformities
	Thyroid nodules (10%)	Hirschprung's disease	Megacolon
		Enlarged peripheral nerves	

MEN, multiple endocrine neoplasia; MTC, medullary thyroid carcinoma; Pheo, pheochromocytoma.

of the three syndromes is given in Table 14-6. Recently, specific genetic mutations have been identified as the likely causal event resulting in the clinical phenotypes associated with the development of the MEN syndromes.

MEN 1 was mapped by linkage analysis to the long arm of chromosome 11 (11q13). In 1997, positional cloning identified the specific gene. The MEN 1 gene encodes a 610-amino acid protein designated *menin*. Menin is principally a nuclear protein known to repress JUN-D–mediated RNA transcription, supporting the hypothesis that MEN 1 is caused by a tumor-suppressor gene.

Conversely, the gene responsible for MEN 2 is a proto-oncogene. It is located on chromosome sub-band 10q11.2 and is known as the RET proto-oncogene. This gene encodes the protein RET (rearranged during transfection), which is a receptor tyrosine kinase.

MEN 1

MEN 1, also known as Wermer's syndrome, has historically been characterized by the development of multigland parathyroid hyperplasia, pancreatic islet cell tumors, and pituitary tumors. Patients with MEN 1 also have a high incidence of foregut carcinoid tumors, adrenocortical tumors, and thyroid adenomas and carcinomas. In addition to endocrine gland abnormalities, patients with MEN 1 often have subtle skin lesions, including lipomas, facial angiofibromas, and skin collagenomas. MEN 1 is found in approximately one of every 30,000 in the general population. Various combinations of tumors develop, with 94% penetrance by age 50 years. The inheritance pattern is autosomal dominant, although the mechanism of tumorigenesis at the cellular level is recessive. A particular individual inherits a germline mutation to one allele at 11q13 (most often encoding truncated, inactive protein); a subsequent somatic mutation to the other allele at the MEN 1 locus results in loss of heterozygosity and eventual phenotypic expression. The clinical manifestations vary and are generally apparent by the third or fourth decade, although with careful screening most known carriers show evidence of tumorigenesis by their mid-twenties.

Hyperparathyroidism

Hyperparathyroidism is the most common endocrine abnormality seen in MEN 1 and is usually the first to develop (in 60%–90% of affected patients). Almost all hyperparathyroidism develops secondary to asymmetric, four-gland hyperplasia. The clinical presentation is similar to that seen in sporadic hyperparathyroidism, with most patients being asymptomatic. Measurement of serum calcium, phosphate, and intact-PTH levels leads to the diagnosis. Increased serum calcium in the face of inappropriately elevated intact-PTH and an elevated 24-hour urinary calcium collection confirm the diagnosis of hyperparathyroidism. As with sporadic hyperparathyroidism, treatment is surgical excision. Pre-excision imaging is of little value prior to initial exploration because of the multi-gland nature of the pathophysiology of MEN 1. In recurrent or persistent hyperparathyroidism, however, noninvasive imaging and often invasive modalities (e.g., angiography and venous sampling) may aid in guiding successful re-exploration. The frequency of synchronous thyroid neoplasms (15%) dictates that a careful evaluation of the thyroid gland be part of any neck exploration in patients with MEN 1.

There continues to be controversy over the appropriate surgical procedure for hyperparathyroidism in the setting of MEN 1. Many surgeons perform a three-and-one-half gland parathyroidectomy, while others advocate total parathyroidectomy with autotransplantation. There is considerable overlap in the reported incidence of recurrent or persistent hyperparathyroidism, as well as permanent hypoparathyroidism with either technique. Theoretically, total parathyroidectomy minimizes the likelihood of recurrent or persistent disease, although adding to the potential risk of permanent hypoparathyroidism. Our preferred technique is to perform a four-gland excision with autotransplantation of pieces of the least hyperplastic gland into the brachioradialis muscle of the non-dominant forearm. Graft-dependent hyperparathyroidism may develop in up to 50% of patients and can be effectively managed by removing several pieces of parathyroid tissue from the forearm under local anesthesia, precluding the need for neck re-exploration and its attendant increased risk of recurrent nerve paresis/paralysis and permanent hypoparathyroidism. Either procedure should include cervical thymectomy because MEN 1 is associated with an increased incidence of supranumery parathyroid glands, which are often located within the thymus, in up to 20% of patients. In general, hyperparathyroidism associated with MEN 2A is much easier to control and is associated with a less frequent recurrence rate after surgery than is MEN 1. Hyperparathyroidism should be addressed before therapy for pancreatic islet cell tumors because control of calcium-dependent hormone release from these tumors may be improved.

Pancreatic Tumors

The second most common neoplasms associated with MEN 1 are the pancreatic islet cell tumors, which occur in approximately 60% of patients with MEN 1. The clinical syndrome associated with these tumors results from the specific hormone secreted by each. The most common islet cell tumors are gastrinomas, followed by insulinomas. Rarely, glucagonomas, VIPomas, and somatostatinomas are found. MEN 1–associated pancreatic endocrine tumors are multifocal and may be located outside the pancreas, as is typical with gastrinomas. It is important to recognize that any particular radiographically demonstrable pancreatic mass may not be specifically responsible for a clinically apparent syndrome. However, the risk of malignancy remains even, and often especially, for clinically silent pancreatic masses. Details of the treatment of these tumors have been discussed previously. One must keep in mind that although biochemical cure is often not a realistic goal, prevention of the lethal consequences of malignant transformation and metastatic disease may be possible by aggressive surgical intervention.

Thompson et al. (1988) have advocated a strategy with this in mind, including the following: distal pancreatectomy at the level of the superior mesenteric vein, regardless of tumor location in the pancreas or duodenum; duodenotomy even without palpable duodenal lesions when faced with elevated serum gastrin and a positive secretin-stimulation test; peripancreatic lymph node dissection for duodenal or pancreatic neuroendocrine masses greater than 3 cm; and enucleation of pancreatic head or uncinate process tumors identified by palpation or intraoperative ultrasound. This aggressive approach remains controversial.

Pituitary Neoplasms

Pituitary neoplasms occur in 30% to 50% of patients with MEN 1; benign prolactin-producing adenomas are most common. Symptoms may be related directly to tumor mass effect (i.e., headache, diplopia, and hypopituitism) or be related to specific hormone overproduction. Excess prolactin causes galactorrhea and amenorrhea in women and impotence in men. Tumors may also produce growth hormone (30%) or ACTH (>10%), leading to acromegaly or Cushing's disease, respectively. Bromocriptine, a dopamine agonist, can be used to treat prolactinomas medically. Transsphenoidal hypophysectomy is reserved for patients who do not respond to bromocriptine and who have nonprolactin-secreting tumors. All patients with MEN 1 should be observed periodically with measurement of serum prolactin and growth hormone levels.

MEN 2

MEN 2 consists of three subtypes, each inherited in an autosomal dominant pattern with 100% penetrance but variable expression; all are marked by the presence of medullary thyroid carcinoma (MTC). MEN 2A and MEN 2B are defined by the presence of MTC and pheochromocytoma. Additionally, in MEN 2A (90% of all cases MEN 2), hyperparathyroidism often develops secondary to four-gland hyperplasia. Patients with MEN 2B (5% of cases of MEN 2) almost invariably have characteristic facies and marfanoid habitus. MEN 2B is also marked by the presence of multiple neuromas on the lips, tongue, and oral mucosa. In addition, patients with MEN 2B have a high incidence of skeletal abnormalities as well as diffuse ganglioneuromatosis of the GI tract, which can lead to a number of GI motility problems, most frequently involving the colon. Megacolon, associated with severe constipation, is the most common GI manifestation. Familial MTC is believed to be the most indolent of the three subtypes and is characterized by the absence of consistent phenotypic manifestations in addition to MTC.

Medullary Thyroid Carcinoma

MTC comprises approximately 5% to 10% of all thyroid malignancies. The vast majority—approximately 80%—of these tumors occur sporadically; the remaining 20% are familial. MTC can occur in the familial setting without any other associated syndromes. Some features of sporadic and familial MTC are shown in Table 14-7. In the setting of MEN 2, MTC is usually the first endocrine abnormality to occur. MTC arises from the parafollicular or C cells of the thyroid gland and as a result can secrete not only calcitonin but also a variety of other hormonally active substances, such as serotonin, ACTH, prostaglandins, melanin, and carcinoembryonic antigen.

CLINICAL PRESENTATION.   MTC is often detected by genetic or biochemical screening when it is clinically occult. Most index cases, or patients who are not identified by screening, present with a palpable neck mass. Approximately 30% of the patients with MTC present with watery diarrhea, usually secondary to the stimulatory effect of high plasma calcitonin levels on intestinal fluid and electrolyte secretion. Symptoms such as hoarseness, dysphagia, and respiratory difficulty may be related to locally advanced disease. Presenting symptoms may also be secondary to metastatic disease, which is most commonly seen in the lungs, liver, and bones.

Table 14-7.   Comparison of features of sporadic versus familial medullary thyroid carcinoma

Feature	Sporadic	Familial
Proportion of cases	80%	20%
Age at onset	40–60 yr	10–30 yr
Location	Unilateral	Bilateral

DIAGNOSIS. Historically, demonstrating elevated calcitonin levels using provocative testing in at-risk individuals has made the diagnosis of MTC. This strategy required multiple tests over many years to establish a diagnosis of MTC, and thus MEN 2. Because of the autosomal-dominant pattern of inheritance, 50% of at-risk patients using this strategy would undergo considerable inconvenience, be subjected to undue anxiety, and be exposed to some degree of risk from provocative testing. The application of genetic screening for the RET proto-oncogene has allowed earlier and more reliable diagnosis of MEN 2 while obviating long-term biochemical screening in those patients lacking the RET gene. Thus, early screening for the RET gene is the preferred method of diagnosis in at-risk patients. The appropriate timing of screening is still a topic of debate, but it is generally accepted that children of patients with MEN 2B should be screened in infancy. Metastatic MTC has been reported in infants less than 1 year old and warrants early and aggressive treatment. Affected children of patients with MEN 2A may have a more indolent disease course, but childhood MTC can develop and should be screened for by age 5 to 6 years.

Otherwise, when patients present with a palpable mass, fine-needle aspiration biopsy should be performed. Histologically, MTC frequently shows sheets of uniformly round or polygonal cells separated by fibrovascular stroma. Immunohistochemical staining for calcitonin in the tumor cells is the most reliable way to confirm the diagnosis. Laboratory measurements for serum calcitonin are also important as a baseline measurement and are usually markedly increased. Patients with clinically occult tumors, however, may have normal or minimally elevated serum calcitonin levels.

Provocative tests still can be useful for follow-up of patients previously treated for MTC. Generally, patients with MTC will have a demonstrable increase in serum calcitonin level; however, up to 30% of patients may have normal levels. By using pentagastrin (with or without calcium infusion) as a calcitonin secretagogue, the diagnosis of recurrence can be made.

TREATMENT. Once the diagnosis of MTC is made, the presence of pheochromocytoma should be excluded before definitive surgical treatment or intervention. Similarly, hyperparathyroidism should be diagnosed, if present, before surgery. If a pheochromocytoma is found, it should be treated first (see Chapter 15). If hyperparathyroidism is diagnosed, it can be treated at the time of neck exploration for the MTC. Important points to keep in mind with regard to treatment of MTC are its aggressive nature relative to well-differentiated thyroid cancer, its inability to concentrate radioactive iodine, the ineffectiveness of radiation and chemotherapy, its frequent multicentricity and the high probability of nodal metastases.

With the above points in mind, the appropriate treatment for MTC is total thyroidectomy and central neck dissection (levels VI and VII). In patients with MEN 2 syndromes, MTC is frequently multicentric and bilateral and metastasizes early to the cervical lymph nodes. The central neck dissection, which removes the lymphatic tissue between the jugular veins laterally, the hyoid bone superiorly, and the innominate vessels inferiorly, helps eradicate microscopic metastatic disease. Some authors argue that in patients with palpable primary tumors, the high frequency of microscopic disease in the lymph nodes bilaterally warrants bilateral functional neck dissections in addition to central nodal dissection. Intraoperative nodal evaluation is believed to be an inadequate predictor of nodal involvement. Others contend that only patients with palpable lymphadenopathy should undergo a concomitant functional neck dissection on the side of the enlarged pathologic nodes.

Intraoperative management of the parathyroid glands is an important consideration during operation for MTC and is controversial as well. Some surgeons are content to identify the glands and leave them in situ, while others advocate four-gland resection with autotransplantation into the non-dominant forearm (MEN 2A [possibility or presence of hyperparathyroidism]) or the sternocleidomastoid muscle (MEN 2B and sporadic MTC).

Patients can be followed postoperatively with provocative testing to identify residual or recurrent MTC. Overall, the prognosis of MTC is good, with 10-year survival rates of 60% to 80% reported for patients with MEN 2A. Patients with MEN 2B usually present with more advanced disease (i.e., extrathyroidal extension or macroscopic nodal metastasis), and long-term survival is less common. In general, the course of the MTC determines the prognosis for patients with MEN 2. The average life expectancy for this group of patients is more than 50 years.

Metastatic Disease

Controversy exists over the appropriate treatment of patients with stimulated elevations of plasma calcitonin levels in the postoperative period. Such a finding implies the presence of residual disease in the neck or mediastinum or undetected metastatic disease. Some clinicians prefer to simply follow these patients with observation because of the relatively slow rate of progression of MTC, while the chances for cure with repeat neck exploration are low and the risks of exploration are increased. Others recommend a repeat neck exploration after selective catheterization of the neck veins and determination of stimulated plasma calcitonin levels. In experienced hands, and with careful patient selection to exclude the presence of distant metastases (often including laparoscopic liver evaluation), a 30% to 40% normalization of plasma calcitonin levels by provocative testing can be achieved after repeat exploration. Radiation therapy may be useful when surgical options are exhausted for residual or recurrent disease in the neck, but such treatment is generally ineffective. Likewise, chemotherapy is generally ineffective in treating metastatic disease; however, doxorubicin, alone or in combination, may result in a partial response. Because of the indolent nature of the tumor, many physicians do not treat metastatic disease aggressively.

Pheochromocytoma

Usually, pheochromocytoma associated with MEN 2 appears between the ages of 10 and 30 years and is diagnosed concurrently with, or shortly after, MTC. The pheochromocytomas associated with MEN 2 are usually bilateral (60%–80% of the time), limited to the adrenal medulla, and almost always benign. The adrenal gland appears to become hyperplastic before the pheochromocytoma develops. Further discussion of pheochromocytoma can be found in the chapter on adrenal tumors (Chapter 15).

The workup and management of pheochromocytoma are discussed in more detail in Chapter 15. MEN 2 is typically diagnosed by catecholamine screening (urinary epinephrine, norepinephrine, and total metanephrines) before the onset of characteristic symptoms. A cross-sectional imaging study (CT or MRI) that demonstrates a unilateral adrenal mass or bilateral adrenal masses is generally adequate for preoperative localization in most cases. When cross-sectional imaging or catecholamine screening is equivocal ^{131}I metaiodobenzylguanidine (MIBG) scanning and additional localizing studies can help confirm the diagnosis. MIBG scintigraphy is also useful to further eliminate the possibility of bilateral pheochromocytomas.

Because many years (10 or more) can separate the appearance of pheochromocytomas in the opposite adrenal gland in patients with MEN 2, if a subsequent tumor develops at all, some controversy exists about the optimal surgical procedure for patients who are initially found to have a unilateral pheochromocytoma. Although some surgeons recommend bilateral adrenalectomy in patients with MEN 2 because bilateral tumors will develop in up to 80% of these patients, a more conservative approach is followed by most to avoid as long as possible the need for lifetime glucocorticoid and mineralocorticoid replacement. This approach involves unilateral adrenalectomy and examination of the contralateral adrenal gland at the time of exploration. If no abnormality is found, the unaffected adrenal gland is left intact and the patient is observed closely for evidence of a contralateral tumor, which develops in approximately 50% of patients after 10 years of follow-up. In the event of bilateral pheochromocytoma, cortical-sparing adrenalectomy has been demonstrated to be an effective alternative to bilateral adrenalectomy, avoiding chronic steroid replacement and the risk of Addisonian crisis. Long-term follow-up is indicated in all patients with MEN syndromes for the recurrence of any endocrine lesion.

Although laparoscopic adrenalectomy has become increasingly popular for benign adrenal lesions, the role of laparoscopy in the surgical treatment of pheochromocytoma has yet to be fully defined. Several groups have demonstrated the safety of laparoscopic adrenalectomy, although patients with pheochromocytoma may experience significant hypertensive crises during laparoscopy, even in the face of adequate preoperative medical treatment. This issue is further discussed in the chapter on adrenal tumors (Chapter 15).

Hyperparathyroidism

Hyperparathyroidism is the third and most variable component of the MEN 2A syndrome. Most often, patients are asymptomatic and the diagnosis is made on routine follow-up laboratory tests. Occasionally, patients present with kidney stones. In patients with MEN 2, a workup for hyperparathyroidism should be undertaken before neck exploration for MTC. In the vast majority of cases, the hyperparathyroidism is secondary to hyperplasia or multiple gland disease. As previously discussed, many surgeons prefer total parathyroidectomy with autotransplantation at the time of thyroidectomy whether or not concurrent hyperparathyroidism exists. However, surgeons who prefer a selective approach may choose not to perform a parathyroidectomy if, at the time of exploration, the calcium levels are normal and the parathyroid glands appear normal. If the calcium and serum PTH levels are elevated, or if the glands appear grossly abnormal or are hyperplastic on biopsy, a total parathyroidectomy should be performed.

Approximately one-half of the most normal-appearing parathyroid gland should be transplanted into the forearm. If normal parathyroid tissue becomes devascularized during total thyroidectomy for MTC in a patient with MEN 2, parathyroid autotransplantation should also be performed. Patients with MEN 2A should have the autotransplant performed into the brachioradialis muscle of the forearm, because the gland could become hyperplastic in the future and this placement facilitates later removal. In patients with MEN 2B, because hyperparathyroidism rarely develops, the devascularized parathyroid glands can be transplanted into the sternocleidomastoid muscle in the neck.

RECOMMENDED READING

Pancreatic Endocrine Tumors

Adams S, Baum RP, Hertel A, et al. Intraoperative gamma probe detection of neuroendocrine tumors. *J Nucl Med* 1998;39:1155.

Alexander HR, Fraker DL, Norton JA, et al. Prospective study of somatostatin receptor scintigraphy and its effect on operative outcome in patients with Zollinger-Ellison syndrome. *Ann Surg* 1998; 228:228.

Arnold R, Simon B, Wied M. Treatment of neuroendocrine GEP tumours with somatostatin analogues. *Digestion* 2000;62(suppl 1):84.

Bieligk S, Jaffe BM. Islet cell tumors of the pancreas. *Surg Clin North Am* 1995;75:1025.

Delcore R, Friesen SR. Gastrointestinal neuroendocrine tumors. *J Am Coll Surg* 1994;178:187.

Doherty GM, Doppman JL, Shawker TH, et al. Results of a prospective strategy to diagnose, localize, and resect insulinomas. *Surgery* 1991;110:989.

Doherty GM, Skögseid B (eds). *Surgical oncology,* Philadelphia: Lippincott Williams & Wilkins, 2001.

Eriksson B, Oberg K, Stridsberg M. Tumor markers in neuroendocrine tumors. *Digestion* 2000;62(suppl 1):33.

Eriksson BK, Larsson EG, Skogseid BM, et al. Liver embolizations of patients with malignant neuroendocrine gastrointestinal tumors. *Cancer* 1998;83:2293.

Evans DB, Skibber JM, Lee JF, et al. Nonfunctioning islet cell carcinoma of the pancreas. *Surgery* 1993;114:1175.

Fraker DL, Alexander HR. The surgical approach to endocrine tumors of the pancreas. *Semin Gastrointest Dis* 1995;6:102.

Gibril F, Doppman JL, Jensen RT. Recent advances in the treatment of metastatic pancreatic endocrine tumors. *Semin Gastrointest Dis* 1995;6:114.

Gibril F, Reynolds JC, Doppman JL, et al. Somatostatin receptor scintigraphy: its sensitivity compared with that of other imaging methods in detecting primary and metastatic gastrinomas. *Ann Intern Med* 1996;125:26.

Gower WR, Fabri PJ. Endocrine neoplasms (non-gastrin) of the pancreas. *Semin Surg Oncol* 1990;6:98.

Grant CS. Surgical aspects of hyperinsulinemic hypoglycemia. *Endocrinol Metab Clin North Am* 1999;28:533.

Harmon JW, Norton JA, Collen MJ. Removal of gastrinomas for the control of Zollinger-Ellison syndrome. *Ann Surg* 1984;200:396.

Heitz PU, Kasper M, Polak JM, et al. Pancreatic endocrine tumors: immunocytochemical analysis of 125 tumors. *Hum Pathol* 1982; 13:263.

Howard TJ, Stabile BE, Zinner MJ, et al. Anatomic distribution of pancreatic endocrine tumors. *Am J Surg* 1990;159:258.

Jensen RT. Zollinger-Ellison syndrome. In: Doherty GM, Skögseid B, eds. *Surgical oncology.* Philadelphia: Lippincott Williams & Wilkins, 2001.

Krejs GJ. Gastrointestinal endocrine tumors. *Scand J Gastroenterol* 1996;220(suppl):121.

Lam KY, Lo CY. Pancreatic endocrine tumour: a 22-year clinicopathological experience with morphological, immunohistochemical observation and a review of the literature. *Eur J Surg Oncol* 1997;23:36.

Lee JE, Evans DB. Advances in the diagnosis and treatment of gastrointestinal neuroendocrine tumors. *Cancer Treat Res* 1997;90: 227.

Legaspi A, Brennan MF. Management of islet cell carcinoma. *Surgery* 1988;104:1018.

Le Treut YP, Delpero JR, Dousset B, et al. Results of liver transplantation in the treatment of metastatic neuroendocrine tumors: a 31 case French multicentric report. *Ann Surg* 1997;225:355.

Mao C, El Attar A, Domenico D, et al. Carcinoid tumors of the pancreas: status report based on two cases and review of the world's literature. *Int J Pancreatol* 1998;23:153.

Maton PN. The use of long-acting somatostatin analogue, octreotide acetate, in patients with islet cell tumors. *Gastroenterol Clin North Am* 1989;18:897.

Maurer CA, Baer HU, Dyong TH, et al. Carcinoid of the pancreas: clinical characteristics and morphologic features. *Eur J Cancer* 1996; 32A:1109.

Meko JB, Norton JA. Endocrine tumors of the pancreas. *Curr Opin Gen Surg* 1994;186.

Nguyen HN, Backes B, Lammert F, et al. Long-term survival after diagnosis of hepatic metastatic VIPoma: report of two cases with disparate courses and review of therapeutic options. *Dig Dis Sci* 1999;44:1148.

Norton JA. Intraoperative methods to stage and localize pancreatic and duodenal tumors. *Ann Oncol* 999;110 (suppl 4):182.

Norton JA. Neuroendocrine tumors of the pancreas and duodenum. *Curr Probl Surg* 1994;31:77.

Norton JA, Doppman JL, Collen MJ, et al. Prospective study of gastrinoma localization and resection in patients with Zollinger-Ellison syndrome. *Ann Surg* 1986;204:468.

Norton JA, Doppman JL, Jensen RT. Curative resection in Zollinger-Ellison syndrome: results of a 10 year prospective study. *Ann Surg* 1992;215:8.

Norton JA, Fraker DL, Alexander HR, et al. Surgery to cure the Zollinger-Ellison syndrome. *N Engl J Med* 1999;341:635.

Oberg K. Neuroendocrine gastrointestinal tumors. *Ann Oncol* 1996;7:453.

Orbuch M, Doppman JL, Jensen RT. Localization of pancreatic endocrine tumors. *Semin Gastrointest Dis* 1995;6:90.

Pasieka JL, McLeod MK, Thompson NW, et al. Surgical approach to insulinomas: assessing the need for preoperative localization. *Arch Surg* 1992;127:442.

Perry RR, Vinik AI. Diagnosis and management of functioning islet cell tumors. *J Clin Endocrinol Metab* 1995;80:2273.

Phan GQ, Yeo CJ, Hruban RH, et al. Surgical experience with pancreatic and peripancreatic neuroendocrine tumors: review of 125 patients. *J Gastrointest Surg* 1998;2:473.

Proye C, Malvaux P, Pattou F, et al. Non-invasive imaging of insulinomas and gastrinomas with endoscopic ultrasonography and somatostatin receptor scintigraphy. *Surgery* 1998;124:1134.

Ricke J, Klose K-J. Imaging procedures in neuroendocrine tumors. *Digestion* 2000;62(suppl 1):39.

Service FJ. Hypoglycemic disorders. *N Engl J Med* 1995;332:1144.

Sloan DA, Schwartz RW, Kenady DE. Surgical therapy for endocrine tumors of abdominal origin. *Curr Opin Oncol* 1993;5:100.

Tanaka S, Yamasaki S, Matsushita H, et al. Duodenal somatostatinoma: a case report and review of 31 cases with special reference to the relationship between tumor size and metastasis. *Pathol Int* 2000;50:146.

Termanini B, Gibril F, Reynolds JC, et al. Value of somatostatin receptor scintigraphy: a prospective study in gastrinoma of its effect on clinical management. *Gastroenterology* 1997;112:335.

Thompson GB, van Heerden JA, Grant CS, et al. Islet cell carcinomas of the pancreas: a twenty-year experience. *Surgery* 1988;104:1011.

Veenhof CHN. Pancreatic endocrine tumors, immunotherapy and gene therapy: chemotherapy and interferon therapy of endocrine tumors. *Ann Oncol* 1999;10(suppl.4):S185.

Venkatesh S, Ordonez NG, Ajani J, et al. Islet cell carcinoma of the pancreas. *Cancer* 1990;65:354.

Weber HC, Venzon DJ, Lin J-T, et al. Determinants of metastatic rate and survival in patients with Zollinger-Ellison syndrome: a prospective long-term study. *Gastroenterology* 1995;108:1637.

Wymenga ANM, Eriksson B, Salmela PI, et al. Efficacy and safety of prolonged-release Lantreotide in patients with gastrointestinal neuroendocrine tumors and hormone-related symptoms. *J Clin Oncol* 1999;17:1111.

Yu F, Venzon DJ, Serrano J, et al. Prospective study of the clinical course, prognostic factors, causes of death, and survival in patients with long-standing Zollinger-Ellison syndrome. *J Clin Oncol* 1999;17:615.

Zollinger RM, Ellison EC, O'Dorisio T, et al. Thirty years' experience with gastrinoma. *World J Surg* 1984;8:427.

Multiple Endocrine Neoplasia

Cance WG, Wells SA. Multiple endocrine neoplasia type IIa. *Curr Probl Surg* 1985;22:1.

Carlson KM, Dou S, Chi D, et al. Single missense mutation in the tyrosine kinase catalytic domain of the RET protooncogene is associated with multiple endocrine neoplasia type 2B. *Proc Natl Acad Sci USA* 1994;91:1579.

Chandrasekharappa SC, Guru SC, Manickam P, et al. Positional cloning of the gene for multiple endocrine neoplasia-type 1. *Science* 1997;276:404.

Clark OH. What's new in endocrine surgery. *J Am Coll Surg* 1997;184: 126.

Eng C. RET proto-oncogene in the development of human cancer. *J Clin Oncol* 1999;17:380.

Gagner M, Breton G, Pharand D, et al. Is laparoscopic adrenalectomy indicated for pheochromocytomas? *Surgery* 1996;120:1076.

Herfarth KK, Bartsch D, Doherty GM, et al. Surgical management of hyperparathyroidism in patients with multiple endocrine neoplasia type 2A. *Surgery* 1996;120:966.

Howe JR, Norton JA, Wells SA. Prevalence of pheochromocytoma and hyperparathyroidism in multiple endocrine neoplasia type 2A: results of long-term follow-up. *Surgery* 1993;114:1070.

Jensen RT. Management of the Zollinger-Ellison syndrome in patients with multiple endocrine neoplasia type 1. *J Intern Med* 1998; 243:477.

Lairmore TC, Ball DW, Baylin SB, et al. Management of pheochromocytomas in patients with multiple endocrine neoplasia type 2 syndromes. *Ann Surg* 1993;217:595.

Lee JE, Curley SA, Gagel RF, et al. Cortical-sparing adrenalectomy for patients with bilateral pheochromocytoma. *Surgery* 1996; 120:1064.

Marx SJ, Agarwal SK, Heppner C, et al. The gene for multiple endocrine neoplasia type 1: recent findings. *Bone* 1999;25:119.

Moley JF, Debenedetti MK, Dilley WG, et al. Surgical management of patients with persistent or recurrent medullary thyroid cancer. *J Intern Med* 1998;243:521.

Moley JF, Debenedetti MK. Patterns of nodal metastases in palpable medullary thyroid carcinoma. *Ann Surg* 1999;229:880.

NIH Conference. Multiple endocrine neoplasia type 1: clinical and genetic topics. *Ann Intern Med* 1998;129:484.

Pipeleers-Mirichal M, Somers G, Willems G, et al. Gastrinomas in the duodenums of patients with multiple endocrine neoplasia type I and the Zollinger-Ellison syndrome. *N Engl J Med* 1990;322:723.

O'Riordain DS, O'Brien T, Crotty TB, et al. Multiple endocrine neoplasia type 2B: more than an endocrine disorder. *Surgery* 1995;118: 936.

Thompson JC, Lewis BG, Wiener I, et al. The role of surgery in Zollinger-Ellison syndrome. *Ann Surg* 1983;197:594.

Thompson NW. Current concepts in the surgical management of multiple endocrine neoplasia type 1 pancreatic-duodenal disease. Results in the treatment of 40 patients with Zollinger-Ellison syndrome, hypoglycemia or both. *J Intern Med* 1998;243:495.

Wolfe MM, Jensen RT. Zollinger-Ellison syndrome: current concepts in the diagnosis and management. *N Engl J Med* 1987;317:1200.

Adrenal Tumors

Hiroomi Tada, Douglas S. Tyler,
and Jeffrey E. Lee

The diagnosis and treatment of adrenal tumors have undergone a significant transformation with recent advances in diagnostic imaging and minimally invasive approaches to surgical resection. However, treatment of the patient with an adrenal mass still requires a thorough understanding of adrenal endocrine physiology as well as sound clinical judgment. Appropriate biochemical evaluation and radiographic assessment of an identified adrenal mass are crucial before surgical intervention. Common nonfunctional adrenal adenomas or "incidentalomas" must be differentiated from functioning adrenal tumors (cortisol-producing adenomas, aldosteronomas, and pheochromocytomas), the occasional metastasis to the adrenal gland, and the rare adrenocortical carcinoma.

ALDOSTERONOMA

Primary hyperaldosteronism (Conn's syndrome) is a clinical syndrome that results from hypersecretion of aldosterone. This condition is caused by bilateral adrenal hyperplasia in approximately 40% of cases and by an adrenal adenoma in approximately 60% of cases. Other rare causes of primary aldosteronism include glucocorticoid-suppressible hyperaldosteronism, adrenocortical carcinoma, and aldosterone-secreting ovarian tumors. Primary hyperaldosteronism is responsible for approximately 0.5% to 1.0% of all cases of hypertension and represents 5% to 10% of surgically correctable cases of hypertension.

Clinical Manifestations

The main problem in diagnosing primary hyperaldosteronism is that the symptoms are usually mild and nonspecific. The most common symptoms are headache, fatigue, polydipsia, polyuria, and nocturia. Hypertension is almost always present but is frequently mild, with diastolic blood pressures less than 120 mm Hg in more than 70% of cases.

Diagnosis

Initial laboratory findings that support a diagnosis of primary hyperaldosteronism include hypertension and spontaneous hypokalemia. Before further biochemical testing, all nonessential medications should be stopped for at least 2 weeks. Diuretics should be discontinued for at least 2 to 4 weeks. Patients should then be placed on a salt-loading diet (100 mmol/day of sodium chloride). Potassium supplementation should be given during salt loading because severe hypokalemia can inhibit aldosterone production in some patients. Measurement of plasma aldosterone and renin activity should be accomplished after 3 hours of upright posture. A plasma aldosterone/plasma renin ratio greater than 20 to 25 (ng/dL:ng/mL/h) is sensitive and specific in the screening and diagnosis of primary hyperaldosteronism. Confirmation of hyperaldosteronism can be obtained using the saline suppression test or the captopril suppression test.

Once the diagnosis of hyperaldosteronism is established, it is critical to differentiate unilateral adrenal adenoma from bilateral hyperplasia of the zona glomerulosa (idiopathic hyperaldosteronism). In patients with an aldosterone-producing adenoma, unilateral adrenalectomy corrects the hypokalemia and decreases the blood pressure in 70% of surgically treated patients. However, surgery is of little value in patients with idiopathic hyperaldosteronism. Patients with a unilateral adenoma usually have more severe hypertension, higher plasma aldosterone levels, and therefore more profound hypokalemia; however, these findings cannot accurately differentiate patients with unilateral adenoma from those with idiopathic hyperaldosteronism. Computed tomography (CT) and magnetic resonance imaging (MRI) can help confirm the presence of a unilateral adrenal nodule, while iodocholesterol (NP-59) imaging and selective venous sampling for aldosterone determinations can localize the hyperfunctioning adrenal tissue to the right or left side. The high frequency of nonfunctioning adenomas in the normal population (2%–8%) means that the finding of a small adrenal mass on CT or MRI is not necessarily diagnostic of a unilateral aldosterone-producing adenoma. Because selective venous sampling is invasive, and cannulation of the right adrenal vein is often difficult and occasionally results in adrenal vein thrombosis with adrenal infarction, we now often combine adrenal imaging (CT or MRI) with iodocholesterol imaging to confirm the presence of a unilateral functioning adrenal mass. Our current approach to the evaluation of patients suspected of having primary hyperaldosteronism is shown in Fig. 15-1.

Treatment

The treatment of primary hyperaldosteronism depends on the cause. Bilateral adrenal hyperplasia is best managed medically using the aldosterone antagonist spironolactone. Most patients can achieve adequate control of their blood pressure with this medication alone or in conjunction with other antihypertensives. When an aldosterone-producing adenoma is diagnosed, the appropriate therapy remains surgical resection. Preoperatively, patients should be placed on spironolactone and given potassium supplementation to help normalize fluid and electrolyte balance over a 3- to 4-week period.

Surgical resection can be performed either through an open or a laparoscopic approach. Since nearly all patients with aldosteronomas have relatively small tumors, they are often excellent candidates for a laparoscopic approach. The early results from surgical resection of an aldosterone-producing adenoma are good, and the long-term cure rate is approximately 70%.

Approximately 2% or less of adrenocortical carcinomas cause isolated hyperaldosteronism. In the very rare situation of a patient presenting with hyperaldosteronism and a large adrenal mass, an open anterior approach should be taken to facilitate complete resection.

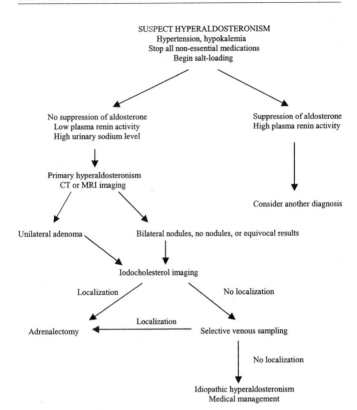

Fig. 15-1.   Algorithm for the evaluation of the patient with suspected primary hyperaldosteronism.

CORTISOL-PRODUCING ADRENAL ADENOMA

Cushing's syndrome is the term used to refer to the state of hypercortisolism that can result from a number of different pathologic processes (Table 15-1). Cortisol regulation involves feedback loops through the pituitary gland and hypothalamus. The most common cause of Cushing's syndrome is exogenous steroid administration. After exclusion of patients taking exogenous steroids, approximately 70% of the remaining cases of hypercortisolism are secondary to hypersecretion of adrenocorticotropic hormone (ACTH) from the pituitary gland, a condition known as Cushing's disease. Most of the time, a small pituitary adenoma is found to be the cause. Ectopic secretion of ACTH, referred to as ectopic ACTH syndrome, is the cause of approximately 15% of cases of Cushing's syndrome. Ectopic ACTH syndrome is usually caused by malignant tumors, with carcinoma of the lung, carcinoma of the pancreas, carcinoid tumors, and malignant thymoma accounting for 80% of such cases. Ectopic secretion of corticotropin-releasing factor is exceedingly rare but has been reported in a few cases.

Table 15-1.   Causes of Cushing's syndrome

Exogenous steroids
Cushing's disease (due to pituitary adenoma)
Adrenal tumors
   Adrenal cortical adenoma
   Adrenal cortical carcinoma
Primary adrenal cortical hyperplasia
Ectopic adrenocorticotropin syndrome
Ectopic corticotropin-releasing factor syndrome

Hypersecretion of cortisol from the adrenal glands accounts for approximately 10% to 20% of cases of Cushing's syndrome. The underlying cause is an adrenal adenoma 50% to 60% of the time and an adrenocortical carcinoma 20% to 25% of the time. Bilateral adrenal hyperplasia accounts for the remaining 20% to 30% of cases.

Clinical Manifestations

Weight gain is the most common feature of hypercortisolism and occurs predominantly in the truncal area. Centripetal obesity combined with muscle wasting in the extremities, fat deposition in the head and neck region ("moon facies"), and a dorsal kyphosis ("buffalo hump") gives the patient a characteristic habitus. Hypertension, abdominal striae, and virilization in females are three other common findings.

Diagnosis

The evaluation for Cushing's syndrome should be aimed at establishing the diagnosis first and then determining the etiology. To establish the diagnosis, a state of hypercortisolism must be documented. The adult adrenal glands secrete on average 10 to 30 mg of cortisol each day. The secretion follows a diurnal variation: cortisol levels tend to be high early in the morning and low in the evening. The most sensitive initial screening test for hypercortisolism in patients with an adrenal mass is an overnight 1-mg dexamethasone suppression test (described below). An alternative first-line screening test is measurement of 24-hour urinary-free cortisol; the normal level is generally below 80 μg/day.

To determine the etiology of an elevated cortisol level, plasma ACTH levels must be checked. ACTH secretion also follows a diurnal variation, preceding that of cortisol by 1 to 2 hours. Suppressed levels of ACTH are seen in patients with adrenal adenomas, adrenocortical carcinomas, or autonomously functioning adrenal hyperplasia. In such cases, autonomous secretion of cortisol by the pathologic process within the adrenal gland inhibits pituitary ACTH release. Patients with Cushing's disease (i.e., a pituitary adenoma secreting ACTH) usually have plasma ACTH levels that are elevated or within the upper limits of normal. When there is an ectopic source of ACTH secretion, for example a metastatic tumor process, the plasma ACTH level is usually markedly increased.

The most sensitive method for detecting hypercortisolism is the overnight low-dose dexamethasone suppression test. One milligram of dexamethasone is taken orally at 11:00 p.m.; normal individuals have a cortisol level less than 5 mg/dL at 8:00 a.m. the following morning. Failure to suppress the 8:00 a.m. cortisol level to less than 5 mg/dL is consistent with hypercortisolism; however, although this test has a false-negative rate of only 3%, the false-positive rate is 30%. Therefore, while a normal overnight dexamethasone suppression test excludes clinically significant hypercortisolism, an abnormal test result requires further investigation. Twenty-four-hour urine collection for urinary-free (unmetabolized) cortisol is somewhat less sensitive than overnight dexamethasone suppression but more specific.

To confirm the presence of Cushing's syndrome, low-dose and high-dose dexamethasone suppression tests can be performed. However, these tests are usually unnecessary in patients with a unilateral adrenal mass with hypercortisolism identified by the overnight 1-mg dexamethasone suppression test and confirmed by 24-hour urine collection. Likewise, while the metyrapone test is occasionally used to differentiate between the various etiologies of Cushing's syndrome, this test is rarely helpful in patients with hypercortisolism and an adrenal mass.

All patients with an incidentally identified adrenal mass should undergo an evaluation to exclude Cushing's syndrome. Initial screening involves the 1-mg overnight dexamethasone suppression test. Patients with suppressed cortisol levels do not have Cushing's syndrome and do not require further evaluation for this condition. Patients without suppressed cortisol levels should undergo a 24-hour urine collection for measurement of free cortisol levels and 17-hydroxy and ketosteroids. In selected cases of patients with hypercortisolism and equivocal abdominal cross-sectional imaging studies, imaging of the adrenal glands with radiolabeled iodocholesterol can help distinguish primary adrenal hyperplasia, which should demonstrate bilateral uptake, from a cortisol-secreting adenoma, which suppresses the contralateral gland and thus limits uptake to only the side containing the adenoma.

Treatment

The appropriate management of Cushing's syndrome depends on the underlying etiology. Patients with Cushing's disease should undergo transsphenoidal hypophysectomy of the pituitary adenoma when it is believed to be resectable. Bilateral adrenalectomy is rarely indicated and should be reserved for patients who fail to respond to hypophysectomy. If bilateral adrenalectomy is performed, patients require not only perioperative steroid coverage (Tables 15-2 and 15-3), but also lifelong replacement of both glucocorticoids and mineralocorticoids. Patients with autonomously functioning bilateral adrenal hyperplasia usually require bilateral adrenalectomy. Patients with ectopic ACTH syndrome should have the underlying malignant lesion identified and resected if possible. Bilateral adrenalectomy should be reserved for the small group of patients whose primary tumor is unresectable and whose symptoms of cortisol excess cannot be controlled medically.

Patients with a neoplasm of the adrenal gland, whether adenoma or carcinoma, should undergo resection of the involved side.

Table 15-2. Recommendations for perioperative glucocorticoid coverage

Surgical Stress	Examples	Hydrocortisone Equivalent (mg)	Duration (d)
Minor	Inguinal herniorraphy	25	1
Moderate	Open cholecystectomy Lower-extremity revascularization Segmental colon resection Total joint replacement Abdominal hysterectomy	50–75	1–2
Major	Pancreaticoduodenectomy Esophagogastrectomy Total proctocolectomy Cardiac surgery with cardiopulmonary bypass	100–150	2–3

Although almost all adenomas can be resected, adrenocortical carcinomas that secrete cortisol are resectable in only 25% to 35% of patients. Chemotherapy has been disappointing in patients with unresectable or metastatic adrenocortical carcinoma. Symptoms related to hypercortisolism can sometimes be minimized with various agents, including mitotane, aminoglutethimide, metyrapone, or ketoconazole.

PHEOCHROMOCYTOMA

Pheochromocytomas represent a potentially curable form of endocrine hypertension that, if undetected, places patients at high risk for morbidity and mortality, particularly during surgery and pregnancy. In large series of hypertensive patients, approximately 0.1% to 0.2% of patients are found to have pheochromocytomas. These neuroectodermal tumors arise from the chromaffin cells of the adrenal medulla. Approximately 10% of

Table 15-3. Comparison of steroid preparations

Steroid	Half-life (hr)	Glucocorticoid Activity (relative to cortisol)	Mineralocorticoid Activity (relative to cortisol)
Cortisol	8–12	1	1
Cortisone	8–12	0.8	0.8
Prednisone	12–36	4	0.25
Prednisolone	12–36	4	0.25
Methylprednisolone	12–36	5	0
Triamcinolone	12–36	5	0
Betamethasone	36–72	25	0
Dexamethasone	36–72	30–40	0

pheochromocytomas are bilateral, with some patients presenting with multiple tumors. Ten percent of pheochromocytomas can be found in extra-adrenal sites, where they are more appropriately called paragangliomas because of their close association with ganglia of the sympathetic nervous system. The most common extra-adrenal sites include the organ of Zuckerkandl (located between the inferior mesenteric artery and the aortic bifurcation), the urinary bladder, the thorax, and the renal hilum.

Histologic evidence of malignancy in pheochromocytomas can be demonstrated approximately 10% of the time; malignancy is more commonly seen with extra-adrenal lesions than with those arising in the adrenal glands. Documenting malignancy can be difficult because invasion of adjacent organs or metastatic disease must be present. Furthermore, both benign and malignant lesions may show tumor penetration of the gland's capsule, invasion of veins draining the gland, cellular pleomorphism, mitoses, and atypical nuclei.

Familial pheochromocytomas account for approximately 10% of cases and are usually benign. The familial syndromes associated with pheochromocytomas include multiple endocrine neoplasia (MEN) types IIA and IIB, in which bilateral tumors are common, as well as the neuroectodermal dysplasias consisting of neurofibromatosis, tuberous sclerosis, Sturge-Weber syndrome, and von Hippel-Lindau disease. Patients with these syndromes require follow-up and periodic screening for pheochromocytoma, especially before any planned surgical procedure.

Clinical Manifestations

The clinical manifestations of pheochromocytoma can be varied and at times quite dramatic. Hypertension, sustained or paroxysmal, is the most common clinical presentation. Paroxysmal elevations in blood pressure can vary markedly in frequency and duration, and can be initiated by a variety of events, including heavy physical exertion and eating foods high in tyramine. Other common symptoms include excessive sweating, palpitations, tremulousness, anxiety, and chest pain. More than half of patients with pheochromocytomas have impaired glucose tolerance, and may have symptoms of diabetes mellitus, including polydipsia or polyuria. These symptoms are secondary to the excess catecholamine secretion by the tumors, and resolve with tumor resection. Patients with functioning tumors are rarely asymptomatic; an exception is patients with hereditary pheochromocytomas. Nonfunctioning pheochromocytomas are rare; extra-adrenal paragangliomas, however, may be non-functioning.

Diagnosis

The diagnosis of pheochromocytoma is made by documenting the excess secretion of catecholamines. Twenty-four-hour urine collections should be tested for free catecholamine levels (dopamine, epinephrine, and norepinephrine) and their metabolites (normetanephrine, metanephrine, vanillylmandelic acid). Increased levels of catecholamines or their metabolites are seen in more than 90% of patients with pheochromocytoma. Plasma levels of free catecholamines are also usually increased. However, because plasma values frequently overlap those seen in essential hypertension, the urinary measurements are accepted as being more specific. The adrenal glands and the organ of Zuckerkandl produce the enzyme phenylethanolamine-*N*-methyl-transferase, which converts norepinephrine to epinephrine. Pheochromocytomas that arise elsewhere do not contain this enzyme and thus do not produce much, if any, epinephrine. As a result, extra-adrenal pheochromocytomas secrete predominantly dopamine and norepinephrine.

Once the diagnosis of pheochromocytoma is made, localization studies can be carried out. A review of preoperative imaging in a large series of histologically confirmed pheochromocytomas found that MRI was the most sensitive modality (98%), followed by CT scans (89%) and ^{131}I-metaiodobenzylguanidine (MIBG) scanning (81%). Our experience indicates that high-quality spiral CT scans can depict up to 95% of adrenal masses larger than 6 to 8 mm and is usually the initial imaging study. MRI may be useful in selected cases because the T2-weighted images can clearly identify chromaffin tissue; the T2-weighted adrenal mass-to-liver ratio of pheochromocytomas or paragangliomas is usually more than three. This ratio is much higher than that of adrenal cortical adenomas, adrenal cortical carcinomas, or metastases to the adrenal gland. Thus the MRI may provide potentially useful functional or biochemical information. MIBG imaging is another procedure that is helpful in localizing extra-adrenal, metastatic, or bilateral pheochromocytomas. This radiolabeled amine is selectively picked up by chromaffin tissue and can identify the majority of pheochromocytomas, regardless of their location. Therefore, MIBG scanning is useful in patients with biochemical evidence of pheochromocytoma whose tumors cannot be localized by CT or MRI and in the follow-up evaluation of patients with suspected or documented recurrent or metastatic disease. Using these techniques, it is rare to have a patient whose pheochromocytoma cannot be localized preoperatively.

Treatment

After diagnosis and localization of the pheochromocytoma, careful preoperative preparation is required to prevent a cardiovascular crisis during surgery caused by excess catecholamine secretion. The main focus of the preoperative preparation is adequate alpha-adrenergic blockade and complete restoration of fluid and electrolyte balance. Phenoxybenzamine is the alpha-adrenergic blocking agent of choice and is usually begun at a dose of 10 mg twice a day. The dosage is gradually increased over a 1- to 3-week period until adequate blockade is reached. The total dosage used should not exceed $1 \text{ mg kg}^{-1} \text{ day}^{-1}$. While use of beta-adrenergic blocking agents has somewhat been controversial, beta blockade following alpha blockade may help prevent tachycardia and other arrhythmias. Beta blockade should not be instituted unless alpha blockade has been established; otherwise, the beta-blocker will inhibit epinephrine-induced vasodilation, leading to more significant hypertension and left heart strain. In addition to requiring pharmacologic preparation, patients with pheochromocytoma require correction of fluid volume depletion as well as any concurrent electrolyte imbalances.

The perioperative treatment of patients with pheochromocytoma can be difficult. Rarely is alpha-adrenergic blockade complete. The anesthesiologist should be prepared to treat a hypertensive crisis with sodium nitroprusside, and tachyarrhythmias with either a beta-blocker or anti-arrhythmics. Surgical exploration has traditionally been performed via an open anterior approach (bilateral subcostal incision) so that both glands can be evaluated and the abdomen examined for metastatic disease. However, if preoperative imaging suggests a modestly sized, benign-appearing pheochromocytoma with a radiographically normal contralateral gland, we currently use a unilateral laparoscopic approach when feasible. The surgeon should manipulate the tumor as little as possible, and ligate the tumor's venous outflow via the adrenal vein as early in the procedure as possible. A laparoscopic approach is particularly appropriate for patients with MEN II or von Hippel-Lindau disease with a small, unilateral pheochromocytoma; for patients with MEN II or von Hippel-Lindau disease with bilateral disease, a bilateral laparoscopic approach may also be appropriate. Cortical-sparing adrenalectomy, either open or laparoscopic, has been performed successfully in patients with MEN II or von Hippel-Lindau disease with bilateral pheochromocytomas, avoiding chronic steroid hormone replacement and the risk of Addisonian crisis in most patients.

Postoperatively, patients should be monitored carefully for 24 hours so they can be observed for arrhythmias, as well as hypotension secondary to compensatory vasodilation that can occur once excess catecholamine stimulation has stopped. Occasionally, hypertension remains a problem postoperatively, especially in those patients who had sustained hypertension preoperatively.

The best currently available palliation for unresectable or metastatic pheochromocytoma is alpha blockade with phenoxybenzamine. Alpha-methyltyrosine can also be used. The most commonly used chemotherapy regimens for pheochromocytoma are high-dose streptozocin and a combination of cyclophosphamide, vincristine, and dacarbazine. The overall response rates with these regimens are approximately 50%. Radiation therapy has been effective only for bony metastases. More recently, there has been some interest in treating metastatic lesions with therapeutic doses of ^{131}I-MIBG. Unfortunately, a high percentage of metastatic pheochromocytomas do not take up ^{131}I-MIBG; therefore, the response rate, as manifested by a reduction in urinary catecholamines, is only approximately 50%. Objective responses as determined by imaging studies are seen even less frequently. The 5-year survival rate for patients with malignant pheochromocytoma is approximately 43%, as compared with a 97% 5-year survival rate for benign lesions.

ADRENAL CORTICAL CARCINOMA

Adrenal cortical carcinoma is a rare malignancy with approximately 150 to 200 new cases reported each year in the United States. There is a bimodal age distribution, with incidence peaking in young children and then again between 40 and 50 years of age.

Clinical Manifestations

Patients with adrenal cortical carcinoma usually present with vague abdominal symptoms secondary to an enlarging retroperitoneal mass or with clinical manifestations of overproduction of one or more adrenal cortical hormones. Most of these tumors are functional as measured by biochemical parameters. Fifty percent secrete cortisol, producing Cushing's syndrome. The workup and treatment of patients with Cushing's syndrome are described in that section in this chapter. Another 10% to 20% of adrenocortical carcinomas produce various steroid hormones, which can cause hypertension and varying degrees of virilization in females and feminization in males.

Diagnosis

The preoperative evaluation of these patients involves a careful biochemical screening, including a 24-hour urine collection to measure levels of cortisol, aldosterone, catecholamines, metanephrine, vanillylmandelic acid, 17-hydroxycorticosteroids, and 17-keto-steroids. The results serve to guide perioperative replacement therapy as well as to exclude pheochromocytoma.

High-resolution abdominal CT and MRI are the best modalities to image the adrenal glands. CT can identify lesions as small as 7 mm. MRI may be especially helpful not only in identifying tumor extension into the inferior vena cava but also in differentiating between various lesions based on the adrenal-to-liver ratio on T2-weighted images. Adenomas usually have ratios of 0.7 to 1.4; malignant lesions, whether primary or metastatic to the adrenal gland, have ratios of 1.4 to 3.0; and pheochromocytomas usually have ratios greater than 3.0. Chest radiography is helpful in ruling out pulmonary metastasis. The various staging systems for adrenocortical carcinomas are shown in Table 15-4.

Treatment

Complete surgical resection is currently the only potentially curative therapy for localized adrenal cortical cancer. Approximately 50% of the tumors are localized to the adrenal gland at the time of initial presentation. We recommend an open transabdominal approach to facilitate maximal exposure for complete resection, minimize the risk of tumor spillage, and allow for vascular control of the inferior vena cava, aorta, and renal vessels when necessary. Radical en bloc resection that includes adjacent organs, if necessary, provides the only chance for long-term survival. Patients who undergo a complete resection of their tumor have a 5-year survival rate of approximately 40%; those who undergo incomplete resection have a median survival duration of less than 12 months. Therefore, the strongest predictor of outcome in this disease is the ability to perform a complete resection.

Common sites of recurrence include lungs, lymph nodes, liver, peritoneum, and bone. Complete resection of recurrent disease, including pulmonary metastases, is associated with prolonged survival in some patients and can control symptoms related to excess hormone production. After a potentially curative resection, patients whose tumors were hormonally active should be monitored with interval urinary steroid profiles as well as abdominal

Table 15-4. Staging systems for adrenal cortical carcinoma

Stage	Macfarlane (1958)	Sullivan (1978)	Icard (1992)	Lee (1995)
I	T1 (≤5 cm), N0, M0	T1 (≤5 cm), N0, M0	T1 (≤5 cm), N0, M0	T1 (≤5 cm), N0, M0
II	T2 (>5 cm), N0, M0	T2 (>5 cm), N0, M0	T2 (>5 cm), N0, M0	T2 (>5 cm), N0, M0
III	T3 (local invasion without involvement of adjacent organs) or mobile positive lymph nodes, M0	T3 (local invasion), N0, M0 or T1–2, N1 (positive lymph nodes), M0	T3 (local invasion) and/or N1 (positive regional lymph nodes), M0	T3/T4 (local invasion as demonstrated by histologic evidence of adjacent organ invasion, direct tumor extension to IVC, and/or tumor thrombus within IVC or renal vein) and/or N1 (positive regional lymph nodes), M0
IV	T4 (invasion of adjacent organs) or fixed positive lymph nodes or M1 (distant metastasis)	T4 (local invasion), N0, M0; or T3, N1, M0; or T1–4, N0–1, M1 (distant metastasis)	T1–4, N0–1, M1 (distant metastasis)	T1–4, N0–1, M1 (distant metastasis)

IVC, inferior vena cava.

and chest imaging studies. Adjuvant therapy for adrenocortical carcinoma (mitotane) has had minimal impact, if any, on disease progression.

Radiation can provide palliation for bony metastases. No chemotherapeutic agent or combination of agents has been shown to be consistently effective against unresectable or metastatic adrenal cortical cancer. Mitotane has been one of the most commonly used systemic agents because of its ability to palliate the endocrine effects of the tumor. This drug is an isomer of dichlorodiphenyltrichloroethane and not only inhibits steroid production but also leads to atrophy of adrenocortical cells. Mitotane is associated with a number of side effects, most notably gastrointestinal and neuromuscular symptoms. In addition, the drug appears to have a narrow therapeutic range and requires close monitoring of serum levels as well as provision of exogenous steroid hormone replacement to avoid symptoms associated with adrenal insufficiency due to suppression of the normal contralateral adrenal gland.

ADRENAL INCIDENTALOMA

With the widespread use of abdominal CT imaging, asymptomatic adrenal lesions are being discovered with increasing frequency. These lesions, termed incidentalomas, are seen in up to 4% of routinely performed abdominal imaging studies and in up to 9% of autopsy series. Although most of these lesions are benign adenomas, some are hormonally active, and a small minority represents an invasive malignancy.

All patients identified with an incidental adrenal mass should be screened to rule out a hormonally active adenoma or pheochromocytoma. Evaluation of patients with an incidentally identified adrenal mass includes measurement of serum electrolyte levels, an overnight 1-mg dexamethasone suppression test (described previously), and a 24-hour urine collection to determine levels of vanillylmandelic acid, metanephrine, and catecholamines (Fig. 15-2). Any hormonally active lesion, regardless of size, should be resected. Furthermore, surgery is indicated if the adrenal mass shows radiographic characteristics suggestive of malignancy, or if the tumor enlarges during follow-up.

If the incidentaloma is nonfunctioning, the risk of malignancy is related to its size and radiographic characteristics. In general, lesions larger than 6 cm should be resected, because as many as 35% may be malignant. Observation and follow-up is generally recommended for nonfunctioning lesions smaller than 3 cm in diameter, but the management of tumors between 3 and 6 cm is more controversial. Data from our own institution and elsewhere have identified patients with adrenal cortical carcinomas arising in tumors smaller than 5 cm. The majority of these small tumors had CT or MRI characteristics suspicious for carcinoma. Based on individual experience and a review of the literature, recent recommendations for resection of nonfunctioning adrenal masses have ranged from 5 cm down to 3 cm. The recent success and advantages of laparoscopic adrenalectomy has led some investigators to suggest operative removal of even small incidentalomas.

At MD Anderson, we recommend adrenalectomy for all biochemically confirmed functioning adrenal tumors and those with suspicious radiographic findings regardless of size. Nonfunctioning tumors between 3 and 6 cm in diameter are most appropriately managed on an individual basis with respect to patient age and general health. For example, a 4 cm tumor in an otherwise healthy 40-year-old patient is probably most appropriately managed by adrenalectomy, whereas the same tumor in a 75-year-old patient with multiple comorbidities might be observed. The following may be helpful in evaluating such patients with intermediate-size nonfunctioning adrenal masses: MRI, a more thorough endocrine evaluation, and consideration of age and comorbidity. Fig. 15-3 provides an overview of our approach to patients with adrenal incidentalomas.

ADRENAL METASTASES

Metastasis of cancers to the adrenal glands is relatively common. Based on autopsy studies, 42% of lung cancers, 16% of gastric cancers, 58% of breast cancers, 50% of malignant melanomas, and a high percentage of renal and prostate cancers have metastasized to the adrenal glands at the time of death. However, only rarely are clinical problems related to these adrenal metastases, such as adrenal insufficiency, encountered. In general, more than 90% of the adrenal gland must be replaced before clinically detectable adrenal cortical hypofunction is appreciated. When adrenal insufficiency does occur, it is usually in the setting of gross enlargement of the adrenal glands as detected by CT.

Surgery for isolated metastases to the adrenal gland may be considered in highly selected patients. These include good-risk individuals in whom there is a prolonged disease-free interval and favorable tumor biology. Evaluation of these patients includes consideration of those who have had a significant progression-free interval, those who have responded to systemic therapy, and those who have a history of isolated metachronous metastases. In particular, a longer disease-free interval from the time of primary cancer therapy to adrenal metastasis is associated with a survival advantage following adrenalectomy. Primary tumor site also appears to affect survival, in that longer median survival times are observed following resection of metastases from primary kidney, melanoma, colon, and lung cancers, and poorer survival in patients with esophageal, liver, unknown primary tumors, and high-grade sarcomas.

Evaluation of the patient with an adrenal mass and a history of malignancy includes an evaluation for hormone production, since some of these patients will have an occult, functioning adrenal tumors unrelated to their prior malignancy, for example a pheochromocytoma (Fig. 15-3). Fine-needle aspiration biopsy may be helpful in selected patients when the results would influence the treatment plan; for example, to confirm a diagnosis of metastasis, particularly in those who are not surgical candidates and in those patients who have not yet had their

Fig. 15-2. **Algorithm for the evaluation of patients with isolated, incidentally identified adrenal tumors.**

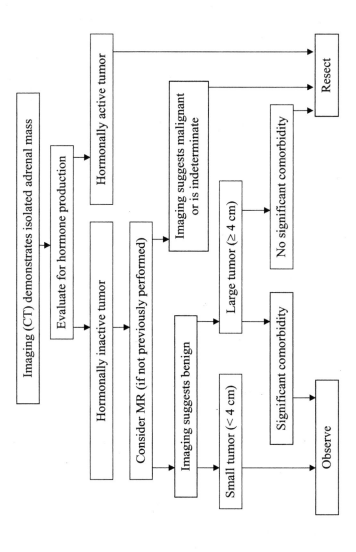

primary cancer resected. In a study of patients with operable non-small cell lung cancer and an adrenal mass, 40% had nonfunctioning adenomas by CT-guided biopsy. In selected patients, however, surgical therapy may be planned solely based on the patient's history and on noninvasive studies, and without preoperative needle biopsy. A history of a malignancy that commonly metastasizes to the adrenal glands, with favorable tumor biology, negative biochemical screening for hormone production, and a mass that either fulfills size criteria for surgical excision or is radiographically suspicious for metastasis

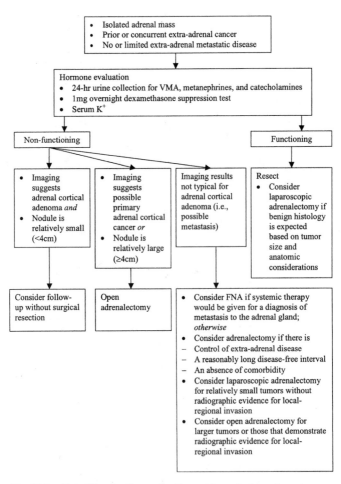

Fig. 15-3. Algorithm for the evaluation and surgical treatment of patients with extra-adrenal cancer presenting with an adrenal mass. VMA, vanillylmandelic acid.

may be considered for resection without preoperative tissue diagnosis.

We emphasize that we do not recommend routine fine needle aspiration of incidentally identified adrenal tumors in patients without a previous diagnosis of cancer. In the absence of signs or symptoms of a solid tumor malignancy, unilateral adrenal metastases are uncommon. Our recent experience with over 1600 patients found that the incidence of metastasis from an occult primary cancer was 0.2% (4 of 1,639). In all four of these patients, malignancy was suspected on the basis of tumor size, bilateral involvement, or symptoms. Therefore, we do not routinely biopsy patients with small nonfunctioning adrenal tumors searching for occult metastatic disease.

RECOMMENDED READING

Primary Hyperaldosteronism

Blumenfeld JC, Sealey JE, Schlussel Y, et al. Diagnosis and therapy of primary hyperaldosteronism. *Ann Intern Med* 1994;121:877.

Lo CY, Tam PC, Kung AWC, et al. Primary aldosteronism: results of surgical treatment. *Ann Surg* 1996;224:125.

Sawka AM, Young WF Jr, Thompson GB, et al. Primary aldosteronism: factors associated with normalization of blood pressure after surgery. *Ann Intern Med* 2001;135(4):258–261.

Vallotton MB. Primary aldosteronism. Parts I and II. *Clin Endocrinol* 1996;45:47.

Weigel RJ, Wells SA, Gunnells JC, et al. Surgical treatment of primary hyperaldosteronism. *Ann Surg* 1994;219:347.

Weinberger MH, Fineberg NS. The diagnosis of primary aldosteronism and separation of two major subtypes. *Arch Intern Med* 1993;153:2125.

Hypercortisolism

Lacroix A, Bolte E, Tremblay J, et al. Gastric inhibitory polypeptide-dependent cortisol hypersecretion: a new cause of Cushing's syndrome. *N Engl J Med* 1992;327:974.

Orth DN. Cushing's syndrome. *N Engl J Med* 1995;332:791.

van Heerden JA, Young WF Jr, Grant CS, et al. Adrenal surgery for hypercortisolism: surgical aspects. *Surgery* 1995;117:466.

Zieger MA, Pass HI, Doppman JD, et al. Surgical strategy in the management of non-small cell ectopic adrenocorticotropic hormone syndrome. *Surgery* 1992;112:994.

Pheochromocytoma

Gagner M, Breton JG, Pharand D, et al. Is laparoscopic adrenalectomy indicated for pheochromocytomas? *Surgery* 1996;120:1076.

Jalil ND, Pattou FN, Combemale F, et al. Effectiveness and limits of preoperative imaging studies for the localization of pheochromocytomas and paragangliomas: a review of 282 cases. *Eur J Surg* 1998;164:23–28.

Lee JE, Curley SA, Gagel RF, et al. Cortical-sparing adrenalectomy for patients with bilateral pheochromocytoma. *Surgery* 1995;120:1064.

Orchard T, Grant CS, van Heerden JA, et al. Pheochromocytoma: continuing evolution of surgical therapy. *Surgery* 1993;114:1153.

Peplinski GR, Norton JA. The predictive value of diagnostic tests for pheochromocytoma. *Surgery* 1994;116:1101.

Werbel SS, Ober KP. Pheochromocytoma: update on diagnosis, localization, and management. *Med Clin North Am* 1995;79:131.

Adrenocortical Masses and Carcinoma

Lenert JT, Barnett CC, Kudelka AP, et al. Evaluation and surgical resection of adrenal masses in patients with a history of extraadrenal malignancy. *Surgery* 2001;130:1060–1067.

Barnett CC, Varma DG, El-Naggar AK, et al. Limitations of size as a criterion in the evaluation of adrenal tumors. *Surgery* 2000;128: 973–982.

Bornstein SR, Stratakis CA, Chrousos GP. Adrenocortical tumors: recent advances in basic concepts and clinical management. *Ann Intern Med* 1999;130:759–771.

Dackiw AP, Lee JE, Gagel RF, Evans DB. Adrenal cortical carcinoma. *World J Surg* 2001;25:914–926.

Demeter JG, De Jong SA, Brooks MH, et al. Long-term results of adrenal autotransplantation in Cushing's disease. *Surgery* 1990; 108:1117.

Doppman JL, Reinig JW, Dwyer AJ, et al. Differentiation of adrenal masses by magnetic resonance imaging. *Surgery* 1987;102:1018.

Graham DJ, McHenry CR. The adrenal incidentaloma: guidelines for evaluation and recommendations for management. *Surg Oncol Clin North Am* 1998;7:749–764.

Herrera MF, Grant CS, van Heerden JA, et al. Incidentally discovered adrenal tumors: an institutional perspective. *Surgery* 1991;110: 1014.

Icard P, Chapuis Y. Andreassian BA, et al. Adrenocortical carcinoma in surgically treated patients: a retrospective study on 156 cases by the French Association of Endocrine Surgery. *Surgery* 1992;112:972.

Lee JE, Berger DH, El-Naggar AK, et al. Surgical management, DNA content, and patient survival in adrenal cortical carcinoma. *Surgery* 1995;118:1090.

Lee JE, Evans DB, Hickey RC, et al. Unknown primary cancer presenting as an adrenal mass: frequency and implications for diagnostic evaluation of adrenal incidentalomas. *Surgery* 1998;124:115–122.

Luton JP, Cerdas S, Billaud L, et al. Clinical features of adrenocortical carcinoma, prognostic factors, and the effect of mitotane therapy. *N Engl J Med* 1990;322:1195.

McFarlane DA. Cancer of the adrenal cortex: the natural history, prognosis and treatment in a study of fifty-five cases. *Ann R Coll Surg Engl* 1958;23:155.

Paul CA, Virgo KS, Wade TP, et al. Adrenalectomy for isolated adrenal metastases from non-adrenal cancer. *Int J Oncol* 2000;17(1):181–187.

Pommier RF, Brennan MF. An eleven-year experience with adrenocortical carcinoma. *Surgery* 1992;112:963.

Ross NS, Aron DC. Hormonal evaluation of the patient with an incidentally discovered adrenal mass. *N Engl J Med* 1990;323:1401.

Salem M, Tainsh RE, Bromberg J, et al. Perioperative glucocorticoid coverage: a reassessment 42 years after emergence of a problem. *Ann Surg* 1994;4:416.

Siren J, Tervahartiala P, Sivula A, et al. Natural course of adrenal incidentalomas: seven-year follow-up study. *World J Surg* 2000;24: 579–582.

Smith CD, Weber CJ, Amerson JR. Laparoscopic adrenalectomy: new gold standard. *World J Surg* 1999;23:389–396.

Sullivan M, Boileau M, Hodges CV. Adrenal cortical carcinoma. *J Urol* 1978;120:660.

Vassilopoulou-Sellin R, Guinee VF, Klein MJ, et al. Impact of adjuvant mitotane on the clinical course of patients with adrenocortical cancer. *Cancer* 1993;71:3119.

Carcinoma of the Thyroid and Parathyroid Glands

Marina E. Jean, Paula M. Termuhlen, and Ana M. Grau

THYROID CANCER

Epidemiology

Thyroid cancer is the most common endocrine malignancy and accounts for approximately 1% of all human malignancies, with an estimated incidence in the United States of 18,400 cases in 2000. The majority of cases—approximately 70%—occur in women. Carcinoma of the thyroid gland is considered an indolent disease; many affected individuals die of other causes. An estimated 1,200 patients die of this disease each year.

The prevalence of thyroid nodules increases linearly with age, with spontaneous nodules occurring at a rate of 0.08% per year beginning early in life and extending into the eighth decade. Clinically apparent nodules are present in 4% to 7% of the adult population and occur more commonly in women. Most nodules are not malignant. Reported malignancy rates are 5% to 12% in patients with single nodules and 3% in patients with multiple nodules. However, a history of radiation exposure has been reported to increase the risk of malignancy in a nodule to 30% to 50%.

Risk Factors

Approximately 9% of thyroid cancers are associated with prior radiation exposure. The risk of cancer from radiation increases linearly with doses up to 20 Gy, with thyroid ablation occurring at higher dose levels. The risk of developing thyroid cancer is inversely related to age at exposure. A history of exposure to ionizing radiation in childhood is a major risk factor for thyroid malignancy, almost always of the papillary type. Individuals 15 years of age or older at exposure do not have a demonstrable radiation-dose–dependent risk of thyroid cancer. In general, radiation-induced thyroid cancer is biologically similar to sporadic thyroid cancer and should be treated in the same manner. However, recent information regarding the high incidence of biologically aggressive thyroid cancer in children exposed to radiation after the Chernobyl nuclear disaster suggests that radiation dose and tumor behavior may be linked. The proportions of less well-differentiated papillary thyroid cancers and of solid-variant papillary thyroid cancers were higher among these children than among patients without radiation exposure. Additional evidence of a link between radiation dose and tumor behavior comes from the finding that exposure to different types of radiation results in different patterns of genetic alterations in thyroid tumors.

Aside from radiation exposure, few environmental risk factors have been confirmed for thyroid carcinoma. Hormonal factors and dietary intake of iodine, retinol, vitamin C, and vitamin E have been suggested to play a role in the etiology of thyroid cancer that has yet to be defined.

Recently, associations have been described between thyroid cancer and several other inherited syndromes, including familial polyposis, Gardner's syndrome, and Cowden disease (familial goiter and skin hamartoma). In addition, papillary thyroid cancer may occur with increased frequency in some families with breast, ovarian, renal, or central nervous system malignancies. Medullary thyroid cancer occurs with a higher frequency in patients who have Hashimoto's thyroiditis. The mechanism underlying these associations is not well understood.

Over the past several years, significant progress has been made in the identification of genes linked to the pathogenesis of thyroid cancer. Studies of the patterns of genetic alterations present in thyroid tumors suggest that there are differences in the pathogenesis of the different thyroid tumor types, which most likely account for the range in biologic behavior observed among thyroid cancers. The *RET* proto-oncogene, which is located on chromosome 10 and encodes a tyrosine kinase receptor, is believed to play a role in the pathogenesis of both hereditary and sporadic medullary thyroid carcinomas (MTC) and papillary thyroid carcinomas (PTC). Activating point mutations in the *RET* proto-oncogene of parafollicular C cells have been detected in virtually all hereditary forms of MTC, including familial MTC, multiple endocrine neoplasia 2A (MEN 2A), and MEN 2B, which account for approximately 25% to 35% of MTC. Mutations in the *RET* proto-oncogene have also been found in sporadic MTC, although different codons of the *RET* proto-oncogene are affected. Rearrangements of the *RET* proto-oncogene in thyroid follicular cells are considered to be an early event in the development of PTCs. Because 90% of patients with autosomal dominant MEN 2A or MEN 2B will develop MTC, screening for germline *RET* mutations has been invaluable in the early identification of patients who have a genetic basis for their disease. The discovery of the *RET* proto-oncogene has had significant clinical impact, affecting the screening and prophylactic treatment of patients who are members of the MEN kindreds.

Somatic mutations in the *Ras* oncogene have been found in both benign and malignant thyroid tumors and thus also seem to be an early event in thyroid tumorigenesis, although some reports suggest that *Ras* mutations are more prevalent in follicular thyroid carcinomas (FTC). The findings of a high prevalence of *p53* mutations in anaplastic carcinomas but not in well-differentiated thyroid carcinomas suggest that *p53* mutations play a role later in thyroid tumor pathogenesis—specifically, in the dedifferentiating transition to the anaplastic phenotype. Numerous other genes (e.g., PTEN, TRK, GSP, and the thyroid-stimulating hormone [TSH] receptor gene) have also been implicated in the pathogenesis of thyroid cancer, although their roles still need to be defined. Currently, very few of the genetic alterations (e.g., p53, ras, RET codon 918, RET/PTC rearrangements) found in thyroid tumors have been shown to have negative implications on prognosis. Much work is still needed to elucidate the molecular biology of thyroid tumors and to translate this knowledge into clinical management.

Pathology

Four tumor types account for more than 90% of thyroid malignancies: PTC, FTC, MTC, and undifferentiated (anaplastic) thyroid carcinoma (UTC). PTC and FTC are further grouped together and referred to as differentiated thyroid carcinoma (DTC), which accounts for approximately 90% of thyroid carcinomas. Differentiated thyroid cancers more commonly occur in women, whereas an equal gender distribution is seen in both MTC and UTC. PTC, FTC, and UTC are derived from the follicular epithelial cells of the thyroid gland, which produce the thyroid hormones. MTC is derived from the calcitonin-secreting parafollicular C cells. Other less common thyroid carcinomas include Hürthle cell carcinoma (a variant of follicular carcinoma), lymphomas, squamous cell carcinomas, sarcomas, and metastatic carcinomas from other sites.

Papillary thyroid carcinoma is the most common thyroid carcinoma, representing 80% of all cases. Patients with PTC usually present during the third to fifth decades. PTC occurs as an irregular solid or cystic mass that arises from follicular epithelium. It is nonencapsulated but sharply circumscribed. Microscopically, the hallmark is papillary fronds of epithelium. Rounded calcific deposits (psammoma bodies) are found in 50% of lesions. Multifocality is a prominent feature of PTC and has been documented in up to 80% of patients. Cervical lymph node metastases are quite common at presentation with a reported frequency of between 30% and 80% in most U.S. and European series. PTC is the predominant tumor type found in patients with a history of radiation exposure. The overall prognosis for patients with PTC is very good: 10-year survival rates are 80% to 95%.

Follicular thyroid carcinoma is the second most common malignancy of the thyroid gland, comprising 10% to 20% of thyroid cancers. Patients with FTC often present a decade later than patients with PTC, during the fifth and sixth decades. Patients with FTC also tend to have slightly larger tumors at presentation than patients with papillary tumors. Cytologic diagnosis of FTC is often difficult due to the similarities between FTC and benign follicular adenomas. Permanent sections showing capsular or vascular invasion are required to confirm diagnosis. FTC is usually encapsulated and consists of highly cellular follicles, most of which are single, solid, and noncystic without central necrosis—not multifocal. Cervical lymph node metastases are less common in FTC and are found in approximately 10% of patients at presentation. FTC has a greater tendency to spread hematogenously to distant sites such as lung and bone and up to 33% of patients have distant metastases at presentation. FTC is often found in association with benign thyroid disorders, such as endemic goiter. A relationship between TSH stimulation and follicular carcinoma has been suggested because of the greater incidence of FTC in iodine-deficient areas. Ten-year survival rates for FTC are 70% to 95%—slightly worse than those for PTC, which is most likely due to later presentation. When patients are matched by age and tumor stage, there is no significant difference in survival between PTC and FTC.

Medullary thyroid carcinomas represent 5% of all thyroid cancers. Eighty percent of tumors are sporadic and 20% occur as part of an autosomal dominant hereditary syndrome. Sporadic MTC often presents in the fifth decade as a unilateral solitary nodule. Patients with familial MTC more commonly present in the fourth decade with multifocal nodules in the upper poles of both thyroid lobes, where there is the greatest concentration of C cells. Bilateral C cell hyperplasia is believed to be a precursor to the development of hereditary MTC. Histologically, MTC is an ill-defined, nonencapsulated, invasive mass composed of spindle-shaped or rounded cells separated by fibrous septa and amyloid deposits. Positive immunohistochemical staining for calcitonin and amyloid aids in the diagnosis of MTC. Medullary carcinomas are slow growing but have a propensity to metastasize early, usually before the primary tumor reaches 2 cm. Fifty percent of patients have regional metastases at the time of diagnosis. Cervical and upper mediastinal lymph nodes are the usual sites involved. Ten-year survival rates for MTC depend on the extent of disease at presentation and are 90% when disease is confined to the thyroid gland, 70% when cervical metastases are present, and 20% when distant metastases are present. The prognosis for patients with MTC falls between that of patients with undifferentiated tumors and patients with well-differentiated tumors. Poor prognostic factors include age greater than 50 years at diagnosis, metastases at the time of diagnosis, and MEN 2B. Seventy percent of patients with MEN 2B have metastases at the time of diagnosis of MTC and of these patients, fewer than 5% survive 5 years.

Undifferentiated (anaplastic) thyroid carcinoma is a rare and highly aggressive tumor that is considered one of the deadliest malignancies. Anaplastic tumors often are inoperable at presentation and account for less than 5% of thyroid cancers. The peak incidence is in the seventh decade and the incidence is the same in men and women. Patients with UTC usually present with a rapidly growing neck mass, often larger than 5 cm that is fixed to underlying structures and causes symptoms of dysphagia, dyspnea, or dysphonia. On pathologic examination, anaplastic tumors are nonencapsulated and often contain areas of extensive necrosis. There are three histologic variants, all of which show high mitotic activity, nuclear pleomorphism, and high vascularity. At the time of diagnosis, 25% of patients have invasion of the trachea, 90% have regional metastases, and 50% have distant metastases—most commonly to the lung. An association between UTC and a history of well-differentiated thyroid cancer has been reported. It has been hypothesized that UTC can develop from within pre-existing differentiated thyroid cancer as a result of dedifferentiation of a clone of tumor cells over time. Despite the use of multimodality regimens, treatment rarely results in cure and 90% of patients die within 6 months of diagnosis often as a result of local progression of disease causing airway obstruction. The 5-year survival rate for UTC is 7%.

Hürthle cell carcinomas represent 5% of thyroid cancers and are considered variants of FTC, although Hürthle cell carcinomas and FTC are thought to be distinct pathologic entities because of differences in their biologic behavior and natural history. As with the diagnosis of FTC, the diagnosis of Hürthle cell carcinomas is difficult to make without the presence of vascular or capsular invasion. Hürthle cell carcinomas are characterized microscopically by polygonal, hyperchromatic cells. The incidence of lymph node metastases at presentation is slightly higher in Hürthle cell carcinomas (approximately 25%) than in FTC. Patients with Hürthle cell carcinomas have been reported to have higher tumor recurrence rates and a worse prognosis when compared to patients with PTC and FTC. Only 10% of Hürthle cell tumors take up radioactive iodine compared to 70% to 80% of papillary and follicular tumors.

Thyroid lymphomas represent fewer than 2% of thyroid cancers. Patients with thyroid lymphomas typically present in the seventh decade. This subtype of thyroid cancer also more commonly affects women and is associated with a history of Hashimoto's thyroiditis. The clinical presentation of thyroid lymphoma may be similar to that of UTC, with a rapidly growing neck mass and symptoms of dysphagia and dysphonia. Lymphomas may be primary or secondary; however, non-Hodgkin's B-cell type lymphomas are the most common primary thyroid lymphomas. Histologically, tumor cells appear monomorphic and noncohesive and stain positive for lymphocyte markers like CD20. It has been reported that 67% of thyroid lymphomas are of mucosa-associated lymphoid tissue (MALT) origin; these tumors are associated with better survival and may be sufficiently treated with radiation therapy alone instead of the multimodality therapy used for non-MALT lymphomas. Prognosis is related to the extent of disease at the time of diagnosis. When lymphoma is confined to the thyroid gland (stage IE), the 5-year survival rate is 75% to 85%. Patients with disease on both sides of the diaphragm (stage IIIE) or disseminated disease (stage IVE) have a 5-year survival rate of less than 35%.

Diagnosis

Most patients with thyroid cancer have no specific symptoms. The most common finding at presentation is a mass or nodule. Less commonly, change in the size of a thyroid nodule or pain from hemorrhage into a nodule will prompt a patient to see a physician. Hoarseness, dysphagia, dyspnea, and hemoptysis are symptoms resulting from invasion of surrounding anatomic structures and are rare in well-differentiated thyroid carcinomas. Occasionally, a patient may present with a palpable cervical lymph node.

A thorough history and physical examination is an important first diagnostic step. Although the history may not be sensitive or specific for detection of a thyroid malignancy, it is important to ascertain whether there is a family history of thyroid cancer, previous radiation exposure, or the presence of symptoms that suggest invasiveness, such as progressive development of hoarseness, dyspnea, and dysphagia. The presence of a single, dominant nodule that is fixed to surrounding tissues and greater than 1 cm in diameter with a hard consistency is suggestive of cancer. The presence of discrete 1- to 2-cm lymph nodes in conjunction with a thyroid nodule is also suggestive of malignancy. Palpable adenopathy is most often found along the middle and lower portions of the jugular vein but may be located lateral to the sternocleidomastoid muscle in the lower portion of the posterior cervical triangle. Other physical findings that suggest invasive malignancy include vocal cord paralysis, fixation of the thyroid nodule, and tracheal deviation or invasion. Cervical spine flexibility should be assessed to ensure that adequate hyperextension of the neck can be achieved in case surgery is needed. Examination of the larynx and vocal cords should be performed either indirectly with a mirror or directly with a flexible fiberoptic scope to document the preoperative condition.

Various diagnostic tests are available to help distinguish benign from malignant disease. The ultimate goal is to avoid operating on benign lesions whenever possible. The initial evaluation of a patient with a single thyroid nodule consists of laboratory thyroid function studies and fine-needle aspiration (FNA) biopsy. Blood tests, such as the measurement of TSH or thyroglobulin, cannot diagnose thyroid carcinoma, but abnormal thyroid function tests argue against the presence of thyroid cancer. The exception is the measurement of serum calcitonin concentrations that can help identify patients with MTC.

Fine-needle aspiration is safe, cost-effective, and the single most useful diagnostic tool in the evaluation of thyroid nodules because it can provide direct information about a lesion. Lesions are classified as benign, malignant, or suspicious for malignancy on the basis of FNA. If an experienced physician performs the FNA and an experienced cytopathologist interprets the cytologic characteristics, the accuracy of FNA in the diagnosis of thyroid cancer can be greater than 90%, with a false-negative rate of less than 5%. Accuracy of FNA is greatest for lesions between 1 and 4 cm; lesions less than 1 cm are difficult to sample, while lesions greater than 4 cm have an increased sampling error as a result of the large area of the lesion. The type of thyroid tumor can also influence the accuracy of FNA. Patients with the diagnosis of follicular neoplasm often require surgical intervention for complete diagnosis. It is difficult to distinguish a follicular adenoma from a follicular carcinoma by FNA because the presence or absence of capsular or vascular invasion is required to make the diagnosis. Patients with inadequate specimens must undergo repeat FNA or surgery to obtain a tissue diagnosis. Individuals with a finding of benign colloid nodule or thyroiditis by FNA are observed with or without thyroid suppression. Growth of a nodule in a patient receiving thyroid suppression is an indication for surgical intervention. Other specific indications for surgical intervention in thyroid abnormalities are listed in Table 16-1.

Ultrasonography of the thyroid is an accurate method for determining the character of a thyroid nodule (solid, cystic, or mixed), the number of thyroid nodules, and the status of cervical lymph nodes, but it cannot differentiate benign from malignant lesions and therefore has limited use in the workup of thyroid nodules. However, ultrasonography may be useful in guiding FNA in patients with lesions that are difficult to palpate and also in increasing the yield from aspirations of small or complex lesions. Ultrasonography is also useful in the long-term follow-up of patients with thyroid nodules.

Radionuclide scintigraphy (^{99}Tc-pertechnetate, ^{125}I or ^{131}I) was previously used as the first diagnostic step in evaluating palpable thyroid masses. Because most thyroid carcinomas and many

Table 16-1. Indications for surgical intervention for thyroid abnormalities

1. FNA of thyroid nodule suspicious for carcinoma or follicular adenoma
2. Thyroid nodule in a patient younger than 20 years, older than 60 years with FNA findings of atypia or in a patient with a history of irradiation
3. Thyroid mass associated with vocal cord paralysis, regional tissue invasion, cervical lymph node metastasis, or fixation to surrounding tissues
4. Hyperfunctioning thyroid nodule in a young patient
5. Solitary cold nodules or dominant nodules in a multinodular goiter that fail to respond to suppressive therapy

FNA, fine needle aspiration.

benign nodules appear cold on scan, the main limitation of radionuclide scanning is that it cannot distinguish between benign and malignant lesions. Approximately 16% of cold (nonfunctioning) nodules, 9% of warm (normal), and 4% of hot (hyperfunctioning) lesions harbor a malignancy. Although a cold lesion has the greatest probability of being malignant, the presence of a hot lesion on a thyroid scan does not exclude malignancy. In general, the use of nuclear thyroid scans has been replaced by FNA for diagnosis.

Other diagnostic imaging studies are seldom needed in the initial evaluation of a patient with a thyroid nodule. Computed tomography (CT) and magnetic resonance imaging (MRI) are useful in the evaluation of large or recurrent cancers suspected of invasion into the surrounding soft tissue. When indicated by the history and physical findings, CT or MRI of the neck and upper mediastinum may be used to delineate extrathyroidal extension and invasion of the trachea or esophagus or to determine the presence of significant cervical or mediastinal metastases. A chest radiograph may be obtained in certain situations to assess for pulmonary metastases and tracheal deviation.

Preoperative laboratory assessments should include thyroid function tests and a serum calcium measurement. Although thyroid function tests do not aid in the diagnosis of thyroid cancer, the presence of hypothyroidism or hyperthyroidism is an important factor to take into account in a patient undergoing general anesthesia. Parathyroid function should be assessed by measuring the serum calcium level, because the incidence of parathyroid adenomas and other hyperfunctioning anomalies of the parathyroid glands is higher in the presence of thyroid nodules or carcinoma. Thyroid antibody tests are important when thyroiditis is a consideration. Serum calcitonin measurements are indicated in patients who have a family history of MTC or a high likelihood of having an MEN syndrome. Patients who have an increased calcitonin level and a preoperative diagnosis of MTC should be screened for pheochromocytoma with a 24-hour urine collection for vanillylmandelic acid, metanephrine, and free catecholamines and for hereditary MTC with *RET* proto-oncogene mutation analysis. Five percent to 7% of patients with apparently sporadic MTC are found to have a mutation consistent with hereditary MTC. Measurement of serum thyroglobulin levels is useful mainly for follow-up studies after treatment of DTC and is not a part of the diagnostic evaluation.

Staging and Prognosis

Several classifications and staging schemes have been proposed for DTC. However, no consensus favoring any one of these systems has emerged. The most commonly used are the AMES (Age, Metastasis, Extent, Size) system, which divides patients into low- and high-risk groups; the TNM (Tumor, Nodes, Metastasis), as used by the American Joint Committee on Cancer; the AGES (Age, Grade, Extent, Size) and MACIS (Metastasis, Age, Completeness of Resection, Invasion, Size) proposed by the Mayo Clinic; the University of Chicago system, which groups patients into four categories—disease limited to the gland (I), lymph node involvement (II), extrathyroidal invasion (III), and distant metastases (IV); and the National Thyroid Cancer Treatment Cooperative Study (NTCTCS) Registry scheme. Analyses comparing the ability of the different classification schemes to stage disease in the same cohort of patients suggest that the TNM (Table 16-2) and NTCTCS (Table 16-3) staging classifications have the best predictive value; therefore, we recommend that clinicians use one of these two staging classifications. The TNM classification stratifies patients into four stages on the basis of tumor size, nodal status, the presence or absence of distant metastases, and age at diagnosis. The NTCTCS scheme also classifies patients into four stages but is based on age at diagnosis, tumor size, tumor type, the presence or absence of nodal or distant metastases, and the presence or absence of capsular or extraglandular invasion.

The prognosis of patients with stage I well-differentiated thyroid carcinoma is excellent, with 20-year survival rates of nearly 100%. Patients with stage IV disease, in contrast, have a 5-year survival rate of only 25%. Within the group of patients with well-differentiated thyroid cancer are a small number who have more aggressive disease and for whom none of the current staging systems apply. As molecular markers of disease are developed, these patients may be able to be identified at earlier stages and offered additional treatment.

In general, the prognosis for patients with PTC is influenced by age, gender, extent of disease, and volume of the primary tumor. Unlike most solid tumors, age at diagnosis may be the most important predictive factor for survival. The significance of gender as a prognostic factor in thyroid cancer is also greater than that for other solid tumors. The prognostic significance of lymph node metastases in differentiated thyroid cancers continues to be debated; in patients with papillary cancer who are less than 40 years of age, the significance is considered negligible. The minimal effect of lymph node metastases on prognosis is reflected in the TNM staging system (Table 16-2), in which lymph node metastases are only factored into the staging of patients greater than 45 years of age. The diminished importance of lymph node metastases is based on data suggesting that microscopic metastases are

Table 16-2. TNM classification system for differentiated thyroid carcinoma

Definition

Primary tumor (T)

TX	Primary tumor cannot be assessed
T0	No evidence of primary tumor
T1	Tumor ≤1 cm, confined to the thyroid
T2	Tumor >1 cm and <4 cm, confined to the thyroid
T3	Tumor >4 cm, confined to the thyroid
T4	Tumor of any size extending beyond the thyroid capsule

Regional lymph nodes (N) (cervical and upper mediastinal)

NX	Regional lymph nodes cannot be assessed
N0	No regional lymph node metastasis
N1	Regional lymph node metastasis
	N1a Metastasis in ipsilateral cervical lymph nodes
	N1b Metastasis in bilateral, midline, or contralateral cervical or mediastinal lymph nodes

Distant metastases (M)

MX	Presence of distant metastasis cannot be assessed
M0	No distant metastasis
M1	Distant metastasis

Stages

Papillary and follicular cancer

	Patient age <45 years	Patients age ≥45 years
Stage I	Any T, any N, M0	T1, N0, M0
Stage II	Any T, any N, M1	T2 or T3, N0, M0
Stage III		T4, N0, M0
		Any T, N1, M0
Stage IV		Any T, any N, M1

Medullary cancer

Stage I	T1, N0, M0
Stage II	T2–T4, N0, M0
Stage III	Any T, N1, M0
Stage IV	Any T, Any N, M1

Undifferentiated cancer

Stage IV (all cases)	Any T, Any N, Any M

present in up to 90% of lymph nodes examined yet clinically significant disease develops in only 10% of patients.

The prognosis of patients with FTC is thought to be poorer than that of patients with PTC, perhaps because of the higher incidence of hematogenous metastases. However, treatment decisions and prognosis are based on well-differentiated thyroid malignancies as a group. Overall 10-year survival rates for patients with thyroid carcinoma are shown in Table 16-4.

Treatment

Controversy continues over the extent of resection necessary in cases of papillary and follicular cancer, the necessity and extent of neck dissection, the role of post-resection thyroid hormone

Table 16-3.   National Thyroid Cancer Treatment Cooperative Study (NTCTCS) Registry Staging[a] classification

Features	Papillary Carcinoma		Follicular Carcinoma	
	Age <45	Age ≥45	Age <45	Age ≥45
Primary tumor size				
<1 cm	I	I	I	II
1–4 cm	I	II	I	III
>4 cm	II	III	II	III
Primary tumor description				
Microscopic multifocal	I	II	I	III
Gross multifocal or gross tumor capsule invasion	I	II	II	III
Microscopic extraglandular invasion	I	II	I	III
Gross extraglandular invasion	II	III	II	III
Poor differentiation	NA	NA	III	III
Metastasis				
Cervical node metastasis	I	III	I	III
Extracervical metastasis	III	IV	III	IV

NA, not applicable.
[a] The disease stage assigned to a patient is the highest stage determined by these clinicopathologic features.

Table 16-4.   Ten-year survival rates for thyroid carcinoma by stage

Stage	10-year Survival (%)
I	95
II	50–95
III	15–50
IV	<15

suppression, and the appropriate use of postoperative therapeutic radioactive [131]I. At this time, no randomized prospective trials have been conducted to clarify these controversies. Certain factors make it unlikely that a prospective trial will be conducted because (a) thyroid cancer is an indolent disease, which would require that patients be followed for long periods of time in order to detect differences in outcome; and (b) given the low incidence of thyroid cancer, Udelsman and colleagues have reported that between 3,000 and 12,000 patients would need to be randomized to conduct a prospective trial. Thus, the majority of treatment decisions for differentiated thyroid cancer have been made based on data from large retrospective series. What follows are the general treatment guidelines used at The University of Texas M.D. Anderson Cancer Center.

Surgical Resection

The principal treatment for thyroid cancer is surgical resection. Accepted surgical management varies from a thyroid lobectomy and isthmectomy to a total thyroidectomy and modified radical neck dissection.

The surgical management of well-differentiated thyroid cancer continues to be controversial, with the debate centering on the extent of thyroidectomy. Proponents of total thyroidectomy argue that this operation can be performed safely by experienced surgeons with a less than 2% incidence of permanent recurrent nerve injury or permanent hypoparathyroidism; foci of papillary carcinoma are found in both thyroid lobes in up to 85% of patients, and 5% to 10% of recurrences occur in the contralateral lobe; the presence of residual thyroid tissue after less than total thyroidectomy hampers the use of thyroglobulin as a marker of persistent or recurrent disease; radioactive iodine can be used to identify and treat residual normal thyroid tissue and recurrent or metastatic disease after total thyroidectomy; there is a lower recurrence rate in patients who have undergone bilateral procedures or total thyroidectomy; and total thyroidectomy minimizes the need for reoperative surgery, which is associated with increased complication rates.

Advocates of more conservative procedures, such as thyroid lobectomy with isthmectomy or near-total thyroidectomy, argue that there is a decreased risk of injury to the recurrent laryngeal nerve and the parathyroid glands with less extensive surgery; it is rare for a total thyroidectomy to remove all of the thyroid gland; occult foci of papillary carcinoma left behind after conservative surgery are rarely of clinical significance; half of clinically significant recurrences after conservative surgery can be safely managed with reoperation; and there is no difference in survival between patients who have undergone more conservative procedures and patients who have undergone total thyroidectomy.

At M.D. Anderson Cancer Center, we perform a total thyroidectomy for all papillary carcinomas larger than 1.0 cm, tumors with extrathyroidal extension or metastases, and tumors in patients 45 years of age or older. Total thyroidectomy is also our treatment of choice for follicular carcinoma and Hürthle cell carcinoma;

however, these diagnoses often cannot be ascertained by frozen-section examination at the time of surgery. If the diagnosis of follicular or Hürthle cell carcinoma is made postoperatively in a patient treated with a thyroid lobectomy, we suggest that a complete thyroidectomy be performed in high-risk patients (i.e., age >45 years, lesions >1 cm, or distant metastases). We consider lobectomy and isthmectomy appropriate treatment for minimal papillary cancers (<1.0 cm in diameter), minimal follicular cancers (<1.0 cm in diameter), and single, well-encapsulated, benign Hürthle cell neoplasms. Patients who have undergone thyroid lobectomy for other reasons and are found to have an incidental microscopic carcinoma on permanent histologic studies also require no further treatment. We combine a therapeutic cervical node dissection with total thyroidectomy in patients with well-differentiated carcinomas and clinical evidence of lymph node metastases.

At M.D. Anderson, patients with sporadic MTC diagnosed preoperatively undergo a total thyroidectomy with in-continuity central compartment dissection and modified radical neck dissection on the side of the lesion. Patients with palpable cervical lymphadenopathy undergo a bilateral modified radical neck dissection at the time of total thyroidectomy. The goals of our aggressive surgical approach are to maximize local-regional tumor control and survival and to minimize the need for reoperation. Our approach is supported by published reports suggesting that patients who undergo total thyroidectomy with compartment-oriented lymphadenectomy have both improved local-regional disease control and improved survival. Our approach is also supported by our knowledge of the biologic behavior of medullary thyroid cancers: these tumors do not concentrate radioiodine, are multifocal, metastasize early, and are not adequately managed with nonsurgical treatments.

Patients who have hereditary MTC as part of the familial MTC or MEN 2 syndromes undergo total thyroidectomy without lymphadenectomy if preoperative studies show a normal basal calcitonin level, normal findings on a cervical sonogram, and positive *Ret* mutational analysis. Patients who have an increased basal calcitonin level or a thyroid nodule detected on physical examination or sonography undergo total thyroidectomy with central compartment lymphadenectomy and bilateral modified neck dissection. Children who are found to carry a hereditary *Ret* proto-oncogene mutation should undergo prophylactic total thyroidectomy. Children in families with the MEN 2A or familial MTC syndromes should undergo surgery at 5 years of age, while children in families with MEN 2B should undergo surgery as early as possible because invasive MTC has been found as early as at birth in these children.

UTC is an aggressive lesion that is usually diagnosed by FNA. Most anaplastic tumors are unresectable at presentation and are thus managed primarily by combination radiation therapy and chemotherapy. Resectable lesions are treated with total thyroidectomy and wide local excision of adjacent soft tissues followed by postoperative adjuvant chemotherapy and radiation therapy. Although different chemotherapy combinations and radiation therapy regimens have been tried, no therapy has been able to improve the outcome of UTC.

Neck Dissection

An understanding of the lymphatic drainage pattern of the thyroid gland is necessary to ensure that the nodal groups at highest risk for metastasis are removed when node dissection is performed. The thyroid gland has an extensive intraglandular network of lymphatic channels that allow for drainage within one lobe and from one lobe to another. The thyroid lymphatics typically drain first into the central compartment (level VI), which contains the pretracheal and paratracheal nodes, and subsequently into the lateral jugular regions (level II–IV). Another route of lymphatic spread for thyroid cancer is along the inferior thyroid artery as it courses behind the common carotid artery and to the lower portion of the posterior triangle of the neck (level V). The superior mediastinal nodes also commonly contain metastases and must be closely examined intraoperatively. The submandibular and submental nodes (level I) rarely contain metastases in patients with DTC. The classic radical neck dissection, which consists of lymphadenectomy of levels II to V as well as removal of the internal jugular vein, sternocleidomastoid muscle, and spinal accessory nerve, is associated with high morbidity and rarely performed. We more commonly perform central compartment node dissection, which removes level VI and superior mediastinal nodes, and modified radical neck dissection, which spares the internal jugular vein, sternocleidomastoid muscle, and spinal accessory nerve, in patients with well-differentiated thyroid cancers.

The necessity and extent of neck dissection, specifically the role of elective node dissection, for differentiated thyroid cancer is another subject of controversy. PTC frequently spreads to cervical lymph nodes, whereas FTC rarely metastasizes to the regional lymph nodes. Although the exact incidence of lymph node metastases in papillary carcinoma is unknown, positive nodes have been found in 30% to 80% of patients who underwent prophylactic neck dissections. Microscopic nodal metastases have been reported in up to 90% of these patients. However, clinically significant nodal disease develops in only approximately 10% of patients with papillary carcinoma. At the heart of the controversy is the issue of whether or not lymph node metastases have an impact on recurrence or survival. The majority of studies in the literature on DTC have reported that positive nodal status influences local-regional recurrence rates, but not patient survival. The majority of studies have also failed to demonstrate a survival benefit in patients with differentiated thyroid tumors who have undergone extensive, prophylactic (elective) node dissection at the time of initial surgery. Whether elective node dissection reduces local-regional recurrence rates is unclear, as there are several conflicting reports in the literature. Of note though, all studies with patients who underwent extensive cervical lymphadenectomy reported higher complication rates.

For patients with papillary cancer, if a total thyroidectomy is performed, then we also perform an en bloc central compartment dissection. If there are clinically palpable nodes in the lateral regions of the neck, an en bloc modified radical neck dissection on the side containing clinically suspicious disease is also performed at the time of total thyroidectomy. In patients with follicular tumors, because of the low incidence of lymph node metastases, we do not perform central compartment lymphadenectomy at the time of total thyroidectomy unless there is palpable adenopathy. At M.D. Anderson, the aggressive use of ultrasound, particularly in high-risk patients, has assisted in the preoperative detection of suspicious nodes and the early determination of the need for lymph node dissection.

A poor prognosis is associated with the presence of lymph node metastases in patients with medullary and anaplastic cancers. We therefore perform a central compartment node dissection and a modified radical neck dissection on the side of the primary lesion at the time of total thyroidectomy in patients with sporadic MTC. A bilateral modified radical neck dissection is also performed if the patient presents with palpable adenopathy.

Surgical Technique

Surgical resection of a possible thyroid carcinoma requires meticulous dissection of the ipsilateral thyroid compartment, identification and preservation of the recurrent laryngeal nerve, and complete resection of the affected lobe and thyroid isthmus. Surgery should be performed with general anesthesia. Identification of the ipsilateral parathyroid glands should be attempted, but preservation of the glands may be impossible if there is extensive invasion by cancer or if there are clinical metastases in the paratracheal area. If the diagnosis of thyroid carcinoma is confirmed intraoperatively by frozen-section histologic examination of the surgical specimen, total thyroidectomy is completed by resecting the opposite lobe with special care taken to identify and spare the parathyroid glands and their blood supply. Once the thyroid gland is removed, the posterior surface is carefully inspected for any possible parathyroid tissue. If suspected parathyroid tissue is identified, a portion is sent for frozen-section examination, with the remnant kept in physiologic solution. If the tissue is confirmed to be parathyroid gland on frozen-section examination, the preserved portion is minced and implanted in a small pocket created in the sternocleidomastoid muscle. Other important structures such as the superior laryngeal nerve, spinal accessory nerve, sternocleidomastoid muscle, esophagus, and trachea should also be preserved unless invasion by tumor is present.

The approach to the thyroid gland itself is through a transverse incision, approximately one or two fingerbreadths above the clavicles. Flaps are elevated superiorly to the level of the thyroid notch and inferiorly to the suprasternal notch in the subplatysmal plane. Separation of the fascia between the strap muscles and the sternocleidomastoid muscles is done to facilitate exposure of the gland and allow inspection of the lower jugular lymph nodes. The strap muscles are separated in the midline and can be divided on the side of the primary tumor if necessary. Portions of the strap muscles adherent to the gland are resected with the specimen. The thyroid compartment may be approached laterally along the anterior border of the sternocleidomast-oid muscle or medially through the midline raphe of the strap muscles.

The thyroid vessels are identified and ligated close to the gland. The thyroid lobe is retracted medially and the middle thyroid vein is identified and divided first. The dissection is continued medially, allowing for identification, dissection, and preservation of the recurrent laryngeal nerve. A nonrecurrent laryngeal nerve on the right side may be recognized as it originates high from the vagus nerve. Nonrecurrent laryngeal nerves may be found in proximity to the superior thyroid vessels or the inferior thyroid artery.

The superior pole vessels are then individually transected with a small curved or right angle hemostat. The superior laryn-geal nerve should be identified between the thyroid vessels as it crosses the constrictor muscle and enters the cricothyroid muscle. The surgeon must exercise caution during dissection of this area as the position of the superior nerve in relation to the vascular pedicle can vary.

The fascia that secures the gland (visceral and suspensory lig-ament) is then incised and the dissection is continued inferiorly along the posterior aspect of the gland. The recurrent laryngeal nerve, if not previously located, is identified in the paratracheal groove inferior to the gland and is dissected superiorly. The infe-rior thyroid artery is then identified and its branches are individ-ually ligated as they enter the thyroid gland, with care taken to avoid injury to the recurrent laryngeal nerve. The anatomic rela-tionship between the nerve and the inferior artery is extremely variable. Also, the nerve may divide into several branches at the level of the inferior thyroid artery. All nerve branches should be preserved during the course of the dissection. Careful dissection is continued up to where the nerve enters the larynx.

Eighty percent of superior parathyroid glands are located within 1 cm of the intersection of the recurrent laryngeal nerve and the inferior thyroid artery, usually within the thyroid fas-cia. Approximately 15% are located within the thyroid capsule, and the remainder is in the retropharyngeal or retroesophageal spaces. The location of the inferior parathyroid glands is far more variable. They are usually anterior and lateral to the recurrent laryngeal nerves. Compromise of the blood supply to the parathy-roid glands is the most common cause of hypoparathyroidism in the postoperative period. Careful attention to dissection of the inferior thyroid vessels and their branches is warranted. Often a small portion of thyroid tissue may have to be spared (subto-tal resection) to preserve the vascular pedicle to the parathy-roid tissue. Meticulous dissection of the parathyroid glands and their vascular supply and autotransplantation of devascular-ized parathyroid tissue are important techniques that have con-tributed to a lower incidence of permanent hypoparathyroidism. All parathyroid-like tissue should be inspected and left attached to individual vascular pedicles. Distinguishing between lymph nodes and parathyroid glands may be difficult. Biopsies should be taken and sent for frozen-section diagnosis if there is any confusion. Histologically confirmed parathyroid glands should be autografted to either the sternocleidomastoid muscle or the brachioradialis muscle of the nondominant arm. Dissection of the opposite lobe, when indicated, proceeds similarly to the dissection of the involved lobe.

Clinically palpable adenopathy, especially in a high-risk patient, requires that a neck dissection be performed. Most lymphoareolar tissue in the thyroid compartment and upper mediastinum to the level of the innominate vein is accessible through a collar incision. Occasionally, because of a patient's anatomy, a sternotomy may be necessary to allow for adequate clearance of upper mediastinal and lower peritracheal nodes. During a central compartment lymphadenectomy, all areolar and lymphatic tissue along the larynx and recurrent laryngeal nerves from the level of the hyoid bone area down to the innominate vessels are removed. The dissection is carried laterally to the internal jugular veins and the tissue is resected in continuity with the tumor specimen. Attention must be paid to identifying the inferior parathyroid glands, which may be difficult to separate from the mass of nodal and fibrofatty tissue that extends inferiorly off the lower pole of the thyroid gland. When the removal of lateral lymph node metastases is indicated, we perform a standard modified radical neck dissection, which removes level II, III, IV, and V lymph nodes and spares the sternocleidomastoid muscle, internal jugular vein, and spinal accessory nerve.

Although extrathyroidal extension of thyroid carcinoma into surrounding tissues is rare, it must be clearly delineated so that judicious resection of invaded structures—including resection of laryngeal nerves, tracheal rings, or portions of the larynx can be performed. Local recurrence is a source of significant morbidity and mortality; therefore, complete surgical extirpation should be performed in order to optimize local control. Fortunately, locally invasive thyroid carcinoma can often be resected with a much narrower margin than other carcinomas that arise in tissues surrounding the thyroid.

Adjuvant Therapy

Controversy exists over the use of adjuvant treatment in the management of well-differentiated thyroid carcinoma. The goal of treatment is to maximize disease-free survival. Retrospective studies of patient cohorts followed postoperatively for many years (often more than 10–20 years) suggest that multimodality adjuvant therapy can decrease local recurrence and may improve survival. The mainstay of adjuvant treatment for well-differentiated thyroid carcinoma is radioactive ^{131}I treatment and TSH suppression. The use of therapeutic radioactive ablation of remnant thyroid tissue after thyroidectomy is well established, but criteria for the use of this treatment vary from institution to institution.

Our practice after total thyroidectomy for follicular or papillary carcinoma of the thyroid is to delay thyroid hormone replacement for 4 to 6 weeks to maximize iodine uptake during scanning. Patients can receive short-acting thyroid hormone replacement (liothyronine) to alleviate symptoms of hypothyroidism for up to 2 weeks after surgery, but all thyroid hormone replacement is stopped until after scanning and radioactive thyroid ablation. A tracer dose (2–5 mCi) of radioactive iodine is then administered, and a whole-body scan is performed. This allows scintigraphic staging of disease and may show the presence and extent of metastases that are minimally recognizable with conventional imaging techniques.

At M.D. Anderson, thyroid remnant ablation is recommended for patients with DTC who are 45 years of age or older, for patients whose primary tumor was greater than 1 cm in diameter or was multifocal, and for patients with extrathyroidal disease due to tissue invasion or metastases. Patients found to have radioiodine uptake in the thyroid bed on the initial postoperative thyroid scan often receive an empiric dose of 100 mCi of radioactive iodine. However, patients who have evidence of residual disease or metastases on their initial postoperative thyroid scan receive higher doses of ^{131}I, in the range of 150 to 200 mCi. The standard ablative dose of ^{131}I for patients with PTC whose tumor was less than 3 cm in diameter without extrathyroidal invasion and few or no lymph nodes involved is 29 mCi, which can be administered as an outpatient. Remnant ablation in all other patients with well-differentiated thyroid carcinoma is 100 mCi, which requires overnight hospitalization. Higher doses may be administered if subsequent thyroid scans demonstrate recurrent or persistent disease. Radioiodine ablation has been associated with a decrease in local-regional relapse rates of up to 50% and a reduction in disease-specific mortality.

After surgery and subsequent ^{131}I ablation therapy, all patients receive hormonal replacement treatment (levothyroxine sodium) at a dose of 100 to 200 mg/day. The dose may vary among patients and is adjusted to reach an appropriate level of TSH suppression for a patient as determined on the basis of the individual patient's disease status and the clinicopathologic features of his or her tumor. TSH suppression and radioactive iodine are of no use in the management of Hürthle cell, medullary, and anaplastic thyroid carcinomas because these tumors do not show consistent uptake of radioactive iodine and generally do not contain TSH receptors, making them insensitive to TSH suppression.

The role of external beam radiation therapy (EBRT) as part of the initial adjuvant treatment regimen for DTC is also controversial. However, several retrospective series have reported that local control can be improved with EBRT, specifically in patients with gross disease following surgical resection or patients considered to be at high risk of relapse (>45 years of age, microscopic residual disease, extensive extrathyroidal invasion). EBRT is currently more often used to palliate metastatic or locally advanced disease, such as bone metastases or thyroid bed recurrences. Patients with MTC who are considered to be at high risk for local-regional recurrence because of microscopic residual disease, extraglandular tumor invasion, and lymph node metastasis are also considered for treatment with adjuvant EBRT. Brierley and colleagues have reported a decrease in the local-regional recurrence rate in patients with MTC who have been treated with postoperative adjuvant EBRT.

Overall, cytotoxic chemotherapy has not been very effective in the treatment of thyroid carcinomas. Chemotherapy has limited use in the treatment of DTC, Hürthle cell carcinomas, and MTC. However, chemotherapy, in combination with EBRT and surgery, is more commonly used to treat UTC, for which there is a lack of effective therapies. Small numbers of patients with UTC have had prolonged survival with different regimens of chemotherapeutic agents, most including doxorubicin, and EBRT.

Surveillance

Most recurrences of well-differentiated thyroid carcinoma occur within the first 5 years after initial treatment, especially in the case of FTC, but recurrences can occur several decades later. Patients with papillary thyroid tumors often recur in the neck, whereas patients with follicular carcinomas more commonly recur at distant sites. Of the patients with PTC with recurrence in the neck, 50% die from thyroid cancer. The most common sites of distant metastases for thyroid cancers are the lungs, bone, soft tissues, brain, liver, and adrenal glands. Lung metastases are more common in young patients, whereas bone metastases are more common in older patients.

A coordinated plan of follow-up for thyroid carcinomas must consider the varied presentations possible for recurrent disease. Most patients are seen every 6 months for 1 to 3 years postoperatively and then yearly. Follow-up visits typically include clinical examination and blood tests measuring the serum thyroglobulin, TSH, and free T4 levels. A chest radiograph is usually obtained on an annual basis. Thyroglobulin values normally drop after thyroidectomy or ablation and serve as a sensitive indicator of recurrent or persistent disease. However, it is important to keep in mind that thyroglobulin production is TSH-dependent; therefore, TSH levels can affect the sensitivity of thyroglobulin measurements in detecting disease. Twenty-five percent of patients with differentiated thyroid cancer have anti-thyroglobulin antibodies, which falsely lower measured thyroglobulin levels. When indicated, a repeat ^{131}I scan is done after temporary (4–6 weeks) cessation of hormonal replacement. Subsequent therapeutic doses of radioactive iodine may be administered. Ultrasonography of the neck may be added to the follow-up regimen, especially in patients who had large tumors or nodal disease. This protocol may vary, depending on the risk group of the patient and special circumstances.

Follow-up for medullary carcinoma differs in that no scanning or thyroglobulin measurements are used. Instead, measurement of calcitonin or pentagastrin-stimulated calcitonin levels is used to observe these patients. Similarly, Hürthle cell, anaplastic carcinoma, and lymphoma cannot be followed by thyroid scanning; therefore, patients require regular follow-up physical examination and radiographic or ultrasound studies.

PARATHYROID CARCINOMA

Epidemiology and Etiology

Primary hyperparathyroidism can be caused by parathyroid adenoma, hyperplasia, and carcinoma. Carcinoma of the parathyroid gland is a rare lesion. The incidence of primary hyperparathyroidism is reported to be one per 2,000, and parathyroid carcinoma is reported to be the cause of primary hyperparathyroidism in only 0.1% to 4% of cases.

The incidences of parathyroid carcinoma are equal in men and women and the tumor is usually diagnosed in the fifth decade. No significant clustering within specific ethnic or income groups or unusual geographic clustering has been observed.

The rarity of parathyroid carcinoma has limited the accumulation of data on its natural history and etiologic factors. Parathyroid carcinoma has been described in association with chronic renal failure and dialysis. It has been proposed that malignant transformation of benign hyperplastic parathyroid tissue occurred in those cases. Associations with familial hyperparathyroidism, including multiple endocrine neoplasia syndromes as well as with sporadic hyperparathyroidism have been described. External irradiation has also been associated with parathyroid neoplasms; however, these neoplasms are more frequently adenomas than carcinomas.

Presentation

Patients with parathyroid carcinoma usually present with severe hypercalcemia. The serum calcium level in parathyroid carcinoma averages more than 14 mg/dL, compared with the lower levels of 10 or 11 mg/dL seen in benign cases of hyperparathyroidism. Intact parathyroid hormone levels in patients with parathyroid carcinoma are at least five times the upper normal limit. As a result, renal (60%) and skeletal (50%) involvement is significantly more common in parathyroid carcinoma than in patients with benign primary hyperparathyroidism, in which renal and skeletal disease occur in 48% and 20% of patients, respectively. Metabolic abnormalities associated with parathyroid cancer include renal disorders (e.g., nephrolithiasis, renal dysfunction, and pyelonephritis), skeletal abnormalities (e.g., osteitis fibrosa cystica), and pancreatitis. Polyuria, polydipsia, or nocturia is observed in 40% of patients and fatigue in 30%. Twenty percent of patients diagnosed with parathyroid cancer are asymptomatic compared with up to 50% of patients with benign hyperparathyroidism.

The presence of a palpable neck mass in a patient with hyperparathyroidism should raise the suspicion of parathyroid carcinoma. A palpable neck mass is observed in 40% of patients with parathyroid cancer but is rare for patients with benign hyperparathyroidism.

Palsy of the recurrent laryngeal nerve in a patient with hyperparathyroidism also suggests parathyroid cancer.

Diagnosis

A high index of suspicion of parathyroid carcinoma should be maintained especially for patients with serum calcium levels over 14 mg/dL and a palpable neck mass.

Preoperative fine needle aspiration biopsy is contraindicated for patients with suspected parathyroid cancer because of the risk of local dissemination. Furthermore, distinguishing parathyroid carcinoma from adenoma is extremely difficult even with histologic examination.

Preoperative localization studies are useful in parathyroid carcinoma. Real-time ultrasound of the neck is effective for localization. Signs of gross invasion and marked irregularity of the tumor margins suggest malignancy.

If the diagnosis has not been suspected before surgery, intraoperative recognition of parathyroid carcinoma is essential. Parathyroid cancer should be suspected in the presence of a gray, firm, adherent parathyroid gland; fibrosis is not seen in normal or adenomatous glands. Local invasion of adjacent tissues and cervical lymph node metastasis further support the diagnosis of parathyroid carcinoma.

Unless the tumor is clinically aggressive, it is difficult to differentiate benign from malignant tumors by pathologic assessment. Invasion of surrounding structures, metastases, or recurrent tumors reflect malignancy. The histologic criteria for a diagnosis of parathyroid malignancy are fibrous capsule or fibrous trabeculae, a trabecular or rosette-like cellular architecture, presence of mitotic figures, and capsular or vascular invasion.

Natural History

Parathyroid carcinoma is a slow-growing, persistent, locally recurrent tumor. Most parathyroid carcinomas are clinically functioning, allowing them to be monitored by measuring intact parathyroid hormone levels. The local recurrence rate has been estimated to range from 36% to 80%, with a wide range in the interval between the initial operation and the manifestation of recurrence; mean 2.6 years (1 month to 19 years). Similarly, recurrence after re-operation presents at variable intervals.

In general, recurrent disease should be treated with surgical resection. Although cure after recurrence is rare, some patients will achieve prolonged disease-free intervals by controlling hypercalcemia, which is the major cause of death. Distant metastases tend to occur late, with lung, liver, bone, and pancreas being frequent sites. The overall 10-year survival rate is less than 50%.

The available data on tumor size and lymph node involvement suggest that neither of these factors are important prognostic markers. A multivariate analysis of prognostic factors in parathyroid carcinoma indicated that the extent of surgery when consisting of tumor resection and en-bloc unilateral or bilateral thyroidectomy correlates most strongly with a longer survival and longer relapse-free period. Hence, it is important to maintain a high level of suspicion for parathyroid cancer during surgery.

Treatment

Surgery is the most effective therapy for carcinoma of the parathyroid glands. Because parathyroid cancer has a propensity for local recurrence and rarely metastasizes to regional nodes, tumors should be resected en bloc with care to preserve the integrity of the parathyroid capsule. En bloc resection requires removal of the ipsilateral central neck contents including the thyroid lobe and tracheoesophageal soft tissues and lymphatics. Structures such as the recurrent laryngeal nerve, esophageal wall, or strap muscles should be removed if the tumor adheres to them; this will reduce the risk of tumor spillage and local recurrence.

The increased local control achieved with resection of the recurrent laryngeal nerve outweighs the complication of vocal cord paralysis, which can be managed if clinically necessary, with Teflon injection of the paralyzed cord. A prophylactic neck dissection is not necessary at the time of the initial procedure unless clinically positive lymph node metastases are detected or there is extensive soft tissue invasion.

As previously mentioned, some patients will achieve prolonged disease-free intervals after one or more surgical procedures for recurrent disease in the neck. Similarly, some patients will benefit from resection of lung metastases. Surgical excision of recurrent carcinoma also offers the best control of hypercalcemia, the principal cause of death in these patients.

Localization of metastatic foci is important for treatment of recurrent parathyroid cancer. Thallium chloride scintiscanning and 99m-technetium sestamibi are useful for locating cervical or upper mediastinal recurrence but frequently fail to detect lung metastases. CT is effective for identification and localization of mediastinal or pulmonary metastases. Venous catheterization and selective venous sampling are helpful when noninvasive studies fail to reveal recurrent tumors. More recently, intraoperative use of a handheld gamma detector after preoperative sestamibi injection has been used to aid in the intraoperative localization of recurrent parathyroid cancer.

Recent reports have challenged the common idea that radiation therapy is not effective in the treatment of parathyroid cancer. This idea was based on anecdotal reports of failure of treatment in patients with advanced unresectable disease. A review of more recent data indicated that radiation therapy might play a role as an adjuvant treatment for patients at high risk for local relapse, such as those with residual microscopic disease and tumor spillage during surgery.

There are no effective chemotherapeutic agents that inhibit parathyroid tumor growth or affect the secretion of parathyroid hormone in parathyroid carcinoma. As a result, medical management is used only to control hypercalcemia.

RECOMMENDED READING

Ain KB. Anaplastic thyroid carcinoma: a therapeutic challenge. *Semin Surg Oncol* 1999;16:64.

Anderson BJ, Samaan NA, Vassilopoulou-Sellin R, et al. Parathyroid carcinoma: features and difficulties in diagnosis and management. *Surgery* 1983;94:906.

Austin JR, El-Naggar AK, Goepfert H. Thyroid cancers II: medullary, anaplastic, lymphoma, sarcoma, squamous cell. *Otolaryngol Clin North Am* 1996;29:611.

Brierley JD, Tsang RW. External-beam radiation therapy in the treatment of differentiated thyroid cancer. *Semin Surg Oncol* 1999;16:42.

Chen H, Udelsman R. Papillary thyroid carcinoma: justification for total thyroidectomy and management of lymph node metastases. *Surg Oncol Clin* 1998;7:645.

Chow E, Tsang RW, Brierley JD, Filice S. Parathyroid carcinoma— the Princess Margaret Hospital experience. *Int J Radiat Oncol Biol Phys* 1998;41:569.

Devine RM, Edis AJ, Banks PM. Primary lymphoma of the thyroid: a review of the Mayo Clinic experience through 1978. *World J Surg* 1981;5:33.

Duh QY, Sancho JJ, Greenspan FS, et al. Medullary thyroid carcinoma: the need for early diagnosis and total thyroidectomy. *Arch Surg* 1989;124:1206.

Evans DB, Fleming JB, Lee JE, et al. The surgical treatment of medullary thyroid carcinoma. *Semin Surg Oncol* 1999;16:50.

Gagel RF, Goepfert H, Callender DL. Changing concepts in the pathogenesis and management of thyroid carcinoma. *CA* 1996;46:261.

Gimm O. Thyroid cancer. *Cancer Letters* 2001;2163:143.

Goldman ND, Coniglio JU. Thyroid cancers I: Papillary, follicular, and Hürthle cell. *Otolaryngol Clin North Am* 1996;29:593.

Hay ID, Grant CS, Taylor WF, et al. Ipsilateral lobectomy versus bilateral lobar resection in papillary thyroid carcinoma: a retrospective analysis of surgical outcome using a novel prognostic scoring system. *Surgery* 1987;102:1089.

Hundahl SA, Fleming ID, Fremgen AM, et al. Two hundred eighty-six cases of parathyroid carcinoma treated in the U.S. between 1985–1995: a National Cancer Data Base Report. The American College of Surgeons Commission on Cancer and the American Cancer Society [see comments]. *Cancer* 1999;86:538.

Kebebew E, Clark OH. Differentiated thyroid cancer: complete rational approach. *World J Surg* 2000;24:942.

Kenady DE, McGrath PC, Schwartz RW. Treatment of thyroid malignancies. *Curr Opin Oncol* 1991;3:128.

Krubsack AJ, Wilson SD, Lawson TL, et al. Prospective comparison of radionucleotide, computed tomographic, sonographic, and magnetic resonance localization of parathyroid tumors. *Surgery* 1989;106:639.

Learoyd DL, Messina M, Zedenius J, et al. Molecular genetics of thyroid tumors and surgical decision making. *World J Surg* 2000;24:922.

Maffioli L, Steens J, Pauwels E, et al. Applications of 99mTc-sestamibi in oncology. *Tumori* 1996;82:12.

Mazzaferri EL, Jhiang SM. Long-term impact of initial surgical and medical therapy on papillary and follicular thyroid cancer. *Am J Med* 1994;97:418.

Mazzaferri EL, Robyn J. Postsurgical management of differentiated thyroid carcinoma. *Otolaryngol Clin North Am* 1996;29:637

McLeod MK, Thompson NW. Hürthle cell neoplasm of the thyroid. *Otolaryngol Clin North Am* 1990;23:441.

Merino MJ, Boice JD, Ron E, et al. Thyroid cancer: a lethal endocrine neoplasm. *Ann Intern Med* 1991;115:133.

Moley JF, Wells SA. Compartment-mediated dissection for papillary thyroid cancer. *Langenbeck's Arch Surg* 1999;384:9.

Nel CJC, van Heerden JA, Goellner JR, et al. Anaplastic carcinoma of the thyroid: a clinicopathologic study of 82 cases. *Mayo Clin Proc* 1985;60:51.

Niederle B, Roka R, Schemper M, et al. Surgical treatment of distant metastases in differentiated thyroid cancer: indication and results. *Surgery* 1986;100:1088.

Norton JA. Reoperative parathyroid surgery: indication, intraoperative decision-making and results. *Prog Surg* 1986;18:133.

Obara T, Fujimoto Y. Diagnosis and treatment of patients with parathyroid carcinoma: an update and review. *World J Surg* 1991; 15:738.

Obara T, Okamoto T, Kanbe M, et al. Functioning parathyroid carcinoma: clinicopathologic features and rational treatment. *Semin Surg Oncol* 1997;13:134.

Pasieka JL. Anaplastic cancer, lymphoma, and metastases of the thyroid gland. *Surg Oncol Clin North Am* 1998;7:707.

Ron E, Saftlas AF. Head and neck radiation carcinogenesis: epidemiologic evidence. *Head Neck Surg* 1996;115:403.

Rosen IB, Sutcliffe SB, Gospodarowicz MK, et al. The role of surgery in the management of thyroid lymphoma. *Surgery* 1988;104:1095.

Samaan NA, Schultz PN, Hickey RC, et al. The results of various modalities of treatment of well differentiated thyroid carcinoma: a retrospective review of 1599 patients. *J Clin Endocrinol Metab* 1992;75:714.

Sandelin K, Thompson NW, Bondeson L. Metastatic parathyroid carcinoma: dilemmas in management. *Surgery* 1991;110:978.

Sandelin K, Auer G, Bondeson L, et al. Prognostic factor in parathyroid cancer: a review of 95 cases. *World J Surg* 1992;16:724.

Shaha AR. Management of the neck in thyroid cancer. *Otolaryngol Clin North Am* 1998;31:823.

Sherman SI. Adjuvant therapy and long-term management of differentiated thyroid carcinoma. *Semin Surg Oncol* 1999;16:30.

Sherman SI. Clinicopathologic staging of differentiated thyroid carcinoma. In: Rose B, ed. *UpToDate in medicine.* CD-ROM. Wellesley, MA: UpToDate, 1997.

Sherman SI. Management of differentiated thyroid carcinoma: an overview. In: Rose B, ed. *UpToDate in medicine.* CD-ROM. Wellesley, MA: UpToDate, 1997.

Sherman SI. Radioiodide treatment of differentiated thyroid cancer. In: Rose B, ed. *UpToDate in medicine.* CD-ROM. Wellesley, MA: UpToDate, 1997.

Sherman SI. Surgery for differentiated thyroid carcinoma. In: Rose B, ed. *UpToDate in medicine.* CD-ROM. Wellesley, MA: UpToDate, 1996.

Sherman SI. Toward a standard clinicopathologic staging approach for differentiated thyroid carcinoma. *Semin Surg Oncol* 1999;16:12.

Shortell CK, Andrus CH. Phillips CE, et al. Carcinoma of the parathyroid gland: a 30-year experience. *Surgery* 1991;110:704.

Thomas CG. Role of thyroid-stimulating hormone suppression in the management of thyroid cancer. *Semin Surg Oncol* 1991;7:115.

Vassilopoulou-Sellin R. Management of papillary thyroid cancer. *Oncology* 1995;145.

Woolam GL. Cancer statistics, 2000. *CA* 2000;50:7.

Wynne AG, van Heerden JA, Carney JA, et al. Parathyroid carcinoma: clinical and pathological features in 43 patients. *Medicine* 1992;71:197.

Hematologic Malignancies and Splenic Tumors

Wayne A.I. Frederick, Jorge A. Romaguera,
James A. Reilly, Jr., and Ana M. Grau

Leukemia and lymphoma account for 6% to 8% of adult cancers and approximately 8% of the deaths from malignancy in the United States. In children younger than 15 years, leukemias are the most common malignancies, with non-Hodgkin's lymphoma (NHL) fourth in frequency. Acute leukemias are the leading cause of cancer deaths in patients younger than 35 years.

Leukemia and lymphoma patients are usually referred to a surgeon with a specific request: diagnostic biopsy, vascular access, and therapeutic splenectomy. Surgeons must be familiar with this group of disorders, both to perform the operation appropriately and to know the procedure's probability of success and risks. At times a major procedure is unlikely to achieve the desired result, or the patient's limited life expectancy makes such an operation unwise.

THE LEUKEMIAS

The chronic proliferative diseases appear to be a spectrum of clonal hematopoietic stem cell disorders ranging in increasing severity from polycythemia vera and essential thrombocythemia to myelogenous metaplasia to chronic myelogenous leukemia (CML). Leukemia ultimately develops in a few patients with polycythemia vera and essential thrombocythemia and a larger percentage of patients with myelogenous metaplasia.

Polycythemia Vera and Essential Thrombocythemia

Polycythemia vera is associated with an autonomous expansion of the red blood cell mass and volume with a variable effect on white blood cells (WBCs) and platelets. The most accepted etiologic mechanism involves the existence of a clone with an abnormally high sensitivity to erythropoietin. Essential thrombocythemia is characterized by an increase in the megakaryocyte lineage, with a greatly increased platelet count and a variable effect on erythrocytes and WBCs. In both diseases there is an increased risk of thrombosis and, paradoxically, of hemorrhage. Three-fourths of patients with polycythemia vera have palpable splenomegaly, and about half have hepatic enlargement. Phlebotomy, low-dose chemotherapy, or a combination of these modalities is the primary treatment for patients with polycythemia vera and essential thrombocythemia. The goal is to obtain a hematocrit of 45% or less. Because of the risk of hemorrhage, any operation should be avoided in these patients until the polycythemia is under control. Rapid phlebotomy to a normal hematocrit and fluid replacement should be performed before emergency surgery. Plateletpheresis has been used to control thrombocytosis.

Although splenectomy has little or no role in the treatment of most patients with polycythemia vera or essential thrombocythemia, condition similar to myelogenous metaplasia develops in a few patients who then require splenectomy. The operative risks are greater and the survival is poorer in this group than in patients with myelogenous metaplasia. Patients with polycythemia vera and essential thrombocythemia should be treated with aggressive nonoperative therapy and offered splenectomy only when pain, anemia, and thrombocytopenia are refractory to other treatment. Splenectomy does not increase the survival rate, but it may improve the quality of life.

Myelogenous Metaplasia

Myelogenous metaplasia is characterized by fibrosis of the bone marrow and extramedullary hematopoiesis, chiefly in the spleen, liver, and lymph nodes. Fibrosis is polyclonal in nature and is thought to be a reactive process to growth factor release from the clonal cells. As the spleen enlarges, the hematopoietic function it serves may be overwhelmed by destructive hypersplenism (excessive destruction of one or more of the blood components, usually by an autoimmune mechanism).

Although some patients are asymptomatic, most present with fatigue, anorexia, and weight loss, or symptomatic splenomegaly. Leukocytosis and thrombocytosis may be present; other hematologic abnormalities such as diminished WBC and platelet counts may result from passive splenic sequestration or active destruction. Active splenic destruction may be humorally mediated (related to specific antibody recognition) or cell mediated (probably by activated macrophages). Peripheral blood smears often demonstrate large platelets, nucleated red cells, anisocytosis, and immature myelogenous elements. The diagnosis is made by bone marrow biopsy. In approximately 5% of cases, myelogenous metaplasia will progress to CML or acute myeloblastic leukemia.

Initial management may include transfusions, steroids, androgens, cytotoxic chemotherapy, and splenic irradiation. If these measures are not effective in treating the complications of hypersplenism, a splenectomy may be indicated. At the University of Texas M.D. Anderson Cancer Center, patients who have myelogenous metaplasia with myelofibrosis are advised to undergo splenectomy under the following conditions: (a) for severe anemia due to hypersplenism when medical management is unsuccessful; (b) for chronically symptomatic splenomegaly; or (c) for the development of worsening congestive heart failure caused by a shunt effect through the spleen. Splenectomy for portal hypertension secondary to increased portal flow associated with splenomegaly has also been reported. Because splenectomy may inadvertently preclude the possibility of performing a splenorenal shunt, it is critical to eliminate hepatic portal hypertension as the cause of the splenomegaly.

Adequate bone marrow activity must be verified before splenectomy is contemplated. If the spleen is the major site of hematopoiesis, splenectomy may result in severe pancytopenia. A bone marrow biopsy and nuclear medicine bone marrow scan may define the hematopoietic productivity of the marrow cavity. Full coagulation studies should be performed and occult disseminated intravascular coagulation should be controlled before surgery.

Splenectomy does not prolong survival but may improve the quality of life. The response rate for anemia varies from 75% to 95% following splenectomy. The morbidity of splenectomy is 35% to 75%, and the mortality rate is 5% to 18%. Low-dose radiation to the spleen may be used in poor candidates for surgery.

Chronic Myelogenous Leukemia

CML, also known as chronic granulocytic leukemia, involves a clonal proliferation of myelogenous stem cells. Approximately 90% of patients will have a translocation of chromosomes 9 and 22; this translocation is called the *Philadelphia chromosome*. The Philadelphia chromosome may be observed clinically to help assess response to therapy.

CML has both a chronic benign phase and a phase of acute blastic transformation. Most patients present with symptoms of the chronic phase, which include fatigue, weakness, night sweats, low-grade fever, and abdominal pain. Splenomegaly may be an isolated finding during physical examination. The WBC and platelet count may be increased; however, the platelets may not function normally. Hypersplenism may result in anemia or thrombocytopenia. Patients with the chronic phase of CML should be evaluated every 3 to 6 months. The median duration of the chronic phase is about 45 months, but some patients may live up to 20 years with this condition. CML will progress from the chronic benign phase to the acute leukemic transformation phase in approximately 80% of patients.

Progressive fatigue, high fevers, increasingly symptomatic splenomegaly, anemia, thrombocytopenia, basophilia, and bone or joint pain may herald the acute or accelerated stage of CML. In addition to the Philadelphia chromosome, other deletions and translocations may be detected. The WBC count may markedly increase and may not be readily controlled by medical means. Increased splenic destruction of blood components may be manifested by more frequent infections or bleeding episodes. Average survival is approximately 6 months, and during this period the disease may become resistant to chemotherapy. Blast crisis is heralded by large numbers of these immature cells in the circulation, with a decrease in other cellular components; this is usually a preterminal event.

Traditional treatment of CML included conventional chemotherapy with hydroxyurea or busulfan. These agents can achieve hematologic remissions, but no significant reduction of Philadelphia chromosome cells has been observed. Interferon alfa (IFN alfa) can achieve hematologic as well as cytogenetic remissions in a significant number of patients and prolong survival in patients who have shown cytogenetic response. Allogenic bone marrow transplant may be curative, but only a limited number of patients qualify for it.

Splenectomy is generally used as palliation for either painful splenomegaly or refractory anemia. Symptoms due to splenomegaly will likely be improved by splenectomy, but the response is variable when splenectomy is performed to correct dyscrasias. Removal of an enlarged spleen before bone marrow transplantation has failed to improve survival or to decrease the relapse frequency. In these patients, though, splenectomy may eliminate a focus of disease or decrease transfusion requirements. Prospective randomized trials will help define the role of splenectomy in the enhancement of bone marrow engraftment. For patients with CML in whom disease becomes resistant to IFN alfa, a splenectomy may improve response to this therapy. Splenectomy does not delay blast transformation, and its effect on survival is controversial. A recent analysis of the M.D. Anderson experience with splenectomy in patients in the accelerated or blastic phase of the disease has shown that although the survival period in these patients may be limited, splenectomy, if indicated, can be performed safely in this phase of the disease and thrombocytopenia can be reliably reversed, minimizing transfusion requirements.

Chronic Lymphocytic Leukemia

Chronic lymphocytic leukemia (CLL) is the most common leukemia in the Western Hemisphere. It is typified by an accumulation of long-lived, mature-appearing but functionally inactive B cells. The median age of onset is in the seventh decade, and the incidence continues to increase beyond that age.

CLL patients may present with enlarged, painless lymph nodes; weakness; weight loss; and anorexia. As the disease progresses, more pronounced lymphadenopathy and splenomegaly may develop. There may be a decrease in red blood cell count due to either bone marrow infiltration with leukemic cells or a Coombs-positive hemolytic anemia. A second malignancy will develop in approximately 20% of patients, most commonly lung cancer, melanoma, or sarcoma. CLL may have either an indolent or an aggressive course, with patient survival ranging from 1 to 20 years. Patients with CLL have a progressive loss of immune function, and infection is the most common cause of death.

Previously, treatment was withheld in the early stages until signs of progression occurred. Currently, at M.D. Anderson, treatment is not generally started in the Rai stage 0 patients (lymphocytosis only), but chemotherapy is used to treat other early stage patients (Rai stage I or II) with poor prognostic signs and all patients with Rai stage III or IV disease (Table 17-1). Fludarabine is used in conjunction with granulocyte-macrophage colony-stimulating factor. Splenectomy may be recommended for patients who are refractory to fludarabine or with symptomatic splenomegaly and for patients with hypersplenism. Experience at M.D. Anderson has shown that splenectomy can provide an excellent hematologic response in patients with either isolated anemia or thrombocytopenia, but this response is relatively poor in patients presenting with both disorders, suggesting that an adequate hematopoietic reserve is required for a significant response. In addition, splenectomy significantly improves survival in selected subgroups of patients with advanced stage CLL when compared with conventional chemotherapy. These subgroups include patients with CLL and hemoglobin levels less than or equal to 10 g/dL or a platelet count less than or equal to 50×10^9L.

Table 17-1.   Rai staging of chronic lymphocytic leukemia

Stage	Criteria
0	Lymphocytosis (WBCs >15,000/mL with >40% lymphocytes in the bone marrow)
I	Lymphocytosis with lymphadenopathy
II	Lymphocytosis with enlarged liver or spleen (lymphadenopathy not necessarily present)
III	Lymphocytosis with anemia. Anemia may be due to hemolysis or to decreased production (lymphadenopathy or hepatosplenomegaly need not be present)
IV	Lymphocytosis with thrombocytopenia (platelet count <100,000/μL) anemia, and lymphadenopathy

WBC, white blood cell.

Hairy Cell Leukemia

Hairy cell leukemia (HCL) is a monoclonal lymphoproliferative disorder of mature B cells. It comprises only 2% to 5% of all leukemias, and there is a 3:1 male predominance. The pathognomonic hairy cells are named for their cytoplasmic projections. These cells may be found in both the bone marrow and the peripheral circulation.

Patients with HCL may complain of weakness and fatigue. Splenomegaly is almost universally present. Approximately 10% of patients with HCL will have such mild symptoms that they never require treatment. Most patients will require therapy for neutropenia, splenomegaly, hypersplenism, or bone marrow failure. Infection related to neutropenia is the most common cause of death.

Early efforts to use chemotherapy to treat HCL were unsuccessful because the degree of associated myelosuppression was not tolerable. Splenectomy became the treatment of choice and was associated with increased survival. Since that time, more effective chemotherapeutic agents have become available. At M.D. Anderson, splenectomy is not used in the routine treatment of patients with HCL. Instead, they are treated with IFN alfa, deoxycoformycin, or chlorodeoxyadenosine. The overall response rate to IFN alfa is between 80% and 90%. If relapse occurs, chlorodeoxyadenosine is usually effective in regaining control of the disease. The few patients who relapse after chlorodeoxyadenosine treatment can achieve second remissions with retreatment. Splenectomy may be considered in the rare cases of pure splenic form of the disease.

Acute Lymphocytic and Myelogenous Leukemia

Except in cases of splenic rupture, splenectomy has no role in the treatment of patients with acute lymphocytic or acute myelogenous leukemia during induction chemotherapy or during relapse. In rare cases, patients in complete remission require splenectomy because of persistent fungal granulomas of the spleen.

Splenic Rupture in Leukemia

Splenic rupture is a rare event in leukemic patients and is almost always associated with some form of trauma. There is no increased risk with any particular type of leukemia, but patients with splenomegaly may be more susceptible to splenic trauma. The reported incidence of rupture from four series was 0.72%. Leukemic patients comprise only 3.5% of those with spontaneous splenic rupture.

Signs and symptoms include abdominal tenderness and rigidity, shifting dullness, and tachycardia. The chest radiograph may demonstrate an elevated hemidiaphragm or a pleural effusion. A high index of suspicion is necessary in evaluating patients with splenomegaly and abdominal pain because the precipitating event may have been so minor as to not be remembered.

Survival rates vary with the rapidity of diagnosis and of performance of splenectomy. Patients who survive splenectomy following rupture have a life expectancy similar to that of other patients with the same type of leukemia.

THE LYMPHOMAS

Hodgkin's Disease

The prognosis of patients with Hodgkin's disease (HD) has improved dramatically over the past 20 years. This advancement is due to increased knowledge of the biology of the disease and more effective use of radiation therapy and multiagent chemotherapy. The role of staging laparotomy continues to evolve as nonoperative staging becomes increasingly accurate and as subsets of patients are identified who are unlikely to benefit from the information laparotomy provides.

HD is characterized by the presence of multinucleated Reed-Sternberg (RS) cells or one of their variants. As opposed to NHL, in which a monoclonal population of malignant lymphocytes usually predominates, in HD the malignant cells are a minority population outnumbered by inflammatory cells.

Patients with HD typically present with nontender lymphadenopathy. The cervical nodes are most commonly involved; other regions, which include the axillary, inguinal, mediastinal, and retroperitoneal nodes are less frequently affected at presentation. The presence or absence of B symptoms should be elucidated from the patient's history. B symptoms include any one of the following: unexplained fever with temperature over 38°C, night sweats significant enough to require changing bed clothes, or weight loss of more than 10% of body weight over 6 months. Although classic for HD, the Pel-Ebstein fever, with progressively shortening intervals between fevers, is a relatively rare phenomenon.

The physical examination should include an evaluation of all lymph node–bearing areas, including Waldeyer's tonsillar ring, and palpation for liver or splenic enlargement. Initial workup should include a complete blood cell count with differential count, liver function tests, and a chest radiograph. A bone marrow biopsy is useful to determine the extent of the disease. Excisional biopsy of the largest node that is likely to provide the diagnosis should be performed. Careful selection of the biopsy site is important because some areas, particularly the inguinal region, frequently contain nondiagnostic inflammatory nodes.

Other clinical staging tools include computed tomography (CT), nuclear medicine scans, and bipedal lymphangiography. CT is used to detect mediastinal and abdominal lymphatic enlargement; however, nodes containing HD often are not enlarged. Gallium scans have been useful in detecting residual disease. Bipedal lymphangiography may detect changes in femoral, inguinal, external iliac, and retroperitoneal nodes. Use of lymphangiography has been questioned in terms of the cost-effectiveness. This procedure can identify lymphatic enlargement as well as changes in the architecture of normal-sized nodes caused by neoplastic involvement.

The prognosis of patients with HD depends on the histologic subtype and stage of disease at presentation. The Rye modification of the Lukes-Butler classification of HD identifies four histologic subtypes: lymphocyte predominant, nodular sclerosis, mixed cellularity, and lymphocyte depleted. These subtypes are determined by the specific variant of RS cell, the ratio of these cells to the normal population, and the degree of sclerosis.

The Ann Arbor staging system (Table 17-2) is used for staging HD based on the extent of disease. Clinical staging includes all data from the history and physical examination and nonoperative diagnostic studies. Pathologic staging includes additional information obtained from a staging laparotomy. The Ann Arbor stages are subclassified to reflect lymphatic disease and involvement of extranodal areas designated by *E,* for involvement of an extralymphatic site (i.e., stomach or small intestine), or *S,* for splenic involvement. Disease is further subclassified according to the presence or absence of systemic symptoms of the disease.

Increasing knowledge of the effect of patient characteristics, histologic subtype, and stage of disease have allowed more individualized treatment of patients, with dramatic improvements in survival. Staging laparotomy was first introduced to define

Table 17-2. Ann Arbor staging system for Hodgkin's disease

Stage	Criteria
I	Involvement of a single lymph node region (I) or a single extralymphatic organ or site (IE)
II	Involvement of two or more lymph node regions on the same side of the diaphragm (II) or of an extralymphatic organ and its adjoining lymph node site (IIE)
III	Involvement of lymph node sites on both sides of the diaphragm (III) or localized involvement of an extra-lymphatic site (IIIE), spleen (IIIS), or both (IIISE)
IV	Diffuse or disseminated involvement of one or more extralymphatic organs with or without associated lymph node involvement
A	Asymptomatic
B	Fever, night sweats, or weight loss of more than 10%

disease extent in all presentations of HD. Subsequently, investigators performed staging by laparotomy to determine which patients had early stage disease that could be treated by local irradiation and which had extensive disease requiring systemic therapy. Previously, up to 40% of patients who underwent staging laparotomy had a change in their clinical stage. Both improvements in the accuracy of radiologic diagnostic procedures and more intensive use of chemotherapeutic and radiation treatments earlier in the course of the disease have decreased the number of patients who require staging laparotomy.

Currently at M.D. Anderson, nonoperative staging and prognostic factors are used to guide therapy in almost all the patients. Patients who require chemotherapy with or without radiation therapy because of extensive disease or poor prognostic factors do not benefit from the additional information gained from a staging laparotomy. Most centers have eliminated staging laparotomy in pediatric patients with HD. This approach is supported by failure of long-term follow-up to show a significant difference in survival between clinical and surgical staging.

Components of a Staging Laparotomy

For staging laparotomy of HD, the abdomen is entered through a midline incision from the xiphoid process to below the umbilicus. A thorough exploration is performed to identify palpable abnormalities. This includes bimanual palpation of the liver, examination of the bowel and mesentery, and exploration of the major nodal groups. Lymph nodes containing disease are often normal in size. The areas most likely to contain disease include the spleen and the splenic, celiac, and portal lymph nodes.

Splenectomy and liver biopsies are performed early in the procedure so that ample time is available to ensure hemostasis. The spleen should routinely be removed because it may contain nonpalpable disease. In children, some surgeons advocate performing a partial splenectomy to prevent a lifetime risk of asplenic sepsis. Splenic nodes, along with the distal 3 cm of the splenic artery and vein, should be removed in continuity with the spleen. The ends of the splenic vessels are marked with titanium clips to guide future radiation therapy if it becomes necessary.

A wedge biopsy specimen is obtained from one or both lobes of the liver, and a deeper biopsy with a Tru-cut core needle is done on both lobes. Additional wedge biopsies should be performed on any grossly abnormal areas of the liver.

As each nodal group is dissected, it is sent as a separate specimen in sterile saline to the pathologist, and the area is marked with titanium clips. The gastrohepatic ligament is incised, and lymph nodes along the hepatic artery leading to the celiac axis are removed. The sentinel node at the junction of the portal vein and the duodenum, along with any other nodes along the porta hepatis, are excised. The transverse colon is retracted superiorly, and the small bowel is reflected to the patient's right to visualize the aorta. The retroperitoneum is incised over the aorta from the left renal vein down to the iliac bifurcation. The nodes between the aorta and the inferior mesenteric vein are excised. Nodes along the iliac vessels and within the mesentery seldom contain disease, but they should be sampled and submitted for review. Any lymph nodes that appeared abnormal on the lymphangiogram should also be removed.

If a bone marrow biopsy specimen has not been obtained preoperatively, one should be obtained from the iliac crest while the patient is under general anesthesia. Oophoropexy was once routinely performed in females of reproductive age, but currently its use is limited to patients with suspected iliac nodal involvement. Some surgeons recommend performing appendectomy during the staging procedure.

The morbidity rate is generally less than 10%, and deaths related to staging laparotomy are rare. Complications include wound problems, atelectasis, pneumonia, pulmonary embolus, and infection. Any complications that delay the initiation of needed systemic therapy or radiation therapy are potentially serious. Long-term complications include small-bowel adhesions, asplenic sepsis, and development of secondary leukemia.

Laparoscopic staging of lymphoma is currently being explored as a modality in the treatment of these patients. Case reports and small series of lymphoma patients staged laparoscopically have been reported in the literature. The indications have been the same as those for open staging, and absolute contraindications are portal hypertension and uncorrectable coagulopathy. The components of laparoscopic staging include percutaneous and wedge liver biopsies, lymph node biopsies, and splenectomy. Because the spleen needs to be removed intact to allow complete pathologic evaluation, a 6- to 8-cm midline incision is made to allow removal of the spleen. This midline incision is then used to complete the lymph node dissection under direct vision. Conversion to open procedure has most frequently been secondary to hemorrhage during splenectomy and varies from 0% to 20%. Diagnostic accuracy has been reported to be close to 90%. Laparoscopic staging of lymphoma may result in a shorter hospital stay and recovery time, but the accuracy and morbidity of this technique cannot be known until more experience is available.

Non-Hodgkin's Lymphoma

Patients in the United States with NHL characteristically have a monoclonal proliferation of lymphocytes, with 80% of cases being of B-cell derivation and the remainder originating from T cells. The diagnosis of various subsets of B-cell NHL depends on the identification of histopathologic markers using monoclonal antibodies and on cellular morphology; criteria assessed are a diffuse versus follicular (nodular) pattern of lymph node involvement, small versus large cell type, and cleaved versus noncleaved nuclear morphology. With this information, the lymphoma can be categorized according to the Working Formulation, which is a modification of the Lukes and Collins schema. Although an in-depth discussion of this classification system is beyond the scope of this chapter, the Working Formulation has simplified our understanding of the behaviors of these subtypes by placing them into one of three categories, depending on whether patients have a low, intermediate, or high risk of death due to the disease. The T-cell NHLs are much more difficult to identify precisely and to place into prognostic groups. More recently, the proposed

European-American classification of lymphoid neoplasms uses morphology, phenotype, and cytogenetics to classify these disorders. The clinical relevance of this classification is under study, but it might offer additional information to the Working Formulation.

Most patients with NHL present with superficial adenopathy, most commonly in the cervical lymph nodes. These nodes are generally enlarged and not tender. The Ann Arbor system (Table 17-2) is used to stage these patients, but it is less helpful in NHL than in HD because more than half of NHL patients present with stage III or IV disease and approximately 20% present with B symptoms. Patients with NHL also are more likely to have hematogenous spread versus lymphatic spread as seen in patients with HD.

Because NHLs do not spread in the orderly manner that HD does, the surgeon is generally asked to perform a diagnostic biopsy, to establish vascular access for chemotherapy, or to treat complications of therapy. Staging laparotomy is not indicated in these patients. Splenectomy is necessary, although rarely, for hypersplenism, massive splenomegaly, or a persistent splenic focus of disease, usually in those with low-grade lymphomas. Although primary splenic lymphoma is unusual, splenectomy may be beneficial for patients with isolated splenic disease. This diagnosis is often made only after splenectomy is performed for hypersplenism or splenomegaly. If the lymphoma is localized to the spleen, the prognosis is similar to that of other stage I patients.

Diagnostic Biopsy for Lymphoma

When lymphoma is suspected, proper planning and execution of the biopsy are crucial to enable the pathologist to make a diagnosis. Because preservation of the architecture aids in histologic diagnosis, efforts should be made to avoid traction or cautery. The largest node found on physical examination should be biopsied. If several nodal areas are enlarged, biopsy of the cervical area is preferred to biopsy of an axillary node, which in turn is superior to biopsy of nodes from the inguinal region. In suspected extranodal disease or in the case of matted nodes, it is important to excise as generous an amount of tissue as possible. Communication with the pathologist is important to guarantee that adequate tissue is sent and that it is delivered in an acceptable fashion. In general, the specimen is sent fresh, is sent in saline, or is wrapped in a saline-soaked sponge. It is important that the specimen be sent directly to the pathologist and that there is an indication that the diagnosis of lymphoma is suspected. Needle biopsies rarely provide an adequate amount of tissue, although they may be helpful in ruling out a carcinoma or sarcoma or in suspected relapse of lymphoma when a tissue diagnosis is needed before treatment.

MISCELLANEOUS SPLENIC TUMORS

Splenic Cysts

A splenic cyst may be confused with a neoplastic process when detected as a palpable abnormality or an unexpected radiologic finding. Patients often present with vague symptoms, possibly due to cyst enlargement. Although parasitic cysts are extremely rare in the United States, they are more common outside this country. Parasitic cysts are most commonly due to an echinococcal infection. Nonparasitic cysts comprise 75% of splenic cysts in the United States and are classified as primary if they have a true cellular lining or secondary if they lack this layer. Primary splenic cysts may be congenital, due to an embryologic remnant, or neoplastic cyst. The neoplastic cysts include epidermoid cysts, dermoid cysts, lymphangiomas, and cavernous hemangiomas. Secondary cysts are the more common type of nonparasitic cyst and are thought to be the result of splenic injury and resultant hematoma.

Splenic cysts rarely require treatment unless they become infected, hemorrhage, or perforate. Treatment may consist of a partial or total splenectomy; marsupialization or drainage procedures should be avoided.

Inflammatory Pseudotumor

Inflammatory pseudotumor, also known as plasma cell granuloma, has histologic features of inflammation and mesenchymal repair. Such masses can be found in various locations in the body, including the respiratory system, gastrointestinal tract, orbit, and lymph nodes. When a pseudotumor is detected in the spleen, it may be mistaken for lymphoma. Pseudotumors are thought to occur at sites of previous trauma or infection. Unfortunately, the definitive diagnosis can be made only after excision. Immunohistochemical stains and flow cytometry studies of the specimen may be useful to rule out a lymphoproliferative disorder.

Nonlymphoid Tumors

The spleen is involved with various benign and malignant nonlymphoid tumors. Benign vascular tumors include hemangioma, lymphangioma, and hemangioendothelioma. Lipoma and angiomyolipoma are also encountered. Angiosarcoma of the spleen confers a poor prognosis; this tumor has been associated with exposure to thorium dioxide, vinyl chloride, and arsenic. Kaposi's sarcoma may be found as an isolated process in the spleen. Other splenic sarcomas, including malignant fibrous histiocytoma, fibrosarcoma, and leiomyosarcoma, are extremely rare.

Splenic Metastasis

Considering the large percentage of the total blood flow that supplies the spleen, it is a surprisingly rare site for metastasis. In autopsy series of cancer patients, the finding of metastasis involving the spleen ranges from 1.6% to 30%. Splenic metastasis is rarely a clinically relevant problem. Melanoma, breast, and lung cancer are the most frequently detected metastases. Splenomegaly is an unusual finding with solitary metastasis. Several small series have reported the use of splenectomy for an isolated splenic metastasis. Resection with curative intent is rarely possible with splenic metastasis, but splenectomy may be necessary for complications such as perforation, splenic vein thrombosis, and growth into adjacent viscera.

SPLENECTOMY

Splenectomy for Hypersplenism

Anemia, neutropenia, and thrombocytopenia may occur for a number of reasons in patients with hematologic malignancies. Because only patients with excessive destruction of a blood component will benefit from a splenectomy, a careful workup should be done to identify the etiology of the process. Patients with hypersplenism may present with a normal-sized spleen, and others may have massive splenomegaly without hypersplenism.

Infusion of the patient's or normal donor platelets tagged with [111]indium is helpful in determining whether the spleen is the site of destruction. Patients with an acquired hemolytic anemia generally have a positive Coombs' test, and the detection of the warm antibody is a good indication that splenectomy will be beneficial. Although chromium-labeled red blood cell scans may be useful in demonstrating decreases in red blood cell survival, they are not as helpful in identifying the site of sequestration. In cases of suspected splenic sequestration, a bone marrow biopsy is important to determine whether adequate precursor cells are available or whether the patient depends on the hematopoietic activity of the spleen.

Splenectomy in patients with CML has been associated with severe bleeding problems. These may be related to impaired clot formation caused by proteases and serases produced by granulocytes. Patients with CML and severe leukocytosis should receive chemotherapy in an attempt to decrease the WBC count to approximately 20,000 cells/mL. Experience at M.D. Anderson suggests that splenectomy is best avoided in patients with CML in whom WBC counts cannot be controlled with chemotherapy. Splenectomy should also be avoided in patients with CML who have had splenic irradiation.

Bleeding and infection are the greatest perioperative risks. Qualitative platelet function should be evaluated rather than relying on a platelet count. The template bleeding time is currently the most widely available laboratory value for identifying adequacy of platelet function. The patient's current and recent medications should be carefully reviewed to identify any drugs that may impair coagulation. Because of potential bleeding problems associated with certain antibiotics, prophylactic coverage must be carefully chosen to avoid increasing the risk of hemorrhage.

Although splenectomy may be performed through either a midline or a subcostal approach, the midline incision is preferred when coagulation defects, thrombocytopenia, or splenomegaly is present. After the splenic pedicle is clamped, thrombocytopenic patients are transfused with fresh single-donor platelets to achieve a platelet count of more than 60,000 cells/mL. Careful hemostasis at the conclusion of the procedure is mandatory. Postoperatively, patients should be monitored closely during the first 48 hours for signs of bleeding. A blood cell count with differential and platelet counts should be obtained every 6 hours for the first 24 hours after the operation. Decreasing platelet and blood counts, despite adequate replacement, suggest an ongoing bleeding process.

Splenectomy for the Massively Enlarged Spleen

Indications for splenectomy in patients with massively enlarged spleens include debilitating symptoms of splenomegaly, excessive destruction of blood components, and concerns of possible splenic rupture. These patients often complain of chronic severe upper abdominal and back pain, impaired respiration, and early satiety. Hypersplenism may be present. Depending on the size of the spleen and the body habitus, the patient may be judged to be at increased risk of splenic trauma.

Preoperatively, it is important to check quantitative and qualitative platelet function values and coagulation studies because hemorrhage is the major complication of splenectomy in this group. Portal venous contrast studies should be performed in patients with possible portal hypertension. If the splenic vein is thrombosed, splenectomy is appropriate, but otherwise it may deprive a patient with portal hypertension of the option of a splenorenal shunt.

Adequate blood products must be available preoperatively. The blood of these patients may be difficult to crossmatch because of numerous past transfusions, and fresh single-donor platelets may be required. Patients should undergo routine bowel preparation, and prophylactic antibiotics should be given.

A midline, rather than subcostal, incision is preferred because the rectus muscles are not severed, which limits bleeding. With increasing size, the spleen becomes more of a midline structure and lends itself to this approach. Before mobilization of the spleen, its vessels should be isolated. The gastrocolic omentum is divided, the lesser sac is entered, and the splenic artery is identified along the posterior-superior surface of the pancreas. The artery is ligated but left intact. The splenic vein is not disturbed yet. The spleen may decrease 20% to 30% in size at this point and allow platelet transfusion without consumption. The splenic flexure of the colon is mobilized, the splenic ligaments are divided, and the spleen is delivered from the splenic fossa. The normally avascular splenic ligaments often contain small vessels in the presence of hematologic malignancies. Dense adhesions between the spleen and the diaphragm may complicate mobilization, and when dissection is particularly difficult, it is better to resect part of the diaphragm with the spleen than to risk hypertrophy of splenic remnants. Such adhesions are formed in areas of splenic infarction and are the most frequent sites of postoperative bleeding in this group of patients.

After the spleen is mobilized, the artery and vein are suture ligated and divided. Liver biopsy may be indicated if involvement by lymphoma is suspected. If an injury to the pancreatic tail is recognized, it should be repaired and drained appropriately. Achieving hemostasis in the splenic bed is crucial and may require suture ligation, cautery, platelet transfusions, and thrombostatic agents. Drains do not reliably warn of postoperative hemorrhage or prevent infection, and except in cases of pancreatic injury, they are not routinely used. Postoperatively, patients should be closely monitored for signs of bleeding or infection.

Laparoscopic Splenectomy

Laparoscopic splenectomy has been used safely in patients with benign hematologic conditions. Recently there has been increasing implementation of this surgical method in splenomegaly in patients with malignant hematologic diseases. The advantages appear to be a quicker recovery and resultant decreased healthcare costs. Prospective randomized trials are required to confirm these observations. To allow adequate pathologic examination of the specimen, the spleen needs to be removed intact through a small incision.

Prophylaxis for Asplenic Sepsis

Patients with hematologic malignancies who undergo splenectomy are at greater risk for asplenic sepsis than are those who have the procedure for other indications. Some patients with hematologic malignancy, especially those with CML and CLL, are at increased risk for sepsis even before splenectomy. The risk of overwhelming postsplenectomy infection (OPSI) is greatest for children. The expected death rate from OPSI in children is one in every 300 to 350 patient-years, and in adults, one in every 800 to 1,000 patient-years. For all patients, the risk is greatest for the first few years following splenectomy, but deaths attributed to OPSI have occurred 30 or more years after splenectomy.

Following splenectomy, there is loss of the opsonins, tuftsin and properdin, a decrease in immunoglobulin M production, impaired phagocytosis, and altered cellular immunity. Poorly opsonized bacteria are best cleared by the spleen, and following the spleen's removal patients are particularly susceptible to the encapsulated bacteria.

Vaccination can decrease the risk of postsplenectomy pneumococcal infection. The 23-valent form of the pneumococcal vaccine should be used. The vaccine is most effective when given several weeks preoperatively. Nevertheless, despite the diminished immunity obtained if the vaccine is given after splenectomy, adequate protection is still achieved in most patients. In patients who are not immunized preoperatively there is no benefit from delaying the immunization for several weeks after surgery, so these patients should be vaccinated without delay. Leukemic patients may not be able to develop antibodies in response to pneumococcal vaccine, but it may still be worthwhile to vaccinate this group. Booster immunizations with the pneumococcal vaccine have no proven benefit, although reimmunization at 3 to 5 years may be required if a decrease in specific antibody levels is documented. Certain subsets of patients are at increased risk of infection with *Haemophilus influenzae* and *Neisseria meningitidis* and, therefore, patients should receive these vaccinations as well. Patients are also instructed to keep a supply of antibiotics such as amoxicillin and Augmentin (amoxicillin; clavulanate potassium) with them, which should be taken at the first sign of a febrile episode. This should also be followed by immediate contact with a physician.

Long-term use of prophylactic oral antibiotics is often recommended in the pediatric population or in patients who may have difficulty reaching a physician. Penicillin is commonly prescribed to these patients. Data have shown benefit of prophylactic penicillin in preventing pneumococcal infection in children with sickle cell disease, but the benefit of this practice has never been proved for other subsets of asplenic patients.

RECOMMENDED READING

Berman RS, Yahanda AM, Mansfield PF, et al. Laparoscopic splenectomy in patients with hematologic malignancies. *Am J Surg* 1999;178:530–536.

Bouroncle BA. Thirty-five years in the progress of hairy cell leukemia. *Leuk Lymphoma* 1994;14:1.

Bouvet M, Babiera GV, Termuhlen PM, et al. Splenectomy in the accelerated or blastic phase of chronic myelogenous leukemia: a single institution, 25-year experience. *Surgery* 1997;122:20.

Brenner B, Nagler A, Tatarsky I, et al. Splenectomy in agnogenic myelogenous metaplasia and postpolycythemic myelogenous metaplasia. *Arch Intern Med* 1988;148:2501.

Canady MR, Welling RE, Strobel SL, et al. Splenic rupture in leukemia. *J Surg Oncol* 1989;41:194.

Carde P, Hagenbeek A, Hayat M, et al. Clinical staging versus laparotomy and combined modality with MOPP versus ABVD in early-stage Hodgkin's disease: the H6 twin randomized trials from the European Organization for Research and Treatment of Cancer Lymphoma Cooperative group. *J Clin Oncol* 1993;11:2258.

Coad JE, Matutes E, Catovsky D. Splenectomy in lymphoproliferative disorders: a report on 70 cases and review of the literature. *Leuk Lymphoma* 193;10:245.

Cortes J, Talpaz M, Kantarjian H. Chronic myelogenous leukemia: a review. *Am J Med* 1996;100:555.

Cusack JC, Seymour JF, Lerner S, et al. The role of splenectomy in chronic lymphocytic leukemia. *J Am Coll Surg* 1997;185:237.

Dawes LG, Malangoni MA. Cystic masses of the spleen. *Am Surg* 1986;52:333.

Edwards MJ, Balch CM. Surgical aspects of lymphoma. *Adv Surg* 1989;22:225.

Farrar WB, Kim JA. Biopsy techniques to establish diagnosis and type of malignant lymphoma. *Surg Oncol Clin North Am* 1993;2:159.

Feldman EJ, Arlin ZA. Modern management of chronic myelogenous leukemia (CML). *Cancer Invest* 1988;6:737.

Fielding AK. Prophylaxis against late infection following splenectomy and bone marrow transplant. *Blood Rev* 1994;8:179.

Flexner JM, Stein RS, Greer JP. Outline of treatment of lymphoma based on hematologic and clinical stage with expected end results. *Surg Oncol Clin North Am* 1993;2:283.

Hagemeister FB, Fuller LM, Martin RG. Staging laparotomy: findings and applications to treatment decisions. In: Fuller L, ed. *Hodgkin's disease and non-Hodgkin's lymphoma in adults and children*. New York: Raven, 1988.

Harris NL. The pathology of lymphomas: a practical approach to diagnosis and classification. *Surg Oncol Clin North Am* 1993;2:167.

Hubbard SM, Longo DL. Treatment-related morbidity in patients with lymphoma. *Curr Opin Oncol* 1991;3:852.

Johnson HA, Deterling RA. Massive splenomegaly. *Surg Gynecol Obstet* 1989;168:131.

Kalhs P, Schwarzinger I, Anderson G, et al. A retrospective analysis of the long-term effect of splenectomy on late infections, graft-versus-host disease, relapse, and survival after allogenic marrow transplantation for chronic myelogenous leukemia. *Blood* 1995; 86:2028.

Kantarjian HM, Smith TL, O'Brien S, et al. Prolonged survival in chronic myelogenous leukemia after cytogenetic response to interferon-a therapy. *Ann Intern Med* 1995;122:254.

Klein B, Stein M, Kuten A, et al. Splenomegaly and solitary spleen metastasis in solid tumors. *Cancer* 1987;60:100.

Kluin-Nelemans HC, Noordijk EM. Staging of patients with Hodgkin's disease: what should be done? *Leukemia* 1991;4:132.

Kraus MD, Fleming MD, Vonderhide RH. The spleen as a diagnostic specimen: a review of 10 year's experience at two tertiary care institutions. *Cancer* 2001;91:11.

Kurzrock R, Talpaz M, Gutterman JU. Hairy cell leukaemia: review of treatment. *Br J Haematol* 1991;79(suppl 1):17.

McBride CM, Hester JP. Chronic myelogenous leukemia: manage ment of splenectomy in a high-risk population. *Cancer* 1977;39: 653.

Morgenstern L, Rosenberg J, Geller SA. Tumors of the spleen. *World J Surg* 1985;9:468.

Mower WR, Hawkins JA, Nelson EW. Postsplenectomy infection in patients with chronic leukemia. *Am J Surg* 1986;152:583.

Noordijk EM, Carde P, Mandard AM, et al. Preliminary results of the EORTC-GPMC controlled clinical trial H7 in early stage Hodgkin's disease. *Ann Oncol* 1994;5(suppl 2):107.

Parker SL, Tong T, Bolden S, et al. Cancer statistics 1997. *CA* 1997;47:5.

Pittaluga S, Bijnens L, Teodorovic A, et al. Clinical analysis of 670 cases in two trials of the European Organization for the Research and Treatment of Cancer Lymphoma Cooperative Group subtyped according to the Revised European-American Classification of lymphoid neoplasms: a comparison with the Working Formulation. *Blood* 1996;10:4358.

Pollock R, Hohn D. Splenectomy. In: Roh MS, Ames FC, eds. *Advanced oncologic surgery*. New York: Mosby-Wolfe, 1994.

Shaw JHF, Print CG. Postsplenectomy sepsis. *Br J Surg* 1989; 76:1074.

Schrenk P, Wayand W. Value of diagnostic laparoscopy in abdominal malignancies. *Int Surg* 1995;80:353.

Styrt B. Infection associated with asplenia: risks, mechanisms, and prevention. *Am J Med* 1990;88:33N.

Tefferi A, Silverstein MN, Noel P. Agnogenic myelogenous metaplasia. *Semin Oncol* 1995;22:327.

Wiernik PH, Rader M, Becker NH, et al. Inflammatory pseudotumor of spleen. *Cancer* 1990;66:597.

Metastatic Cancer of Unknown Primary Site

Rosa F. Hwang and Barry J. Roseman

Patients with metastatic cancer of unknown primary site comprise fewer than 5% of patients with newly diagnosed cancer. The diagnostic evaluation and treatment of these patients can be challenging, and although care of these patients is coordinated largely by the medical oncologist, the surgeon may play an important role in these patients' care. In particular, a surgeon often is asked to evaluate a patient with cancer that has spread to a lymph node, the liver, or the peritoneal cavity. This chapter will define the problem of metastatic cancer of unknown primary site, outline a logical and practical approach to the diagnostic evaluation of these patients, and discuss the role of surgery in several clinical scenarios.

DEFINITION AND GENERAL CONSIDERATIONS

The syndrome of metastatic cancer of unknown primary site has multiple synonyms in the clinical literature (Table 18-1). These tumors often are grouped according to histologic subtype. The major subtypes include squamous cell cancer, adenocarcinoma, and undifferentiated neoplasms, the name given to a heterogeneous group of tumors of various cell origins.

In large series, the most common locations of metastases of unknown primary site are the lymph nodes, bones, lungs, and liver. Other metastatic sites include the brain, meninges, pleura, subcutaneous tissues, adrenal glands, peritoneum, kidney, and pancreas.

In most patients, the site of origin of the metastatic disease is never discerned. In others, however, the primary site from which the metastases are derived is identified eventually through exhaustive search while the patient is living, at surgery, or at autopsy. In only 25% of cases of unknown primary cancers is the primary site identifiable during the patient's lifetime. At autopsy, the primary tumor will be identified in 70% of cases. This body of data clearly reveals that metastases from squamous cell cancers typically originate in the head and neck region or the lungs, whereas metastatic adenocarcinomas most frequently originate in the lungs, breasts, or thyroid gland in the case of metastases above the diaphragm or from the pancreas, liver, stomach, colon, or rectum in the case of metastases below the diaphragm.

Defining therapeutic goals is important when treating a patient with metastatic cancer of unknown primary site. This is particularly true for patients with metastatic adenocarcinoma or undifferentiated carcinoma, whose median survival duration is less than 6 months. In a recent series by Abbruzzese et al. (2000) that evaluated 1,109 consecutive patients with unknown primary cancers, the median survival time was 11 months. They found

---

Table 18-1. Synonyms for metastatic cancer of unknown primary site

Metastasis of unknown origin
Tumors of unknown origin
Metastasis from undetected primary cancers
Cancer of unknown primary
Metastatic carcinoma of unknown primary
Metastatic cancer without detectable primary
Carcinoma of unknown primary
Metastatic adenocarcinoma of unknown primary

---

that the number of organ sites involved correlates with survival: for one, two, or three or more sites, the median survival was 14, 11, and 8 months, respectively.

Specific subgroups of patients with metastatic cancer of unknown primary site have a considerably better prognosis than the group as a whole, when given appropriate therapy. This includes patients with squamous cell cancer metastatic to cervical lymph nodes, women with metastatic adenocarcinoma in axillary lymph nodes, men with undifferentiated cancer and elevated β-human chorionic gonadotropin or α-fetoprotein levels, women with peritoneal carcinomatosis, and patients with neuroendocrine cancer of unknown primary site. These specific subgroups are discussed later in more detail.

The goals in evaluating patients with metastatic cancer of unknown primary site should be to identify those tumor types in which a cure or good disease control is possible, to determine if the tumor is locally confined or broadly metastatic, and to identify any symptoms for which local therapy may be effective.

HISTORY AND PHYSICAL EXAMINATION

In patients with metastatic cancer of unknown primary site, as with all patients with cancer, a careful history and physical examination are essential in establishing several important facts that have an impact on choice of therapy. The history of a malignancy or a family history of cancer may guide the surgeon in establishing the site of an occult primary tumor. Often, symptoms related to an unknown primary cancer are of relatively recent onset (<3 months) with rapid progression of disease. A complete systems review may help to determine the degree of symptoms and extent of the patient's disease. The general functional status of the patient is also a crucial factor, one that must be clarified before an individualized treatment decision can be made.

In the physical examination, several areas warrant particular attention. The head and neck should be examined thoroughly, particularly when a diagnosis of squamous cell cancer has been made. This includes examination of the oropharynx, hypopharynx, and nasopharynx as well as the larynx, typically assisted by indirect or fiberoptic laryngoscopy. The thyroid gland should be examined for enlargement or asymmetry. All nodal basins, including those of the head and neck and the supraclavicular, axillary, and inguinal regions, should be examined for palpable or enlarged lymph nodes.

In women, a careful breast examination should be performed, and a thorough bimanual pelvic examination, including a rectal examination, is essential. For men, the testicular and prostate examinations are particularly important, as is a careful rectal examination. All patients should undergo a thorough skin examination.

LABORATORY AND RADIOGRAPHIC EVALUATION

Routine complete blood cell count, blood chemistry studies, liver function tests, and urinalysis should be performed in all patients, and stool should be checked for occult blood. Beyond these basic tests, the clinical laboratory has limited usefulness in the diagnostic evaluation of the patient with cancer of unknown primary site.

Radiographic studies in patients with cancer of unknown primary site should focus on identifying the primary tumor and delineating the extent of metastatic disease. A chest radiograph is indicated in all patients to assess the presence of pulmonary metastases and for preoperative evaluation. Women of childbearing age or older, particularly those with metastatic adenocarcinoma, should undergo mammography. Unfortunately, identifying subtle radiographic abnormalities is difficult in younger women, who often have extremely dense breast tissue. Directed computed tomography (CT) may be helpful. These include a CT scan of the neck for patients with squamous cell cancer and of the chest, abdomen, and pelvis for patients with metastatic adenocarcinoma.

The role of magnetic resonance imaging (MRI) in identifying the primary tumor has not been studied well for most cases of unknown primary cancer, except for suspected occult breast carcinoma. In a recent study of 22 women with malignant axillary lymph nodes and negative findings on mammography and physical examination, MRI revealed a primary breast cancer in 86%. More recently, the utility of positron emission tomography (PET) has been evaluated in identifying the unknown primary tumor site. When fluorodeoxyglucose (FDG)-PET was performed on 27 patients with metastatic lymph nodes in the neck, the primary tumor was identified in 7 patients (26%). Similarly, a recent series of patients with cervical as well as extracervical metastases without a known primary tumor showed that FDG-PET was able to image the primary site in one third of patients.

In general, exhaustive pursuit of the primary site in these patients by radiographic studies is not helpful. This endeavor can be expensive, inconvenient, and traumatic for patients and often has no significant impact on patients' therapy or the ultimate course of the disease.

BIOPSY AND PATHOLOGIC EVALUATION

The next step in evaluating the patient with metastatic cancer of unknown primary site is to perform a tissue biopsy. This is particularly true for patients who present with lymphadenopathy. Fine-needle aspiration (FNA) largely has replaced core biopsy as a first technique. In some instances, such as for subtyping of lymphoma, open biopsies are needed to obtain larger tissue specimens that exhibit tissue architecture. FNA is recommended initially; this can be followed by core biopsy, incisional biopsy, or excisional biopsy as needed for specific cases. Once a tissue specimen has been obtained, fresh, unfixed tissue is sent to the pathology laboratory for routine microscopy (hematoxylin and eosin staining), electron microscopy, immunohistochemical studies, and hormone receptor studies. Close communication between the clinician and the pathologist is important, because details of the history and physical examination can influence the pathologic review and facilitate submission of additional tissue if necessary for an accurate diagnosis.

Light microscopy is ordinarily sufficient to determine the cell of origin; for difficult cases, electron microscopy may be helpful, as different tumor types have characteristic electron microscopic findings. For example, desmosomes and intracellular bridges are associated with squamous cell cancer, whereas tight junctions, microvilli, and acinar spaces are associated with adenocarcinoma. Premelanosomes are associated with melanoma, and neurosecretory granules are associated with small cell or neuroendocrine tumors. Lymphoma typically is characterized by an absence of junctions between the cells under electron microscopy.

Immunohistochemical studies are sometimes useful as an adjunct to microscopy and have become a routine histologic technique. Several markers can be stained by monoclonal antibodies and then visualized through a secondary labeling technique. For example, prostatic acid phosphatase and prostate-specific antigen are associated with prostate cancer, whereas neuron-specific enolase and chromogranin are associated with small cell lung cancer and carcinoid tumors. Germ cell tumors often stain for β-human chorionic gonadotropin and α-fetoprotein. α-Fetoprotein also is associated with hepatocellular carcinoma. Monoclonal immunoglobulins are indicative of lymphoma or plasmacytoma, and the presence of estrogen receptor or progesterone receptor is associated with breast and ovarian cancers.

Several tumor-derived mucins purportedly can help identify the source of the cancer in patients with cancer of unknown primary site. The best known of these are CA-125 in ovarian and uterine cancer; CA 15-3 in breast, ovarian, and pancreatic cancer; and CA 19-9 in pancreatic and gastrointestinal tract tumors. Table 18-2 lists several such proteins and other tumor markers used in helping to identify the source of metastases from an unknown primary site.

Unfortunately, patients with carcinoma of unknown primary site typically have a nonspecific overexpression of many of these tumor markers, and in such patients routine screening for elevations of serum tumor marker levels offers no diagnostic or prognostic assistance. None of these markers has been found to have adequate specificity or sensitivity to consistently identify a primary tumor, nor predictive value for either response to chemotherapy or survival.

Another recently developed tool is genetic analysis of the biopsy specimen to look for specific oncogenes that are expressed erroneously or at abnormally high levels in human cancer cells. Examples of these include the *HER-2/neu* oncogene, which is associated with breast cancer, the *bcr/abl* oncogene, which is associated with chronic myelogenous leukemia and B-cell lymphoma,

Table 18-2. Clinical role of selected tumor markers

Tumor Marker	Role in Differential Diagnosis	Role in Staging and Prognosis
AFP	Identification of hepatocellular carcinoma or germ cell tumors	Serum levels correlate with tumor burden and response to therapy
β-hCG	Identification of trophoblastic and germ cell tumors	Serum levels correlate with tumor burden and response to therapy
β2-microglobulin	Not very useful	Serum levels correlate with response to therapy for myeloma and lymphoma
CA 15-3	Identification of possible breast carcinoma, but elevated serum levels also noted in ovarian, lung, and GI carcinomas	High serum levels associated with metastatic carcinoma
CA 19-9	Identification of possible pancreatic cancer or other GI cancer	High serum levels helpful in determining response to treatment and detecting recurrence
CA 125	Identification of possible ovarian or uterine cancer, but elevated serum levels may be noted in breast, lung, or GI cancers	Serum levels helpful in determining response to treatment and detecting recurrence
Calcitonin	Screening and diagnosis of medullary carcinoma of thyroid	Minimal role
CEA	Distinction of carcinoma from mesothelioma	High serum levels correlate with liver metastasis
Cytokeratin	Distinction of carcinoma from lymphoma or melanoma by immunohistochemistry	Minimal role
Epithelial membrane antigen	Distinction of carcinoma from melanoma by membrane immunohistochemistry	Minimal role
LCA	Identification of lymphoma or leukemia by immunohistochemistry	Minimal role
PSA	Identification of prostate carcinoma	Serum levels correlate with stage and response to therapy

AFP, alpha-fetoprotein; CEA, carcinoembryonic antigen; GI; gastrointestinal; hCG, human chorionic gonadotropin; LCA, leukocyte common antigen; PSA, prostate-specific antigen.

and various other oncogenes that are related to specific cancers. Whether using such sophisticated molecular techniques will be beneficial in evaluating patients with metastatic cancer of unknown primary site is not known.

SPECIFIC DISEASE SITES

Metastatic Cancer to Cervical Lymph Nodes

The presence of an enlarged cervical lymph node often leads to a biopsy demonstrating metastatic cancer. The group of patients with metastatic squamous cell cancer to cervical lymph nodes and unknown primary tumor site has a better prognosis than the unknown primary tumor group as a whole.

The neck comprises more than 25 nodal basins. These nodes have been grouped into six specific levels to standardize the pathologic evaluation of patients. The classification of cervical lymph nodes is shown in Table 18-3. The most common site of metastasis in patients with head and neck squamous cell cancer is the jugulodigastric or level II upper internal jugular chain nodes, followed by the midjugular nodes. Metastasis to the other cervical nodal groups occurs with less frequency.

In those patients with cervical lymph nodes from an occult squamous cell primary cancer, a careful head and neck examination is particularly important. Adequate lighting and mirrors must be used to visualize the entire oropharynx, hypopharynx, nasopharynx, and larynx. A chest radiograph is always indicated, and a CT scan of the head and neck usually is indicated in these patients to determine the primary site and to obtain complete staging information.

If no primary tumor is found with physical examination and radiographic studies, panendoscopy is a common next step. This normally is done in the operating room with the patient under general anesthesia. Esophagoscopy, laryngoscopy, bronchoscopy, and nasopharyngoscopy are performed in an attempt to visualize and obtain a biopsy specimen of the most common sites of occult squamous cell cancer in the head and neck region. Random biopsies of the most probable tumor site locations are performed, based on the location of the adenopathy.

Typical occult primary tumor sites in squamous cell cancer are the nasopharynx, the midbase of the tongue, the pyriform sinus, and the tonsils. Table 18-4 shows the common pattern of cervical

Table 18-3.   Classification of cervical lymph nodes

Level	Nodes
I	Submental nodes
II	Upper internal jugular chain nodes
III	Middle internal jugular chain nodes
IV	Lower internal jugular chain nodes
V	Spinal accessory nodes
	Transverse cervical nodes
VI	Tracheoesophageal groove nodes

Table 18-4.   Probable site of the primary tumor according to the location of the cervical metastases

Location of Nodes	Primary Tumor Site
Submental	Floor of the mouth, lips, or anterior tongue
Submaxillary	Retromolar trigone or glossopalatine pillar
Jugulodigastric	Hypopharynx, base of the tongue, tonsil, nasopharynx, or larynx
Low jugular	Thyroid, hypopharynx, or nasopharynx
Supraclavicular	Lung (40%), thyroid (20%), GI (12%), GU (8%)
Posterior triangle	Nasopharynx

GI, gastrointestinal; GU, genitourinary.

metastasis from different squamous cell tumors in the head and neck region. Based on the location of the nodal metastases, extrapolation of the likely source of the occult primary often is possible, and the endoscopic examination can be focused on these locations.

Following this evaluation, a subgroup remains of patients in whom the primary tumor site is not identified. The standard approach to these patients is a combination of lymphadenectomy and radiation therapy directed to the most likely primary sites. Based on large series, expected 5-year survival in this group of patients is from 32% to 55%, and overall rate of control of neck disease is 75% to 85% with this combined therapy. Patients with extranodal extension or lymph nodes larger than 6 cm (N3 disease) have higher rates of both local recurrence and distant metastases.

Patients with metastatic adenocarcinoma in cervical lymph nodes from an occult primary tumor have a less favorable outcome. Retrospective series have shown that attempts to treat these patients with lymphadenectomy and radiation therapy are much less effective than in squamous cell carcinoma; the rate of local recurrence in cases so treated is nearly 100% and the 5-year survival rate is 0% to 10%.

Of particular interest in patients undergoing surgery is the presence of an enlarged Virchow (supraclavicular) node, common in patients with metastatic adenocarcinoma. One study retrospectively reviewed 152 FNA biopsies of supraclavicular lymph nodes, comparing the sites of primary tumor when the metastasis was in the right versus the left supraclavicular node. Sixteen of 19 primary pelvic tumors metastasized to the left supraclavicular node, and six of six primary abdominal malignancies metastasized to the left supraclavicular node. However, thoracic, breast, and head and neck malignancies showed no differences in patterns of metastasis to the right and left supraclavicular nodes. On the basis of this information, the investigation for the source of primary tumor in patients who present with adenocarcinoma in a left-sided Virchow node should focus on the abdomen and pelvis.

Metastatic Cancer to Axillary Lymph Nodes

The histologic type of the tumor should guide the evaluation of patients with cancer metastatic to axillary lymph nodes. For example, when a biopsy of axillary lymph nodes yields lymphoma, a complete staging evaluation should be performed to determine whether systemic chemotherapy or radiation therapy is the appropriate treatment. Patients with melanoma should be examined carefully for a primary site in the ipsilateral extremity. Patients with squamous cell cancer metastatic to the axillary lymph nodes should have a careful skin examination, a chest radiograph to rule out a lung primary tumor, a detailed head and neck examination, and CT scans of the head and neck and the chest to look for an occult squamous cell primary tumor.

Men with adenocarcinoma metastatic to an axillary lymph node and an unknown primary tumor source should be evaluated for lung, gastrointestinal, and genitourinary primary tumors. Women with adenocarcinoma metastatic to the axillary lymph nodes should be evaluated similarly, although in women the likelihood of an occult breast primary tumor is high. These patients should be examined carefully for a breast tumor, and every woman should have a mammogram. Ultrasonography of the breast can be used if the mammogram does not identify a lesion, especially in younger patients with dense breasts. As discussed previously, MRI has shown promise in identifying primary breast carcinomas.

Several large studies demonstrate that if no extramammary primary tumor or systemic metastases are found, the most likely diagnosis is cancer of the ipsilateral breast. Women with occult breast cancer presenting with axillary metastases constitute approximately 0.5% of all women with breast cancer. When large numbers of such patients are treated for a presumptive diagnosis of breast cancer, the recurrence and survival results are similar to those of patients with a similar stage of breast cancer and a known primary tumor. Retrospective review of the mastectomy specimens from patients with occult primary tumors shows that, in 50% to 65% of cases, a primary tumor ultimately can be identified in the surgical specimen. The remainder of the tumors is probably too small to be detected by the standard sampling techniques that pathologists use to study breast specimens.

The pathologic pattern of an axillary lymph node with occult breast cancer may be different from that of a typical mammary cancer. A review by Haupt et al. (1985) demonstrated that 65% of lymph nodes in occult breast cancers exhibited a pattern of infiltration with diffuse sheets of large apocrine-like cells, which also can be seen in renal cell carcinoma, melanoma, and lymphoma. Only 23% showed the usual features of a breast adenocarcinoma. Distinguishing a primary breast cancer in the axillary tail of the breast and an involved axillary lymph node can be extremely difficult. While a primary breast cancer should demonstrate normal breast tissue in the specimen and a lymph node metastasis would contain some normal lymphoid architecture, occasionally a lymph node may be replaced completely by tumor with extracapsular extension into the axillary fat. Differentiating metastasis of a breast cancer to an axillary lymph node versus axillary soft tissue is important, because upstaging from stage II breast cancer with an involved axillary lymph node to stage IV with metastatic disease in soft tissues significantly influences prognosis and thus therapy for the patient. The biopsy specimen from the lymph node should be subjected to routine histologic and immunohistochemical evaluation for estrogen and progesterone receptors. Although neither highly sensitive nor highly specific, the presence of estrogen or progesterone receptors in this clinical scenario strongly suggests a breast primary tumor.

The treatment for women with adenocarcinoma metastatic to axillary lymph nodes has evolved dramatically over the past several years. The three general approaches are immediate mastectomy, watchful waiting, and radiation therapy. Immediate mastectomy has been the traditional therapy for women with isolated metastatic adenocarcinoma in axillary lymph nodes and is associated with good long-term survival rates and low risk of local recurrence. A large series by Ashikari et al. in 1976 showed a 10-year survival rate of 79% in these patients. The majority of cancers found in mastectomy specimens were T1 lesions. As the use and quality of mammograms has increased, the rate of detection of primary cancers within mastectomy specimens has decreased from as high as 92% to 8% to 45% because previously "occult" primary tumors are now detectable with mammography.

Watchful waiting is another option, in which axillary dissection alone is followed by observation of the breast. The principal drawback of this approach is that 25% to 75% of patients will have a recurrence in the breast, requiring further therapy. Although salvage treatment with mastectomy is successful in most of these patients, metastases may develop in a small subgroup of patients that might have been prevented by more aggressive local therapy.

The third approach to women with axillary metastases from an unknown primary site is breast-conservation therapy. This approach has been studied at The University of Texas M.D. Anderson Cancer Center, and the results are encouraging. In patients who have undergone axillary lymph node dissection alone, the incidence of local recurrence is 65% at 10 years, whereas a combination of axillary lymph node dissection and radiation therapy reduces the local recurrence rate to 25%. With this treatment, the overall survival rate was no different from that of patients with the same nodal stage of disease who underwent mastectomy. Addition of adjuvant chemotherapy to surgery and radiation therapy increased the survival rate from 60% to 85% at 10 years. Tamoxifen should be part of therapy for women of any age whose primary tumor (if identified) or axillary nodal metastases express estrogen and/or progesterone receptors.

Several studies have confirmed that survival rates associated with breast-conservation therapy are equivalent to those associated with mastectomy in patients with occult primary breast cancer. Most patients who initially present with clinically evident positive nodes need both local and regional lymph node irradiation and should be given the same treatment options as are given patients with known breast cancer of similar nodal stage. Recently, a review at M.D. Anderson Cancer Center analyzed 45 female patients with isolated axillary nodal metastases without a known primary tumor. Median follow-up duration was 7 years. Patients underwent either mastectomy or breast-conservation surgery; external beam radiation therapy was used in 71% of patients and systemic chemotherapy was given to 73%. No significant difference was found between mastectomy and breast conservation in locoregional recurrence, distant metastases, or 5-year survival rate. Regardless of surgical treatment used, the number of involved nodes was the only determinant of survival.

Metastatic Cancer to the Inguinal Nodes from an Unknown Primary Site

A relatively infrequent presentation of metastatic cancer of unknown primary site is metastases to the inguinal lymph nodes. Excluding melanoma, which is discussed separately, the most common histologic type is unclassified carcinoma. The second most common type is squamous cell carcinoma, and a small number of patients will have adenocarcinoma. In evaluating patients with inguinal metastases, a thorough investigation for the primary tumor should include examination of the skin of the lower extremities, perineum, and buttocks and an examination for a primary tumor of the perineal or pelvic region. After evaluation for other metastatic disease, inguinal lymph node dissection typically is performed to obtain additional pathologic specimens and for regional disease control. Patients are then considered for treatment with systemic therapy on the basis of the tissue diagnosis.

Metastatic Melanoma of Unknown Primary Site

One area of clear interest to the surgical oncologist is metastatic melanoma of unknown primary site. Approximately 5% of patients with melanoma present with metastatic disease of the lymph nodes from an unknown primary tumor. Several studies have compared these patients with similar cohorts of patients who have equivalent nodal status and a known primary site in terms of recurrence and survival. Although patients with unknown primary tumors historically were thought to have a worse prognosis, several recent large studies have contradicted these early findings.

Patients with metastatic melanoma and an unknown primary tumor must be examined carefully from scalp to toes for a potential primary tumor site. For the purpose of studying this subgroup of patients, strict criteria have been established in the course of retrospective analysis to exclude patients with potential sites of an occult primary tumor that may have been missed (Table 18-5).

In an important study from Memorial Sloan-Kettering Cancer Center, published by Chang and Knapper in 1982, 166 patients with metastatic melanoma of unknown primary site were reviewed retrospectively. This group comprised 4.4% of all the melanoma cases followed during the review period. These patients were compared on several parameters with a control group of patients who had known primary tumors. All patients had clinical stage II disease according to the older staging criteria in which patients with suggestive palpable lymph nodes were defined as having clinical stage II disease.

The distribution of metastases in patients with unknown primary tumors was similar to that in patients with known primary

Table 18-5. Metastatic melanoma of unknown primary: stringent definition of patient population

Exclude patients with any of the following:
1. History of having had a mole, birthmark, freckle, chronic paronychia, or skin blemish previously excised, electrodesiccated, or cauterized
2. Metastatic melanoma in one of the node-bearing areas and presentation with a scar indicating previous local treatment in the skin area drained by this lymphatic basin
3. No recorded physical examination of anus and genitalia
4. Previous orbital enucleation or exenteration

tumors. Most tumors were found in the axillary lymph nodes, and many were found in the groin and cervical regions. Patients with clinical stage II disease had a 46% 5-year survival rate and a 41% 10-year survival rate, a finding similar for men and women. Patients who had residual disease in the lymphadenectomy specimen, indicating the presence of more extensive lymph node involvement, had lower survival rates. Finally, patients who had prompt lymphadenectomy had a substantially better prognosis than those who had a delay in treatment, with a threefold improvement in the 5- and 10-year survival rates.

A second large series from the John Wayne Cancer Center reviewed 188 patients with lymph node metastases from unknown primary melanoma and compared these with a group of patients with a known primary tumor. Several variables—such as age, gender, anatomic site, and treatment with adjuvant immunotherapy—were similar in the two groups. In this group of patients with clinical stage II melanoma, those with lymph node metastases from an unknown primary melanoma had no significant improvement in 5- and 10-year survival rates than patients with a known primary melanoma. More recently, a retrospective analysis from the University of Pennsylvania of 40 patients with melanoma of unknown primary site revealed that overall 4-year survival rate for these patients was significantly higher than that for patients with equivalent nodal disease and a known concurrent primary melanoma (57% vs. 19%). Similarly, patients with melanoma of unknown primary site with visceral metastases had longer median survival than those with known primary tumors.

Because patients with melanoma metastatic to the lymph nodes from an unknown primary tumor have as favorable an outlook as patients with a known primary melanoma, the nodal basin in patients with unknown primary tumors should be approached in a standard fashion. Patients should be offered radical lymph node dissection, followed by adjuvant immunotherapy for patients with disease localized to the nodal basin.

Peritoneal Carcinomatosis of Unknown Primary Site in Women

Another subgroup of patients with a particularly favorable prognosis is women with peritoneal carcinomatosis of unknown primary site. Several studies have shown that women who present with peritoneal carcinomatosis should be treated in a similar fashion to those with known advanced ovarian cancer. This would include maximal surgical cytoreduction at initial laparotomy followed by platinum-based combination chemotherapy. These patients are characterized by an indolent disease course, high rates of response to systemic therapy, and a chance for long-term, disease-free survival. Median survival is typically 16 months to 2 years. Men with isolated peritoneal carcinomatosis and other patients whose tumor histologic types do not resemble ovarian carcinoma have much poorer overall survival rates.

Unknown Primary Tumor with Metastatic Liver Disease

The surgeon occasionally is involved in the evaluation of a patient who presents with metastatic liver disease from an unknown primary tumor. The liver tumor may be discovered when the patient presents with symptoms on routine physical examination or incidentally on a radiologic study such as an abdominal sonogram or CT scan.

When patients present with metastatic liver disease from an unknown primary tumor, the cell type is most often adenocarcinoma. However, anaplastic or poorly differentiated carcinoma, small cell carcinoma, squamous cell carcinoma, gastrinoma, insulinoma, and sarcomas such as hemangiosarcoma and leiomyosarcoma also are found. When the diagnosis is adenocarcinoma of unknown primary site metastatic to the liver, the most likely primary tumor is a gastrointestinal tract malignancy, followed by a lung or breast tumor.

Patients with adenocarcinoma of unknown primary site metastatic to the liver should be evaluated with a comprehensive history and physical examination, as discussed earlier in this chapter, with particular attention paid to the breast and gynecologic examination in women and the genital and rectal examination in men. A chest radiograph, mammogram, and barium study of the colon and rectum or colonoscopy can be performed to look for the most likely sources of the primary tumor. CT scan of the abdomen is useful to quantify the liver disease and may help to identify the primary tumor. An exhaustive search for the primary tumor that includes thyroid scan, upper endoscopy, upper gastrointestinal series with small bowel follow-through, intravenous pyelogram, or other such studies usually is not productive unless the patient has significant symptoms, such as pain or gastrointestinal tract bleeding or obstruction. At M.D. Anderson, the studies most likely to identify a primary site were the combination of pathologic analysis, chest radiograph, and CT scan of the abdomen and pelvis. The number of primary cancers found by other procedures, including gastrointestinal endoscopy, was small; thus these studies are recommended only for patients with symptoms specific to the stomach, small bowel, or colorectum.

Patients with suspected liver metastases and an unknown primary tumor should have a liver biopsy so that a specific tissue diagnosis can be obtained. The predominant histologic type is adenocarcinoma (57%–67%), followed by carcinoma, neuroendocrine and squamous features. The overall survival of patients with unknown primary tumor and liver metastases is poor (median,

7 months), which may persuade physicians to provide only supportive care for this group of patients. A review of 365 patients at M.D. Anderson found that those who were treated with some type of chemotherapy did better than untreated patients (median survival, 12 vs. 5 months), although this difference may reflect a selection bias to offer chemotherapy only to patients with better performance status at the time of diagnosis.

One group of patients with unknown primary tumor and liver metastases that has been found to have longer survival than the group as a whole consists of those patients with histologic features associated with neuroendocrine carcinoma. Survival is threefold to fivefold longer for this group than for patients with other histologic types and thus electron microscopy and special immunohistochemical stains should be performed to differentiate this subgroup of tumors from other less favorable histologic types.

Chemotherapy for Metastatic Cancer of Unknown Primary Site

In studying the effects of chemotherapy on patients with cancer of unknown primary site, several uncontrolled factors limit comparison of patients within and between series. Among these factors are variations in clinical and pathologic evaluation, inclusion of patients with the primary site identified, presence of visceral versus nodal metastases, age, performance status, and whether the studies were performed in a single institution or multiple institutions.

When chemotherapy is given to unselected groups of patients with metastatic cancer of unknown primary site, an overall 5% to 10% 5-year survival rate can be anticipated. No effective therapy is known for metastatic adenocarcinoma or poorly differentiated carcinoma. Several cisplatin-based regimens have produced complete response rates of 10% to 25%, but these regimens produce 5-year disease-free survival rates of only 5% to 15%. Greco et al evaluated the addition of paclitaxel to a regimen of carboplatin and etoposide in a phase II trial of 71 patients. This combination produced major responses or stable disease status in 80% of patients, whose tumor histologic types were mostly adenocarcinomas or poorly differentiated carcinomas. Responses were probably short-lived, because median survival duration was 11 months, similar to that for other regimens using doxorubicin, 5-fluorouracil, or cisplatin. Patients with squamous cell cancer or neuroendocrine cancer have a significantly better response to chemotherapeutic agents than patients with other tumor types.

Given the poor results of chemotherapy in patients with poorly differentiated carcinoma or adenocarcinoma metastatic to lymph nodes or viscera, keeping a perspective on the overall disease process is important while treating such patients. The benefits of therapy must be compared with the toxic effects of a given chemotherapy regimen.

Although cure is an unrealistic goal for many patients with metastatic cancer of unknown primary site, the surgeon often is involved in the palliative care of such patients. Examples of palliation in such patients include debulking of tumors causing pain or obstruction, enteral tubes for decompression, thoracentesis for patients with respiratory compromise from pleural effusions, and radiation therapy for painful bone metastases. Patients should be offered adequate analgesics to ensure that they are comfortable, and both patients and their families should be provided adequate emotional support and access to resources that optimize their quality of life.

RECOMMENDED READING

Abbruzzese JL, Lenzi R, Raber MN. Carcinoma of unknown primary. In: Abeloff MD, Armitage JD, Lichter AS, eds. *Clinical oncology,* 2nd ed. New York: Churchill Livingstone, 2000.

Albers CA, Johnson RH, Mansberger AR. The management of patients with metastatic cancer from an unknown primary site. *Am Surg* 1981;47:162.

Anbari K, Schuchter L, Bucky L, et al. Melanoma of unknown primary site. *Cancer* 1997;79:9.

Ayoub JP, Hess KR, Abbruzzese MC, et al. Unknown primary tumors metastatic to liver. *J Clin Oncol* 1998;16:6.

Cervin JR, Silverman JF, Loggie BW, et al. Virchow's node revisited. *Arch Pathol Lab Med* 1995;119:727.

Chang P, Knapper WH. Metastatic melanoma of unknown primary. *Cancer* 1982;49:1106.

deBraud F, Al-Sarraf M. Diagnosis and management of squamous cell carcinoma of unknown primary tumor site of the neck. *Semin Oncol* 1993;20:273.

Ellerbroek N, Holmes F, Singletary E, et al. Treatment of patients with isolated axillary nodal metastases from an occult primary carcinoma consistent with breast origin. *Cancer* 1990;66:1461.

Glynne-Jones RG, Anand AK, Young TE, et al. Metastatic adenocarcinoma in the cervical lymph nodes from an occult primary. *Clin Oncol* 1989;1:19.

Greco FA, Burris HA, Erland JB, et al. Carcinoma of unknown primary site-long term follow-up after treatment with paclitaxel, carboplatin and etoposide. *Cancer* 2000;89:12.

Greco FA, Vaughn WK, Hainsworth JD. Advanced poorly differentiated carcinoma of unknown primary site: recognition of a treatable syndrome. *Ann Intern Med* 1986;104:547.

Greenberg BR, Lawrence HJ. Metastatic cancer with unknown primary. *Med Clin North Am* 1988;72:1055.

Haupt HM, Rosen PP, Kinne DW. Breast carcinoma presenting with axillary lymph node metastases. *Am J Surg Pathol* 1985;9:165.

Holmes FF, Fouts TL. Metastatic cancer of unknown primary site. *Cancer* 1970;4:816.

Jackson B, Scott-Conner C, Moulder J. Axillary metastasis from occult breast carcinoma: diagnosis and management. *Am Surg* 1995;61:431.

Jakobsen J, Aschenfeldt P, Johansen J, et al. Lymph node metastases in the neck from unknown primary tumour. *Acta Oncol* 1992;31:653.

Kambhu SA, Kelsen DP, Fiore J, et al. Metastatic adenocarcinomas of unknown primary site. *Am J Clin Oncol* 1990;13:55.

Le Chevalier TL, Cvitkovic E, Caille P, et al. Early metastatic cancer of unknown primary origin at presentation. *Arch Intern Med* 1988;148:2035.

Lenzi R, Hess KR, Abbruzzese MC, et al. Poorly differentiated carcinoma and poorly differentiated adenocarcinoma of unknown origin: favorable subsets of patients with unknown-primary carcinoma? *J Clin Oncol* 1997; 15:1.

Lenzi R, Abbruzzese MC, Raber MN, et al. Clinical outcomes of patients with metastatic carcinomas of unknown primary presenting with peritoneal carcinomatosis (abstract). *Proc Am Soc Clin Oncol* 1997;16:295.

Leonard RJ, Nystrom JS. Diagnostic evaluation of patients with carcinoma of unknown primary tumor site. *Semin Oncol* 1993;20:244.

Lleander VC, Goldstein G, Horsley JS. Chemotherapy in the management of metastatic cancer of unknown primary site. *Oncology* 1972;26:265.

McCunniff AJ, Raben M. Metastatic carcinoma of the neck from an unknown primary. *Int J Radiat Oncol Biol Phys* 1986;12:1849.

Muggia FM, Baranda J. Management of peritoneal carcinomatosis of unknown primary tumor site. *Semin Oncol* 1993;20:268.

Nesbit RA, Tattersall MH, Fox RM, et al. Presentation of unknown primary cancer with metastatic liver disease: management and natural history. *Aust NZ J Med* 1981;11:16.

Pacini P, Olmi P, Cellai E, et al. Cervical lymph node metastases from an unknown primary tumour. *Acta Radiol Oncol* 1981;20:311.

Pavlidis N, Kalef-Ezra J, Braissoulis E, et al. Evaluation of six tumor markers carcinoma of unknown primary. *Med Pediatr Oncol* 1994;22:162.

Read NE, Strom EA, McNeese MD. Carcinoma in axillary nodes in women with unknown primary site: results of breast-conserving therapy. *Breast J* 1996;2:403.

Reintgen DS, McCarty KS, Woodard B, et al. Metastatic malignant melanoma with an unknown primary. *Surg Gynecol Obstet* 1983;156:335.

Roseman BJ, Clark O. Common clinical problems: evaluation of the patient with a neck mass. In: Wilmore DW, Cheung LY, Harken AH, et al, eds. *Scientific american surgery.* Vol. II. New York: Scientific American, 1996.

Ruddon RW, Norton SE. Use of biological markers in the diagnosis of cancers of unknown primary tumor. *Semin Oncol* 1993;20:251.

Schwarz D, Hamberger AD, Jesse RH. The management of squamous cell carcinoma in cervical lymph nodes in the clinical absence of a primary lesion by combined surgery and irradiation. *Cancer* 1981;48:1746.

Steckel RJ, Kagan AR. Diagnostic persistence in working up metastatic cancer with an unknown primary site. *Radiology* 1980;134:367.

Stewart JF, Tattersall MH, Woods RL, et al. Unknown primary adenocarcinoma: incidence of overinvestigation and natural history. *BMJ* 1979;1:1530.

Strnad CM, Grosh WW, Baxter J, et al. Peritoneal carcinomatosis of unknown primary site in women. *Ann Intern Med* 1989;11:213.

Vijuk G, Coates AS. Survival of patients with visceral metastatic melanoma from an occult primary lesion: a retrospective matched cohort study. *Ann Oncol* 1998;9:419–422.

Wallack MK, Reynolds B. Cancer to the inguinal nodes from an unknown primary site. *J Surg Oncol* 1981;17:39.

Wolff AC, Lange JR, Davidson NE. Occult primary cancer with axillary nodal metastases. In: Singletary SE, Robb GL, eds. *Adjuvant therapy of breast disease.* Hamilton, Ontario: BC Decker, 2000.

Wong JH, Cagle LA, Morton DL. Surgical treatment of lymph nodes with metastatic melanoma from unknown primary site. *Arch Surg* 1987;122:1380.

Yang ZY, Hu YH, Yan JH, et al. Lymph node metastases in the neck from an unknown primary. *Acta Radiol Oncol* 1983;22:17.

Genitourinary Cancer

Samuel F. Huang and Colin P.N. Dinney

Global cancer statistics reveal that in 1998 genitourinary cancers represented approximately 10% of new cancers diagnosed worldwide. These cancers occur in approximately 300,000 patients within the United States each year, and prostate cancer is now the most common malignancy in U.S. men. Recognizing these facts, practicing physicians require an essential understanding of the diagnosis and treatment of these diseases. In this chapter we review the current management of prostate, bladder, renal, and testicular neoplasm.

PROSTATE CANCER

Epidemiology and Etiology

In men, prostate cancer is the most common malignancy and the second leading cause of solid cancer mortality. Average mortality rates (1990–1997) are estimated to be 54.1 per 100,000 in African-American males and 23.3 per 100,000 in white males. Prostate cancer screening was introduced in the United States during the mid to late 1980s. Since this introduction, the pattern of disease incidence has changed. From 1988 to 1992, the annual percent increase of prostate cancer incidence was estimated at 17.5% per year. From 1992 to 1995, the incidence decreased 10.3% per year. This decrease has leveled off and from 1995 to1997, the average annual decrease in incidence was 2.1% and the average annual incidence was 149.7 cases per 100,000. These cancer trends are not equivalent between whites and African-Americans. Prostate cancer incidence among African-Americans has increased an average of 0.7% annually from 1990 to 1997. Furthermore, although the average annual mortality rates have decreased 2.2% per year (1990–1997) overall, African-Americans have only experienced an average mortality rate decrease of 1.1% per year throughout 1990 to 1997.

Prostate cancer rarely occurs before age 50 years, and the incidence increases through the ninth decade of life; however, some of this increase may be attributable to an increase in prostate cancer screening in the later decades. It is estimated that 30% to 50% of men older than 50 years have histologic evidence of prostate cancer at autopsy, while at age 75 or older, it is estimated that this figure increases to 50% to 70%.

Many factors have been proposed to be associated with the development of prostate cancer. The presence of an intact hypothalamic-pituitary-gonadal axis and advanced age are the most universally accepted risk factors. Migration studies support a role for environmental influences on prostate cancer. Higher rates of prostate cancer have been found amongst populations with higher amounts of fat in the diet. Beneficial dietary associations include isoflavinoids, lycopenes, selenium, and vitamin E; however, additional prospective randomized trials are needed to confirm the beneficial effects of these factors. It is unclear whether the increased mortality rate of prostate cancer in African-Americans is due to unique racial biologic factors, as opposed to dietary influences and access to health care issues. Occupational exposure to cadmium has been associated with increased risk of prostate cancer, but this relationship is not yet proven to be causal.

Evidence has shown that a man with one, two, or three first-degree relatives affected with prostate cancer has a two, five, or 11 times greater risk, respectively, of the development of prostate cancer than the general population. A Mendelian pattern of autosomal dominant transmission of prostate cancer accounts for 43% of disease occurring before age 55 years and 9% of all prostate cancers occurring by age 85 years.

Anatomy

The normal prostate gland weighs 15 to 20 g and is divided into three major glandular zones. The *peripheral zone* constitutes 70% of the prostate gland and is the area palpated during digital rectal examination (DRE). The area around the ejaculatory ducts is called the *central zone* and accounts for 25% of the gland. The *transitional zone* makes up 5% of the prostate gland around the urethra. In a pathologic review of 104 prostate glands from patients who underwent radical prostatectomy, 68% of the cancers were located in the peripheral zone, 24% in the transitional zone, and only 8% in the central zone. Almost all stage A (nonpalpable) cancers in that study were found in the transitional zone, the area most susceptible to benign prostatic hyperplasia.

Screening

Although good screening methods for prostate cancer are available, controversy surrounds the concept of screening for this disease. It is estimated that less than 10% of men with prostate cancer die because of the disease. This leads to a lack of consensus on the optimal management of early stage disease and to questions regarding the cost-effectiveness of a national screening effort for all men older than 50 years. Currently, the American Cancer Society recommends a DRE and measurement of prostate-specific antigen (PSA) starting at age 50 years old. For African-American men or men with a family history of prostate cancer, screening should begin at 40 years old.

Diagnosis

Patients with low-volume, clinically localized prostate cancer are typically asymptomatic; abnormalities are detected by DRE or increased serum PSA level. Advanced prostate cancer can be asymptomatic; present as local symptoms of urinary hesitancy, frequency, and urgency; or present as systemic symptoms of weight loss, fatigue, and bone pain.

PSA is a serine protease produced by the epithelium of the prostate. PSA is not specific for prostate cancer and can be increased in benign conditions of the prostate such as prostatitis, prostatic infarction, and prostatic hyperplasia. Transurethral resection of the prostate (TURP) and prostatic needle biopsy significantly increase the serum PSA level above baseline for up to 8 weeks. DRE, cystoscopy, and transrectal ultrasound (TRUS) do not alter serum PSA to a clinically significant degree. The positive predictive value of a PSA level greater than 4 ng/mL for the detection of prostate cancer is 34.4%, while the positive predictive value for an abnormal DRE is 21.4%. Detection rates demonstrate that DRE and PSA together (5.8%) are superior to either DRE (3.2%) or PSA (4.6%) alone. Free PSA is a form of PSA not conjugated to protease inhibitors in the serum. Decreased percentage-free PSA (<25%) is associated with prostate cancer, and measurement of free PSA is performed to improve the specificity of PSA testing in the range of 4 to 10 ng/mL and thus eliminate unnecessary biopsies.

TRUS is performed using real-time imaging with a 7-MHz transducer, which allows both transverse and sagittal imaging of the prostate gland. Prostate cancer typically appears as a hypoechoic region within the prostate. TRUS can also be used to measure the dimensions of the prostate gland to calculate the glandular volume.

Lymphatic metastases can be detected by computed tomography (CT), lymphangiography, and magnetic resonance imaging (MRI). However, the only reliable method for staging pelvic lymph nodes is a pelvic lymphadenectomy.

Radionuclide bone scan remains the most sensitive test to detect skeletal metastases. However, Oesterling (1993) found the yield of a bone scan was 2% if a patient has a PSA level less than 20 ng/mL and evidence of skeletal metastasis, while no patients had a positive bone scan with a PSA less than 8 ng/mL. Therefore, based on this data, radionuclide bone scans are not necessary for staging prostate cancer patients who have a low serum PSA level and no skeletal symptoms. When bone metastases are present, 80% are osteoblastic, 15% are mixed osteoblastic-osteolytic, and 5% are osteolytic. A chest radiograph is performed to detect the presence of pulmonary metastases.

The diagnosis of prostate cancer is made by the histologic finding of prostate cancer in a prostatic biopsy, in a prostatic needle aspiration, or in tissue obtained from prostatectomy for benign disease. Adenocarcinoma is the predominant cell type of prostate cancer and is the only type discussed in this chapter.

Grading and Staging

The Gleason grading system is the most widely used grading system. It recognizes five histologic patterns of prostate cancer. The scores of the predominant and secondary patterns are added to yield a range of tumor grades from 2 to 10.

The biologic behavior of the tumor can be further categorized by stage, which accounts for tumor volume and location. Prostate cancer typically spreads to the pelvic lymph nodes, bone, and lungs. The 1997 American Joint Committee on Cancer/International Union against Cancer TNM staging classification is shown in Table 19-1.

Table 19-1.   Staging systems for prostate cancer

Primary tumor clinical (T)

TX	Primary tumor cannot be assessed
T0	No evidence of primary tumor
T1	Clinically inapparent tumor not palpable or visible by imaging
	T1a: Tumor incidental histologic finding in 5% or less of tissue resected
	T1b: Tumor incidental histologic finding in more than 5% of tissue resected
	T1c: Tumor identified by needle biopsy because of increased PSA
T2	Tumor confined within the prostate gland
	T2a: Tumor involves one lobe
	T2b: Tumor involves both lobes
T3	Tumor extends through the prostate capsule
	T3a: Extracapsular extension (unilateral or bilateral)
	T3b: Seminal vesicle invasion
T4	Invasion of bladder or rectum

Regional lymph nodes (N)

NX	Regional lymph nodes cannot be assessed
N0	No regional lymph node metastasis
N1	Metastasis in regional lymph node or nodes

Distant metastases (M)

MX	Distant metastasis cannot be assessed
M0	No distant metastasis
M1	Distant metastasis
	M1a: Nonregional lymph nodes
	M1b: Bone(s)
	M1c: Other site(s)

PSA, prostate specific antigen.

Management of Early Disease

In 1987, the National Cancer Institute published a consensus statement on the treatment of early stage prostate cancer. The report concluded: "Radical prostatectomy and radiation therapy are clearly effective forms of treatment in the attempt to cure tumors limited to the prostate for appropriately selected patients ... What remains unclear is the relative merit of each in producing lifelong freedom from cancer recurrence ... Properly designed and completed randomized trials that evaluate both disease control and quality of life after modern radiation therapy compared with radical prostatectomy are essential." These criteria have yet to be fulfilled; however, there appears to be little difference in clinical and biochemical outcomes between the two modalities when similar patient groups are compared.

Surgery

The surgical excision of prostate cancer by complete removal of the prostate gland, seminal vesicles, and ampullae of the vasa deferentia was first performed in the early 1900s. This procedure, known as a *radical prostatectomy*, can be performed using a perineal or retropubic approach.

Zincke et al. (1994) reported their experience with radical prostatectomy in 1,143 patients with 10- and 15-year cause-specific survival rates of 90% and 83% and metastasis-free survival of 83% and 77%, respectively. Complication rates are low. Mortality is less than 0.7% and the incidence of severe incontinence is 1.4%. Leandri et al. (1992) reported on 620 patients and found a 6.9% early complication rate, 1.3% late complication rate, and 0.2% mortality rate. Sexual potency was maintained in 71% in whom a nerve-sparing technique was used, and 5% experienced stress incontinence after 1 year.

Radiation Therapy

External beam radiation therapy is used for the definitive treatment of localized and regionally extensive prostatic adenocarcinoma. At M.D. Anderson, 60 to 70 Gy was given to 114 patients with localized prostate cancer as primary therapy. The 5- and 10-year uncorrected survival rates are comparable to radical surgery (89% and 68%, respectively). In this series there was no difference in survival between patients with stages A and B disease. Skeletal metastases were the most common site of relapse. Serious complications developed in only 1.8% of treated patients. Conformal radiation therapy is currently used to decrease adverse local side effects of radiation therapy and increase total dosage. Larger doses are used in select patients; however, longer follow-up is needed to fully define the role of dose escalation. At M.D. Anderson, we recommend radical prostatectomy for the treatment of early-stage prostate cancer. Primary radiation therapy is reserved for patients with significant comorbid medical illnesses.

Management of Locally Advanced Prostate Cancer/Lymph Node Metastasis

Locally advanced prostate cancer involves areas outside the prostatic capsule, such as fat, seminal vesicles, levator muscles, or other adjacent structures. Locally advanced prostate cancer is associated with a 53% incidence of lymph node metastases and decreased overall survival rate compared to early stage disease. At M.D. Anderson, locally advanced disease with or without lymph node metastasis is treated with primary radiation therapy and androgen ablation with a 6-year biochemical failure rate of 13%. Longer follow-up is still needed. Our experience with locally advanced disease treated with primary radiation therapy demonstrated 5-, 10-, and 15-year uncorrected actuarial survival rates of 72%, 47%, and 17%, respectively. The local control rate was 75% at 15 years of follow-up.

Treatment modalities other than radiation therapy used for locally advanced disease include radical prostatectomy, TURP, and hormonal therapy. Tumor grade, stage, bulk of tumor, and seminal vesicle involvement in locally advanced disease are associated with the interval between radical prostatectomy and disease progression. The actuarial 5-year survival rate for patients with locally advanced disease who have undergone TURP is 64%, making TURP an option for patients with short life expectancies, such as the very elderly and those with serious coexisting medical problems.

Systemic Prostate Cancer

Patients with metastatic prostate cancer have a median survival duration of 30 months, with an estimated 5-year survival rate of 20%. The treatment of metastatic prostate cancer is androgen ablation therapy. The hypothalamus produces luteinizing hormone–releasing hormone (LHRH) and corticotropin-releasing factor, which stimulate the anterior pituitary gland to release adrenocorticotropic hormone (ACTH) and luteinizing hormone (LH). LH stimulates testosterone production by the testes, and ACTH stimulates the adrenal glands to produce androstenedione and dehydroepiandrosterone, precursors of testosterone and dihydrotestosterone (DHT). Although the testes are the major source of testosterone, the adrenal glands can supply up to 20% of the DHT found in the prostate gland.

Androgen ablation therapy consists of either bilateral orchiectomy or LHRH agonists, which chronically stimulate the pituitary gland, resulting in a decrease in LH release. Decrease in LH leads to castrate levels of testosterone production by the testes. Flutamide, an antiandrogen, works by blocking uptake or binding of androgen in target tissues. Combination of flutamide with either surgical or medical androgen ablation is termed total androgen blockade.

Bilateral orchiectomy and LHRH agonists appear to have equal efficacy when used as monotherapy for metastatic prostate cancer. The Medical Research Council of the United Kingdom performed a randomized prospective trial with 934 patients and found that immediate androgen ablation delays disease progression and decreases pathologic fractures. We recommend immediate androgen suppression for select patients. Total androgen ablation with an LHRH agonist plus an antiandrogen is controversial. Many studies have shown no benefit of combined therapy with an antiandrogen versus LHRH agonist monotherapy. Intermittent androgen therapy has been demonstrated to improve quality of life, but its long-term effects on survival are unknown. The options for hormonally resistant metastatic prostate cancer are limited to palliation or chemotherapy as part of a clinical trial. The use of radiopharmaceutical agents such as strontium-89 is for palliation of metastatic bone disease only. The combination of estramustine plus taxanes are currently demonstrating activity against hormone-refractory prostate cancer, but their use has not advanced past the investigative stage.

BLADDER CANCER

Epidemiology and Etiology

Bladder cancer is the second most common genitourinary malignancy in the United States. It is the fourth most common cancer in men and the tenth most common cancer in women. In 2000, 53,200 new cases were reported and approximately 12,000 deaths were attributed to bladder cancer. The incidence is lowest in African-American females (6 per 100,000) and highest in white males (31 per 100,000). White males also have the highest mortality rate: 5.8 deaths per 100,000.

The etiology of urothelial cancers, of which bladder cancer is the most common, is well established. Cigarette smoking has been linked to 30% to 40% of all cases of bladder cancer. The chemicals 1-naphthylamine, 2-naphthylamine, benzidine, and 4-aminobiphenyl have been shown to promote urothelial carcinogenesis. Workers in the textile, leather, aluminum refining, rubber, and chemical industries who are exposed to high levels of these chemicals have an increased incidence of bladder cancer. Other chemicals that have been linked to urothelial cancer are MBUCCA (plastics industry), phenacetin, and the antineoplastic agent cyclophosphamide. In addition, recurrent bladder infections, as well as infections with the parasite *Schistosoma haematobium* have been associated with squamous cell carcinoma of the bladder.

Pathology

The urinary bladder is a hollow viscus that functions in both the storage and evacuation of urine. Histologically, the bladder is composed of mucosa, lamina propria, muscularis, and serosa (limited to the dome). Localized bladder cancer is classified as *superficial disease,* which is limited to the mucosa and lamina propria, or *invasive disease,* which extends into the muscularis and beyond. Approximately 70% of newly diagnosed bladder cancers are superficial, whereas the remaining 30% are invasive or metastatic. Once a bladder cancer extends through the basal layer of the mucosa, it may invade blood vessels and lymphatics, thereby providing a route of metastasis. Carcinoma *in situ,* an aggressive form of superficial disease, is composed of anaplastic cells limited to the mucosal layer.

The World Health Organization (WHO) classifies epithelial tumors of the bladder into four histologic types: transitional cell carcinoma (TCC) (91%), squamous cell carcinoma (7%), adenocarcinoma (2%), and undifferentiated carcinoma (<1%). However, up to 20% of TCCs contain areas of squamous differentiation, and up to 7% contain areas of adenomatous differentiation. The remainder of this section discusses TCC.

Clinical Presentation

Eighty percent of all patients who present with bladder carcinoma have gross or microscopic hematuria, typically painless and intermittent. Approximately 20% of patients complain of symptoms of vesical irritability, including urinary frequency, urgency, and dysuria. Other symptoms include pelvic pain, flank pain (from ureteral obstruction), and lower-extremity edema. Patients with systemic disease may present with anemia, weight loss, and bone pain.

Diagnosis

A patient who presents with hematuria or other symptoms of bladder cancer should undergo a thorough urologic evaluation consisting of a history, physical examination, urinalysis, intravenous urogram, and cystoscopic examination of the urinary bladder with barbotage of urine for cytologic examination. The most useful of these steps is the examination of the bladder using a rigid or flexible cystoscope. Papillary and sessile tumors are easily visualized through the cystoscope; carcinoma *in situ,* however, can appear as normal mucosa. Fewer than 60% of bladder tumors can be seen on an intravenous urogram, but this examination will also identify other abnormalities that may be present in the genitourinary tract. Urine cytology is reported as positive in 30% of patients with grade 1 tumors, 50% of patients with grade 2 tumors, and from 65% to 100% of patients with high grade tumors or carcinoma *in situ* (see next section for definition of grades).

Grading and Staging

The WHO uses a grading system based on the cytologic features of the tumor. Grade 1 represents a well-differentiated tumor; grade 2, a moderately differentiated tumor; and grade 3, a poorly differentiated bladder cancer.

Once a bladder tumor is diagnosed, the urologist must accurately stage the tumor. The initial transurethral resection of the bladder tumor (TURBT) will determine the histologic depth of invasion of the tumor as well as the presence or absence of dysplasia or carcinoma *in situ*. A bimanual examination should be performed at the time of resection to determine whether a mass is present and, if so, whether it is fixed or mobile.

Further workup for detecting metastasis consists of a CT scan, liver function tests, a chest radiograph, and a bone scan (if the alkaline phosphatase level is elevated or the patient's symptoms suggest systemic disease). American Joint Committee on Cancer International Union Against Cancer (TNM) staging systems are listed in Table 19-2.

Management

Superficial Bladder Cancer

Approximately two thirds of bladder cancers present as superficial disease (e.g., Ta, T1, or Tis). An estimated 70% of these superficial cancers are Ta and 30% are T1. Ten percent of all bladder cancers present with Tis or carcinoma in situ (CIS). After the initial treatment of superficial bladder cancer, the cancer can be cured, can recur with the same stage and grade, or can recur with progression of stage or grade. Risk factors associated with both disease recurrence and progression include a high tumor grade, lamina propria invasion, dysplasia elsewhere in the bladder, positive urinary cytology findings, tumor diameter larger than 5 cm, vascular or lymphatic invasion, multicentricity, and expression of either epidermal growth factor or transforming growth factor-alpha.

Initial treatment of superficial bladder cancer focuses on eradication of the existing disease and prophylaxis against disease recurrence or progression. TURBT has been the standard treatment for existing stage Ta and T1 tumors as well as visible stage Tis tumors. Laser fulguration is another therapeutic option that results in fewer bleeding complications. The advantage of transurethral

Table 19-2. Staging systems for bladder cancer

Primary tumor clinical (T)

TX	Primary tumor cannot be assessed
T0	No evidence of primary tumor
Ta	Noninvasive papillary carcinoma
Tis	Carcinoma in situ
T1	Tumor invades subepithelial connective tissue
T2	Tumor invades muscle
	T2a: Tumor invades superficial muscle
	T2b: Tumor invades deep muscle
T3	Tumor invades perivesical tissue
	T3a: Microscopically
	T3b: Macroscopically
T4	Invasion of any of the following: prostate gland, uterus, vagina, pelvic wall, or abdominal wall
	T4a: Tumor invades prostate, uterus, or vagina
	T4b: Tumor invades pelvic or abdominal wall

Regional lymph nodes (N)

NX	Regional lymph nodes cannot be assessed
N0	No regional lymph node metastasis
N1	Metastasis in single lymph node 2 cm or less in the largest dimension
N2	Metastasis in single lymph node greater than 2 cm in the largest dimension but less than 5 cm, or multiple lymph nodes, none larger than 5 cm in greatest dimension
N3	Metastasis in a lymph node larger than 5 cm in greatest dimension

Distant metastases (M)

MX	Distant metastasis cannot be assessed
M0	No distant metastasis
M1	Distant metastasis

resection over laser fulguration is that it provides tissue for histologic examination.

Patients with Tis, high-grade Ta or T1 lesions, multiple tumors, recurrent tumors, tumors larger than 5 cm, or persistently positive cytology findings may be candidates for adjuvant intravesical therapy. Intravesical agents can be used as therapeutic, adjuvant, or prophylactic treatment for bladder cancer. Thiotepa, mitomycin C, doxorubicin, and epirubicin are the chemotherapeutic agents used most frequently. Bacille Calmette-Guerin (BCG), a live attenuated tuberculosis organism, has become the most widely used intravesical agent in superficial bladder cancer. BCG enhances the patient's own immune response against the tumor, providing resistance to disease recurrence and progression. Although specific dose scheduling varies, most treatment regimens include intravesical treatment weekly for 4 to 8 weeks, followed by an optional series of maintenance treatments administered over many months. BCG has been shown to eliminate CIS in 80% of patients at a 5-year follow-up, reduce tumor recurrence rate for patients with T1 disease to 30% at 4 years, and eliminate residual tumor in up to 59% of patients. Maintenance therapy is controversial. Lamm et al. (2000) randomized 384 patients with superficial bladder cancer to receive induction and maintenance BCG or just induction BCG therapy only. Median recurrence-free survival time was longer for those who received induction and maintenance therapy; however, at 5-year follow-up there was no difference in survival.

There is good evidence that T1 high-grade cancer has a high rate of progression and therefore confers a high risk of death. Therefore, we recommend early radical cystectomy for select patients with high-grade T1 bladder cancer.

Invasive Bladder Cancer

Tumors that have penetrated the muscularis propria are considered invasive. Several options are available for treatment of patients with invasive tumors. A small subset of patients may be eligible for bladder-sparing therapy. Herr (2001) demonstrated a 76% overall survival rate, with 57% of the patients preserving their bladders in 45 patients treated with aggressive transurethral re-resection of invasive bladder tumors (median follow-up 61 months). Patients with a muscle-invasive tumor that is primary and solitary, does not have surrounding urothelial atypia, and allows for a 2-cm surgical margin may be candidates for partial cystectomy. At M.D. Anderson, data have shown that approximately 5% of patients are actually suitable for bladder-sparing surgery; 5-year survival rates have been comparable to those achieved with radical cystectomy.

Primary external beam radiation therapy has been used to treat invasive bladder cancer. Treatment protocols advocate doses of 65 to 70 Gy. Five-year survival rates range from 21% to 52% for stage B2 and from 18% to 30% for stage C. Local recurrence occurs in 50% to 70% of these patients. Stage T4 lesions fare worse, with 5-year survival rates consistently below 10%. Our experience at M.D. Anderson found a 26% 5-year survival rate with primary external beam radiation. Thus external beam radiation therapy may be useful in patients who do not wish to have surgery or for whom radical surgery is medically contraindicated; however, the survival rate for radiation therapy is less than that for radical surgery.

In an attempt to improve survival and bladder preservation rates, multimodality strategies have combined TURBT, chemotherapy, and radiation. Kachnic et al. from Massachusetts General Hospital (1997) reported on 106 patients with stages T2 to T4 bladder cancers who were treated with TURBT, 2 cycles of MCV, and 40 Gy radiation therapy plus concurrent cisplatin. Overall 5-year survival was 52% and overall 5-year survival rate with the bladder intact was 43%. These results are comparable to contemporary radical cystectomy series; however, this regimen involves significant morbidity and patient investment in complex treatment schedules. Moreover, patients are subjected to a considerable risk of eventual cystectomy and superficial bladder cancer recurrence.

Radical cystectomy with pelvic lymphadenectomy is performed with the intent of removing all localized and lymphatic disease. At M.D. Anderson, the 5-year actuarial survival rates for patients

with invasive bladder carcinoma after radical cystectomy alone
are 79% for stage B, 46% for stage C, 54% for stage D with nodal
spread, and 32% for stage D with visceral metastases. The local
recurrence rate is 7% and the operative mortality rate is 1.1%.
Fourteen percent of patients undergoing cystectomy with lymphadenectomy are found to have unsuspected metastases to the
pelvic lymph nodes. The majority of these cases involve one or
two nodes limited to an area below the bifurcation of the common
iliac arteries and medial to the external iliac artery.

Once a patient undergoes cystectomy, the ureters must be di-
verted into an alternate drainage system. The most common urinary diversion used today is the orthotopic urinary diversion with
an ileal segment used for bladder substitution. Patients who are
unable to undergo an orthotopic diversion include patients with
elevated serum creatinine, evidence of lymph node metastasis,
prostatic urethral invasive TCC or CIS, or inflammatory bowel
disease. Furthermore, these patients must be willing and able
to undergo a vigorous voiding re-education program. Radiation
therapy may render continence difficult; therefore, some patients
may not benefit from this type of diversion. In the end, if they are
unable to fulfill these criteria, then a cutaneous ileal conduit is
recommended.

Metastatic Disease

Cisplatin appears to be the single agent with the greatest activity against TCC of the bladder; however, single-agent therapy
response rates are only in the range of 10% to 30%. Traditionally,
chemotherapy for bladder cancer included cisplatin, methotrexate, vinblastine, and doxorubicin (M-VAC). In the M.D. Anderson
trial of M-VAC, a complete response rate of 35% and a partial response rate of 30% were observed. Other trials have documented
similar response rates, with median survival of approximately
1 year. Newer regimens using gemcitabine and cisplatin have
demonstrated no significant difference in survival when compared to M-VAC, but adverse side effects are less with the newer
regimen.

At M.D. Anderson, adjuvant and neoadjuvant chemotherapy is
used for select patients with unfavorable disease characteristics.
Unfavorable features include resected nodal metastases, extrave-
sical involvement, lymphovascular permeation, or involvement
of pelvic viscera. Previously, treatment in select patients with adjuvant chemotherapy at M.D. Anderson resulted in a 70% 5-year
survival rate, which is comparable to patients without unfavorable features. Randomized prospective trials are now being completed to confirm these results for neoadjuvant chemotherapy.

RENAL CANCER

Epidemiology and Etiology

Tumors of the renal and perirenal tissues comprise 3% of cancer incidence and mortality in the United States. Renal cell carcinoma (RCC) represents 85% of all renal parenchymal tumors
and is the only renal tumor discussed in this chapter. In 2000, an
estimated 31,200 people were diagnosed with kidney cancer and
11,900 people died of this disease. From 1975 to 1995, both the

incidence and mortality rates of RCC have increased. The upward trend in mortality rates suggests that the increased incidental diagnosis of early stage asymptomatic tumors does not fully account for the overall increase in incidence. Males are affected twice as often as females. RCC most frequently occurs in the fifth to sixth decades of life.

Several risk factors have been identified to be associated with RCC. Case-control studies have found strong correlations with smoking and obesity. Hypertension and diuretic use have also been found to be associated with RCC; however, it is unclear if this is a causal relationship. RCC can occur either sporadically or genetically. Hereditary RCC tends to occur at an earlier age of onset and tends to be bilateral and multifocal. A well-described familial syndrome is von Hippel-Lindau (VHL) disease, which is characterized by cerebellar hemangioblastoma, retinal angiomata, bilateral RCC, and islet cell tumors of the pancreas. Both sporadic and VHL disease types have a common genetic mechanism that includes loss of a region of chromosome 3. Hereditary nonpapillary RCC is an autosomal dominant syndrome associated with the same chromosome 3 abnormalities, while hereditary papillary RCC is an autosomal dominant syndrome associated with abnormalities of the *met* gene on chromosome 7. RCC is also associated with polycystic kidney disease, "horseshoe kidneys," and acquired renal cystic disease.

Pathology

Most RCCs originate in the proximal tubular cells of the kidney. The tumor is multifocal in 6.5% to 10% of cases. The renal capsule and Gerota's fascia surrounding the kidney limit local extension of the tumor. The predominant cell type is clear cell, but granular and spindle-shaped cells also may be present. The tumor cells are typically rich in glycogen and lipid, giving the tumor a clear cell appearance microscopically and a characteristic yellow appearance grossly.

Clinical Presentation

RCC was traditionally called the "internist's tumor" because of its subtle presentation. Now more than 40% of clinically unsuspected tumors are found incidentally by abdominal imaging done for other reasons. Gross or microscopic hematuria, the most common presenting symptom, is present in more than half of patients with RCC. The classic triad of hematuria, abdominal mass, and flank pain occurs in approximately 19% of patients. Paraneoplastic syndromes occur in 10% to 40% of cases and consist of pyrexia, anemia, erythrocytosis, hypercalcemia, liver dysfunction (Stauffer's syndrome), and hypertension. Other symptoms can include bone pain and central nervous system abnormalities, as up to 30% of patients present with bone and brain metastases.

Diagnosis

The workup of a patient with the preceding symptoms should include a history, physical examination, complete blood cell count, serum chemistry panel, urinalysis, urine culture, and a contrast-enhanced CT scan. In most cases, the CT scan will define the nature of the mass. If any of the studies obtained suggests involvement of the renal vein or vena cava, an MRI should be obtained to assess the extent of the tumor thrombus. In contrast to the management of other renal tumors, RCC may be treated surgically without preoperative histologic diagnosis of the tumor.

If a mass suggests RCC, a metastatic workup consisting of a chest radiograph, CT scan (if not already obtained), and liver function tests should be performed. The most common sites of metastases of RCC in decreasing order are the lung, bone, and regional lymph nodes. If the patient does not have an increased alkaline phosphatase level or skeletal pain, a bone scan is usually not required. A CT scan of the brain can be performed if there is any suspicion of brain metastases; however, this is not done routinely.

Grading and Staging

The most widely used grading system for RCC is the Fuhrman system, which is based on nuclear morphology. Recently, the WHO classified the sarcomatoid variant separately as spindle cell carcinoma. Patients with this classification seem to fare slightly worse than those with the granular or clear cell type, and it is generally agreed that the sarcomatoid cell type is found in more aggressive tumors.

The TNM system is the most commonly used for staging in the United States. Please refer to Table 19-3.

Table 19-3. Staging systems for renal cell cancer

Primary tumor clinical (T)

TX	Primary tumor cannot be assessed
T0	No evidence of primary tumor
T1	Tumor 7 cm or less in greatest dimension, limited to the kidney
T2	Tumor 7 cm or more in greatest dimension, limited to the kidney
T3	Tumor extends into major veins or invades adrenal gland or perinephric tissues but not beyond Gerota's fascia
	T3a: Tumor invades adrenal gland or perinephric tissues but not beyond Gerota's fascia
	T3b: Tumor grossly extends into renal vein(s) or vena cava below diaphragm
	T3c: Tumor grossly extends into vena cava above diaphragm
T4	Tumor invades beyond Gerota's fascia

Regional lymph nodes (N)

NX	Regional lymph nodes cannot be assessed
N0	No regional lymph node metastasis
N1	Metastasis in single regional lymph node
N2	Metastasis in multiple regional, contralateral, or bilateral nodes

Distant metastases (M)

MX	Distant metastasis cannot be assessed
M0	No distant metastasis
M1	Distant metastasis

Management

Localized Renal Cell Carcinoma

Surgical excision is the only effective treatment of localized RCC. In a radical nephrectomy, the kidney, ipsilateral adrenal gland, and surrounding Gerota's fascia are all resected en bloc. Although no randomized study has proved its benefit over simple nephrectomy, radical nephrectomy has the theoretical advantage of removing the lymphatics within the perinephric fat. Up to 20% of patients have evidence of regional lymphatic metastases without distant disease. The 5-year survival rates for patients with positive lymph nodes range from 8% to 35%. Extended lymphadenectomy has never been proved to be of benefit in patients who undergo radical nephrectomy, and many surgeons prefer a limited node dissection, which has limited morbidity, for prognostic information.

The surgical approach to radical nephrectomy is determined by the size and location of the tumor as well as the surgeon's preference. A modified flank, midline, or subcostal (chevron) incision can be used. Large upper-pole tumors may be approached through a thoracoabdominal incision for greater exposure. Because the incidence of ipsilateral adrenal metastasis in lower-pole tumors is rare, not to removing the adrenal gland at the time of nephrectomy for a lower-pole lesion is accepted.

Approximately 15% to 20% of RCCs invade the renal vein and 8% to 15% invade the vena cava. Involvement of RCC in the renal vein usually does not pose a significant problem. Vena caval involvement, however, may require additional extensive procedures. Vena caval thrombi have been divided by many authors into three groups. Type 1 thrombi (50%) are completely infrahepatic, type 2 (40%) are intrahepatic, and type 3 (10%) extend up into the right atrium of the heart. In cases with vena caval involvement, it is imperative that the surgeon be familiar with techniques of vascular surgery, and consideration should be given to consulting with a cardiothoracic surgeon, especially for type 3 thrombi.

There are situations in which nephron-sparing surgery is indicated for patients with RCC. For example, in cases of bilateral tumor involvement, renal insufficiency, solitary kidney, or VHL, a parenchyma-sparing procedure may be indicated. In this procedure, the renal artery is temporarily occluded, the kidney cooled down, and partial nephrectomy or wedge resection performed. Frozen sections of the surgical margins are typically analyzed to ensure adequacy of resection. After restoration of arterial blood flow, the renal capsule is closed or, alternatively, omentum or perirenal fat is sutured to the defect to promote healing. Five-year survival rates after partial nephrectomy for patients with stage I or II disease are approximately 70% and 60%, respectively.

Although radical nephrectomy remains the standard treatment in patients with localized RCC and a normal contralateral kidney, nephron-sparing surgery for patients with a tumor 4 cm or less yields 5-year cancer-specific survival rates of 92% to 97%. The incidence of tumor recurrence within the renal remnant is reported to be from 0% to 6%. Therefore, nephron-sparing surgery and radical nephrectomy provide equally effective curative treatments for single, small, well-localized tumors.

Advanced Renal Cell Carcinoma

Approximately 10% of patients present with locally advanced disease that has invaded adjacent structures. In general, the 3-year survival rate for these patients after surgery is less than 10%. Nephrectomy in this situation is done to improve the quality of life for symptomatic patients rather than to prolong survival. Nephrectomy has also been performed in the presence of metastatic disease to as part of clinical protocols that require removal of the primary lesion.

Distant metastatic disease can be categorized as a solitary metastasis or bulky metastatic disease. Several studies have shown higher 3-year survival rates, ranging from 20% to 60%, after radical nephrectomy with removal of a solitary metastasis. Solitary lung metastases appear to be associated with better survival rates than metastases to other organ sites.

Cytotoxic chemotherapy is ineffective in RCC; the highest objective response rate for single-agent therapy is only 16%. Interleukin-2 (IL-2) has yielded durable response rates of 15% to 19% in various trials. Whether nephrectomy will augment this response is unclear. Given the poor response rates to stimulate the immune systems of patients with metastatic renal cell carcinoma, new biologic therapies have shifted toward transplantation of either dendritic cells or bone marrow from suitable donors.

TESTICULAR CANCER

Epidemiology and Etiology

Malignant tumors of the testis are rare. It is estimated that 6,900 cases of testis cancer were diagnosed in 2000, but only 300 men will die of this disease. Ninety-five percent of these tumors are of germ cell origin. Although testis tumors can occur at any age, specific tumor types tend to occur at different ages. Choriocarcinomas tend to occur between 24 and 28 years of age, embryonal carcinomas from 26 to 34 years of age, seminomas from 32 to 42 years of age, and lymphomas and spermatocytic seminomas after the age of 50 years.

The most well known etiologic factor in the development of testis cancer is cryptorchidism. Between 3% and 11% of all cases of testis cancer occur in cryptorchid testes. Although trauma to the testis has been linked to testis cancer, there is no evidence of a definite relationship.

Carcinoma in situ is a precursor of testicular germ cell cancer. Five percent to 6% of men with a unilateral germ cell tumor have CIS in the contralateral testis and a germ cell tumor will develop in 50% of these men. Other men with a high risk of CIS are individuals with intersex, cryptorchidism, infertility, or an extragonadal germ cell tumor.

Clinical Presentation

Testicular cancer typically presents as a painless testicular enlargement. Advanced disease can present as back pain, flank pain, or systemic symptoms. The differential diagnosis includes varicocele, hydrocele, hematoma, epididymitis, orchitis, and inguinal hernia.

Diagnosis

Although the diagnosis is usually evident at physical examination to an experienced clinician, scrotal ultrasound can be useful in establishing the diagnosis. Any solid testicular mass is considered a testicular tumor until proved otherwise. Once a testicular tumor is suspected, the patient's levels of the tumor markers alpha-fetoprotein (AFP) and human chorionic gonadotropin (hCG) should be tested. Following this, he should undergo a radical (inguinal) orchiectomy. There is no role for fine-needle aspiration or Tru-cut biopsy in the workup of this disease.

After radical orchiectomy, a CT scan of the chest, abdomen, and pelvis should be performed. If they were initially elevated, tumor markers should be reanalyzed following orchiectomy, after allowing the appropriate time for each marker to return to baseline.

Staging

The American Joint Committee on Cancer and International Union Against Cancer TNM testicular cancer staging system is outlined in Table 19-4. In terms of biologic behavior and therapy, testicular tumors can be categorized as seminomatous or nonseminomatous germ cell tumors (NSGCT). Seminomas are radiation-sensitive and chemosensitive tumors that undergo lymphatic spread in an orderly fashion. In contrast, NSGCT are less radiation-sensitive and have a higher metastatic rate than seminomas.

Management

Seminomatous Germ Cell Tumors

After radical orchiectomy, stage I and IIA seminomas are typically treated with radiation therapy to the ipsilateral iliac and periaortic areas up to the level of the diaphragm after radical orchiectomy. Using radiation therapy, the cure rate for stage I disease approaches 100%. Although 10% to 15% of patients with stage IIA disease have relapses, more than half of these respond successfully to salvage therapy, yielding a survival rate of 95% for patients with stage IIA disease.

Stage IIB or III disease is usually treated with cisplatin- or carboplatin-based chemotherapy. Surgery is generally reserved for lymphatic disease that does not respond to chemotherapy or radiation therapy. Using this approach, 5-year disease-free survival rates of 86% and 92% have been obtained for patients with stages IIB and III disease, respectively.

Nonseminomatous Germ Cell Tumors

The optimal therapy for stage I disease is controversial; options include surveillance, retroperitoneal lymph node dissection (RPLND), and primary systemic chemotherapy. Overall, approximately 20% to 30% of patients with stage I disease who undergo surveillance experience relapse. Wishnow et al. (1989) at M.D. Anderson Cancer Center found that patients with vascular invasion in their tumor, AFP levels greater than 80 ng/mL, or more than 80% embryonal elements in their tumor were at high risk for relapse. High-risk patients have been offered two courses of carboplatin, etoposide, and bleomycin (CEB). Low-risk patients are offered observation. At 30 months follow-up, no patients treated with CEB experienced relapse.

Table 19-4. AJCC/IUAC systems for testicular cancer

Primary tumor clinical (T)

pTX	Primary tumor cannot be assessed
pT0	No evidence of primary tumor (scar in testis)
pTis	Intratubular germ cell neoplasia (carcinoma in situ)
pT1	Tumor limited to the testis and epididymis and no vascular/lymphatic invasion
	Tumor may invade into the tunica albuginaea but not the tunica vaginalis
pT2	Tumor limited to the testis and epididymis with vascular/lymphatic invasion or tumor invading into the tunica albuginaea with involvement of the tunica vaginalis
pT3	Tumor invades the spermatic cord with or without vascular/lymphatic invasion
pT4	Tumor invades the scrotum with or without vascular/lymphatic invasion

Regional lymph nodes (N)

NX	Regional lymph nodes cannot be assessed
N0	No regional lymph node metastasis
N1	Lymph node mass 2 cm or less in greatest dimension; or multiple lymph nodes masses, none more than 2 cm in greatest dimension.
N2	Lymph node mass, more than 2 cm but not more than 5 cm in greatest dimension; or multiple lymph node masses, any one mass greater than 2 cm but not more than 5 cm in greatest dimension.
N3	Lymph node mass more than 5 cm in greatest dimension.

Distant metastases (M)

MX	Distant metastasis cannot be assessed
M0	Nonregional nodal or pulmonary metastasis
M1	Nonpulmonary viseral metastases

Serum tumor markers

Stage	LDH	hCG (mIU/mL)	AFP (ng/mL)
S0	$\leq$ Normal	$\leq$ N	$\leq$ N
S1	< 1.5 X Normal	< 5,000	< 1,000
S2	1.5–10 X Normal	5,000–50,000	1,000–10,000
S3	> 10 X Normal	> 50,000	> 10,000

Stage		LDH	hCG (mIU/mL)	AFP (ng/mL)
Stage 0		pTis	N0	M0	S0
Stage I					
	IA	T1	N0	M0	S0
	IB	T2–T4	N0	M0	S0
	IS	Any T	N0	M0	S1–S3
Stage II					
	IIA	Any T	N1	M0	S0–1
	IIB	Any T	N2	M0	S0–1
	IIC	Any T	N3	M0	S0–1
Stage III					
	IIIA	Any T	Any N	M1	S0–1
	IIIB	Any T	Any N	M0–1	S2
	IIIC	Any T	Any N	M0–1	S3

AFP, alpha-fetoprotein; AJCC, American Joint Committee on Cancer; hCG, human chorionic gonadotropin; IUAC, International Union Against Cancer; LDH, lactic dehydrogenase.

The recurrence rate after RPLND for low-volume stage II disease is less than 20%. Thus both RPLND and primary systemic chemotherapy have been used to treat low-volume retroperitoneal disease. Survival rates of 97% or better have been associated with both forms of therapy. At M.D. Anderson, patients with stage II disease are treated with primary chemotherapy, and RPLND is used to remove residual disease.

Because of the high recurrence rates associated with RPLND for stage IIB, IIC, and III NSGCTs, primary systemic chemotherapy is the treatment of choice for this disease. RPLND is used to remove any residual disease that may be present after primary chemotherapy and to determine the need for further therapy. Recent experience with chemotherapy for advanced NSGCT at M. D. Anderson has shown 5-year survival rates of 96% and 76% for low- and high-volume stage III disease, respectively.

Because a majority of NSGCTs produce either AFP or β-hCG, these markers are helpful in monitoring the patient for treatment response and recurrent disease.

Despite the relatively early age of onset of testis cancer, this disease remains one of the most curable cancers in humans.

RECOMMENDED READING

Prostate Cancer

Brawn PN, Ayala AG, von Eschenbach AC, et al. Histologic grading study of prostate adenocarcinoma: the development of a new system and comparison of other methods—a preliminary study. *Cancer* 1982;49:525.

Catalona WJ, Richie JP, Ahmann FR, et al. Comparison of DRE and serum PSA in the early detection of prostate cancer. *J Urol* 1994;151:1283–1290.

Catalona WJ, Partin AW, Slawin KM, et al. Use of percentage of free prostate specific antigen to enhance the differentiation of prostate cancer from benign prostatic disease: a prospective multicenter clinical trial. *JAMA* 1998;297:1542–1547.

Chybowski FM, Keller JJ, Bergstralh EJ, et al. Predicting radionucleotide bone scan findings in patients with newly diagnosed untreated prostate cancer: prostate specific antigen is superior to all other clinical parameters. *J Urol* 1991;145:313.

Cooner WH, Mosley BR, Rutherford JR, et al. Prostate cancer detection in a clinical urological practice by ultrasonography, digital rectal examination and prostate specific antigen. *J Urol* 1990;143:1146.

Laufer M, Denmeade SR, Sinibaldi J, et al. Complete androgen blockade for prostate cancer: what went wrong? *J Urol* 2000;164(1): 3–9.

Leandri P, Rossignol G, Gautier JR, et al. Radical retropubic prostatectomy: morbidity and quality of life. Experience with 620 consecutive cases. *J Urol* 1992;147:883.

McNeal JE, Redwine EA, Freiha FS, et al. Zonal distribution of prostatic adenocarcinoma. *Am J Surg Pathol* 1988;12:897.

The Medical Research Council Prostate Cancer Working Party Investigations Group. Immediate versus deferred treatment for advanced prostate cancer: initial results of the Medical Research Council Trial. *Br J Urol* 1997;79:235.

National Institutes of Health. Consensus development conference on the management of clinically localized prostate cancer (1987: Bethesda, MD). NCI monograph no. 7, NIH publication no. 88-3005. Washington, DC: US Government Printing Office, 1988:3–6.

Oesterling JE. Using PSA to eliminate the staging radionuclide bone scan. Significant economic implications. *Urol Clin North Am* 1993; 20(4):671–680.

Osterling JE, Martin SK, Bergstrlh EJ, et al. The use of prostate specific antigen in staging patients with newly diagnosed prostate cancer. *JAMA* 1993;269:57–60.

Ries LAG, Wingo PA, Miller DS, et al. The annual report to the nation on the status of cancer, 1973–1997, with a special section on colorectal cancer. *Cancer* 2000;88(10):2398–2422.

Scardino PT, Frankel JM, Wheeler TM, et al. The prognostic significance of post-irradiation biopsy results in patients with prostate cancer. *J Urol* 1986;135:510.

Stamey TA, McNeal JE. Adenocarcinoma of the prostate. In: Walsh PC, Retik AB, Stamey TA, et al., eds. *Campbell's urology,* 8th ed. Philadelphia: Saunders, 1998.

Vogelzang NJ, Scardino PT, Shipley WU, et al. *Comprehensive textbook of genitourinary oncology,* 2nd ed. Philadelphia: Lippincott Williams & Wilkins, 2000.

Zagars GK, von Eschenbach AC, Johnson DE, et al. The role of radiation therapy in stages A2 and B adenocarcinoma of the prostate. *Int J Radiat Oncol Biol Phys* 1988;14:701.

Zagars GK, Pollack A, von Eschenbach AC. Management of unfavorable locoregional prostate carcinoma with radiation and androgen ablation. *Cancer* 1997;80(4):764–772.

Zinke H, Bergstralh EJ, Blute ML, et al. Radical prostatectomy for clinically localized prostate cancer, long term results of 1,143 patients from a single institution. *J Clin Oncol* 1994;12(11):2254–2263.

Bladder Cancer

Catalona WJ. Bladder cancer. In: Gillenwater JY, Grayhack JT, Howards SS, et al., eds. *Adult and pediatric urology.* Chicago: Year Book Medical Publishers, 1987.

Cummings KB, Barone JG, Ward WS. Diagnosis and staging of bladder cancer. *Urol Clin North Am* 1992;19:429.

Heney NM, Ahmad S, Flanagan MJ, et al. Superficial bladder cancer: progression and recurrence. *J Urol* 1983;130:1083.

Herr HW. Transurethral resection of muscle invasive bladder cancer. *J Clin Oncol* 2001;19(1):81–93.

Herr HW. Tumour progression and survival in patients with T1G3 bladder tumors: 15 year outcome. *Br J Urol* 1997;80(5):762–765.

Kachnic LA, Kaufman DS, Heney NM, et al. Bladder preservation by combined modality therapy for invasive bladder cancer. *J Clin Oncol* 1997;15:1022.

Lamm DL. Long term results of intravesical therapy for superficial bladder cancer. *Urol Clin North Am* 1992;19:573.

Lamm DL, Blumenstein BA, Crissman JD, et al. Maintenance bacillus Calmette-Guerin immunotherapy for recurrent TA, T1 and carcinoma in situ transitional cell carcinoma of the bladder: a randomized Southwest Oncology Group Study. *J Urol* 2000;163(4): 1124–1129.

Logothetis CJ, Dexeus FH, Finn L, et al. A prospective randomized trial comparing MVAC and CISCA chemotherapy for patients with metastatic urothelial tumors. *J Clin Oncol* 1990;8:1050.

Logothetis CJ, Johnson DE, Chong C, et al. Adjuvant cyclophosphamide, doxorubicin, and cisplatin chemotherapy for bladder cancer: an update. *J Clin Oncol* 1988;6:1590–1596.

Logothetis C, Swanson D, Amato R, et al. Optimal delivery of perioperative chemotherapy: preliminary results of a randomized, prospective, comparative trial of preoperative and postoperative chemotherapy for invasive bladder carcinoma. *J Urol* 1996;155(4):1241–1245.

Pollack A, Zagars GK, Swanson DA. Muscle-invasive bladder cancer treated with external beam radiotherapy: prognostic factors. *Int J Radiat Oncol Biol Phys* 1994;30:267–277.

Stockle M, Wellek S, Meyenburg W, et al. Radical cystectomy with or without adjuvant polychemotherapy for non-organ-confined transitional cell carcinoma of the urinary bladder: prognostic impact of lymph node involvement. *Urol* 1996;48(6):868–875.

Vogelzang NJ, Scardino PT, Shipley WU, et al. *Comprehensive textbook of genitourinary oncology,* 2nd ed. Philadelphia: Lippincott Williams & Wilkins, 2000.

Renal Cancer

Couillard DR, deVere White RW. Surgery of renal cell carcinoma. *Urol Clin North Am* 1993;20:263.

Kletcher BA, Qian J, Bostwick DG, et al. Prospective analysis of multifocality in renal cell carcinoma: influence of histological pattern, grade, size, number, volume, and DNA ploidy. *J Urol* 1995;153:904–906.

Ries LAG, Kosay CL, Hankey BF, et al., eds. *SEER cancer statistics review, 1973–1995.* Bethesda, MD: National Cancer Institute, 1998.

Williams RD. Renal, perirenal, and ureteral neoplasms. In: Gillenwater JY, Grayhack JT, Howards SS, et al., eds. *Adult and pediatric urology.* Chicago: Year Book Medical Publishers, 1987.

Wirth MP. Immunotherapy for metastatic renal cell carcinoma. *Urol Clin North Am* 1993;20:283.

Testis Cancer

Amato R. Chemotherapy for stage I and II testis cancer. In: Vogelzang NJ, Scardino PT, Shipley WU, et al., eds. *Comprehensive textbook of genitourinary oncology,* 2nd ed. Philadelphia: Lippincott Williams & Wilkins, 2000.

Amato R, Banks E, Ro J, Swanson DA. Post-ochiectomy adjuvant chemotherapy for patients with stage I non-seminomatous germ cell tumors of the testis (NGCTT) at high risk of relapse. *Proc AUA* 1999;161[S]:157[abst 604].

Logothetis CJ. The case for relevant staging of germ cell tumors. *Cancer* 1990;65:709.

Sternberg CN. Role of primary chemotherapy in stage I and low-volume stage II non-seminomatous germ-cell testis tumors. *Urol Clin North Am* 1993;20:93.

Wishnow KI, Johnson DE, Swanson DA, et al. Identifying patients with low-risk clinical stage I non-seminomatous testicular tumors who should be treated by surveillance. *Urol* 1989;34:339.

Gynecologic Cancers

Michael W. Bevers, Diane C. Bodurka Bevers,
and Judith K. Wolf

The surgical oncologist and the gynecologic oncologist share a common territory—the abdomen. The surgical oncologist must at a minimum maintain a familiarity with all oncologic processes affecting the abdominal cavity. Unfortunately, the subspecialization of medicine not only challenges physicians to keep pace with advances in their own fields, but also makes learning about advances and trends in other fields a Herculean task. This chapter discusses the basics of gynecologic oncology so that these disease processes are considered when examining patients and appropriate management occurs when encountering these neoplasms unexpectedly. Emphasis is placed on diagnosis, staging, and surgical management.

VULVAR CANCER

Incidence

Vulvar cancer accounts for 3% to 5% of all female genital malignancies and 1% of all malignancies in women. Between 2,000 and 3,000 new cases are diagnosed annually. The average age at diagnosis is 65, with the trend toward younger age at time of diagnosis.

Risk Factors

The cause of vulvar cancer appears to be multifactorial; this disease is not as strongly associated with human papillomavirus as is cervical cancer. Risk factors include advanced age, low socioeconomic status, hypertension, diabetes mellitus, prior lower genital tract malignancy (cervical cancer), and immunosuppressed status.

Pathology

Eighty-five percent of vulvar malignancies are squamous cell carcinomas; 6% of cases are malignant melanomas.

Routes of Spread

Vulvar cancer spreads by direct extension, embolization to regional lymphatics (groin), and hematogenous spread to distant sites.

Clinical Features

Symptoms
Chronic pruritus, ulceration, and the presence of nodules are symptoms of this disease.

Physical Findings

Lesions arise from the labia majora (40%), labia minora (20%), periclitoral area (10%), and perineum/posterior fourchette (15%). Lesions may appear as a dominant mass, warty area, ulcerated area, or thickened white epithelium.

Diagnosis

Five percent of cases are multifocal. It is critical to biopsy any suspicious area. Use a Keye's punch biopsy and lidocaine without epinephrine for anesthesia. Most patients tolerate mild discomfort well.

Pretreatment Workup

Careful physical examination, including pelvic examination and measurement of the lesion, is required. Other components of the pretreatment workup include complete blood cell count, serum glucose, blood urea nitrogen, creatinine, and liver function tests; chest radiograph; mammogram; and cystoscopy or proctoscopy, depending on site and extent of lesion. Barium enema, computed tomography (CT), or magnetic resonance imaging (MRI) should be performed if indicated. Preoperative medical clearance is necessary for patients with chronic disease or other appropriate indications.

Staging

Since 1988, vulvar cancer has been surgically staged using a system that incorporates the TNM (tumor, node, metastasis) classification; modifications to the TNM system were added in 1995 (Table 20-1).

Treatment of Vulvar Cancer by Stage

Stage I

Wide local excision should be performed if the lesion is microinvasive (<1 mm invasion). Radical wide excision with a traditional 2-cm gross margin (measured with ruler) and superficial dissection of the ipsilateral groin is appropriate for all other stage I lesions. Bilateral superficial groin dissection should be performed if the lesion is within 1 cm of the midline.

Stage II

Radical vulvectomy with bilateral node dissection, including superficial and deep inguinal nodes, is the standard approach to stage II disease. A more conservative approach used at M.D. Anderson Cancer Center is radical wide excision instead of radical vulvectomy; local recurrence rates are similar. Adjuvant radiation therapy may be indicated if the tumor-free margin of resection is less than 8 mm, tumor thickness is greater than 5 mm, or lymphovascular space invasion is present.

Stage III

Treatment must be individualized for each patient with stage III disease. Options include surgery, radiation, or a combination of treatment modalities, again depending on each patient's case. A

Table 20-1. Surgical staging of vulvar cancer

Stage	Classification	Description
IA	T1N0M0	Tumor confined to the vulva and/or perineum; lesion is 2 cm or less in diameter with stromal invasion no greater than 1 mm; negative nodes.
IB	T1N0M0	Tumor confined to the vulva and/or perineum; lesion is 2 cm or less in diameter with stromal invasion greater than 1 mm; negative nodes.
II	T2N0M0	Tumor confined to the vulva and/or perineum; lesion is greater than 2 cm in diameter; negative nodes.
III	T3N0M0 T1N1M0 T3N1M T2N1M0	Tumor of any size with adjacent spread to the lower urethra and/or vagina, the anus, or unilateral regional lymph node metastasis.
IVA	T1N2M0 T3N2M0 T4, any N, M0	Tumor invades the upper urethra, bladder mucosa, rectal mucosa, pelvic bone, and/or bilateral regional metastasis.
IVB	Any T or N, M1	Any distant metastasis, including pelvic nodes.

modified radical vulvectomy (radical wide local excision is used in some institutions) with inguinal and femoral node dissection can be performed; pelvic and groin radiation therapy are administered with positive groin nodes. Preoperative radiation therapy (with or without radiation-sensitizing chemotherapy) can be given to increase the operability and decrease the extent of resection. This is followed by radical excision with bilateral superficial and deep groin node dissection. Radiation therapy alone is an option if the patient or extent of lesion is deemed unsuitable for radical surgery.

Stage IV

Treatment of stage IV disease must also be individualized for each patient. Options include radical vulvectomy and pelvic exenteration, radical vulvectomy followed by radiation therapy, preoperative radiation therapy (with or without radiation-sensitizing chemotherapy) followed by radical surgical excision, and radiation therapy (with or without radiation-sensitizing chemotherapy) if the patient is not eligible for surgery or the lesion is deemed inoperable.

Recurrent Disease

Treatment of recurrent disease depends on the site and extent of the recurrence. Options include radical wide excision with or without radiation therapy (depending on prior treatment and extent of recurrence), groin node debulking followed by radiation

Table 20-2. Five-year survival rates for vulvar cancer (by stage)

Stage I	95%
Stage II	75%–85%
Stage III	5%
Stage IVA	20%
Stage IVB	5%

therapy (depends on prior treatment), and pelvic exenteration. Patients with regional or distant metastasis are more difficult to treat; often palliative therapy is the only option.

Prognostic Factors

There are a variety of prognostic factors for vulvar carcinoma. Inguinal node metastasis appears to be the single most important prognostic variable (Table 20-2). Other factors include lymphovascular space invasion, and stage, including lesion size, site of lesion, histologic grade, and depth of invasion.

Recommended Surveillance

Physical and pelvic examinations should be performed every 3 months the first year, every 4 months in years 2 and 3, every 6 months in years 4 and 5, and once a year thereafter. A Papanicolaou smear should be performed annually.

VAGINAL CANCER

Incidence

Primary vaginal cancer represents 1% to 2% of malignancies of the female genital tract. The average age at diagnosis is 60 years. Most vaginal neoplasms represent metastases from another primary source.

Risk Factors

A variety of risk factors are associated with vaginal cancer, including low socioeconomic status, history of human papillomavirus infection, chronic vaginal irritation, and prior abnormal Papanicolaou smear with cervical intraepithelial neoplasia. Other factors are prior hysterectomy (59% of patients with primary vaginal cancer), prior treatment for cervical cancer, and in utero exposure to diethylstilbestrol during the first half of pregnancy. Diethylstilbestrol was used to prevent complications of pregnancy such as threatened abortion and prematurity from 1940 to 1971; clear cell carcinoma of the vagina develops in approximately 1 in 1,000 women exposed to diethylstilbestrol in utero. The peak age at diagnosis is 19 years.

Pathology

Eighty-five percent of vaginal cancers are squamous cell neoplasms. Other histologic subtypes include adenocarcinomas (9%), sarcomas (6%), melanomas, clear cell carcinoma, and other rare histologies.

Routes of Spread

Vaginal cancer metastasizes via direct extension to adjacent structures. It can also spread through a well-established lymphatic drainage distribution. Lesions of the upper two thirds of the vagina metastasize directly to pelvic lymph nodes. Lesions of the lower one third of the vagina metastasize primarily to the inguinofemoral nodes and secondarily to pelvic nodes. Hematogenous spread represents late occurrence because disease is confined primarily to the pelvis in the majority of cases.

Clinical Features

Symptoms

Painless vaginal bleeding and vaginal discharge are the primary symptoms associated with vaginal cancer. Bladder symptoms, tenesmus, and pelvic pain, which is usually indicative of locally advanced disease, are less commonly seen.

Physical Findings

Lesions are located primarily in the upper one third of the vagina, usually on the posterior wall. The appearance of lesions varies, ranging from exophytic to endophytic. Surface ulceration is usually not present except in advanced cases.

Visualization of lesions identified by Papanicolaou smear may require colposcopy.

Pretreatment Workup

Careful physical examination, including pelvic examination with colposcopy, is required, unless the lesion is visible. Other components of the pretreatment workup include complete blood cell count, serum glucose, blood urea nitrogen, creatinine, and liver function tests; chest radiograph; mammogram; and cystoscopy or proctoscopy, depending on site and extent of lesion. Barium enema, CT, or MRI should be performed if indicated. Preoperative medical clearance is necessary for patients with chronic disease or other appropriate indications.

Staging

The clinical staging scheme for vaginal cancers is outlined in Table 20-3.

Treatment of Vaginal Cancer by Stage

Stage 0

Stage 0 disease may be treated by surgical excision, laser ablation, and, in some cases, topical 5-fluorouracil.

Stage I

Lesions of the upper vaginal fornices may be treated with radical hysterectomy and lymphadenectomy or radiation therapy alone. All stage I lesions (including lesions of the upper vaginal fornices) may be treated with radiation therapy, usually in the form of an intracavitary cylinder.

Table 20-3. Clinical staging of vaginal cancer

Stage	Description
0	Carcinoma in situ, intraepithelial carcinoma
I	Carcinoma limited to vaginal wall
II	Carcinoma involves subvaginal tissue but does not extend to pelvic wall
III	Extension to pelvic wall
IV	Extension beyond the true pelvis or involvement of bladder or rectal mucosa
IVA	Spread to adjacent organs and/or direct extension beyond the pelvis
IVB	Spread to distant organs

Stages II–IV

External-beam radiation therapy and intracavitary or interstitial therapy are used for stage II to IV disease. The groin should be treated if the lower one third of the vagina is involved with tumor.

Recurrent Disease

Treatment of recurrent disease depends on the extent of recurrence. Options include wide local excision, partial vaginectomy, and exenteration. Chemotherapy may be given for distant metastatic disease; however, the role of chemotherapy is unclear because of the rarity of the disease.

Prognostic Factors

The most important prognostic factor for vaginal cancer is the stage of disease (Table 20-4).

Recommended Surveillance

Physical and pelvic examinations should be performed every 3 months the first year, every 4 months in years 2 and 3, every 6 months in years 4 and 5, and once a year thereafter. A Papanicolaou smear should be performed annually.

CERVICAL CANCER

Incidence

Approximately 15,000 new cases of cervical cancer are reported annually, and there are approximately 4,000 to 5,000 annual associated deaths.

Table 20-4. Five-year survival rates for vaginal cancer (by stage)

Stage I	80%
Stage II	45%
Stage III	35%
Stage IV	10%

Risk Factors

Cervical cancer is a sexually transmitted disease, and the first solid tumor to be linked to a virus. Infection with human papillomavirus, specifically types 16 and 18, is associated with the development of this disease. Other risk factors include early age at first intercourse, multiple sexual partners, multiparity, sexual contact with men at high risk for penile cancers or men who have had partners with cervical cancer, and smoking. One half of the women with newly diagnosed invasive cervical cancer have never had a Papanicolaou smear, and another 10% have not had a Papanicolaou smear in the previous 5 years.

Pathology

Eighty-five percent of cervical cancers are squamous cell carcinomas, and 10% to 15% are adenocarcinomas, including the less common adenosquamous type. The remainder of cases is rarer histologies, including small cell tumors, sarcomas, lymphomas, and melanomas.

Routes of Spread

Cervical cancer spreads by a variety of mechanisms. It can directly invade surrounding structures, including the parametria, corpus, and vagina. Lymphatic metastases are relatively ordered and predictable, sequentially involving parametrial, pelvic, iliac, and paraaortic nodes. Hematogenous metastases and intraperitoneal implantation can also occur.

Clinical Features

Symptoms

Discharge and abnormal bleeding—including postcoital, intermenstrual, and postmenopausal bleeding, and menorrhagia—are often the first signs of cervical cancer. Urinary frequency and pain can also occur and may indicate advanced disease.

Physical Findings

Examination varies, depending on the site of the lesion (endocervix or ectocervix). Careful inspection and palpation, including bimanual and rectovaginal examinations, are required to identify the size and extent of the lesion.

Pretreatment Workup

Careful physical examination must be performed, including pelvic examination and biopsy of the lesion. Other components of the pretreatment workup include complete blood cell count, serum glucose, blood urea nitrogen, creatinine, and liver function tests; chest radiograph; and mammogram. The following additional studies should be performed for patients with symptoms and disease stages IB2 to IV: cystoscopy, proctoscopy, barium enema (as indicated), and CT scan. MRI may be useful, especially when attempting to delineate endometrial lesions from endocervical lesions. According to the guidelines established by the International Federation of Gynecology and Obstetrics (FIGO), staging procedures are limited to physical examination, cervical

Table 20-5. Clinical staging of cervical cancer

Stage	Description
I	In general, lesions are confined to the cervix; uterine involvement is disregarded.
IA	Preclinical cervical cancers diagnosed by microscopy alone
IA1	Stromal invasion ≤3 mm deep and ≤7 mm wide
IA2	Stromal invasion >3 mm but ≤5 mm deep and ≤7 mm wide
IB	Lesions larger than stage IA lesions, whether seen clinically or not
IB1	Clinical lesions ≤4 cm
IB2	Clinical lesions >4 cm
II	Extension beyond the cervix, but no extension to the pelvic sidewall or the lower one-third of the vagina
IIA	No obvious parametrial involvement
IIB	Parametrial involvement
III	Extension to the pelvic wall with no cancer-free space between the tumor and the pelvic wall; tumor involves the lower one-third of the vagina. All cases of hydronephrosis or nonfunctioning kidney, unless secondary to unrelated cause.
IIIA	Involvement of the lower one-third of the vagina; no extension to the pelvic sidewall
IIIB	Extension to the pelvic wall, hydronephrosis, or nonfunctioning kidney
IV	Extension beyond the true pelvis or clinical involvement of the mucosa of the bladder or rectum
IVA	Spread to adjacent organs
IVB	Spread to distant organs

conization, intravenous pyelogram, barium enema, cystoscopy, proctoscopy, and chest radiograph.

Staging

The clinical staging scheme for classifying cervical cancer is outlined in Table 20-5. The term *microinvasive cervical cancer* is sometimes applied to stage IA lesions. This diagnosis must be made from either a cone biopsy or a hysterectomy specimen. The following definitions have been derived by two different medical associations and are referred to when considering therapy:

FIGO definition. See the definition under FIGO stage IA, Table 20-5.

Society of Gynecologic Oncologists (SGO) definition. Microinvasion with depth of invasion in one or more foci of less than 3 mm and no lymphovascular space involvement.

Treatment of Cervical Cancer by Stage

Stage IA

Lesions that satisfy the SGO definition of microinvasion may be treated conservatively with any of the following modalities:

simple hysterectomy, cervical conization in cases where maintenance of fertility is an issue, and intracavitary radiation therapy
for patients who do not qualify for surgery.

Lesions that do not satisfy the SGO definition of microinvasion
(lymphovascular space invasion or invasion >3 mm) are significantly more likely to recur when treated conservatively; therefore, radical hysterectomy and lymph node dissection or radiation
therapy should be performed.

Stages IB, IIA

Surgery and radiation therapy result in similar cure rates when
patients are carefully selected; squamous lesions 4 to 5 cm and
adenocarcinomas less than 3 cm are potential surgical candidates. The standard treatment options are radical hysterectomy
and pelvic lymph node dissection and radiation therapy with 40 to
45 Gy external-beam irradiation and two intracavitary systems.
Patients with risk factors for recurrence on pathologic evaluation
(i.e., two or more positive nodes) also receive adjuvant radiation
therapy. Simple hysterectomy after pelvic radiation therapy is
indicated primarily in a patient whose tumor responds slowly to
radiation therapy or when vaginal anatomy precludes optimal
intracavitary placement.

Stages IIB to IVA

Radiation therapy is the treatment of choice for locally advanced
disease. Surgery may be used as adjuvant therapy for stage IVA
disease without parametrial involvement and in cases of persistent central disease following radiation therapy.

Stage IVB

Stage IVB disease is primarily treated with chemotherapy because the disease is disseminated. Radiation therapy can be used
for local control and palliation of symptoms. Cisplatin is the most
studied active agent; other options include ifosfamide and mitomycin C. Current clinical trials using vinorelbine (Navelbine)
have also demonstrated some activity in cervix cancer.

Recurrent Disease

The treatment of recurrent disease depends on disease location
and original treatment modality. Central recurrence may be managed with pelvic exenteration if no contraindicating factors are
present. Patients who have had prior radiation therapy and extensive pelvic recurrence or distant metastatic disease are treated
similarly to those patients with stage IVB disease.

Prognostic Factors

The most important prognostic factors for stage I disease include
lymphovascular space involvement, tumor size, depth of invasion,
and presence of lymph node metastases (Table 20-6). For stages II
to IV disease, stage, presence of lymph node metastases, tumor
volume, age, and the patient's performance status are key prognostic factors. The overall survival rates for cervical cancer are
highlighted in Table 20-7.

Table 20-6.   Incidence of nodal metastasis by stage

Stage	Positive Pelvic Nodes (%)	Positive Paraaortic Nodes (%)
IA1	0	0
IA2 (1–3 mm)	0.6	0
IA2 (3–5 mm)	4.8	<1
IB	15.9	2.2
IIA	24.5	11
IIB	31.4	19
III	44.8	30
IVA	55	40

Recommended Surveillance

Greater than 50% of all recurrences are diagnosed in the first year following treatment. Seventy-five percent are diagnosed by year 2 following treatment, and 95% within 5 years of treatment.

ENDOMETRIAL CANCER

Incidence

Endometrial cancer is the most common malignancy of the female genital tract and the fourth most common malignancy in women (following breast, lung, and colon cancers). Approximately 35,000 new cases are diagnosed annually, and approximately 6,000 women die yearly from this disease. The median age at onset is 63 years; however, up to 25% of patients are premenopausal.

Risk Factors

Risk factors for endometrial cancer reflect a chronic estrogenized state. These factors include nulliparity, early menarche, late menopause, obesity, unopposed estrogen therapy, and chronic disease (i.e., diabetes mellitus and hypertension).

Pathology

Ninety percent of endometrial cancers are adenocarcinomas (70% grade 1, 15% grade 2, and 15% grade 3), 5% to 7% are papillary serous carcinomas, and the remaining 2% to 3% are clear cell carcinomas. The latter two cell types represent a more aggressive histologic type.

Table 20-7.   Five-year survival rates for cervical cancer (by stage and histology)

Stage I	Squamous, 65%–90%
	Adenocarcinoma, 70%–75%
Stage II	Squamous, 45%–80%
	Adenocarcinoma, 30%–40%
Stage III	Squamous up to 60%
	Adenocarcinoma, 20%–30%
Stage IV	Squamous and adenocarcinoma, <15%

Routes of Spread

Endometrial cancer metastasizes by myometrial invasion and direct extension to adjacent structures. Transtubal passage of exfoliated cells, lymphatic embolization, and hematogenous dissemination can also occur.

Clinical Features

Symptoms

Ninety percent of patients present to their physicians complaining of abnormal uterine bleeding or postmenopausal bleeding; approximately 15% of patients with postmenopausal bleeding have uterine cancer. Patients may also experience pelvic pressure and pelvic pain. Associated findings include pyometra, hematometra, an abnormal Papanicolaou smear (the presence of atypical glandular cells on a Papanicolaou smear requires that an endometrial biopsy be performed to rule out malignancy), heavy menses, and intermenstrual bleeding.

Pretreatment Workup

Careful physical examination, including pelvic examination, is required. Pathologic confirmation of disease by endometrial biopsy or dilatation and curettage is essential. Other components of the pretreatment workup include complete blood cell count, serum glucose, blood urea nitrogen, creatinine, and CA-125; chest radiograph; and mammogram. Diagnostic tests—including CT, barium enema, intravenous pyelogram, proctosigmoidoscopy, cystoscopy, and, in some cases, MRI—should be performed as indicated by symptoms or examination findings.

Staging

The staging schema for endometrial cancer is described in Tables 20-8 and 20-9.

Treatment

The most active chemotherapeutic agents in the treatment of endometrial cancer are cisplatin, doxorubicin, and Taxol. Alone these agents produce a 30% response rate; when combined, the response rate is approximately 50%. Progestin therapy may be used to treat metastatic tumors with progesterone receptors; response is seen in 25% to 30% of cases. Hormone therapy with tamoxifen produces a response in approximately 20% of cases.

Prognostic Factors

Surgical stage is the most important prognostic variable (Table 20-10). Other prognostic factors are myometrial invasion, lymphovascular space invasion, nuclear grade, histologic type, tumor size, patient age, positive peritoneal cytologic findings, hormone receptor status, and type of primary treatment used (surgery vs. radiation therapy).

UTERINE SARCOMAS

Incidence

Uterine sarcomas account for approximately 3% to 5% of uterine cancers.

Table 20-8.   Surgical staging of endometrial cancer

Stage	Description
I	Carcinoma confined to the uterine corpus IA: Tumor limited to the endometrium IB: Invasion of one-half or less of the myometrium IC: Invasion of more than one-half of the myometrium
II	Extension of cancer to cervix but not outside uterus IIA: Endocervical glandular involvement only IIB: Cervical stromal invasion
III	Extension of the tumor outside the uterus but confined to the true pelvis or paraaortic area IIIA: Tumor invades serosa and/or adnexa, with or without positive cytology IIIB: Vaginal metastases IIIC: Metastases to pelvic and/or paraaortic lymph nodes
IV	Distant metastases or involvement of adjacent pelvic organs IVA: Tumor invasion of the bowel or bladder mucosa IVB: Distant metastases including intra-abdominal and/or inguinal lymph nodes

Risk Factors

Most patients have no known risk factors. A small number of patients have a history of pelvic irradiation.

Pathology

The disease arises from mesodermal derivatives that include uterine smooth muscle, endometrial stroma, and blood and lymphatic vessel walls. The number of mitoses per 10 high-power fields, degree of cytologic atypia, and presence of coagulative necrosis are the most reliable predictors of biologic behavior. Uterine sarcomas are classified according to the types of elements involved (pure [only mesodermal elements present] or mixed [both mesodermal and epithelial elements present]) and whether malignant mesodermal elements are normally present in the uterus (homologous [only smooth muscle and stroma present] or heterologous [striated muscle and cartilage present]) (Table 20-11).

Table 20-9.   FIGO definitions for tumor grading

Grade	Definition
1	5% or less of a nonsquamous or nonmorular solid growth pattern
2	6% to 50% of a nonsquamous or nonmorular solid growth pattern
3	More than 50% of a nonsquamous or nonmorular solid growth pattern

FIGO, International Federation of Gynecology and Obstetrics.

Table 20-10. Five-year survival rates for endometrial cancer (by stage)

Stage I	90%
Stage II	75%
Stage III	40%
Stage IV	10%

Routes of Spread

Sarcomas demonstrate a propensity for early hematogenous dissemination and lymphatic spread (one third of patients).

Histologic Frequencies

One half of endometrial sarcomas are malignant mixed müllerian tumors. Other histologic types include leiomyosarcomas (40%), endometrial stromal sarcomas (8%), adenosarcomas, pure heterologous sarcomas, and other variants (1%–2%).

Pretreatment Workup

Careful physical examination, including pelvic examination, is required (Table 20-12). Endometrial biopsy, dilatation and curettage, or both are essential to providing pathologic confirmation of disease. Other components of the pretreatment workup include complete blood cell count, serum glucose, blood urea nitrogen, creatinine, and liver function tests; chest radiography; mammogram; and cystoscopy or proctoscopy, depending on site and extent of lesion. Preoperative medical clearance is necessary for patients with chronic disease or other appropriate indications.

Staging

No official staging system exists for sarcomas; therefore the FIGO staging system for uterine corpus carcinoma is used. (See Table 20-8.)

Table 20-11. Classifications of uterine sarcomas

Type	Homologous	Heterologous
Pure	Leiomyosarcoma Stromal sarcoma	Rhabdomyosarcoma Chondrosarcoma Osteosarcoma Liposarcoma
Mixed	Mixed mesodermal (müllerian) sarcoma or malignant mixed mesodermal (müllerian) tumors with homologous components (also called carcinosarcomas)	Mixed mesodermal (müllerian) sarcomas or malignant mixed mesodermal (müllerian) tumors with heterologous components

Table 20-12.   Clinical features of uterine sarcomas

Cell Type	Patient's Age (yr)	Signs and Symptoms	Diagnosis
Endometrial stromal sarcoma	42–53	Vaginal bleeding Uterine enlargement Lower abdominal pain or pressure	EMB or D&C
Leiomyosarcoma	45–55	Vaginal bleeding Rapid uterine enlargement Lower abdominal pain or pressure	Difficult preoperative diagnosis; only 15% diagnosed by EMB or D&C
Malignant mixed mesodermal tumors	65–75	Several factors in common with endometrial cancer (nulliparity, obesity, and diabetes) Vaginal bleeding Enlarged uterus	EMB or D&C (In up to 50% of cases, the tumor protrudes through the cervix.)
Adenosarcoma	Any age; most common in the 5th decade of life	Vaginal bleeding Uterine enlargement	EMB or D&C (In up to 50% of cases, the tumor protrudes through the cervix.)

D&C, dilatation and curettage; EMB, endometrial biopsy.

Table 20-13.   Five-year survival rates for uterine sarcomas (by stage)

Stage I	50%
Stages II–IV	15% or less

Treatment

Surgical excision is the only treatment of curative value. Pelvic radiation therapy has a role in local control of tumor; however, because of the propensity for early hematogenous spread, this treatment does not affect outcome. Leiomyosarcomas generally do not respond to radiation therapy. Cisplatin, doxorubicin, and ifosfamide have shown some activity against uterine sarcomas; leiomyosarcomas are more sensitive to doxorubicin. There may be some benefit to hormonal therapy with megestrol acetate; tamoxifen is recommended in cases where hormone receptors have been identified. Hormonal therapy is the treatment of choice for low-grade endometrial stromal sarcoma.

Prognostic Factors

The most important prognostic factor is surgical stage of disease (Table 20-13). The presence of sarcomatous overgrowth and deep myometrial invasion must be considered in cases of adenosarcoma because it adds to an adverse prognosis.

Recommended Surveillance

Physical and pelvic examinations should be performed every 3 months the first year, every 4 months in years 2 and 3, every 6 months in years 4 and 5, and once a year thereafter. A Papanicolaou smear and chest radiograph should be obtained annually.

EPITHELIAL OVARIAN CANCER

Incidence

Epithelial ovarian cancer occurs in 1 in 70 women. Approximately 27,000 new cases are diagnosed annually, and approximately 15,000 women will die each year from this disease. Epithelial ovarian cancer comprises 90% of all ovarian cancers. The median age at diagnosis is 61 years. Less than 10% of cases are due to transmission of an autosomal dominant gene. Three hereditary forms of ovarian cancer have been identified: site-specific familial ovarian cancer, breast-ovarian familial cancer syndrome (associated with an abnormality in *BRCA-1*, or *BRCA-2*, the breast-ovarian cancer susceptibility genes), and Lynch II syndrome (nonpolyposis colon cancer, endometrial cancer, breast cancer, and ovarian cancer clusters in first- and second-degree relatives).

Risk Factors

A variety of factors are thought to increase the risk of developing ovarian cancer. These include increased age (peak age is 70 years), nulliparity, early menarche, late menopause, delayed childbearing, and Ashkenazi Jewish descent. There may be an association with use of fertility drugs, but this has not been conclusively

Table 20-14.   Major histologic types of epithelial ovarian carcinomas

Histologic Type	Percent of Ovarian Tumors	Percent Bilaterality
Serous	46	73
Mucinous	36	47
Endometrioid	8	33
Clear cell	3	13
Transitional	2	—
Mixed	3	—
Undifferentiated	<2	53
Unclassified	<1	—

demonstrated. The use of oral contraceptives appears to have a protective effect against the development of epithelial ovarian cancer; this effect may last up to 10 years.

Pathology

There is a 15% to 30% incidence of concomitant endometrial carcinoma in cases of endometrioid ovarian carcinoma. Cases of synchronous appendiceal and ovarian mucinous tumors have also been reported; however, it is not unusual for appendiceal cancer to spread to the ovaries, and this often makes it difficult to determine the site of the primary disease (Table 20-14).

Routes of Spread

The most common route of spread is transcoelomic, as exfoliated cells tend to assume the circulatory path of the peritoneal fluid and implant along this path. Ovarian cancer may also metastasize to the lymph nodes, but hematogenous spread is uncommon.

Clinical Features

General

The interval from onset of disease to diagnosis is often prolonged because of a lack of specific symptoms during the early stages; therefore, diagnosis is often not made until patients have disseminated disease. Approximately 65% of cases are stage III or stage IV disease at diagnosis.

Symptoms

Symptoms that may be suggestive of ovarian cancer include abdominal fullness, early satiety, dyspepsia, urinary frequency, constipation, unexplained pelvic pain, and increased flatulence.

Physical Findings

An adnexal mass noted on routine pelvic examination and a palpable fluid wave are often found in patients with ovarian cancer. Five percent of patients with presumed ovarian cancer have another primary that has metastasized to the ovary. The most common primary sites that metastasize to the ovary are the breast, gastrointestinal tract, and pelvic organs.

Pretreatment Workup

Careful physical examination, including pelvic examination, is required. Other components of the pretreatment workup include complete blood cell count, serum glucose, blood urea nitrogen, creatinine, liver function tests, serum albumin, CA-125 (elevated in approximately 80% of cases), chest radiograph, and mammogram. Imaging studies may be helpful but most often do not change the planned staging procedure. CT may help determine the extent of disease. Barium enema is useful in examination of the colon. In older patients, barium enema can be particularly helpful in diagnosing a colonic primary, which may present similarly to ovarian cancer. Intravenous pyelography is also helpful in certain clinical situations.

Staging

The staging schema for epithelial ovarian cancer is outlined in Table 20-15.

Treatment

The initial step in treatment is surgical cytoreduction with appropriate intraoperative staging procedures, including abdominal and pelvic cytology, careful exploration of all abdominal and pelvic structures and surfaces, total abdominal hysterectomy and bilateral salpingo-oophorectomy (exceptions include concern about fertility and early stage disease), infracolic omentectomy with or without appendectomy, and selective pelvic and paraaortic lymph node sampling. Primary cytoreduction is a key component in advanced cases; survival is directly correlated to the amount of residual tumor remaining. Optimal tumor reductive surgery is loosely defined as the diameter of the largest residual tumor implant being less than 2 cm. If the residual mass is greater in size, the cytoreduction is deemed suboptimal. At the M.D. Anderson Cancer Center, routine "second-look" operations are no longer performed. A "second-look" operation may be included as part of an investigational trial. There are certain exceptions to the use of surgical exploration and cytoreduction as initial treatment. Primary chemotherapy may be used, followed by interval debulking, in certain subsets of patients such as those with advanced disease (i.e., patients with pleural effusions that reaccumulate rapidly after thoracentesis), those with bulky disease, and those who did not undergo appropriate primary cytoreductive surgery. The impact this approach has on survival, however, is unproven in those patients with advanced and bulky disease.

Prognostic Factors

Prognostic histopathologic factors include histologic type, histologic grade, and DNA ploidy (Table 20-16). Clinical factors that are of prognostic significance include surgicopathologic stage, extent of residual disease remaining following primary cytoreduction, volume of ascites, patient age, and patient performance status.

Survival Based on Performance Status

Patients with poor performance status before treatment (Karnofsky status <70%) have significantly shorter survival.

Table 20-15.   Surgical staging of epithelial ovarian cancer

Stage	Description
I	Growth limited to the ovaries
	IA Growth limited to one ovary, no ascites, no tumor on the external surfaces, capsules intact
	IB Growth in both ovaries, no ascites, no tumors on external surfaces, capsule intact
	IC Stage IA or IB characteristics, but with tumor on the surface of one or both ovaries, ruptured capsule(s), or malignant ascites with positive peritoneal cytology
II	Growth involving one or both ovaries with pelvic extension
	IIA Extension and/or metastases to the uterus and/or tubes
	IIB Extension to other pelvic tissues
	IIC Stage IIA or IIB characteristics, but with tumor on the surface of one or both ovaries, ruptured capsule(s), or malignant ascites with positive peritoneal cytology
III	Growth involving one or both ovaries with peritoneal implants outside the pelvis and/or positive retroperitoneal or inguinal nodes; superficial liver metastasis equals stage III; tumor limited to the true pelvis but with histologically proved malignant extension to small bowel or omentum
	IIIA Tumor grossly limited to the true pelvis with negative nodes but histologically confirmed microscopic seeding of abdominal peritoneal surfaces
	IIIB Tumor involving one or both ovaries with histologically confirmed implants of abdominal peritoneal surfaces, none exceeding 2 cm in diameter; nodes are negative
	IIIC Abdominal implants greater than 2 cm in diameter and/or positive retroperitoneal or inguinal nodes
IV	Growth involving one or both ovaries with distant metastases; positive cytology from pleural effusion or pathologic confirmation of parenchymal liver metastases

OVARIAN TUMORS OF LOW MALIGNANT POTENTIAL

Incidence

These tumors comprise as many as 5% to 15% of all ovarian malignancies. The highest incidence is among white women, with a mean age at diagnosis of 39 to 45 years (approximately 10 years younger than the mean age at diagnosis of epithelial ovarian cancer).

Risk Factors

No significant risk factors have been identified, and there does not appear to be a protective effect associated with pregnancy

Table 20-16. Five-year survival rate for epithelial ovarian cancer

Stage	Serous Carcinoma by Stage and Grade			
	All Grades(%)	Grade 1(%)	Grade 2(%)	Grade 3(%)
IA	85	92.5	86	63
IB	69	85	90	79
IC	59	78	49	51
IIA	62	64	65	39
IIB	51	79	43	42
IIC	43	68	46	20
IIIA	31	58	38	20
IIIB	38	73	42	21
IIIC	18	46	22	14
IV	8	14	8	6

Residual disease, all stages, following primary cytoreductive surgery

Amount of Residual Disease	Survival (%)
Microscopic (residual disease)	40–75
Macroscopic (optimal debulking)	30–5
Macroscopic (suboptimal debulking)	5

Status at second look, all stages by disease status

Disease Status	Survival (%)
No evidence of disease	50
Microscopic disease	35
Macroscopic disease	5

or exogenous hormones. There is no apparent association with family history.

Pathology

The main histologic categories are serous and mucinous. Secondary categories include transitional, endometrioid, clear cell, and mixed. Diagnosis of tumors of low malignant potential requires the absence of frank stromal invasion (there is a subcategory for microinvasive tumor implants) and the presence of any two of the following factors: nuclear atypia, mitotic activity, multilayering of epithelium, and epithelial budding.

Routes of Spread

As with epithelial ovarian cancer, low malignant potential tumors spread via a transcoelomic route. Lymphatic metastases may also occur.

Clinical Features

Ovarian tumors of low malignant potential present in a manner similar to that of epithelial ovarian cancer. The most common symptoms are low abdominal pain or discomfort, early satiety, dyspepsia, sense of abdominal enlargement, and discovery of an adnexal mass on routine pelvic examination. The CA-125 may be elevated in serous tumors.

Pretreatment Workup

Careful physical examination, including pelvic examination, is required. Other components of the pretreatment workup include complete blood cell count, serum glucose, blood urea nitrogen, creatinine, liver function tests, serum albumin, CA-125 (may be elevated), chest radiograph, and mammogram. Imaging studies may be helpful but most often do not change the planned staging procedure. CT may help determine the extent of disease. Barium enema is useful in examination of the colon. In older patients, barium enema can be particularly helpful in diagnosing a colonic primary, which may present similarly to ovarian cancer. Intravenous pyelography is also helpful in certain clinical situations.

Staging

The surgical staging scheme for ovarian tumors of low malignant potential is identical to that used for epithelial ovarian cancer (see Table 20-15). Their distribution is outlined in Table 20-17.

Treatment

Recommended treatment for all patients is primary surgery; fertility-sparing procedures should be performed if fertility is a factor in patients with stage I disease.

Stages I and II

Surgical cytoreduction is the essential element with close surveillance postoperatively. No role for adjuvant chemotherapy or radiation therapy has been documented.

Stages III and IV

Surgical cytoreduction is the key element. Platinum-based chemotherapy may be of benefit for residual disease following cytoreduction, but adjuvant therapy is unproved to date.

Recurrent Disease

Tumors of low malignant potential typically have an indolent clinical course and may recur late. Cytoreduction as outlined for stages III and IV can be considered in select patients.

Table 20-17.   Distribution of ovarian tumors of low malignant potential by stage

	Histologic Type	
Stage	Serous (%)	Mucinous (%)
I	65	89.5
II	14	1
III	20	9
IV	1	0.5

Table 20-18. Five-year survival rate for ovarian cancer (by stage)

Stage I	95%
Stage II	75%–80%
Stage III	65%–70%

Proposed Prognostic Factors

Proposed prognostic factors include stage at diagnosis, residual tumor volume, and presence of invasive implants (Table 20-18).

SEX CORD STROMAL TUMORS

Incidence

Sex cord stromal tumors account for 5% to 8% of all ovarian malignancies and represent 5% of childhood malignancies. These tumors are uncommon before menarche; occurrence before menarche is associated with precocious puberty.

Pathology

As their name suggests, these tumors are derived from sex cords or stroma. Derivatives include granulosa cells, theca cells, stromal cells, Sertoli cells, Leydig cells, and cells resembling embryonic precursors of these cell types (Table 20-19). These tumors are also referred to as "functioning tumors" because as many as 85% synthesize steroids (estrogen, progesterone, testosterone, and corticosteroids).

Routes of Spread

The pattern of metastatic spread is analogous to that of epithelial ovarian cancers.

Clinical Features

Granulosa Cell Tumors

Granulosa cell tumors comprise 1% to 2% of all ovarian tumors. Adult-type tumors (95% of all granulosa cell tumors)

Table 20-19. Major classifications

Granulosa cell tumors
    Adult
    Juvenile
Thecomas and fibromas
    Thecomas
    Fibromas-fibrosarcomas
Stromal tumors with minor sex cord elements
Sertoli stromal cell tumors
    Sertoli cell
    Leydig cell
    Sertoli-Leydig cell tumors
Gynandroblastomas
Sex cord tumors with annular tubules
Unclassified

are characterized by secretion of excess estrogen. Patients may experience menstrual irregularities or postmenopausal bleeding. Five percent of patients present with an acute abdomen caused by tumor hemorrhage. Patients with juvenile-type granulosa cell tumors (5% of granulosa cell tumors) can also present with menstrual abnormalities, abdominal pain, and, rarely, postmenopausal bleeding. Associated pathosis includes coexisting endometrial hyperplasia (5%), coexisting endometrial carcinoma (6%–30%), leiomyomata, and virilizing features in rare tumors producing testosterone. Granulosa cell tumors produce estrogen and rarely may also produce testosterone.

Thecomas

Thecomas are responsible for 1% of all ovarian tumors and are one third as common as granulosa cell tumors. The mean age at diagnosis is 53 years, and 2% to 3% of these tumors are bilateral. Menstrual abnormalities and postmenopausal bleeding are the most common presenting symptoms. Associated pathosis includes leiomyomata, endometrial hyperplasia, and coexisting endometrial cancer. Thecomas produce estrogen.

Fibromas and Fibrosarcoma

Fibromas and fibrosarcoma are the most common sex cord stromal tumors and comprise 4% of all ovarian neoplasms. The mean age at diagnosis is 46 years; 10% of these lesions are bilateral. Symptoms include ascites in 50% of patients with tumors greater than 6 cm, increased abdominal girth, Meig's syndrome (right pleural effusion and ascites), and Gorlin's syndrome with basal nevi. These tumors are primarily inert but may secrete small amounts of estrogen.

Sertoli Cell Tumors

The average age of women with Sertoli cell tumors is 27 years, but these tumors can occur at any age. Sertoli cell tumors are unilateral. Seventy percent of patients have symptoms related to excess estrogen, whereas 20% exhibit signs of virilization. Rarely, hyperaldosteronemia may develop, manifested as hypertension and hyperkalemia. Seventy percent of these tumors produce both estrogen and androgens, whereas 20% produce androgens alone.

Leydig Cell Tumors

Leydig cell tumors occur at an average age of 50 to 70 years but can occur at any age. Tumors are unilateral, and patients experience symptoms related to the peripheral effects of hormone products. Thyroid disease and familial occurrence are associated with these tumors. Eighty percent of Leydig cell tumors produce androgens, 10% produce estrogen, and 10% are inert.

Sertoli-Leydig Cell Tumors

Sertoli-Leydig cell tumors occur at an average age of 25 to 40 years but can occur at any age. These tumors are rarely bilateral. Symptoms include virilization in one third to one half of patients and amenorrhea. Most of these tumors produce testosterone, and some may produce alpha-fetoprotein.

Gynandroblastomas

Gynandroblastomas are unilateral tumors that can occur at any age. Patients may experience either estrogenic effects or virilization secondary to the hormone products of these tumors. Histologically, both granulosa cell and Sertoli-Leydig cell components may be present in these tumors. These tumors may produce androgens, may produce estrogen, or may be inert.

Sex Cord Tumors with Annular Tubules

The average age of patients with sex cord tumors with annular tubules is 25 to 35 years. Sixty-six percent of the tumors associated with Peutz-Jeghers syndrome are bilateral; the remaining is predominantly unilateral. Patients exhibit symptoms of excess estrogen when these tumors are associated with Peutz-Jeghers syndrome. Excess estrogen is present in only 40% of those without Peutz-Jeghers syndrome. Associated pathosis includes Peutz-Jeghers syndrome and endocervical adenocarcinoma. Sex cord tumors with annular tubules produce estrogen.

Pretreatment Workup

Careful physical examination, including pelvic examination, is required. Other components of the pretreatment workup include complete blood cell count, serum glucose, blood urea nitrogen, creatinine, liver function tests, serum albumin, CA-125, chest radiography, and mammography. Evaluation of levels of serum estradiol, dehydroepiandrosterone, testosterone, 17-OH-progesterone, and hydrocortisone may be helpful in diagnosis. CT and ultrasound should be performed to evaluate the adrenal glands and ovaries. Imaging studies may be helpful but most often do not change the planned staging procedure.

Staging

In general, surgical staging can be accomplished by unilateral salpingo-oophorectomy if there is a desire to maintain fertility, peritoneal cytology, infracolic omentectomy, selective biopsies of nodes and abdominal structures, and appropriately targeted biopsies. Dilatation and curettage, and endocervical curettage should be performed to evaluate any coexistent pathologic process. These tumors are surgically staged according to the staging scheme for epithelial ovarian cancer (see Table 20-15).

Treatment

Tumors of stromal origin (thecomas, fibromas) and Leydig cell tumors generally follow a benign course; surgery is the only treatment. Sertoli or granulosa types are generally of low malignant potential, tend to recur late, and rarely metastasize. Chemotherapy should be considered for advanced disease. Postoperative adjunctive therapy with bleomycin, etoposide, and cisplatin or other platinum-based chemotherapy should be considered in patients with Sertoli or Leydig cell tumors with poor differentiation and heterologous components and in patients with advanced or recurrent stromal tumors; pelvic radiation therapy can also play a role in treatment of these patients. Survival rates are described in Table 20-20.

Table 20-20.   Five-year survival rate (by tumor type)

Granulosa cell tumors
  85%–90% for tumors confined to the ovary
  55%–60% for tumors with extraovarian extension

Sertoli or Leydig cell tumors with poor differentiation have a poor
    prognosis

Other tumors of sex cord stromal origin have survival rates
    consistent with benign processes and low-grade malignancies

OVARIAN GERM CELL TUMORS

Incidence

Germ cell tumors comprise 15% to 20% of all ovarian neoplasms
and are the second most common type of ovarian tumor. In the
first two decades of life, 70% of ovarian tumors are of germ cell
origin and one third are malignant. The mean age at diagnosis is
19 years; germ cell tumors rarely occur after the third decade of
life. Sixty percent to 75% of cases are stage I at diagnosis.

Pathology

The seven types of germ cell tumors and the percentage of occurrence are:

Dysgerminoma (40%)
Endodermal sinus tumor (yolk sac tumor; 22%)
Immature teratoma (20%)
Embryonal carcinoma (rare)
Choriocarcinoma (rare)
Polyembryoma (rare)
Mixed forms (10%–15%)

Routes of Spread

See the discussion of epithelial ovarian cancer.

Clinical Features

Germ cell malignancies grow rapidly and are often characterized by pain secondary to torsion, hemorrhage, or necrosis (Table
20-21). Germ cell malignancies may also cause bladder, rectal,
or menstrual abnormalities. Dysgerminomas account for 20% to
30% of malignant ovarian tumors diagnosed during pregnancy.
Embryonal carcinomas may produce estrogen and cause precocious puberty.

Pretreatment Workup

Careful physical examination, including pelvic examination, is
required. Other components of the pretreatment workup include
complete blood cell count, serum glucose, blood urea nitrogen,
creatinine, liver function tests, serum albumin, and chest radiography. Serum markers, including alpha-fetoprotein, human
chorionic gonadotropin, and lactic dehydrogenase, should be measured. It is important to check the karyotype in premenopausal
women with ovarian masses due to an increased incidence of dys-
genic gonads in patients with these tumors.

Table 20-21. **Clinical features of ovarian germ cell tumors**

Tumor	Bilaterality	hCG	AFP	LDH
		Tumor Markers		
Dysgerminoma	10%–15%	±	−	+
Endodermal sinus tumor	Rare; dermoids common in contralateral ovary	−	+	±
Immature teratoma	Rare; dermoids common in contralateral ovary	−	±	±
Embryonal carcinoma	Rare	+	+	±
Choriocarcinoma	Rare	+	−	−
Polyembryoma	Rare	±	±	±

AFP, Alpha-fetoprotein; hCG, human chorionic gonadotropin; LDH, lactate dehydrogenase.

Staging

In general, surgical staging can be accompanied by unilateral salpingo-oophorectomy if there is a desire to preserve fertility, peritoneal cytology, infracolic omentectomy, and selective biopsies of nodes and abdominal structures. In patients who are inadequately staged, there are two options: surgical re-exploration and appropriate staging, or initiation of chemotherapy without reexploration. It is most prudent not to delay chemotherapy by reexploration and staging, because these tumors are highly chemosensitive. These tumors are surgically staged according to the staging schema for epithelial ovarian cancer (see Table 20-15).

Treatment

The primary treatment component is chemotherapy; this is recommended for all patients with germ cell tumors except those with stage I tumors. Chemotherapy should begin 7 to 10 days after surgical exploration because of rapid tumor growth. The first-line regimen is bleomycin, etoposide, and cisplatin administered for three or four cycles in 21-day intervals. Patients who experience a recurrence less than 6 weeks after chemotherapy are said to be "platinum resistant"; those who experience a recurrence more than 6 weeks after the last cycle of chemotherapy are said to be "platinum sensitive." Bleomycin, etoposide, and cisplatin may be restarted in patients who are platinum sensitive.

High-dose chemotherapy with autologous bone marrow rescue is a viable option in patients who are platinum resistant. Ifosfamide has shown some activity in patients with testicular cancer and may be useful for patients who are platinum resistant. Radiation therapy may have a limited role in treatment of dysgerminomas.

Table 20-22. Survival rate (by tumor type and time interval)

Dysgerminoma (5 yr)	
Stage I	90%–95%
All stages	60%–90%
Endodermal sinus tumors (2 yr)	
Stages I and II	90%
Stages III and IV	50%
Immature teratoma (5 yr)	
Stage I	90%–95%
All stages	70%–80%
Grade 1	82%
Grade 2	62%
Grade 3	30%
Embryonal carcinoma (5 yr)	
All stages	39%

Choriocarcinoma has a poor prognosis. Polyembryoma has a poor prognosis. Mixed tumor has a variable survival and is dependent on the tumor composition.

Prognostic Factors

Dysgerminomas greater than 10 to 15 cm in diameter or with a high mitotic index and anaplasia tend to recur most often. Prognostic factors for immature teratomas include grade of lesion, extent of disease at diagnosis, and amount of residual tumor; tumor grade is determined by the presence of immature neural elements (Table 20-22).

MANAGEMENT OF THE UNSUSPECTED OVARIAN MASS FOUND AT LAPAROTOMY

The finding of an unsuspected ovarian mass at the time of exploratory laparotomy or at laparotomy for an unrelated condition can pose a therapeutic dilemma to the surgeon. Appropriate treatment depends on several factors, including the patient's age, the size and consistency of the mass, possible bilaterality, and gross involvement of other structures.

OVARIAN MASSES IN WOMEN OF CHILDBEARING AGE

An unsuspected mass in a young patient is most likely benign. Among the most frequently found benign masses involving the adnexa are the nonneoplastic or functional cysts, which are related to the process of ovulation. These cysts are significant primarily because they cannot be easily distinguished from true neoplasms on clinical grounds alone. If ovulation does not occur, a clear, fluid-filled follicular cyst up to 10 cm in diameter may develop. This functional cyst usually resolves spontaneously within several days to 2 weeks. When a patient ovulates, a corpus luteum is formed that may become abnormally large because of hemorrhage within the corpus luteum or cyst formation. A patient with a hemorrhagic corpus luteum may present with an acute abdomen necessitating laparotomy. Often the bleeding area may be oversewn without performing a cystectomy or salpingo-oophorectomy. It is critical to check a pregnancy test in a premenopausal woman who presents with an acute abdomen, because surgery may result in loss of function of the corpus luteum, which sustains pregnancy during the first trimester. In pregnant patients, postoperative support with progesterone therapy can be used to help carry the pregnancy through the critical period.

Ovulating patients can also present with functional ovarian cysts. These are usually asymptomatic but can cause lower abdominal or pelvic pain; however, signs of an acute abdomen are rare. A simple cyst up to 5 cm in diameter found incidentally at the time of surgery in an ovulating patient can be observed safely. If it is only a functional cyst, it should disappear after the patient's next menstrual period. Resolution can be evaluated with physical examination alone or in conjunction with pelvic ultrasound. Functional cysts are more common in patients who have anovulatory cycles, such as patients with polycystic ovarian syndrome or obese patients.

Dermoid cysts, or benign cystic teratomas, are the most common ovarian tumors in women in the second and third decades of life. These cystic masses may be of any size, and up to 15% are bilateral. Torsion is the most frequent complication and commonly occurs in children, young women, and pregnant women. Severe acute abdominal pain is usually the initial symptom, and this condition is considered to be an emergency. Treatment is cystectomy, with close inspection of the other ovary. A cystectomy can usually be performed even for large lesions. The remainder of the ovary should be re-approximated with an absorbable suture; it will usually continue to function normally.

Other common benign neoplasms that occur in young patients include serous and mucinous cystadenomas. These are treated with unilateral salpingo-oophorectomy if the other ovary appears normal. Endometriomas, or the so-called chocolate cysts of endometriosis, can also occur in young women. These patients may have a history of endometriosis or chronic pelvic pain. Often other endometriotic implants may be seen in the pelvis or abdominal cavity, which may be helpful in establishing the diagnosis. The treatment of endometriomas may be cystectomy or unilateral oophorectomy, again depending upon the degree of normal-appearing ovarian tissue that remains. Every effort should be made to salvage the normal-appearing portion of ovary.

If, upon opening the abdomen, ascites is present, the ascites should be evacuated and submitted for cytologic analysis. After careful inspection and palpation, if the tumor appears to be confined to one ovary and malignancy is suspected, unilateral salpingo-oophorectomy is appropriate in most circumstances. If the ovarian mass is thought to be benign, ovarian cystectomy may be preferable. The ovarian capsule should be inspected for any evidence of rupture, adherence, or excrescence. Once removed, the ovarian specimen should be sent for frozen-section examination. If malignancy is diagnosed, surgical staging is appropriate, with biopsy of the omentum, peritoneal surfaces of the pelvis and upper abdomen, and retroperitoneal lymph nodes (including both the paraaortic and bilateral pelvic regions).

If the contralateral ovary appears normal, existing information suggests that random biopsy or wedge resection is not indicated because of the potential for future infertility caused by peritoneal adhesions or ovarian failure. One should also not rely too heavily on frozen-section diagnosis in making the decision to perform hysterectomy and bilateral salpingo-oophorectomy in a young patient. If the histologic diagnosis is questionable, it is always preferable to wait for permanent section results. General criteria for conservative management include the following:

1. Young patient desirous of future childbearing.
2. Patient and family consent and agree to close follow-up.
3. No evidence of dysgenetic gonads.
4. Any unilateral malignant germ cell tumor.
5. Any unilateral stromal tumor.
6. Any unilateral borderline tumor.
7. Stage Ia invasive epithelial tumor.

The advent of in vitro fertilization technology should also have an impact on intraoperative management. Convention has dictated that, if a bilateral salpingo-oophorectomy is indicated, a hysterectomy should also be performed. However, current technology for donor oocyte transfer and hormonal support allows a woman without ovaries to sustain a normal intrauterine pregnancy. Similarly, if the uterus and one tube and ovary are resected because of tumor involvement, current techniques allow for retrieval of oocytes from the patient's remaining ovary, in vitro fertilization with sperm from her partner, and implantation of the embryo into a surrogate's uterus.

To summarize, in any patient for whom the diagnosis is unclear by examination or after consultation with a gynecologic oncologist, the most prudent procedure is removal of the involved ovary with frozen-section diagnosis to rule out malignancy. Again, this assumes that the operator does not feel the mass is benign. The most frequently seen malignant tumors in young women and girls are those of germ cell or stromal origin. These are usually unilateral, may be multicystic, or may contain solid components. Treatment of these tumors has been described earlier. Malignant epithelial tumors are particularly uncommon in young women; however, if a multiseptated or solid mass is found at laparotomy, suggesting an epithelial tumor, the involved ovary should be removed and frozen-section diagnosis obtained. Management of epithelial ovarian cancer has been addressed previously.

OVARIAN MASSES IN POSTMENOPAUSAL WOMEN

The risk of an ovarian mass being malignant begins to increase at 40 years of age and rises steadily thereafter. Therefore the finding of an unsuspected ovarian mass in a postmenopausal woman is a more ominous sign. The most common malignant neoplasms in this age group are malignant epithelial tumors; germ cell and stromal cell tumors rarely occur. Note that benign lesions, such as epithelial cystadenomas and dermoid cysts, can still occur in this population, although at a much less frequent rate than in younger patients. Treatment of an unanticipated ovarian mass in a postmenopausal patient includes salpingo-oophorectomy and frozen-section diagnosis. Appropriate staging biopsies should also be performed. A gynecologic oncologist should be consulted if at all possible.

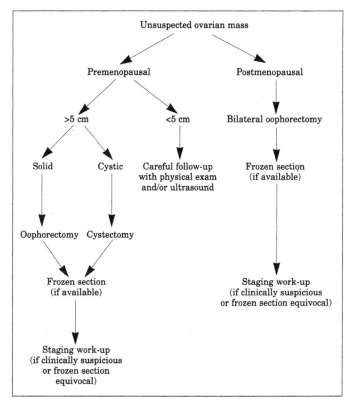

Figure 20-1. Management of the unsuspected ovarian mass found at the time of laparotomy.

CONCLUSIONS

An unsuspected mass on the ovary at the time of surgery should be considered a significant finding, and appropriate consultation or removal of the tumor with frozen-section diagnosis should be undertaken in all cases except for simple functional cysts in young premenopausal patients. If frozen-section analysis is not immediately available, the lesion should still be removed and sent for permanent section pathologic diagnosis (assuming the remainder of the pelvic and abdominal organs are normal). It must be understood that the patient may need additional definitive surgery at a later time if the lesion is ultimately found to be malignant (Fig. 20-1).

FALLOPIAN TUBE CANCER

Incidence

Fallopian tube cancer accounts for 0.1% to 0.5% of all gynecologic malignancies. The average age at diagnosis is 55 years.

Risk Factors
No known risk factors exist for developing this disease.

Pathology
The most common histologic type is adenocarcinoma, and the most common tumors of the fallopian tube are metastatic lesions from other sites. To establish a diagnosis of primary fallopian tube cancer, the following criteria (Hu's criteria) must be met: the main tumor must be in the tube; the mucosa should be involved microscopically and should exhibit a papillary pattern; the transition between benign and malignant tubal epithelium should be demonstrated if the tubal wall is significantly involved with tumor.

Routes of Spread
Fallopian tube cancer metastasizes in a manner similar to that of epithelial ovarian cancer. Lymphatic spread tends to play more of a role in fallopian tube cancer, likely due to the presence of significant lymphatics in the fallopian tubes. One third of patients with fallopian tube cancer exhibit evidence of nodal metastases.

Clinical Features
The classic triad of primary fallopian tube cancer, although present in less than 15% of patients, includes a watery vaginal discharge, pelvic pain, and a pelvic mass. Watery discharge and vaginal bleeding are the most commonly reported symptoms.

Pretreatment Workup
Careful physical examination, including pelvic examination, is required. Other components of the pretreatment workup include complete blood cell count, serum glucose, blood urea nitrogen, creatinine, liver function tests, serum albumin, CA-125, chest radiography, and mammography. Imaging studies may be helpful but most often do not change the planned staging procedure. CT may help determine the extent of disease. Barium enema is useful in examination of the colon. In older patients, barium enema can be particularly helpful in diagnosing a colonic primary, which may present similarly to ovarian and fallopian tube cancers. Intravenous pyelography is also helpful in certain clinical situations.

Staging
There is no official FIGO staging for fallopian tube cancer; by convention, the staging criteria used for epithelial ovarian cancer are used (see Table 20-15).

Treatment
Treatment of fallopian tube cancer is analogous to that of epithelial ovarian cancer (see page 394).

Prognostic Factors
Although prognostic factors are unclear because of the rarity of this tumor, they are most likely similar to those of epithelial ovarian cancer. Overall survival is estimated to be 40%, which

**Table 20-23. Five-year survival rate
for ovarian germ cell tumors (by stage)**

Stage I	72%
Stage II	38%
Stage III	18%
Stage IV	0%

is higher than the 5-year survival rate for patients with epithelial ovarian cancer. This survival rate is likely related to diagnosis at earlier stages (Table 20-23).

GESTATIONAL TROPHOBLASTIC DISEASE

Definition

Gestational trophoblastic disease (GTD) is characterized by an abnormal proliferation of trophoblastic tissue; all forms develop in association with pregnancy. Malignant gestational trophoblastic disease can be subdivided into two categories: nonmetastatic or locally invasive gestational trophoblastic disease and metastatic gestational trophoblastic disease.

Incidence

Because this category of interrelated diseases is associated with a gestational event, the age of occurrence spans the entire reproductive spectrum. Hydatidiform moles occur in 1/600 therapeutic abortions and in 1/1,000 to 1/2,000 pregnancies in the United States; of these, approximately 20% develop malignant sequelae, including invasive moles, placental site trophoblastic tumors, and gestational choriocarcinoma. Choriocarcinoma is estimated to occur in 1 in 20 to 40,000 pregnancies, with half of the cases following term gestations, 25% following molar gestations, and 25% following other gestational events.

Pathology

Gestational trophoblastic disease is divided into the following categories: hydatidiform mole (Table 20-24), invasive mole, choriocarcinoma, and placental site trophoblastic tumor. Nonmetastatic disease following molar evacuation may histologically be that of hydatidiform (invasive) mole or choriocarcinoma. Persistent gestational trophoblastic disease following a nonmolar pregnancy is predominantly choriocarcinoma and in rare instances may be placental site trophoblastic tumor. Metastatic gestational trophoblastic disease diagnosed in the early months after molar evacuation may be hydatidiform mole or choriocarcinoma. When gestational trophoblastic disease is found remote from a gestational event, it is most characteristically choriocarcinoma.

Risk Factors for Hydatidiform Mole

Various well-established risk factors are associated with hydatidiform mole (Table 20-25). These include age (increased risk is associated with age <20 years and >40 years); previous molar pregnancy (women who have had one molar pregnancy have a 0.5% to 2.5% risk of a second occurrence; women who have had two molar

Table 20-24. Classifications of hydatidiform mole

Feature	Partial Mole	Complete Mole
Hydatidiform swelling of villi	Diffuse	Focal
Trophoblast	Cyto-and syncytial hyperplasia	Syncytial
Embryo	Absent	Present
Villous capillaries	No fetal RBCs	Many fetal RBCs
Gestational age at diagnosis	8–16 wk	10–22 wk
β-hCG	Usually >50,000 mIU/mL	Usually >50,000 mIU/mL
Malignant potential	15%–25%	5%–10%
Karyotype	46XX (95%) 46XY (5%)	Triploid (80%)
Size for dates		
Small	33%	65%
Large	33%	10%

β-hCG, beta subunit of human chorionic gonadotropin; RBCs, red blood cells.

Table 20-25. Clinical features of molar pregnancy and the associated risk for development of malignant gestational trophoblastic disease

Clinical Feature	Percent Malignant GTD
Delayed postmolar evacuation hemorrhage	75
Theca lutein cyst > 5 cm	60
Acute pulmonary insufficiency following mole evacuation	58
Uterus large for dates	45
Serum β-hCG > 100,000 mIU/mL	45
Second molar gestation	40
Maternal age > 40 yr	25

β-hCG, beta subunit of human chorionic gonadotropin; GTD, gestational trophoblastic disease.

pregnancies have a 33% risk of a third occurrence); previous spontaneous abortion (risk of a molar gestation increases with each subsequent spontaneous abortion), and race (increased incidence among Asian women; decreased risk among black women).

Routes of Spread

Malignant gestational trophoblastic disease spreads primarily by a hematogenous route.

Clinical Features

Hydatidiform Mole

Vaginal bleeding, uterine size larger than dates, and the presence of prominent theca lutein ovarian cysts are all characteristic clinical features of hydatidiform mole. Other associated findings include toxemia, hyperemesis, hyperthyroidism, and respiratory symptoms such as dyspnea, respiratory distress, and oral pain.

Partial Mole

Patients with partial moles may present in the same manner as those with missed or incomplete abortions, exhibiting vaginal bleeding and the passage of tissue per vagina.

Pretreatment Workup For Molar Pregnancy

Careful physical examination, including pelvic examination, is required. Other components of the pretreatment workup include complete blood cell count, serum glucose, blood urea nitrogen, creatinine, liver function tests, serum albumin, thyroid function tests, β-human chorionic gonadotropin (serum), and chest radiography.

Metastatic Workup for Malignant/ Persistent Gestational Trophoblastic Disease

Metastatic workup for malignant/persistent gestational trophoblastic disease consists of all the preceding tests described for molar pregnancy, as well as pelvic sonography, CT scan of abdomen/pelvis, CT scan or MRI of brain, and CT scan of chest. Measurement of cerebrospinal β-human chorionic gonadotropin by lumbar puncture should be performed if any metastatic disease is present and findings of CT scan or MRI of the brain is negative. The plasma-to-cerebrospinal fluid β-human chorionic gonadotropin ratio is usually less than 60 in cases with cerebral metastases. Metastatic lesions should not be biopsied (i.e., a vaginal nodule) because these lesions are very vascular, and patients have exsanguinated from such biopsies.

Common Metastatic Sites

Malignant gestational trophoblastic disease may metastasize to a wide variety of sites, including the lungs (80%); vagina (30%); pelvis (20%); brain (10%); liver (10%); bowel, kidney, spleen (<5%); and other locations (<5%). In less than 5% of cases, the β-hCG titer may remain elevated without clinical or radiographic evidence of disease. The staging of this disease progression is outlined in Table 20-26.

Table 20-26. FIGO staging

Stage I	Confined to the uterine corpus
Stage II	Metastasis to pelvis and vagina
Stage III	Metastasis to the lung
Stage IV	Distant metastasis to the brain, liver, kidneys, or gastrointestinal tract

FIGO, International Federation of Gynecology and Obstetrics.

Treatment

Molar Pregnancy

Dilation and curettage is the standard treatment of molar pregnancy. Hysterectomy may be performed if fertility is not an issue.

Nonmetastatic Gestational Trophoblastic Disease (FIGO Stage I)

If preservation of fertility is not desired, hysterectomy is recommended for stage I disease. If preservation of fertility is desired, adjuvant single-agent chemotherapy with methotrexate or dactinomycin should be administered for at least one menstrual cycle past a normal β-hCG level. If there is resistance (demonstrated β-hCG level that increases or remains at a plateau), the patient should be crossed over to the agent that was not initially administered. If resistance persists, combination chemotherapy with EMA-CO (etoposide, methotrexate, dactinomycin, cyclophosphamide, and vincristine) or MAC (methotrexate, actinomycin, and cyclophosphamide) should be administered.

Metastatic Gestational Trophoblastic Disease
(FIGO Stages II–IV)

LOW-RISK GESTATIONAL TROPHOBLASTIC DISEASE (WORLD HEALTH ORGANIZATION RISK SCORE OF 0 TO 4). As initial treatment, patients should receive methotrexate or dactinomycin. If there is resistance, the patient should be crossed over to the agent that was not initially administered. If resistance persists, combination chemotherapy with EMA-CO or MAC should be administered. If there is resistance to EMA-CO and MAC, salvage therapy includes the combination of cisplatin, bleomycin, and vinblastine. Ifosfamide also may have a role in refractory cases.

INTERMEDIATE RISK (WORLD HEALTH ORGANIZATION RISK SCORE OF 5 TO 7). Variable treatment regimens exist for intermediate-risk GTD. Single agents can be given, but the failure rate is 20%. Combination chemotherapy is often administered as first-line therapy.

HIGH RISK (WORLD HEALTH ORGANIZATION RISK SCORE OF 8 OR MORE). Combination chemotherapy is treatment of choice for high-risk disease. EMA-CO is the initial chemotherapeutic regimen, with cisplatin, bleomycin, and vinblastine used as salvage treatment.

Special Considerations

Patients with brain metastases may be treated with radiotherapy for local control and prophylaxis against hemorrhage. Patients

Table 20-27. Factors affecting prognosis and response to therapy based on World Health Organization Prognostic Index Score

| Factor | World Health Organization Index Score | | | |
	0	1	2	4
Age (yr)	< 39	> 39		
Antecedent pregnancy	Hyd mole	Abortion	Term	—
Interval between antecedent pregnancy and start of chemotherapy (mon)	< 4	4–6	7–12	>12
β-hCG (mIU/mL)	< 10^3	10^3–10^4	10^4–10^5	>10^5
ABO blood groups (female × male)		O × A A × O	B, AB	—
Largest tumor (cm)		3–5	> 5	—
Site of metastasis	Lung, vagina, pelvis	Spleen, kidney	GI tract, liver	Brain
Number of metastases identified	0	1–4	4–8	> 8
Prior chemotherapy			Single drug	≥ 2 drugs

β-hCG, Beta subunit of human chorionic gonadotropin; GI, gastrointestinal; Hyd, hydatidiform.

with residual solitary liver or lung lesions may be candidates for surgical resection.

Prognostic Factors

Factors that may affect a patient's prognosis and response to treatment are outlined in Table 20-27.

Survival

The cure rate for stage I to III disease is greater than 80%. The cure rate for stage IV disease is approximately 50%.

Recommended Surveillance

Post-treatment surveillance is essentially the same for all cases of gestational trophoblastic disease, with the exception of patients with stage IV disease, because they require a longer period of surveillance. Weekly measurements of β-hCG levels are drawn until levels are normal for 3 consecutive weeks. Monthly β-hCG values are then drawn until levels are normal for 12 consecutive months, except with stage IV disease, which requires 24 months of surveillance. Contraception is mandatory throughout the follow-up period.

GENE THERAPY

During the past decade, advances in molecular biology and technology have opened the door to novel treatment strategies. The ability to modify genetic material and transfer it into cells to either replace a missing or malfunctioning gene or provide a new function to a cell has opened a new spectrum of potential therapeutic possibilities in the treatment of gynecologic malignancies.

In broad, general terms, gene therapy involves the production of genetic material (DNA or RNA) and subsequent injection into the host via a delivery system followed by integration into the host genome and its subsequent effect. Currently, the gene transfer systems under study use liposomes, retroviruses, or adenoviruses as delivery vehicles to integrate the gene sequences into the host genome and exert one of the following antitumor or protective effects:

1. Immunoregulatory gene alteration and antitumor vaccines. This approach may involve the manipulation of cytokine and immunosuppressive expression, redirection of tumor infiltrating lymphocytes, or stimulation of dendritic cells.
2. Antioncogene and tumor suppressor gene alterations. These include the oncogenes *erbB-2,* c-*myc, jun, fos,* k-*ras,* and the suppressor gene *p-53.*
3. Pro-drug therapy that uses cancer cells transfected with a gene that encodes an enzyme capable of converting a normally nontoxic substance into a toxic metabolite. Upon presentation of the substrate, the toxic metabolite produced in the transgene expressing tumor cells induces its death. A current example of this approach is the HSV-TK/ganciclovir system.

Another unique approach to gene therapy involves the *MDR1* gene, which is known to confer immunity from certain chemotherapeutic agents. Research is currently evaluating the transfer of the *MDR1* gene to the host's bone marrow to theoretically allow higher doses of chemotherapy to be given with less bone marrow suppression.

At present there are ongoing phase I trials, primarily in ovarian cancer, that have shown that the genetic modification of cancer cells and subsequent expression of transgenes is feasible. The current clinical trials are promising and indicate that gene therapy may be further refined as our knowledge of immunomodulatory factors, cancer genetics, and improvement of delivery systems evolves. At present, gene therapy is still in its infancy, but one day it may be a truly effective treatment alternative for patients.

RECOMMENDED READING

Vulvar Cancer

Anderson JM, Cassady JR, Shimm DS, et al. Vulvar carcinoma. *Int J Radiat Oncol Biol Phys* 1995;32:1351.

Berek JS, Heaps JM, Fu YS, et al. Concurrent cisplatin and 5-fluorouracil chemotherapy and radiation therapy for advanced-stage squamous carcinoma of the vulva. *Gynecol Oncol* 1991;2: 197.

Binder SW, Huang I, Fu YS, et al. Risk factors for the development of lymph node metastasis in vulvar squamous cell carcinoma. *Gynecol Oncol* 1990;37:9.

Boyce J, Fruchter RG, Kasambilides E, et al. Prognostic factors in carcinoma of the vulva. *Gynecol Oncol* 1985;20:364.

Burke TW, Stringer CA, Gershenson DM, et al. Radical wide excision and selective inguinal node dissection for squamous cell carcinoma of the vulva. *Gynecol Oncol* 1990;38:328.

Chung AF, Woodruff JW, Lewis JL, Jr. Malignant melanoma of the vulva: a report of 44 cases. *Obstet Gynecol* 1975;45:638.

Creasman WT. New gynecologic cancer staging. *Gynecol Oncol* 1995;58:157.

Hacker NF, Van der Velden J. Conservative management of early vulvar cancer. *Cancer* 1993;71[suppl]:1673.

Heaps JM, Fu YS, Montz FJ, et al. Surgical-pathologic variables predictive of local recurrence in squamous cell carcinoma of the vulva. *Gynecol Oncol* 1990;38:309.

Homesley HD, Bundy BN, Sedlis A, et al. Assessment of current International Federation of Gynecology and Obstetrics staging of vulvar carcinoma relative to prognostic factors for survival (a Gynecologic Oncology Group study). *Am J Obstet Gynecol* 1991;164:997.

Homesley HD, Bundy BN, Sedlis A, et al. Prognostic factors for groin node metastasis in squamous cell carcinoma of the vulva (a Gynecologic Oncology Group study). *Gynecol Oncol* 1993;49:279.

Hopkins MP, Reid GC, Morley GW. The surgical management of recurrent squamous cell carcinoma of the vulva. *Obstet Gynecol* 1990;75:1001.

Keys H. Gynecologic Oncology Group randomized trials of combined technique therapy for vulvar cancer. *Cancer* 1993;71[suppl]:1691.

Malfetano JH, Piver MS, Tsukada Y, et al. Univariate and multivariate analyses of 5-year survival, recurrence, and inguinal node metastases in stage I and II vulvar carcinoma. *J Surg Oncol* 1985;30:124.

Perez CA, Grigsby PW, Galakatos A, et al. Radiation therapy in management of carcinoma of the vulva with emphasis on conservation therapy. *Cancer* 1993;71:3707.

Podratz KC, Symmonds RE, Taylor WF, et al. Carcinoma of the vulva: analysis of treatment and survival. *Obstet Gynecol* 1983;61:63.

Russell AH, Mesic JB, Scudder SA, et al. Synchronous radiation and cytotoxic chemotherapy for locally advanced or recurrent squamous cancer of the vulva. *Gynecol Oncol* 1992;47:14.

Sedlis A, Homesley H, Bundy BN, et al. Positive groin lymph nodes in superficial squamous cell vulvar cancer: a Gynecologic Oncology Group study. *Am J Obstet Gynecol* 1987;156:1159.

Shimm DS, Fuller AF, Orlow EL, et al. Prognostic variables in the treatment of squamous cell carcinoma of the vulva. *Gynecol Oncol* 1986;24:343.

Stehman FB, Bundy BN, Dvoretsky PM, et al. Early stage I carcinoma of the vulva treated with ipsilateral superficial inguinal lymphadenectomy and modified radical hemivulvectomy: a prospective study of the Gynecologic Oncology Group. *Obstet Gynecol* 1992;79:490.

Thomas GM, Dembo AJ, Bryson SC, et al. Changing concepts in the management of vulvar cancer. *Gynecol Oncol* 1991;42:9.

Vaginal Cancer

Berek JS, Hacker NF. *Practical gynecologic oncology,* 2nd ed. Baltimore: Williams and Wilkins, 1994.

Delclos L, Wharton JT, Rutledge FN. Tumors of the vagina and female urethra. In: Fletcher GH, ed. *Textbook of radiotherapy,* 3rd ed. Philadelphia: Lea and Febiger, 1980.

Herbst AL, Robboy SJ, Scully RE, et al. Clear cell adenocarcinoma of the vagina and cervix in girls: analysis of 170 registry cases. *Am J Obstet Gynecol* 1974;119:713.

Kucera H, Vavra N. Primary carcinoma of the vagina: clinical and histopathological variables associated with survival. *Gynecol Oncol* 1991;40:12.

Kucera H, Vavra N. Radiation management of primary carcinoma of the vagina: clinical and histopathological variables associated with survival. *Gynecol Oncol* 1991;40:12.

Morrow CP, Curtin JP, Townsend DE. *Synopsis of gynecologic oncology,* 4th ed. New York: Churchill Livingstone, 1993.

Perez CA, Camel HM, Galakatos AE, et al. Definitive irradiation in carcinoma of the vagina: long-term evaluation of results. *Int J Radiat Oncol Biol Phys* 1988;15:1283.

Stock RG, Chen AS, Seski J. A 30-year experience in the management of primary carcinoma of the vagina: analysis of prognostic factors and treatment modalities. *Gynecol Oncol* 1995;56:45.

Cervical Cancer

Alberts DS, Kronmal R, Baker LH, et al. Phase II randomized trial of cisplatin chemotherapy regimens in the treatment of recurrent or metastatic squamous cell cancer of the cervix: a southwest oncology group study. *J Clin Oncol* 1987;5:1791.

American Cancer Society. *Cancer facts and figures.* Atlanta: American Cancer Society, 1995.

Artman LE, Hoskins WJ, Bibro MC, et al. Radical hysterectomy and pelvic lymphadenectomy for stage IB carcinoma of the cervix: 21 years' experience. *Gynecol Oncol* 1987;28:8.

Coia L, Won M, Lanciano R, et al. The patterns of care outcome study for cancer of the uterine cervix: results of the Second National Practice Survey. *Cancer* 1990;66:2451.

Coleman RE, Harper PG, Gallagher C, et al. A phase II study of ifosfamide in advanced and relapsed carcinoma of the cervix. *Cancer Chemother Pharmacol* 1986;18:280.

Creasman WT. New gynecologic cancer staging. *Gynecol Oncol* 1995;58:157.

Creasman WF, Fetter BF, Clarke-Pearson DL, et al. Management of stage IA carcinoma of the cervix. *Am J Obstet Gynecol* 1985;153:164.

Dembo AJ, Balogh JM. Advances in radiotherapy in the gynecologic malignancies. *Semin Surg Oncol* 1990;6:323.

Eifel PJ, Burke TW, Delclos L, et al. Early stage I adenocarcinoma of the uterine cervix: treatment results in patients with tumors ~4 cm in diameter. *Gynecol Oncol* 1991;41:199.

Fletcher GH, Rutledge FN. Overall results in radiotherapy for carcinoma of the cervix. *Clin Obstet Gynecol* 1967;10:958.

Grigsby PW, Perez CA. Radiotherapy alone for medically inoperable carcinoma of the cervix: stage IA and carcinoma in situ. *Int J Radiat Oncol Biol Phys* 1991;21:375.

Hopkins MP, Morley GW. Squamous cell cancer of the cervix: prognostic factors related to survival. *Int J Gynecol Cancer* 1991;1:173.

Morrow CP, Curtin JP, Townsend DE. *Synopsis of gynecologic oncology*, 4th ed. New York: Churchill Livingstone, 1993.

Perez CA, Grigsby PW, Nene SM, et al. Effect of tumor size on the prognosis of carcinoma of the uterine cervix treated with irradiation alone. *Cancer* 1992;69:2796.

Rutledge FN, Smith JP, Wharton JT, et al. Pelvic exenteration: analysis of 296 patients. *Am J Obstet Gynecol* 1977;129:881.

Sevin BU, Nadji M, Averette HE, et al. Microinvasive carcinoma of the cervix. *Cancer* 1992;70:2121.

Stehman FB, Bundy BN, DiSaia PJ, et al. Carcinoma of the cervix treated with radiation therapy: a multivariate analysis of prognostic variables in the gynecologic oncology group. *Cancer* 1991;67:2776.

Thomas G, Dembo A, Fyles A, et al. Concurrent chemoradiation in advanced cervical cancer. *Gynecol Oncol* 1990;38:446.

Vermorken JB. The role of chemotherapy in squamous cell carcinoma of the uterine cervix: a review. *Int J Gynecol Cancer* 1993;3:129.

Endometrial Cancer

American Cancer Society. *Cancer facts and figures*. Atlanta: American Cancer Society, 1995.

Axelrod JH, Gynecologic Oncology Group. Phase II study of whole-abdominal radiotherapy in patients with papillary serous carcinoma and clear cell carcinoma of the endometrium or with maximally debulked advanced endometrial carcinoma (summary last modified 05/91), GOG-94, clinical trial, closed, 02/24/92.

Boring CC, Squires TS, Tong T. Cancer statistics, 1991. *Cancer* 1991;41:19.

Burke TW, Munkarah A, Kavanagh JJ, et al. Treatment of advanced or recurrent endometrial carcinoma with single-agent carboplatin. *Gynecol Oncol* 1993;51:397.

Burke TW, Stringer CL, Morris M, et al. Prospective treatment of advanced or recurrent endometrial carcinoma with cisplatin, doxorubicin, and cyclophosphamide. *Gynecol Oncol* 1991;40:264.

Creasman WT. New gynecologic cancer staging. *Obstet Gynecol* 1990;75:287.

Creasman WT, Morrow CP, Bundy BN, et al. Surgical pathologic spread patterns of endometrial cancer: a Gynecologic Oncology Group study. *Cancer* 1987;60:2035.

Gusberg SB. Virulence factors in endometrial cancer. *Cancer* 1993;71[suppl]:1464.

Hancock KC, Freedman RS, Edwards CL, et al. Use of cisplatin, doxorubicin, and cyclophosphamide to treat advanced and recurrent adenocarcinoma of the endometrium. *Cancer Treat Rep* 1986;70:789.

Homesley HD, Zaino R. Endometrial cancer: prognostic factors. *Semin Oncol* 1994;21:71.

Lanciano RM, Corn BW, Schultz DJ, et al. The justification for a surgical staging system in endometrial carcinoma. *Radiother Oncol* 1993;28:189.

Lentz SS. Advanced and recurrent endometrial carcinoma: hormonal therapy. *Semin Oncol* 1994;21:100.

Marchetti DL, Caglar H, Driscoll DL, et al. Pelvic radiation in stage I endometrial adenocarcinoma with high-risk attributes. *Gynecol Oncol* 1990;37:51.

Morrow CP, Bundy BN, Kurman RJ, et al. Relationship between surgical-pathological risk factors and outcome in clinical stage I and II carcinoma of the endometrium: a gynecologic oncology group study. *Gynecol Oncol* 1991;40:55.

Morrow CP, Curtin JP, Townsend DE. *Synopsis of gynecologic oncology,* 4th ed. New York: Churchill Livingstone, 1993.

Nori D, Hilaris BS, Tome M, et al. Combined surgery and radiation in endometrial carcinoma: an analysis of prognostic factors. *Int J Radiat Oncol Biol Phys* 1987;13:489.

Piver MS, Hempling RE. A prospective trial of postoperative vaginal radium/cesium for grade 1 to 2 less than 50% myometrial invasion and pelvic radiation therapy for grade 3 or deep myometrial invasion in surgical stage I endometrial adenocarcinoma. *Cancer* 1990;66:1133.

Potish RA, Twiggs LB, Adcock LL, et al. Role of whole abdominal radiation therapy in the management of endometrial cancer: prognostic importance of factors indicating peritoneal metastases. *Gynecol Oncol* 1985;21:80.

Quinn MA, Campbell JJ. Tamoxifen therapy in advanced/recurrent endometrial carcinoma. *Gynecol Oncol* 1989;32:1.

Roberts JA, Gynecologic Oncology Group. Phase III randomized evaluation of adjuvant postoperative pelvic radiotherapy vs no adjuvant therapy for surgical stage I and occult stage II intermediate-risk endometrial carcinoma (summary last modified 08/95), GOG-99, clinical trial, closed, 07/03/95.

Rutledge F. The role of radical hysterectomy in adenocarcinoma of the endometrium. *Gynecol Oncol* 1974;2:331.

Seski JC, Edwards CL, Herson J, et al. Cisplatin chemotherapy for disseminated endometrial cancer. *Obstet Gynecol* 1982;59:225.

Uterine Sarcomas

Berek JS, Hacker NF. *Practical gynecologic oncology,* 2nd ed. Baltimore: Williams and Wilkins, 1994.

Gershenson DM, Kavanagh JJ, Copeland LJ, et al. Cisplatin therapy for disseminated mixed mesodermal sarcoma of the uterus. *J Clin Oncol* 1987;5:618.

Harlow BL, Weiss NS, Lofton S. The epidemiology of sarcomas of the uterus. *J Natl Cancer Inst* 1986;76:399.

Hornback NB, Omura G, Major FJ. Observations on the use of adjuvant radiation therapy in patients with stage I and II uterine sarcoma. *Int J Radiat Oncol Biol Phys* 1986;12:2127.

Major FJ, Blessing JA, Silverberg SG, et al. Prognostic factors in early-stage uterine sarcoma: a gynecologic oncology group study. *Cancer* 1993;71[suppl]:1702.

Morrow CP, Curtin JP, Townsend DE. *Synopsis of gynecologic oncology,* 4th ed. New York: Churchill Livingstone, 1993.

Norris HJ, Taylor HB. Postirradiation sarcomas of the uterus. *Obstet Gynecol* 1965;26:689.

Olah KS, Dunn JA, Gee H. Leiomyosarcomas have a poorer prognosis than mixed mesodermal tumours when adjusting for known prognostic factors: the result of a retrospective study of 423 cases of uterine sarcoma. *Br J Obstet Gynaecol* 1992;99:590.

Omura GA, Blessing JA, Lifshitz S, et al. A randomized clinical trial of adjuvant adriamycin in uterine sarcomas: a gynecologic oncology group study. *J Clin Oncol* 1985;3:1240.

Omura GA, Blessing JA, Major F, et al. A randomized clinical trial of adjuvant adriamycin in uterine sarcomas: a gynecologic oncology group study. *J Clin Oncol* 1985;3:1240.

Silverberg SG, Major FJ, Blessing JA, et al. Carcinosarcoma (malignant mixed mesodermal tumor) of the uterus: a gynecologic oncology group pathologic study of 203 cases. *Int J Gynecol Pathol* 1990;9:1.

Sutton GP, Blessing JA, Barrett RJ, et al. Phase II trial of ifosfamide and mesna in leiomyosarcoma of the uterus: a gynecologic oncology group study. *Am J Obstet Gynecol* 1992;166:556.

Sutton GP, Gynecologic Oncology Group. Phase II master protocol study of chemotherapeutic agents in the treatment of recurrent or advanced uterine sarcomas—IFF plus mesna (summary last modified 04/93), GOG-87B, clinical trial, completed, 12/28/94.

Sutton GP, Gynecologic Oncology Group. Phase III study of IFF and the uroprotector mesna administered alone or with CDDP in patients with advanced or recurrent mixed mesodermal tumors of the uterus (summary last modified 08/95), GOG-108, clinical trial, active, 02/15/89.

Wheelock JB, Krebs H-B, Schneider V, et al. Uterine sarcoma: analysis of prognostic variables in 71 cases. *Am J Obstet Gynecol* 1985;151:1016.

Epithelial Ovarian Cancer

Berek JS, Hacker NF. *Practical gynecologic oncology,* 2nd ed. Baltimore: Williams and Wilkins, 1994.

Cannistra SA. Cancer of the ovary. *N Engl J Med* 1993;329:1550.

Dembo AJ, Davy M, Stenwig AE. Prognostic factors in patients with stage I epithelial ovarian cancer. *Obstet Gynecol* 1990;75:263.

Einzig AI, Wiernik PH, Sasloff J, et al. Phase II study and long-term follow-up of patients treated with taxol for advanced ovarian adenocarcinoma. *J Clin Oncol* 1992;10:1748.

Eisenhauer EA, ten Bokkel Huinink WW, Swenerton KD, et al. European-Canadian randomized trial of paclitaxel in relapsed ovarian cancer: high-dose versus low-dose and long versus short infusion. *J Clin Oncol* 1994;12:2654.

Flam F, Einhorn N, Sjovall K. Symptomatology of ovarian cancer. *Eur J Obstet Gynecol Reprod Biol* 1988;27:53.

Gershenson DM, Mitchell MF, Atkinson N, et al. The effect of prolonged cisplatin-based chemotherapy on progression-free survival in patients with optimal epithelial ovarian cancer: "maintenance" therapy reconsidered. *Gynecol Oncol* 1992;47:7.

Goodman HM, Harlow BL, Sheets EE, et al. The role of cytoreductive surgery in the management of stage IV epithelial ovarian carcinoma. *Gynecol Oncol* 1992;46:367.

Hakes TB, Chalas E, Hoskins WJ, et al. Randomized prospective trial of 5 versus 10 cycles of cyclophosphamide, doxorubicin, and cisplatin in advanced ovarian carcinoma. *Gynecol Oncol* 1992;45:284.

Heintz APM, Hacker NF, Lagasse LD. Epidemiology and etiology of ovarian cancer: a review. *Obstet Gynecol* 1985;66:127.

Hogberg T, Kagedal B. Long-term follow-up of ovarian cancer with monthly determinations of serum CA 125. *Gynecol Oncol* 1992; 46:191.

Hoskins WJ. Surgical staging and cytoreductive surgery of epithelial ovarian cancer. *Cancer* 1993;71[suppl]:1534.

Hoskins WJ, Bundy BN, Thigpen JT, et al. The influence of cytoreductive surgery on recurrence-free interval and survival in small-volume stage III epithelial ovarian cancer: a gynecologic oncology group study. *Gynecol Oncol* 1992;47:159.

Hoskins WJ, McGuire WP, Brady MF, et al. The effect of diameter of largest residual disease on survival after primary cytoreductive surgery in patients with suboptimal residual epithelial ovarian carcinoma. *Am J Obstet Gynecol* 1994;170:974.

Kohn EC, Sarosy G, Bicher A, et al. Dose-intense taxol: High response rate in patients with platinum-resistant recurrent ovarian cancer. *J Natl Cancer Inst* 1994;86:18.

Krag KJ, Canellos GP, Griffiths CT, et al. Predictive factors for long term survival in patients with advanced ovarian cancer. *Gynecol Oncol* 1989;34:88.

Lynch HT, Watson P, Lynch JF, et al. Hereditary ovarian cancer: heterogeneity in age at onset. *Cancer* 1993;71[suppl]:573.

Martinez A, Schray MF, Howes AE, et al. Postoperative radiation therapy for epithelial ovarian cancer: the curative role based on a 24-year experience. *J Clin Oncol* 1985;3:901.

McGuire WP, Hoskins WJ, Brady MF, et al. Cyclophosphamide and cisplatin compared with paclitaxel and cisplatin in patients with stage III and stage IV ovarian cancer. *N Engl J Med* 1996; 334:1.

Morris M, Gershenson DM, Wharton JT, et al. Secondary cytoreductive surgery for recurrent epithelial ovarian cancer. *Gynecol Oncol* 1989;34:334.

NIH Consensus Conference. Ovarian cancer: screening treatment, and follow-up. *JAMA* 1995;273:491.

Omura GA, Brady MF, Homesley HD, et al. Long-term follow-up and prognostic factor analysis in advanced ovarian carcinoma: the gynecologic oncology group experience. *J Clin Oncol* 1991;9:1138.

Omura GA, Bundy BN, Berek JS, et al. Randomized trial of cyclophosphamide plus cisplatin with or without doxorubicin in ovarian carcinoma: a gynecologic oncology group study. *J Clin Oncol* 1989;7:457.

Pecorelli S, Bolis G, Colombo N, et al. Adjuvant therapy in early ovarian cancer: results of two randomized trials. *Gynecol Oncol* 1994;52:102.

Pettersson F. *Annual report of the results of treatment in gynecologic cancer.* International Federation of Gynecology and Obstetrics (FIGO), vol. 20. Stockholm: Panoramic Press, 1988.

Piver MS, Baker TR, Jishi MF, et al. Familial ovarian cancer: a report of 658 families from the Gilda Radner familial ovarian cancer registry 1981 to 1991. *Cancer* 1993;71[suppl]:582.

Piver MS, Malfetano J, Baker TR, et al. Five-year survival for stage IC or stage I, grade 3 epithelial ovarian cancer treated with cisplatin-based chemotherapy. *Gynecol Oncol* 1992;46:357.

Potter ME, Partridge EE, Hatch KD, et al. Primary surgical therapy of ovarian cancer: how much and when? *Gynecol Oncol* 1991;40: 195.

Sigurdsson K, Alm P, Gullberg B. Prognostic factors in malignant ovarian tumors. *Gynecol Oncol* 1983;15:370.

Trimble EL, Arbuck SG, McGuire WP. Options for primary chemotherapy of epithelial ovarian cancer: taxanes. *Gynecol Oncol* 1994;55:S114.

van der Burg ME, van Lent M, Buyse M, et al. The effect of debulking surgery after induction chemotherapy on the prognosis in advanced epithelial ovarian cancer. *N Engl J Med* 1995;332:629.

Williams L. The role of secondary cytoreductive surgery in epithelial ovarian malignancies. *Oncology* 1992;6:25.

Young RC, Gynecologic Oncology Group. Phase III randomized study of CBDCA/TAX administered for 3 vs 6 courses for selected stages IA-C and stages IIA-C ovarian epithelial cancer (summary last modified 10/95), GOG-157, clinical trial, active, 03/20/95.

Young RC, Walton LA, Ellenberg SS, et al. Adjuvant therapy in stage I and stage II epithelial ovarian cancer: results of two prospective randomized trials. *N Engl J Med* 1990;322:1021.

Zaino RJ, Unger ER, Whitney C. Synchronous carcinomas of the uterine corpus and ovary. *Gynecol Oncol* 1984;19:329.

Ovarian Tumors of Low Malignant Potential

Bell DA, Scully RE. Serous borderline tumors of the peritoneum. *Am J Surg Pathol* 1990;14:230.

Casey AC, Bell DA, Lage JM, et al. Epithelial ovarian tumors of borderline malignancy: long-term follow-up. *Gynecol Oncol* 1993;50:316.

de Nictolis M, Montironi R, Tommasoni S, et al. Serous borderline tumors of the ovary. *Cancer* 1992;70:152.

Fort MG, Pierce VK, Saigo PE, et al. Evidence for the efficacy of adjuvant therapy in epithelial ovarian tumors of low malignant potential. *Gynecol Oncol* 1989;32:269.

Gershenson DM, Silva EG. Serous ovarian tumors of low malignant potential with peritoneal implants. *Cancer* 1990;65:578.

Hopkins MP, Kumar NB, Morley GW. An assessment of pathologic features and treatment modalities in ovarian tumors of low malignant potential. *Obstet Gynecol* 1987;70:293.

Koern J, Trope CG, Abeler VM. A retrospective study of 370 borderline tumors of the ovary treated at the Norwegian Radium Hospital from 1970 to 1982. *Cancer* 1993;71:1810.

Kurman RJ, Trimble CL. The behavior of serous tumors of low malignant potential: Are they ever malignant? *Int J Gynecol Pathol* 1993;12:120.

Leake JF, Currie JL, Rosenshein NB, et al. Long-term follow-up of serous ovarian tumors of low malignant potential. *Gynecol Oncol* 1992;47:150.

Michael H, Roth LM. Invasive and noninvasive implants in ovarian serous tumors of low malignant potential. *Cancer* 1986;57:1240.

Rice LW, Berkowitz RS, Mark SD, et al. Epithelial ovarian tumors of borderline malignancy. *Gynecol Oncol* 1990;39:195.

Sutton GP, Bundy BN, Omura GA, et al. Stage III ovarian tumors of low malignant potential treated with cisplatin combination therapy (a gynecologic oncology group study). *Gynecol Oncol* 1991;41:230.

Trimble EL, Trimble CL. Epithelial ovarian tumors of low malignant potential. In: Markman M, Hoskins WJ, eds. *Cancer of the ovary.* New York: Raven Press, 1993.

Trope C, Kaern J, Vergote IB, et al. Are borderline tumors of the ovary overtreated both surgically and systematically? A review of four prospective randomized trials including 253 patients with borderline tumors. *Gynecol Oncol* 1993;51:236.

Yazigi R, Sandstad J, Munoz AK. Primary staging in ovarian tumors of low malignant potential. *Gynecol Oncol* 1988;31:402.

Sex Cord Stromal Tumors

Berek JS, Hacker NF. *Practical gynecologic oncology,* 2nd ed. Baltimore: Williams and Wilkins, 1994.

Bjorkholm E, Silversward C. Prognostic factors in granulosa-cell tumors. *Gynecol Oncol* 1981;11:261.

Bjorkholm E, Silversward C. Theca cell tumors. Clinical features and prognosis. *Acta Radiol* 1980;19:241.

Evans AT III, Gaffey TA, Malkasian GD, Jr. Clinicopathologic review of 118 granulosa and 82 theca cell tumors. *Obstet Gynecol* 1980;55:231.

Fox H, Agarical K, Langley FA. A clinicopathologic study of 92 cases of granulosa cell tumors of the ovary with special reference to the factors influencing prognosis. *Cancer* 1975;35:231.

Gershenson DM. Management of early ovarian cancer: germ cell and sex cord-stromal tumors. *Gynecol Oncol* 1994;55:S62.

Lappohn RE, Burger HG, Bouma J, et al. Inhibin as a marker for granulosa-cell tumors. *N Engl J Med* 1989;321:790.

Meigs JV, Armstrong SH, Hamilton HH. A further contribution to the syndrome of fibroma of the ovary with fluid in the abdomen and chest, Meig's syndrome. *Am J Obstet Gynecol* 1943;46:19.

Norris HJ, Taylor HB. Prognosis of granulosa-theca tumors of the ovary. *Cancer* 1968;21:255.

Roth LM, Anderson MC, Govan AD, et al. Sertoli-Leydig cell tumors: a clinicopathologic study of 34 cases. *Cancer* 1981;48:187.

Scully RE. Ovarian tumors: A review. *Am J Pathol* 1977;87:686.

Young RH, Scully RE. Ovarian sex cord-stromal tumors: recent progress. *Int J Gynecol Pathol* 1982;1:101.

Young RH, Scully RE. Ovarian sex cord stromal and steroid cell tumors. In: Roth LM, Czernobilsky B, eds. *Tumors and tumor-like conditions of the ovary.* New York: Churchill Livingstone, 1985.

Young RH, Welch WR, Dickersin GR, et al. Ovarian sex cord tumor with annular tubules. Review of 74 cases including 27 with Peutz-Jeghers syndrome and four with adenoma malignum of the cervix. *Cancer* 1982;50:1384.

Ovarian Germ Cell Tumors

Gershenson DM. Update on malignant ovarian germ cell tumors. *Cancer* 1993;71[suppl]:1581.

Gershenson DM, Morris M, Cangir A, et al. Treatment of malignant germ cell tumors of the ovary with bleomycin, etoposide, and cisplatin. *J Clin Oncol* 1990;8:715.

Kurman RJ, Norris HJ. Malignant germ cell tumors of the ovary. *Hum Pathol* 1977;8:551.

Morrow CP, Curtin JP, Townsend DE. *Synopsis of gynecologic oncology,* 4th ed. New York: Churchill Livingstone, 1993.

Munshi NC, Loehrer PJ, Roth BJ, et al. Vinblastine, ifosfamide and cisplatin (VeIP) as second line chemotherapy in metastatic germ cell tumors (GCT). *Proceed Am Soc Clin Oncol* 1990;9:134.

Romero R, Schwartz PE. Alpha-fetoprotein determinations in the management of endodermal sinus tumors and mixed germ cell tumors of the ovary. *Am J Obstet Gynecol* 1981;141:126.

Schwartz PE, Morris JM. Serum lactic dehydrogenase: a tumor marker for dysgerminoma. *Obstet Gynecol* 1988;72:511.

Serov SF, Scully RE, Robin IH. *International histologic classification of tumours,* no. 9. *Histological typing of ovarian tumours.* Geneva: World Health Organization, 1973.

Slayton RE, Park RC, Silverberg SG, et al. Vincristine, dactinomycin, and cyclophosphamide in the treatment of malignant germ cell tumors of the ovary. *Cancer* 1985;56:243.

Williams SD, Birch R, Einhorn LH, et al. Treatment of disseminated germ-cell tumors with cisplatin, bleomycin, and either vinblastine or etoposide. *N Engl J Med* 1987;316:1435.

Williams SD, Blessing JA, Hatch KD, et al. Chemotherapy of advanced dysgerminoma: Trials of the Gynecologic Oncology Group. *J Clin Oncol* 1991;9:1950.

Williams S, Blessing JA, Liao SY, et al. Adjuvant therapy of ovarian germ cell tumors with cisplatin, etoposide, and bleomycin: a trial of the gynecologic oncology group. *J Clin Oncol* 1994;12:701.

Williams SD, Blessing JA, Moore DH, et al. Cisplatin, vinblastine, and bleomycin in advanced and recurrent ovarian germ-cell tumors: a trial of the gynecologic oncology group. *Ann Intern Med* 1989;111:22.

Williams SD, Gershenson DM. Management of germ cell tumors of the ovary. In: Markman M, Hoskins WJ, eds. *Cancer of the ovary.* New York: Raven Press, 1993.

Williams SD, Gynecologic oncology group. Phase II combination chemotherapy with BEP (CDDP/VP-16/BLEO) as induction followed by VAC (VCR/DACT/CTX) as consolidation in patients with incompletely resected malignant ovarian germ cell tumors (summary last modified 10/95), GOG-90, clinical trial, active, 09/15/86.

Fallopian Tube Cancer

Eddy GL, Copeland LJ, Gershenson DM, et al. Fallopian tube carcinoma. *Obstet Gynecol* 1984;64:156.

Hu CY, Taymor ML, Hertig AT. Primary carcinoma of the fallopian tube. *Am J Obstet Gynecol* 1950;59:58.

Morris M, Gershenson DM, Burke TW, et al. Treatment of fallopian tube carcinoma with cisplatin, doxorubicin and cyclophosphamide. *Obstet Gynecol* 1990;76:1020.

Rose PG, Piver MS, Tsukada Y. Fallopian tube cancer. *Cancer* 1990; 66:2661.

Sedlis A. Carcinoma of the fallopian tube. *Surg Clin North Am* 1978; 58:121.

Gestational Trophoblastic Disease

Azab M, Droz JP, Theodore C, et al. Cisplatin, vinblastine, and bleomycin combination in the treatment of resistant high-risk gestational trophoblastic tumors. *Cancer* 1989;64:1829.

Bagshawe KD. High-risk metastatic trophoblastic disease. *Obstet Gynecol Clin North Am* 1988;15:531.

Berek JS, Hacker NF. *Practical gynecologic oncology,* 2nd ed. Baltimore: Williams and Wilkins, 1994.

Lurain JR. Gestational trophoblastic tumors. *Semin Surg Oncol* 1990;6:347.

Morrow CP, Curtin JP, Townsend DE. *Synopsis of gynecologic oncology,* 4th ed. New York: Churchill Livingstone, 1993.

Mutch DG, Soper JT, Babcock CJ, et al. Recurrent gestational trophoblastic disease: experience of the southeastern regional trophoblastic disease center. *Cancer* 1990;66:978.

Newlands ES, Bagshawe KD, Begent RH, et al. Results with the EMA/CO (etoposide, methotrexate, actinomycin D, cyclophosphamide, vincristine) regimen in high risk gestational trophoblastic tumours, 1979 to 1989. *Br J Obstet Gynaecol* 1991;98:550.

Surwit EA. Management of high-risk gestational trophoblastic disease. *J Reprod Med* 1987;32:657.

World Health Organization Scientific Group. Gestational trophoblastic diseases. *WHO Tech Rep Ser* 1983;692:1.

Gene Therapy

Dorigo O, Berek JS. Gene therapy for ovarian cancer: development of novel treatment strategies. *Int J Gynecol Cancer* 1997;7:2.

Sobol RE, Shawler DL, Dorigo O, et al. Immunogene therapy of cancer. In: Sobol RE, Scanlon KJ, eds. *The internet book of gene therapy.* Norwalk: Appleton and Lange, 1995.

Vile R, Russell SJ. Gene transfer technologies for the gene therapy of cancer. *Gene Therapy* 1995;1:88.

Oncologic Emergencies

Jeffrey D. Wayne and Richard J. Bold

True oncologic emergencies are rare, and often do not require surgery, such as superior vena cava (SVC) syndrome, spinal cord compression, and paraneoplastic syndromes. However, surgeons are often asked to consult on how to manage patients with malignancies who have complications from tumor progression, or from cytotoxic therapies. This chapter first describes some of the more common extra-abdominal problems among surgical patients with cancer, and then focuses specifically on the acute abdominal conditions for which surgical consultation is obtained.

EXTRAABDOMINAL EMERGENCIES

Superior Vena Cava Syndrome

Obstruction of the SVC results in a constellation of signs and symptoms collectively known as the superior vena cava syndrome (SVCS). Impedance of outflow from the SVC may result from external compression by neoplastic disease, fibrosis secondary to inflammation, or thrombosis. In up to 97% of patients with SVCS, this condition is caused by malignancy. Lung cancer and lymphoma are the most frequent causes. An increasingly common etiology of SVCS is thrombosis secondary to indwelling central venous catheters. The underlying source of obstruction of the SVC must be established, as this information is used to guide therapy and to determine prognosis. In the past, patients with SVCS were emergently treated with mediastinal irradiation. However, because radiation-induced tissue necrosis often frustrates later attempts at tissue diagnosis, empiric radiation therapy is no longer advocated. Therapy based on the specific type of tumor can often provide substantial palliation and even a cure for patients presenting with SVCS.

The SVC is the primary conduit for venous drainage of the head, neck, upper extremities, and upper thorax. This thin-walled, compliant vessel is surrounded by more rigid structures, including the mediastinal and paratracheal lymph nodes, the trachea and right mainstem bronchus, the pulmonary artery, and the aorta. It is therefore susceptible to external compression by any space-occupying lesion. Obstruction of outflow from the SVC results in venous hypertension of the head, neck, and upper extremities, which in turn manifests as SVCS. In most cases, obstruction of the SVC is not an acute event, and the signs and symptoms of SVCS develop gradually. The most common symptoms include dyspnea, which occurs in 63% of patients with SVCS and facial fullness in 50% of patients. Physical findings commonly associated with SVCS include facial edema, venous engorgement of the neck and chest wall, cyanosis, and plethora. Symptoms worsen when the patient bends forward or reclines. Obstruction of the SVC becomes a true emergency when associated laryngeal edema nial pressure is elevated.

Patients with SVCS should be thoroughly evaluated, beginning with a directed history and physical examination. A history of malignancy, heavy smoking, or symptoms such as cough, fever, and night sweats should be noted. It is important to examine all lymph node basins and to note the presence of a central venous catheter. Chest radiography reveals an abnormality in 84% of patients with SVCS, although the findings are often nonspecific. A computed tomography (CT) scan of the chest is the initial test of choice and will determine whether the obstruction is due to external compression, or to thrombosis. CT scans also provide anatomic detail of tumor masses, and can be used as a guide for percutaneous biopsy. Magnetic resonance imaging (MRI) is an alternative for patients with renal insufficiency or an allergy to contrast. Minimally invasive techniques of tissue diagnosis include sputum cytology, CT-guided percutaneous biopsy, bronchoscopy, lymph node biopsy, and bone marrow biopsy. Invasive procedures, such as mediastinoscopy and thoracotomy, should be considered if all initial measures fail to establish a diagnosis. These invasive procedures can be performed safely in most patients with SVCS. Using these techniques to guide individualized treatment is preferable to proceeding with nonspecific therapy.

When the etiology of SVCS is malignancy, treatment is based on tumor type. Using diuretics and elevation of the head mitigate the symptoms of SVCS, and using steroids reduces inflammation. Only those patients with evidence of impending airway obstruction or elevated intracranial pressure should be considered for emergent radiation therapy. Even in such cases, intubation, mechanical ventilation, and osmotic diuretics can suspend the progression of symptoms for a period sufficient to allow for a tissue diagnosis. Once the diagnosis is made, tumor-specific therapy should be initiated. Small cell lung cancer and lymphoma are best treated with combination chemotherapy; radiation therapy may be used for consolidation. In a series of 56 patients with small cell lung cancer, SVCS was resolved in all 23 patients treated with chemotherapy alone, in 64% of those treated with radiation therapy alone, and in 83% of those treated with combination therapy. Non–small cell lung cancer is most often treated with radiation therapy. One commonly used fractionation schedule provides high-dose treatment (3–4 Gy/day) for 3 days followed by conventional dose fractionation (1.8–2.0 Gy/day) to a total of 50 to 60 Gy. About 70% of patients on such a treatment schedule respond within 2 weeks.

Patients with SVCS secondary to catheter-induced thrombosis may be successfully treated with thrombolytic agents followed by systemic anticoagulation. Thrombolytic agents are most effective when patients are treated within 5 days after the onset of symptoms. Alternatively, catheter removal followed by systemic anticoagulation often results in gradual recanalization of the SVC and resolution of symptoms. For SVCS refractory to such measures, balloon angioplasty and expandable stents are palliative modalities. Surgical intervention consisting of innominate vein-right atrial bypass is generally reserved for patients in whom the SVCS arises from causes other than malignancy.

Spinal Cord Compression

Spinal cord compression is the second most common neurologic complication of cancer with an estimated 20,000 new cases annually in the United States alone. Autopsy studies suggest that 5% of patients with malignancies have evidence of spinal cord involvement. Early recognition and diagnosis are essential, as spinal cord compression can produce paralysis and loss of sphincter control if left untreated. Patients in whom symptoms present early and in whom neurologic deficits are minimal have the most favorable prognosis. Unfortunately, nearly 80% of patients are unable to walk at the time of presentation.

Spinal cord compression in patients with cancer usually involves extradural metastatic lesions of the vertebral body or neural arch. Tumors expand posteriorly, resulting in anterior compression of the dural sac. Rarely, metastasis can occur in intradural locations without bony involvement. Paraspinal tumors can also cause spinal cord compression by penetrating the intervertebral foramen.

Most of the data on spinal cord compression in malignancy are from animal models. If spinal cord compression develops gradually, decompression can be delayed without impairing the return of neurologic function; however, in cases of rapid compression of the spinal cord, therapeutic intervention must be performed immediately to avoid irreversible neurologic deficits. Spinal cord edema also plays an important role in the development of neurologic injury.

Although spinal cord compression can occur as the initial manifestation of disease, most patients who present with spinal cord compression due to malignancy have been previously diagnosed with cancer. The interval from initial diagnosis to epidural spinal cord compression varies with the type of primary tumor involved. Lung cancer may have an aggressive presentation, with epidural spinal cord compression developing within a few months after diagnosis of the primary lesion. Conversely, patients with carcinoma of the breast have been reported to manifest spinal cord compression up to 20 years after initial presentation of disease.

The incidences of involvement of the three spinal cord segments (cervical, 10%; thoracic, 70%; lumbosacral, 20%) reflect the number of vertebrae in each anatomic segment. More than 90% of patients with spinal cord compression due to malignancy present with localized back pain, which may be exacerbated by movement, recumbency, coughing, sneezing, or straining. The pain due to spinal cord compression can be radicular in distribution. Pain is usually present for several weeks before neurologic symptoms develop. Left untreated, weakness and numbness occur, usually beginning in the toes and ascending to the level of the lesion. Autonomic dysfunction usually occurs late in the disease process. The onset of urinary retention and constipation represents an ominous sign, indicating possible progression to irreversible paraplegia.

Physical examination may reveal tenderness, upon palpation, over the involved vertebrae. Straight leg raise and neck flexion may produce pain at the level of the involved vertebrae. Weakness, spasticity, abnormal reflexes, and extensor plantar response

(Babinski's sign) may be evident on physical examination. A palpable urinary bladder or decreased anal sphincter tone may be present.

Patients with signs of impending neurologic deficits should undergo immediate evaluation and treatment. Depending on the history and physical examination, patients should be treated with dexamethasone 10 mg IV followed by 4 mg IV or PO every 6 hours. Rapid radiographic assessment should be performed simultaneously. In more than two thirds of patients with spinal cord compression, plain films of the spine show evidence of bony abnormalities. Radiographic findings suggestive of a spine metastasis include erosion or loss of vertebral pedicles, partial or complete collapse of vertebral bodies, and paraspinal soft-tissue masses. However, normal spine radiographs do not exclude the possibility that epidural metastases are present. In fact, patients with lymphoma typically have normal spine radiographs even when epidural tumors are present.

Currently, MRI is the study of choice for evaluating patients with suspected spinal cord compression after plain radiographs have been obtained. MRI has several advantages over CT myelogram. Lumbar puncture, which is required for a myelogram, is associated with substantial morbidity in patients who have a space-occupying lesion and with potential bleeding complications in patients who have coagulopathies. MRI is useful in defining the extent of tumor involvement, designing portals for radiation therapy, and planning surgical intervention. MRI also distinguishes extradural from intradural lesions. Gadolinium contrast is usually not required for extradural lesions, but optimal imaging of extramedullary and intramedullary intradural lesions requires the use of this agent. If MRI results in equivocal or negative findings, then CT myelography should be performed.

Early intervention is essential in the management of malignant spinal cord compression. The functional status at the time of presentation clearly correlates with the post-treatment outcome. For example, fewer than 10% of patients who present with paraplegia become ambulatory after treatment. Radiotherapy and/or surgical intervention are the standard treatment modalities. Typically, 3,000 cGy is given in dose fractions of 300 to 500 cGy, with excellent resolution of pain and neurologic symptoms. Laminectomy is effective in managing patients with epidural masses but has limited use if the tumor is growing in a direction anterior to the spinal cord. In select cases, surgical resection may provide symptomatic relief, but careful patient selection is essential. Chemotherapy may help in managing patients with epidural spinal cord compression due to lesions that are sensitive to certain agents; however, a role for chemotherapy as an adjuvant or a primary treatment has not been clearly defined.

Pericardial Tamponade

Tamponade in patients with cancer most often results from malignant obstruction of pericardial lymphatics, leading to the accumulation of fluid within the pericardial sac. While both primary neoplasms of the heart and metastatic lesions can incite the development of pericardial effusions, metastatic disease to the pericardium is the most frequent etiology. Lung cancer, breast cancer, lymphoma, leukemia, and melanoma are the malignancies most commonly implicated in pericardial tamponade. Alternatively, pericardial effusions in the cancer patient can also occur as a result of radiation therapy.

The pericardial sac normally contains 20 mL of fluid at a mean pressure below the values of the right and left ventricular end-diastolic pressures. As pericardial fluid accumulates, this pressure rises until the intrapericardial pressure equals or surpasses the ventricular end-diastolic pressure. At this point, diastolic filling is compromised and cardiac output falls. The development of symptoms depends on the rate of accumulation and the volume of pericardial fluid, as well as on the compliance of the pericardial sac. A pericardial effusion as small as 150 mL may induce hemodynamically significant tamponade. In cases of more gradual accumulation, effusions may reach volumes up to 2 liters.

The symptoms of pericardial tamponade are often vague. Frequent complaints include chest pain, anxiety, and dyspnea. Clinical signs include tachycardia, diminished heart sounds, jugular venous distention, pulsus paradoxus, and ultimately, shock. The electrocardiogram reveals low voltage throughout all leads, with sinus tachycardia. Two-dimensional echocardiography best demonstrates the presence of pericardial fluid and is the test of choice for stable patients with suspected pericardial tamponade.

The treatment of pericardial tamponade is removal of the pericardial effusion, which may be accomplished via needle pericardiocentesis. A drainage catheter may then be inserted into the pericardial space over a guidewire. If readily available, echocardiography will help minimize complications. Removal of a small amount of fluid results in a dramatic and immediate improvement for the patient in extremis. Without additional treatment, malignant pericardial effusions often recur. Thus, a drainage catheter should be left in place so that the rate of fluid accumulation can be monitored. The options for preventing reaccumulation include tetracycline sclerosis, surgery, and radiation therapy. The instillation of 500 to 1,000 mg of tetracycline into the pericardial sac induces an inflammatory response, with subsequent fibrosis and obliteration of the pericardial space. Multiple instillations are usually necessary. Treatment should be repeated until the drainage is less than 25 mL per 24 hours. Successful control of effusions is obtained in 86% of patients who undergo needle pericardiocentesis.

Surgical options to resolve pericardial tamponade include subxiphoid pericardiotomy, window pericardectomy, and complete pericardectomy. The subxiphoid approach is usually preferred, as it avoids the thoracotomy required by the other procedures and can be performed under local anesthesia. Multiple series have documented a recurrence rate of 7% after this technique. Complete pericardiectomy is reserved for patients with radiation-induced effusions. Radiation therapy is useful in stable patients with a malignant effusion secondary to lymphoma; treatment is given in dose fractions of 2 to 3 Gy to a total dose of 20 to 40 Gy.

Outcome after treatment of pericardial tamponade depends in part on tumor type. The median survival times range from 3.5 months for patients with lung cancer to as long as 18.5 months in patients with breast cancer.

Paraneoplastic Crises

Some tumors retain the biochemical characteristics of their cell type of origin and secrete biologically active substances. Other tumors can develop the ability to synthesize and produce hormones that have a wide range of biologic effects. The secretion of these substances is often unregulated, thus disrupting homeostasis. These states have been termed paraneoplastic syndromes. In patients with cancer, these syndromes may cause severe symptoms that require emergent treatment. The full spectrum of paraneoplastic syndromes is extensive; this section describes the more common syndromes, highlighting the physiologic manifestations, pathophysiology, and treatment of each.

Hypercalcemia

Hypercalcemia is the most common metabolic complication of malignancy, occurring in approximately 10% to 20% of cancer patients. Tumors most commonly associated with hypercalcemia include carcinomas of the breast, lung, and kidney, as well as multiple myeloma. Patients with parathyroid carcinoma characteristically present with intractable hypercalcemia. Although more than 80% of patients with hypercalcemia have bone metastasis, there is no correlation between the extent of bone involvement and the degree of hypercalcemia, nor between the presence of bony metastasis and the development of hypercalcemia. Current data suggest that the hypercalcemia of malignancy is mediated by tumor-induced humoral factors. Parathyroid hormone-related protein (PTHRP), osteoclast-activating factor (OAF), prostaglandins, and numerous other cytokines may play a role in the development of hypercalcemia in patients with malignancies.

Calcium homeostasis is normally a tightly controlled process. Parathyroid hormone (PTH), 1,25-dihydroxyvitamin D_3, and calcitonin are the primary regulators of the serum calcium level. These hormones ensure that the net absorption of calcium by the gastrointestinal tract is balanced by the amount excreted by the kidney. Under normal conditions, the serum calcium level is maintained between 8.5 mg/dL and 10.5 mg/dL. Approximately 45% of calcium exists in the ionized, metabolically active form, and the other 55% is protein-bound. Most cases of hormonally mediated hypercalcemia in cancer patients result from the activity of PTHRP, which like PTH, enhances renal tubular resorption of calcium. Unlike patients with hyperparathyroidism, patients with hypercalcemia secondary to PTHRP have impaired production of 1,25-dihydroxyvitamin D_3 and show no evidence of renal bicarbonate wasting. This mechanism is particularly prevalent in solid tumors, especially epidermoid carcinomas.

OAF is responsible for hypercalcemia in patients with multiple myeloma and lymphoma. This osteolytic polypeptide stimulates osteoclast proliferation and the release of lysosomal enzymes and collagenase. Despite the potent osteolytic activity of OAF in vitro, patients with elevated OAF levels do not develop hypercalcemia unless there is associated renal insufficiency. Transforming growth factor, epidermal growth factor, interleukin-1, platelet-derived growth factor, tumor-derived hematopoietic colony-stimulating factors, tumor necrosis factor (TNF) (particularly TNF-β), and lymphotoxin are all potent inducers of bone resorption in vitro and may have a role in the hypercalcemia of malignancy.

Multiple organ systems are involved in the constellation of symptoms caused by hypercalcemia. These symptoms are nonspecific, and their severity is directly related to the degree of calcium elevation. Neuromuscular symptoms often predominate. If left untreated, initial manifestations of fatigue, weakness, lethargy, and apathy can progress to profound mental status changes and psychotic behavior. Nausea, vomiting, anorexia, obstipation, ileus, and abdominal pain are among the gastrointestinal symptoms that may accompany hypercalcemia. Renal tubular dysfunction can occur and is manifested by the development of polydipsia, polyuria, and nocturia. Severe volume contraction occurs, potentiating serum calcium elevation. Without prompt therapy, prolonged hypercalcemia may progress to permanent renal tubular damage.

Because calcium acts as a neurotransmitter, the myocardium is particularly prone to hypercalcemia-induced toxicity. Acute hypercalcemia can slow the heart rate and shorten ventricular systole. With moderate elevation of the calcium level, the QT interval is shortened, and atrial and ventricular arrhythmias may occur. Electrocardiographic changes seen with elevated serum calcium levels include bradycardia, prolonged PR interval, shortened QT interval, and widened T waves. Under extreme circumstances, an acute rise in serum calcium can result in sudden death from cardiac arrhythmias.

Laboratory studies critical in the work-up of patients with hypercalcemia include serum calcium, phosphate, alkaline phosphatase, PTH, electrolytes, blood urea nitrogen, total protein, albumin, and creatinine levels. In patients with severe hypoalbuminemia, the ionized calcium level is more accurate than the serum calcium level. Also, abnormal binding of calcium to paraprotein without an elevation in the ionized calcium level can be seen in patients with multiple myeloma. Elevated immunoreactive PTH levels in association with hypophosphatemia suggest ectopic PTH secretion. Hypercalcemia secondary to malignancy usually has an acute onset, a high serum calcium level (>14 mg/dL), a low serum chloride level, and elevated or normal serum phosphate and bicarbonate levels. These laboratory findings help differentiate hypercalcemia caused by cancer from that secondary to hyperparathyroidism, which is associated with an elevated serum calcium level in the presence of decreased serum phosphate and bicarbonate levels.

Prompt identification and treatment of hypercalcemia are essential. Symptomatic patients and those patients with a serum calcium level of 12 mg/dL or greater require urgent treatment. Intravenous hydration with restoration of intravascular volume increases glomerular filtration rate and is the mainstay of initial management. Diuretics that block calcium resorption in the ascending loop of Henle and augment renal calcium excretion (e.g., furosemide) may be helpful after intravascular volume has been repleted. The initial dose of furosemide in patients without renal impairment is 40 mg IV, followed by 40 to 80 mg every 2 to 4 hours as needed.

Bisphosphonates block osteoclastic bone resorption and substantially reduce serum calcium levels. Etidronate disodium was the first biphosphonate approved for use in the United States. A typical dose regimen is 7.5 mg/kg per day IV for several days, followed by 20 mg/kg per day orally. Pamidronate, a "second-generation" biphosphonate, is more effective than etidronate and has the advantage of inhibiting bone resorption caused by osteoclast activity while leaving bone mineralization unimpaired. Furthermore, pamidronate has a faster onset, a longer effect, and a more durable response. The dose of pamidronate is 60 to 90 mg given IV. Patients usually begin to notice relief of symptoms within hours, and the effect usually lasts for 2 to 3 weeks. Maintenance therapy can be given via intermittent IV infusion every 3 to 4 weeks, or continuous oral administration. Oral dosages between 400 and 1,200 mg/day in divided doses have achieved fairly good response rates.

The antibiotic plicamycin (Mithracin), an effective inhibitor of bone resorption, generally induces a decline in serum calcium within 6 to 48 hours. Plicamycin has limited antineoplastic activity; however, when used at doses of 25 mg/kg per day by IV infusion, the drug provides a marked reduction in bone resorption. Toxicities of plicamycin include thrombocytopenia, hypotension, and hepatic and renal insufficiency. These adverse effects are rare when the dosage is restricted to less than 30 mg/kg per day.

Gallium nitrate is another potent inhibitor of bone resorption. Administration of this agent to patients with malignant disease and hyperparathyroidism causes profound reductions in serum calcium. Incorporation of gallium nitrate into bone causes hydroxyapatite to become less soluble and more resistant to cell-mediated resorption. In addition, gallium nitrate impairs osteoclast acidification of bone matrix by decreasing transmembrane proton transport. This agent may also enhance bone formation by stimulating bone collagen synthesis and increasing calcium incorporation into bone. These actions result in a net reduction of serum calcium. When given at a dosage of 100 to 200 mg/kg per day via continuous IV infusion, for 5 to 7 days, normal serum calcium levels are achieved in 80% to 90% of patients. Nephrotoxicity, the dose-limiting factor, may be minimized by pretreatment IV hydration prior to treatment.

Hyponatremia/Syndrome of Inappropriate Antidiuretic Hormone

Considerable neurologic dysfunction can occur when the serum sodium level falls abruptly or decreases to levels below 115 to 125 mg/dL. Mental status changes, seizures, coma, and, ultimately, death may result if therapeutic intervention is not urgently instituted. The syndrome of inappropriate antidiuretic hormone (SIADH) may be associated with cancers of the prostate, adrenal glands, esophagus, pancreas, colon, and head and neck as well as with carcinoid tumors and mesotheliomas. Small cell carcinoma of the lung is the most common malignancy associated with SIADH.

Dilutional hyponatremia is caused by excessive water resorption in the collecting ducts. This increase in intravascular volume leads to increased renal perfusion along with a substantial decrease in proximal tubular absorption of sodium. In the presence of renal insufficiency, there is increased ADH secretion and excessive water reabsorption from the collecting ducts, resulting in dilutional hyponatremia.

Patients with mild hyponatremia frequently complain of anorexia, nausea, myalgia, headaches, and subtle neurologic symptoms. When the onset of hyponatremia is rapid or the absolute serum sodium level falls below 115 mg/dL, patients develop severe neurologic dysfunction. Alterations in mental status can range from lethargy to confusion and can ultimately progress to coma. Seizures and psychotic behavior can occur at low serum sodium levels as well. Physical findings in patients with profound hyponatremia include alterations in mental status, abnormal reflexes, papilledema, and, occasionally, focal neurologic signs.

Laboratory data and diagnostic studies aid clinicians in determining the etiology of hyponatremia. Pseudo-hyponatremia is due to hyperproteinemia, hyperglycemia, or hyperlipidemia. Serum protein electrophoresis, glucose, and lipid determinations can rule this out. The possibility of drug-induced hyponatremia should also be considered. Such chemotherapeutic agents as vincristine and cyclophosphamide, as well as mannitol, morphine and diuretics, may contribute to hyponatremia, as may the abrupt withdrawal of corticosteroids.

A detailed history and physical examination, along with careful evaluation of the patient's fluid intake and output is often sufficient to determine a patient's intravascular volume and can eliminate water toxicity as a possible cause of hyponatremia. Laboratory investigation should include measurement of serum and urine electrolytes and creatinine. A typical finding in patients with SIADH is that the urine sodium concentration is inappropriately high for the level of hyponatremia. Also, the urine osmolality is often greater than the plasma osmolality, and the urine is never maximally diluted. Other findings indicative of SIADH include a low BUN, hypouricemia, and hypophosphatemia, which result from decreased renal proximal tubular resorption. A chest radiograph and head CT scan should be done to exclude unsuspected pathology of the pulmonary or central nervous system (CNS).

Ideally, therapy for SIADH should be directed toward the underlying cause. In the case of small cell lung cancer, effective multi-drug chemotherapy usually results in resolution of hyponatremia. SIADH resulting from CNS metastasis may improve with the use of corticosteroids and radiation therapy. If the etiology of SIADH cannot be identified, then the therapy for patients with severe hyponatremia is water restriction: a restriction of free water to 500 to 1,000 mL/day should correct the hyponatremia within 5 to 10 days. If the serum sodium level does not improve after restriction of free water for this period, demeclocycline should be used. Demeclocycline is an ADH antagonist that produces a dose-dependent, reversible nephrogenic diabetes insipidus. The recommended initial dose of demeclocycline is 600 mg daily (given in two or three divided doses). The potential adverse effect of nephrotoxicity with demeclocycline is usually seen only when extremely high doses are used (1,200 mg/day). Because this agent is secreted in urine and bile, dose adjustments must be made in patients with renal or hepatic insufficiency.

When severe hyponatremia produces seizures or coma, 3% hypertonic saline or normal saline infusion with IV furosemide should be used. The rate of correction of the serum sodium level should be limited to 0.5 to 1.0 mEq per hour to minimize the risk of CNS toxicity.

Hypoglycemia

Insulin-producing islet cell tumors (insulinomas) are the prototypical lesions associated with hypoglycemia. However, other tumors that often result in hypoglycemia include hepatomas, adrenocortical tumors, and tumors of mesenchymal origin. Mesenchymal tumors comprise more than 50% of non-islet cell neoplasms seen in association with hypoglycemia. Of these, mesothelioma, fibrosarcoma, neurofibrosarcoma, and hemangiopericytoma are the most common.

The mechanism of hypoglycemia resulting from insulinomas involves the unregulated and inappropriate secretion of excess insulin. In contrast, the serum insulin level is normal in cases of non-islet cell tumors. Substances with non-suppressible insulin-like activities (NSILAs) have been detected in patients with malignancy-associated hypoglycemia. Two classes of compounds have been isolated based on molecular weight and ethanol solubility. The low-molecular-weight compounds consist of Insulin Growth Factor (IGF)-I, IGF-II, somatomedin A, and somatomedin C. IGF-I and IGF-II have amino acid sequences similar to proinsulin but do not react with anti-insulin antibodies. The metabolic activity of these compounds is only 1%-2% that of insulin. Approximately 40% of cancer patients with symptomatic hypoglycemia have elevated plasma levels of NSILAs.

Increased glucose use may account for the hypoglycemia seen in association with large tumors. Hepatic glucose production (700 g/day) may fall short of daily glucose requirements in the presence of tumors weighing more than 1 kg, which use 50 to 200 g/day of glucose. Defects in the usual counter-regulatory mechanism of glucose control may also account for malignancy-induced hypoglycemia. Cancer-related hypoglycemia usually develops gradually and does not allow the usual increase in counter-regulatory hormones seen with hypoglycemia arising from nonmalignant etiologies.

Symptoms of hypoglycemia include excessive fatigue, weakness, dizziness, and confusion. In malignancy-associated hypoglycemia, neurologic symptoms usually predominate and may progress to seizures and coma if left untreated. These more severe neurologic complications are usually associated with serum glucose levels below 40 to 45 mg/dL.

Before cancer is determined to be the etiology of hypoglycemia, all other potential causes must be excluded. Exogenous insulin or oral hypoglycemic agents, adrenal insufficiency, pituitary insufficiency, ethanol abuse, and malnutrition are among the common causes of hypoglycemia. In cases of cancer, measurement of fasting serum glucose and insulin levels will aid in determining whether hypoglycemia is due to an islet cell tumor or to a non-islet cell tumor. Patients with insulinomas have increased insulin levels, with fasting glucose levels below 50 mg/dL. In contrast, cases of non-islet cell tumors are marked by a normal or low insulin level associated with hypoglycemia. Also, because insulinomas produce large amounts of proinsulin, they tend to have an elevated proinsulin-to-insulin ratio.

Under ideal circumstances, complete extirpation of the tumor is the optimal therapeutic intervention for hypoglycemia secondary to solid tumors. In cases of an insulinoma, simple enucleation or subtotal pancreatectomy frequently provides a cure. About 90% of these tumors are benign. Diazoxide may benefit patients with insulin-secreting tumors by inhibiting insulin secretion. This drug is not effective in the treatment of non-islet cell tumors. In some cases, radiation therapy reduces tumor bulk and provides palliation of hypoglycemia. Diet modification should be used as the second line of therapy, i.e., when resection is not possible. Frequent feedings can reduce hypoglycemic attacks. Corticosteroids and growth hormone may provide temporary relief. Subcutaneous glucagon injections can also be used to aid in glucose regulation.

Tumor Lysis Syndrome

Tumor lysis syndrome is a critical complication of cytotoxic therapy that requires a team approach in the intensive care unit to prevent the sequelae of permanent renal failure and death. The syndrome is triggered by rapid cell turnover and increased release of intracellular contents into the bloodstream, and is characterized by hyperuricemia, hyperkalemia, hyperphosphatemia, and hypocalcemia. Occasionally, this syndrome occurs spontaneously in patients with lymphomas and leukemia; however, it is more common after cytotoxic chemotherapy-induced rapid cell lysis. The rapid release of intracellular contents can overwhelm the excretory ability of the kidneys, and electrolyte levels can become dangerously elevated. Patients with large, bulky tumors that are sensitive to cytotoxic chemotherapy are particularly prone to this syndrome, as are patients undergoing treatment for Burkitt's or non-Hodgkin's lymphoma, acute lymphoblastic leukemia, acute nonlymphoblastic leukemia, or chronic myelogenous leukemia in blast crisis. Tumor lysis syndrome can also occur after treatment of small cell lung cancer, metastatic breast cancer, and metastatic medulloblastoma. Tumor lysis syndrome occurs not only with cytotoxic chemotherapy but also following radiation therapy, hormonal therapy (e.g., tamoxifen), and cryotherapy of primary and metastatic tumors of the liver.

Metabolic abnormalities associated with tumor lysis syndrome include hyperuricemia, hyperkalemia, and hyperphosphatemia with hypocalcemia. The pathologic processes seen with this syndrome are due to the propensity of uric acid, xanthine, and phosphate to precipitate in the renal tubules. This precipitation can impair renal excretory function and cause further elevation of these metabolites in the serum. Renal insufficiency typically does not develop from the metabolic derangements alone; a combination of low urine flow rates and elevated serum metabolites is usually required to precipitate renal dysfunction. Thus, oliguric patients are at significantly higher risk of developing renal failure during rapid cellular lysis.

Hyperkalemia results from the release of intracellular contents and is further perpetuated by renal insufficiency. Potassium elevation can have life-threatening consequences and requires immediate intervention. Cardiac toxicity is evidenced by the characteristic electrocardiographic changes seen with potassium levels above 6 mEq/dL. These changes include loss of P waves, peaked T waves, a widened QRS complex, and depressed ST segments. Heart block and diastolic cardiac arrest may result if hyperkalemia is left untreated.

Rapid tumor lysis can also cause hyperphosphatemia, which is usually accompanied by hypocalcemia. Hypocalcemia in tumor lysis syndrome is thought to be due to the formation of calcium-phosphate salts that precipitate in soft tissues. Hyperphosphatemia is further exacerbated by the formation of these calcium-phosphate complexes in renal tubules, causing progressive renal insufficiency.

Preventive measures can be taken to minimize the toxicities of tumor lysis. Patients should undergo vigorous IV hydration before treatment with potentially toxic chemotherapeutic agents is begun. Another important preventive measure is to alkalinize the urine during the first 1 to 2 days of cytotoxic treatment. These measures counteract hyperuricemia by increasing the solubility of uric acid. Allopurinol has also been shown to effectively decrease the formation of uric acid and to reduce the incidence of uric acid nephropathy. In patients with large, bulky tumors that are known to have a high growth fraction, allopurinol should be administered before planned chemotherapeutic intervention.

An electrocardiogram should be obtained in all patients with hyperkalemia or hypocalcemia, and continuous cardiac monitoring should be instituted. Hyperkalemia should be treated with the standard measures for acutely lowering the serum potassium level. These measures include IV administration of insulin and glucose, loop diuretics, and sodium bicarbonate. Calcium should be given to stabilize the myocardium. Regardless of measures used to acutely lower the serum potassium, a sodium-potassium exchange resin should be given to lower the total body potassium load (15 g sodium polystyrene sulfonate [Kayexalate] orally or by rectum every 6 hours). If there is evidence of worsening renal function with poor resolution of the metabolic abnormalities, hemodialysis should be considered.

Central Venous Catheter Sepsis

The use of indwelling vascular access catheters is widespread in modern cancer care. Catheter-based infection is a major source of morbidity. When catheter infection is suspected, the access site should be carefully examined. Erythema, induration, and suppuration are signs of site infection, which require immediate catheter removal. Bacteremia and sepsis from catheter infection should be documented by drawing blood cultures from both the catheter and peripheral sites. Coagulase-negative staphylococci are the most common pathogens isolated in catheter-based infection, although numerous gram-positive, gram-negative, and fungal species may also be responsible. More than 80% of catheter-based infections can be treated effectively with a 10- to 14- day course of IV antibiotics. Antibiotic therapy should be given through the infected catheter and rotated between ports when multilumen catheters are present. Persistence of positive blood cultures or signs of systemic sepsis, particularly in neutropenic patients, necessitates immediate catheter removal. In patients with vascular grafts or implanted prostheses, immediate catheter removal is indicated once an infection has been documented.

ABDOMINAL EMERGENCIES

Intestinal Obstruction

Bowel obstruction continues to be a considerable source of morbidity and mortality in patients with cancer. The decisions regarding the timing and the extent of surgery remain difficult, and few studies offer much guidance. Approximately two thirds of patients with ovarian cancer present with at least one episode of bowel obstruction, and nearly all patients with carcinomatosis suffer some sort of intestinal complication. In up to one third of all patients with a history of cancer who present with a bowel obstruction, the cause of the obstruction is a benign source (e.g., adhesions, hernias, and radiation enteritis). In the other two thirds of these patients, either primary or metastatic disease is the source of their intestinal obstruction. The intra-abdominal malignancies most often associated with obstruction of the gastrointestinal tract are carcinomas of the ovary, colon, and stomach. Extra-abdominal malignancies may metastasize to the peritoneal cavity and cause obstruction; in such cases, the most common sources are carcinomas of the lung, breast, and melanoma.

Functional obstruction of the bowel without a mechanical cause (colonic "pseudo-obstruction" or Ogilvie's Syndrome) is a common problem in patients with cancer. Narcotic analgesics, electrolyte abnormalities, radiation therapy, malnutrition, and prolonged bedrest may all contribute to delayed intestinal motility. The treatment consists of correcting the underlying cause and decompressing the bowel with a nasogastric tube. Colonoscopic decompression should be considered when the size of the cecum reaches 10 cm. Surgery is indicated if the degree of intestinal dilatation progresses to the point of impending perforation or if the patient shows any evidence of peritonitis. Tube cecostomy is the procedure of choice in these often-debilitated patients, with resection and ileostomy formation reserved for cases of frank perforation. Another measure that has been recently described involves the administration of neostigmine (2.0–2.5 mg IV). This therapy has shown promise in a number of small series, but should only be considered for patients in a closely monitored setting.

The evaluation of intestinal obstruction in patients with cancer should be similar to that in patients with benign disease. After a complete history, physical examination, and evaluation of laboratory and radiologic data, the degree and site of obstruction should be delineated. Immediate laparotomy is indicated for those patients who have signs or symptoms of intestinal ischemia, necrosis, or frank perforation (abdominal tenderness, leukocytosis, fever, or tachycardia). Nearly 10% of patients will have concurrent small- and large-bowel obstruction. To exclude the possibility of colonic obstruction before laparotomy, a Gastrografin enema may be obtained, particularly in patients with multiple sites of intra-abdominal tumor. Either an upper gastrointestinal series with small-bowel follow-through or enteroclysis may be useful in patients with recurrent partial small-bowel obstructions. Finally, a CT scan of the abdomen and pelvis using oral and rectal contrast may help identify the location and etiology of the obstruction. Before laparotomy, all patients should undergo standard resuscitation including IV fluid administration, correction of electrolyte abnormalities, and placement of a nasogastric tube.

In patients with a partial small-bowel obstruction, a trial of medical management is worthwhile. Up to 50% of patients respond to conservative treatment, which may require up to 2 weeks of intestinal decompression. Surgery is advocated for patients who do not respond to medical management or whose condition progresses to complete obstruction. Medical management is rarely successful in patients with a complete obstruction at any level, and these patients should undergo exploration. The goal of surgery is to provide relief of the obstruction, although this goal cannot always be accomplished. The surgeon should fully explore the abdomen and attempt to identify the cause of the obstruction. Benign adhesions should be lysed with care. In cases of radiation enteritis, gentle handling of the bowel is essential. Resection may be adequate for short segments of intestine but long segments are best treated by internal bypass. A similar approach should be taken in relieving bowel obstruction caused by malignancy, although occasionally the extent of the malignant disease is too extensive to allow for any of these options. In such cases, placement of a venting gastrostomy for symptomatic relief is all that is indicated. A gastrostomy provides considerable relief from continued emesis and avoids the need for prolonged placement of a nasogastric tube.

Exploration related to a malignant bowel obstruction is associated with substantial morbidity and mortality. Almost 10% of patients die because of surgery, and another 30% suffer operative complications. Furthermore, patients have a mean survival of only about 6 months following laparotomy for a malignant bowel obstruction. Bowel obstruction from benign disease is rare in patients with known residual or recurrent intra-abdominal tumor. Therefore, bowel obstruction in patients with documented intra-abdominal disease can be viewed as a premorbid event, with prolonged survival unlikely despite any intervention. Given such a poor prognosis, it is often more appropriate to pursue nonsurgical options (e.g., placement of a percutaneous endoscopic gastrostomy tube).

Another recently employed management strategy for malignant obstruction of the rectum is the use of self-expanding metal stents. These stents may be used either as a definitive measure or as an adjunct to allow for bowel decompression and cleansing in preparation for surgery. While colonic perforation is a potential complication, these devices may allow patients with near-complete obstructions to avoid an ostomy and thus enjoy better quality of life.

Intestinal Perforation

Perforation of the gastrointestinal tract in patients with cancer may occur at nearly any time in the course of the disease. Indeed, the condition may be the presenting sign of cancer, such as in cases of perforated primary colorectal carcinoma. The perforation may occur during treatment (either chemotherapy or radiation therapy), or it may be the result of metastatic tumor later in the course of the disease. Most perforations of the gastrointestinal tract of cancer patients are from benign causes (e.g., peptic ulcer disease, diverticulitis, and appendicitis) and should be treated according to standard surgical principles. Surgery is associated with significant morbidity and mortality but is often the only therapeutic option available for this life-threatening complication. Patients must be well informed of the risks of surgery and must understand that an ostomy is a possibility before an emergency laparotomy. Nonsurgical treatment, comfort care, or both may be appropriate, depending on the patient's wishes, prognosis, and overall medical status.

Intestinal perforation is the presenting symptom of disease in a small group of patients with undiagnosed colorectal carcinoma. However, on further questioning, these patients usually state that they have had some symptoms, whether related to obstruction or to bleeding, attributable to the tumor. The perforation may be the result of full-thickness colonic involvement with the tumor and subsequent necrosis of a region of the intestinal wall. A carcinoma that nearly or completely obstructs the lumen of the colon may also present with perforation proximal in the intestinal tract, usually the cecum. In general, patients who present with either perforated or obstructing colorectal cancer have a poorer overall prognosis, stage for stage, than do patients without these presentations. Furthermore, the operative mortality rate associated with emergency laparotomy for perforated colorectal cancer approaches 30%.

Perforation of the gastrointestinal tract following chemotherapy for metastatic solid tumors is a potentially fatal complication. The rate of operative mortality has been reported to be as high as 80% for an emergency laparotomy in patients with metastatic cancer receiving chemotherapy. Factors associated with a high rate of complications include chemotherapy-induced myeloid toxicity, protein malnutrition, and immunosuppression. Furthermore, traditional signs of an acute surgical abdomen may be masked in these patients, leading to a delay in diagnosis. Finally, because the prognosis of these patients is poor, the decision to proceed with exploratory laparotomy is difficult and is often made late in the clinical course.

Most cases of gastrointestinal perforation related to malignant disease are caused by hematologic malignancies, with solid tumors, such as ovarian carcinoma, being an extremely uncommon cause. Lymphoma with intestinal involvement is the malignancy most likely to lead to gastrointestinal perforation following systemic chemotherapy. In such cases, perforation is often related to transmural involvement of the intestine, resulting in full-thickness necrosis following chemotherapy. Furthermore, because of the extensive involvement of the gastrointestinal tract by lymphoma and the relative chemosensitivity of this neoplasm, perforation is not uncommon following chemotherapy. Conversely, metastases from solid organ tumors are often limited to the serosal surface and therefore do not lead to full-thickness necrosis following chemotherapy.

Radiation therapy directed at the abdomen may damage the gastrointestinal tract. The extent of injury depends on the dose of radiation delivered, the radiation fields utilized, the energy of the ionizing radiation, and the use of adjunctive methods to shield the intestines. Immediate effects include damage and subsequent sloughing of the mucosal layer of the intestinal tract. Most of the immediate effects lead to substantial nausea and vomiting, which are usually temporary. Most patients can be managed as outpatients, and oral agents can be used to palliate symptoms. However, a small but significant fraction of patients require hospitalization for intravenous administration of fluid and antiemetics. Finally, in its severest form, radiation-induced injury leads to full-thickness injury of the intestinal tract with subsequent perforation. Such an injury usually occurs later in the course of the radiation therapy or follows the completion of treatment. Once the diagnosis is made, the management of this condition is similar to that of any intestinal perforation.

Upon abdominal exploration, the area of perforation should be resected, if possible. A conservative approach to reestablishing gastrointestinal continuity should be used, especially for patients with poor nutritional status, altered host immune response or impending shock. Ostomies should be used liberally and may be reversed at a subsequent procedure, if appropriate. Furthermore, strong consideration should be given to the placement of gastrostomy and feeding jejunostomy tubes. Such devices obviate the need for prolonged nasogastric intubation and allow for early enteral feeding.

Biliary Obstruction

Biliary obstruction by metastases to the hilum of the liver or portal lymph nodes is an uncommon but troublesome problem in patients with cancer. Such obstructions may be caused by a variety of tumor types, including lymphoma, melanoma, and carcinoma of the breast, colon, stomach, lung, or ovary. Obstruction of the biliary tree due to primary carcinomas of the common bile duct and pancreas is discussed elsewhere. Evaluation is best performed with CT scan, which provides information on the site of obstruction, reveals the degree of biliary obstruction, allows evaluation of the remainder of the abdomen, and often gives clues as to the cause of obstruction. When necessary, endoscopic ultrasound or CT-guided fine-needle aspiration can be performed in this region to obtain a tissue diagnosis.

The prognosis for patients with biliary obstruction from metastatic disease is poor. In one published series of 12 patients with biliary obstruction from metastases, 11 patients had disease either in other intra-abdominal sites or in extra-abdominal locations. The 60-day mortality rate in this group has been reported to be as high as 67%. Thus, treatment should aim to palliate jaundice and to prevent cholangitis. Endoscopic retrograde cholangiopancreatography and stent placement best accomplish drainage of the biliary tree. If this approach is unsuccessful, percutaneous transhepatic drainage is indicated. External-beam irradiation, with or without chemotherapy, may also provide substantial palliation, especially in cases of obstruction due to primary biliary or pancreatic carcinoma. Surgery should be reserved for patients who are at low-risk–that is patients for whom the risk of metastatic disease is low and the chance for long-term survival is high.

Neutropenic Enterocolitis

The terms neutropenic enterocolitis, typhlitis, necrotizing enteropathy, and ileocecal syndrome have all been used to describe a clinical entity characterized by febrile neutropenia, abdominal distension, right-sided abdominal pain, tenderness, and diarrhea. The syndrome most often occurs in patients undergoing chemotherapy for a hematologic malignancy, but may also occur in patients with solid tumors. Signs and symptoms characteristically develop after neutropenia lasting 7 days or more. The initial presentation consists of right-sided abdominal pain, tenderness, and fever and may mimic appendicitis. The diagnosis is made clinically, often by exclusion of other pathologic causes. Serial examinations by the same examiner are critical for proper diagnosis and treatment. Abdominal films characteristically reveal a nonspecific ileus pattern with some dilation of the cecum. Pneumatosis is an inconsistent finding. The CT findings for neutropenic enterocolitis are also nonspecific, consisting mainly of bowel-wall thickening and edema. However, CT scans are invaluable to rule out other pathologic conditions. Complete work-up should include stool cultures for bacteria and *Clostridium difficile* toxin.

The severity of neutropenic enterocolitis varies, and therapy must be individualized. Medical management, which includes bowel rest, nasogastric suction, broad-spectrum antibiotics, and IV hyperalimentation, is successful in most cases. Although granulocyte transfusion has never been proven to be effective, granulocyte colony-stimulating factors, which shorten the neutropenic period, likely improve outcome. Surgical intervention is indicated in cases of perforation, uncontrolled hemorrhage, sepsis, and progression of symptoms on medical therapy. Right hemicolectomy with or without ileostomy is the surgery of choice in most cases.

Hemorrhage

Malignant tumors are rarely the source of significant intra-abdominal hemorrhage, even in patients with known cancer. Peptic ulcer disease and gastritis, the most common causes of bleeding in unselected series, are the leading etiologies in 54% to 75% of patients with cancer. Gastrointestinal lymphomas and metastatic tumors are the lesions that most commonly initiate massive hemorrhage. Because spontaneous hemorrhage caused by tumors rarely occurs, individuals with cancer should receive the same systematic approach to diagnosis and treatment as do those without malignant disease. While resuscitation with crystalloid and blood products is under way, the diagnostic work-up to define the site and etiology of bleeding should begin. Bleeding proximal to the ligament of Treitz is marked clinically by hematemesis or blood per nasogastric aspirate. Upon the finding of such signs, upper endoscopy should be performed promptly.

Bright red blood per rectum should initiate investigation of a colonic or rectal source. In such cases, either proctoscopy or sigmoidoscopy serves as an expedient initial diagnostic maneuver. Angiography and nuclear red cell scans are often useful to localize bleeding sites in the colon and small bowel. Mild blood loss due to a colonic neoplasm can usually be treated endoscopically with electrocautery or placement of topical hemostatic agents if the lesion is within the rectum. Some patients require urgent surgical resection of a colonic neoplasm for continued bleeding, but this procedure can usually be delayed to allow for localization of the site of bleeding and until the bowel has been mechanically cleansed to allow for a primary anastomosis. If the bleeding cannot be localized and the hemorrhage is massive, immediate exploration with intraoperative endoscopy should be considered. Exploration, endoscopy, or both may allow localization of the bleeding site so that surgical resection may be directed; however, total abdominal colectomy may be needed if the hemorrhage cannot be precisely localized. Small-bowel tumors rarely present with massive gastrointestinal hemorrhage, although gastric carcinoma may occasionally present with acute bleeding. The evaluation and treatment approaches are nearly identical to those for similar conditions arising from a colonic source, with endoscopy as the first line of treatment and surgical resection reserved for a more elective setting.

Extraluminal, intra-abdominal hemorrhage should be suspected when there is significant blood loss without hematemesis, melena, or hematochezia. The retroperitoneum is the most frequent site of occult intra-abdominal hemorrhage. If this condition is suspected, CT scan is the best method of evaluation. Therapy for intra-abdominal hemorrhage is initially directed at resuscitation and correction of any existing coagulopathy. A history of aspirin or nonsteroidal anti-inflammatory use within 1 week must raise suspicion of platelet dysfunction, and a bleeding time should be obtained. After the site and source of bleeding have been identified, specific therapy is instituted. Under controlled conditions, invasive therapies, such as angiographic embolization, may be attempted. The timing of surgical intervention is based on the rate and volume of blood loss, the underlying pathology, and the patient's overall prognosis.

RECOMMENDED READING

Arrambide K, Toto RD. Tumor lysis syndrome. *Semin Nephrol* 1993;13:273–280.

Aurora R, Milite F, Vander Els NJ. Respiratory emergencies. *Semin Oncol* 2000;27:256–269.

Camunez F, Echenagusia A, Simo G, et al. Malignant colorectal obstruction treated by means of self-expanding metallic stents: effectiveness before surgery and in palliation. *Radiology* 2000;216:492–497.

Chen HS, Sheen-Chen SM. Obstruction and perforation in colorectal adenocarcinoma: an analysis of prognosis and current trends. *Surgery* 2000;127:370–376.

Ciezki JP, Komurcu S, Macklis RM. Palliative radiotherapy. *Semin Oncol* 2000;27:90–93.

Chisolm MA, Mulloy AL, Taylor AT. Acute management of cancer-related hypercalcemia. *Ann Pharmacother* 1996;30:507–513.

Hoegler D. Radiotherapy for palliation of symptoms in incurable cancer. *Curr Probl Cancer* 1997;21:129–183.

Ibrahim NK, Sahin AA, Dubrow RA, et al. Colitis associated with docetaxel-based chemotherapy in patients with metastatic breast cancer. *Lancet* 2000;355:281–283.

Lefor AT. Perioperative management of the patient with cancer. *Chest* 1999;115[5 suppl]:165S–171S.

Makris A, Kunkler IH. Controversies in the management of metastatic spinal cord compression. *Clin Oncol* 1995;7:77–81.

Miller M. Inappropriate antidiuretic hormone secretion. *Curr Ther Endocrinol Metab* 1997;6:206–209.

Nussbaum SR. Pathophysiology and management of severe hypercalcemia. *Endocrinol Metab Clin North Am* 1993;22:343–362.

Ostler PJ, Clarke DP, Watkinson AF, et al. Superior vena cava obstruction: a modern management strategy. *Clin Oncol* 1997;9:83–89.

Ponec RJ, Saunders MD, Kimmey MB. Neostigmine for the treatment of acute colonic pseudo-obstruction. *N Engl J Med* 1999;341:137–141.

Reed CR, Sessler CN, Glauser FL, et al. Central venous catheter infections: concepts and controversies. *Intensive Care Med* 1995;21:177–183.

Reyes CV, Thompson KS, Massarani-Wafai R, et al. Utilization of fine-needle aspiration cytology in the diagnosis of neoplastic superior vena cava syndrome. *Diagn Cytopathol* 1998;19:84–88.

Schindler N, Vogelzang RL. Superior vena cava syndrome. Experience with endovascular stents and surgical therapy. *Surg Clin North Am* 1999;79:683–694.

Tang E, Davis D, Silberman H. Bowel obstruction in cancer patients. *Arch Surg* 1995;130:832–836.

Theriault RL. Hypercalcemia of malignancy: pathophysiology and implications for treatment. *Oncology* 1993;7:47–50.

Wade DS, Nava HR, Douglass HO Jr. Neutropenic enterocolitis. *Cancer* 1992;69:17–23.

Biologic Cancer Therapy

Daniel Albo and Thomas N. Wang

Biologic therapy is cancer treatment that produces antitumor effects primarily through the manipulation of natural defense mechanisms of the host. Biologic therapy induces, uses, or modifies the host's immune system to efficiently recognize and destroy cancer cells. Biologic therapy has emerged as an important fourth modality for the treatment of cancer, joining surgery, radiation therapy, and chemotherapy in our armamentarium against cancer. The increasing application of biologic therapy is the result of a better understanding of the basic concepts of host defense mechanisms. Basic science research on the immune system has taken biologic therapy out of its infancy and into clinical trials. This chapter will discuss biologic therapies that have shown promise in the treatment of human cancers including cytokines, vaccines, cellular therapies, monoclonal antibodies (MAbs), and gene therapies.

THE IMMUNE SYSTEM AND CYTOKINES

Immunotherapy for cancer is entering a new phase of active investigation at both the preclinical and clinical levels. This is due to exciting developments in basic immunology and tumor biology that have tremendously increased our understanding of the mechanisms of interactions between the immune system and tumor cells. The immune system is made up of a wide array of cell types, but lymphocytes provide the specificity of the immune response. The immune system can largely be divided into the cellular branch and the humoral branch. These branches differ in both effector cell type and mechanism of antigen recognition. T lymphocytes (T cells) are responsible for many of the functions of the cellular branch, such as delayed-type hypersensitivity and rejection of grafts and tumors. The humoral branch is largely associated with B lymphocytes (B cells) and the production of antibodies (Abs).

Cellular Immunity

T cells are $CD3^+$ cells that recognize antigens via T-cell receptors (TCRs). TCRs have a specificity analogous to that of immunoglobulins (Igs). T cells can be divided into two major types: $CD8^+$ cytotoxic T lymphocytes (CTLs), which are capable of direct cellular killing, and $CD4^+$ T helper lymphocytes (T_H cells), which produce cytokines. CTLs interact with human leukocyte antigen (HLA) class I molecules on the surface of target cells. The HLA class I molecules (HLA-A, HLA-B, and HLA-C) are expressed on all cells and present short (8- to 10-amino acid) peptides that have been processed from degraded endogenous self proteins or viral proteins. The TCR/CD3 complex of CTLs specifically recognizes a single peptide/HLA complex on the surface of a target cell and then is triggered to destroy that cell by granule exocytosis. This process involves the release of cytolysin (perforin) and granzymes (serine protease-containing granules), which lead to apoptosis.

T$_H$ cells interact with specialized antigen-presenting cells (APCs), such as macrophages, dendritic cells (DCs), and B cells, that express HLA class II molecules. HLA class II molecules present longer (12- to 20-amino acid) peptides that have been taken up from exogenous proteins and processed by APCs. When a T$_H$ cell's specific TCR has been activated, the cell begins to produce cytokines that enhance B-cell Ab production, support T-cell responses, and activate other immune cells. T$_H$ cells can be further divided into subtypes on the basis of their pattern of cytokine production, the antigens that stimulate them, and the immune responses the cells support. T$_H$1 cells promote cytotoxic cellular responses, delayed-type hypersensitivity, and macrophage activation, by secreting interleukin-2 (IL-2), interferon-γ (IFN-γ), and tumor necrosis factor-β (TNF-β). T$_H$2 cells support B-cell responses and the production of IgG, IgA, and IgE Abs by secreting IL-4, IL-5, IL-6, and IL-10. Both subsets of T$_H$ cells produce TNF-α, IL-3, and granulocyte-macrophage colony-stimulating factor (GM-CSF). T$_H$1 cells are usually stimulated by infectious agents such as viruses and bacteria, whereas T$_H$2 cells respond to allergens and parasites.

Costimulatory signals can be delivered by cytokines or by specific costimulatory molecules. The latter are typically but not exclusively present on APCs like macrophages, monocytes, B cells and DCs. Presentation of antigen to naive T cells without costimulation may lead to T-cell tolerance. In fact, the adequate antigen presentation to a naive immune system occurs through these APCs. With the possible exception of B-cell lymphoma, tumor cells seldom express costimulatory molecules. The most potent APC subset in terms of antitumor CTL induction is the subset known as DC. Through endocytosis, DCs take up antigenic substances ranging from soluble antigen to apoptotic cells. Subsequently, the antigens are endogenously processed by the DC. This results in epitopes presented on the surface of DCs in the context of the autologous HLA alleles and costimulatory molecules. DCs feature high amounts of the HLA molecules that are essential to CTL recognition. The vast expression of adhesion and co-stimulatory molecules, and the production of T-cell–specific chemokines are of essential importance for the microenvironment in which an effective immune response can be initiated: tumor cells that by themselves induce tolerance evoke a potent immune response once fused with DCs. This essential difference caused by presentation through DCs is also confirmed by in vivo experiments. To activate this process of antigen presentation by DCs, the antigen has to be present along with signals of tissue damage, the so-called danger signals. Heat shock proteins (HSPs), which chaperone the important epitopes of a cell (discussed in more detail in the section HSP vaccination later in this chapter), can be regarded as such a signal. From the available evidence it may be concluded that HSPs constitute an important source of antigen for processing and presentation by DCs under natural conditions. Apart from their role in presentation of antigen to CTLs, DCs are also important in the induction of T$_H$ cell and natural killer (NK) cell responses. This makes DCs a critical component of the antitumor response and implies great promise for clinical applications of DCs.

NK cells are large, granular cytotoxic lymphocytes that are distinct from T and B cells. NK cells participate in the host's first line of defense and are nonspecific. These cells are CD3$^-$ and do not express TCRs. NK cells express the CD56 molecule, which promotes cellular adhesion, and the receptor for Igs. These cells participate in antibody-dependent cellular cytotoxicity (ADCC). NK cells are not target-cell specific but demonstrate target cell selectivity, the mechanisms of which are unknown. Clearly, NK cells are more cytotoxic for tumor cells and virally infected cells than for normal cells.

Humoral Immunity

B cells are the major cell type of the humoral branch of the immune system. Although T cells are restricted to recognizing processed antigens that come from protein sources and are presented in the context of "self" HLA molecules, B cells can recognize unprocessed antigens and, without the context, other molecules. Moreover, B cells can recognize not only proteins but also polysaccharides and nucleic acids. Antibodies (Abs) on the surface of B cells act first as cell surface receptors, forming tight, noncovalent complexes with specific antigens. Once the binding of a cell-surface Ab to its specific target antigen activates a B cell, the cell undergoes maturation to a plasma cell, producing a specific Ab. The Abs produced are soluble, secreted molecules that bind the target fixing complement, marking it for phagocytosis or initiating ADCC.

All Abs are composed of two identical chains, the heavy and light chains, which are covalently bound by disulfide bonds, forming a Y-shaped molecule. There are five major classes of Abs that differ in structure and function, IgG, IgM, IgA, IgD, and IgE. IgG Abs are monomers with a γ-heavy chain and four subclasses. IgG Abs fix complement, cross the placenta, bind monocytes and neutrophils, and are the predominant Abs involved in secondary immune responses. IgM Abs are pentamers with a mu-heavy chain and two subclasses. IgM Abs fix complement, are involved in primary immune responses, and function as lymphocyte surface receptors and as accessory secretory Abs. IgA Abs are monomers with an α heavy chain and two subclasses. IgA Abs predominate in secretions. IgD Abs are monomers with a δ heavy chain. IgD Abs are thought to act as lymphocyte receptors. IgE Abs are monomers with ϵ-heavy chains. IgE Abs bind basophils and mast cells and are effectors of allergic and anaphylactic reactions.

The specificity of an Ab is determined by gene rearrangement in the variable domains of the heavy and light chains. Within these variable regions are three distinct widely separated areas that are hypervariable. These segments are called collectively the complementary determining regions. When the polypeptide is folded, these regions are brought together to form the antigen binding site. The diversity of Abs is generated by gene rearrangements within complementary determining regions and in the D and J joining genes of both the heavy and light chains. The specificity and diversity of the TCRs are similarly determined.

Cytokines

Cytokines are immunobiologically active molecules produced by defined cell populations that either enhance or suppress specific immunologic functions. Certain cytokines enhance the expression of target antigens, major histocompatibility complex (MHC) molecules, or APCs. Other cytokines (e.g., IL-1, TNF, IL-6, IL-7, IL-12) facilitate antigen presentation by providing accessory signals that enhance the ability of lymphocytes to respond to mitogenic stimuli. The absence of such accessory signals can lead to immunologic anergy. The cytokines IL-2 and IL-4 may augment T-cell proliferation and overcome the requirement for cellular cooperation in the generation of CTL responses. Finally, lymphocytes and some tumors may produce cytokines, such as IL-10, that suppress immune responses.

RATIONALE FOR IMMUNOTHERAPY

The immune system plays an active role against neoplastic diseases. It has long been known that animals cured of cancer through excision of a primary tumor appear to be protected against that cancer type in subsequent tumor challenge experiments. Moreover, patients with drug-induced prolonged immunosuppression after organ transplantation and patients with severe immunodeficiency syndromes have a higher incidence of several tumors. Melanoma is the human malignancy studied in greatest detail from an immunologic standpoint.

MHC class I expression, which allows recognition of the tumor by the immune system, in melanoma, is associated with a better clinical prognosis. Loss or defect of MHC class I expression is associated with a worse prognosis. Moreover, brisk lymphocytic infiltration of a primary melanoma is an independent good prognostic factor, and the development of vitiligo as a consequence of an immune reaction to melanoma differentiation antigens has been reported to correlate with a better clinical response.

Other tumors in which immunogenicity is far less accepted also appear to be able to provoke protective responses. In colorectal cancer, CTL infiltration of tumors is associated with a much better prognosis. In addition, T-cell profile (impaired CD4+ counts) correlates with progression of disease. Moreover, also in colorectal cancer, HLA class II expression by tumor cells, which is essential for the induction of T_H cell responses, appears to be associated with improved prognosis.

IMMUNOTHERAPY STRATEGIES

Many strategies have emerged in the course of the development of cancer immunotherapy. The oldest approach was an effort to nonspecifically boost the general function of the immune system (a strategy termed active nonspecific immunostimulation), initiated by Coley (1986). He injected patients with bacterial toxins and observed regression of solid neoplasms, probably as a result of activation of cytokines. Some of these bacterial toxins are still in clinical use today.

Most efforts to modulate the immune system have focused on the cellular immunity. Three different approaches have been devised. The first approach attempts to improve the function of the immune system in general without actually altering the target or specific effector cells themselves. Examples of this approach are the administration of cytokines such as IL-2, IFN alfa, and IFN gamma. The second approach aims at activating the immune system by optimizing the presentation of antigen: vaccination or active specific immunotherapy. Examples range from the application of synthetic peptides that represent single epitopes to vaccination with viable whole tumor cells, the antigens of which can then be endogenously processed by professional APCs. The third strategy, known as adoptive immunotherapy, uses the infusion of effector cells that have been stimulated to act against the tumor, expanded in vitro, or both, (e.g., antitumor CTLs or allogeneic lymphocytes after bone marrow transplantation). But even lymphocytes stimulated in vitro with IL-2 in the absence of tumor antigens (lymphokine-activated killer [LAK] cells) can be used for adoptive immunotherapy. This implies that adoptive transfer can be antigen specific (antitumor CTLs) or nonspecific (LAK cells).

Nonspecific Stimulation

Agents used for nonspecific simulation of the immune system have been evaluated for more than a century. In 1986, Coley introduced the idea of stimulating the immune system as a whole by introducing bacterial agents. Since then most other studies of nonspecific immune stimulation have also used bacterial agents, including bacillus *Calmette-Guerin* (BCG) and *Corynebacterium parvum*. Material of viral origin and various chemical substances have also been applied.

With the exception of BCG in superficial bladder cancer, immunostimulants have not been found to be effective as single agents. However, a number of immunostimulants have demonstrated promise as adjuvant therapy with other forms of immunotherapy or chemotherapy. A possible explanation for the reported benefit of immunostimulants in combination with other adjuvant therapy may lie in the nonspecific immune stimulation that counteracts the immunologically depressing effect of major surgical trauma and helps the patient cope with the microbiologic hazards associated with the perioperative period. However, the mechanism of this effect has not been studied in treated patients.

Bacillus Calmette-Guerin

BCG is undoubtedly the best known of the agents used for nonspecific immunostimulation. BCG injection results in cytokine secretion and activation of DCs, which may explain its antitumor effect. The use of BCG as single-agent therapy for superficial bladder cancer is widespread. Phase III studies have shown that administration of BCG after bladder resection reduces the recurrence risk by 45%, similar or superior to results seen with mitomycin C. Among patients with recurrent disease, BCG improved the 5-year disease-free survival rate from 17% to 37% in infiltrating tumors and from 18% to 45% in carcinoma in situ. In many other malignancies, however, including melanoma, single agent BCG proved to have no effect in prospectively randomized phase III trials. In malignant melanoma, adjuvant BCG after surgery is not beneficial in patients with AJCC stages I or III, but the effect in patients with stage II disease remains controversial. Oral BCG monotherapy and intralesional BCG injections are effective, mainly against cutaneous metastases, but have no impact on overall survival.

Levamisole

Another agent widely used for nonspecific immune stimulation is levamisole. Although levamisole as single agent adjuvant therapy in colorectal carcinoma was ineffective, the combination of levamisole and 5-fluorouracil (5-FU) reduced the risk of recurrence by 41% and reduced the overall death rate by 33%. These results compare favorably with outcomes achieved with the combination of 5-FU and folinic acid, and the toxicity of the 5-FU-levamisole regimen was identical to that of 5-FU alone. Subsequently, 5-FU-levamisole has been substituted by 5-FU-leucovorin as standard of care in the adjuvant treatment of colon cancer. No antitumor activity of levamisole was found in patients with melanoma.

Other Immunostimulating Agents

In addition to BCG and levamisole, other immunostimulating agents of various origins have been described and used. Picibanil (OK-432) is a lyophilized preparation of inactivated *Streptococcus pyogenes* that is known to augment nonspecific T-cell cytotoxicity, LAK cell activity, and tumoricidal activation of macrophages. In an analysis of the combined results of two phase III studies for a total of 330 gastric cancer patients, the addition of picibanil to standard surgery and chemotherapy resulted in a 5-year survival rate (45%) almost double that seen with surgery alone (24%) or with surgery plus chemotherapy (29%). However, a more detailed evaluation of this treatment at a 5-year follow-up study casts doubts on its clinical impact. The influences on cytokine levels responsible for the effect of picibanil were investigated only recently in melanoma patients and were found to involve IL-1, TNF, and IFN γ.

In a placebo-controlled prospective randomized trial in 64 patients with high-risk nonmetastatic breast cancer, the addition of sodium dithiocarbonate to adjuvant treatment with 5-FU, doxorubicin, and cyclophosphamide (FAC) after modified radical mastectomy resulted in improved overall survival compared with surgery plus FAC alone (81% vs. 55%). Disease-free survival improved from 55% to 76%. These results, however, have not been confirmed by additional prospective randomized trials.

Preoperative administration of *Propionibacterium avidum* (OK 42) to patients with colorectal carcinoma resulted in increased survival time and decreased rates of recurrence and metastasis in patients with stage I and II disease only. Postoperative quality of life was reported improved too. Additional studies are needed to confirm these results.

CYTOKINES

Many of the known human cytokines are now readily available at reasonable cost thanks to recombinant technology. Because the administration and evaluation of cytokines are essentially identical to the administration and evaluation of any pharmaceutical preparation and clinical use of cytokines is much less labor-intensive than most other immunotherapeutic options, cytokines are attractive agents for clinical research and implementation. Trials of cytokines in cancer patients largely outnumber trials of any other form of immunotherapy in this population, even though the studied malignancies are often relatively rare, for example, renal cancer and melanoma. Cytokines are also used in combination treatment strategies.

Insufficient concentration of appropriate cytokines is one of the reasons proposed for failure of the immune system to recognize and destroy tumors. The efficacy of adoptive transfer of effector cells and tumor vaccination is also believed to depend on cytokine levels. This is the rationale behind combinations of cytokine treatment and vaccination or adoptive transfer. Although systemic toxicity is a problem with many cytokines, their activity is mainly locoregional. This implies that locoregional application would allow much higher tissue concentrations in the targeted tissue resulting in better clinical outcomes. A recent report has suggested that cytokines such as TNF-α and IFN gamma may cause tumor-restricted disruption of the tumor vasculature in isolated limb perfusion through reduced activation of the aVb3 integrin that is expressed selectively on the proliferating tumor endothelium. This forms the rationale for isolated limb and liver perfusion therapy, one of the important applications of cytokines. Biologic systems to obtain local secretion of cytokines have also been developed.

The functions of cytokines are generally complex. Frequently, the effect of a cytokine involves several other cytokines. The cytokines most frequently tested in a clinical setting are IL-2, IFN-α, IFN-γ, TNF-α, and GM-CSF. The use of cytokines known to have accessory function in the generation of T-cell–mediated immunity (e.g., TNF, IL-1, IL-6, IL-7, and IL-12) is a logical approach to cancer immunotherapy that has been studied in some detail. The hypothesis is that such signals could be lacking or deficient in the tumor-bearing host. Because T-cell recognition of antigen in the absence of accessory signals can lead to immunologic anergy, this pathway is of extreme importance. Systemic administration of such cytokines or, more elegantly, vaccination with cells expressing such cytokines, would be expected to be beneficial. In addition to modifying the in vivo inflammatory environment, cytokine transduction may cause other phenotypic changes in tumors. An autocrine action of cytokines may be linked to cell growth, secondary cytokine production, and the secreted extracellular matrix.

Inflammatory/T-Cell Reactive Cytokines

Interleukin-2

IL-2 is the most extensively studied cytokine to date. It is a lymphocyte-secreted, 15-kDa glycoprotein produced in response to several stimuli. In addition to stimulating the proliferation of T cells, it activates T and B cells, NK cells, and macrophages and induces the production of other cytokines, such as TNF, IFN γ, and GM-CSF. Systemic administration of IL-2 alone and in combination with other cytokines has been studied in several trials, principally in patients with melanoma and renal cell carcinoma. Because IL-2 has been studied longer than any other cytokine, data regarding IL-2 responses are substantial. Most protocols involve high-dose bolus regimens of 720,000 international units (IU) per kilogram every 8 hours for days 1 to 5 and 15 to 19, repeated every 4 to 6 weeks. Trials involving lower doses (72,000 IU/kg) or continuous-infusion therapy have demonstrated results similar to those for high-dose treatment schemes. The lower dosing schedules substantially reduce the toxicity associated with higher-dose therapy, side effects of which include capillary leak syndrome, hypotension, azotemia, and metabolic acidosis. The toxicity of IL-2 seems related to induction of TNF-α, and the magnitude of this response appears to be genetically determined, resulting in individual variation in the toxicity of IL-2.

Overall response rates of approximately 20% (approximately 20% of responses are complete) have been achieved with a variety of doses and schedules. Meta-analyses reveal that IL-2 may confer in patients with excellent performance status, compared with standard nonbiologic therapy. Combinations of IL-2 and IFN-α have been used in the treatment of renal cell carcinoma and melanoma and have produced response rates similar to those seen with IL-2 alone. Adding cisplatin to the IL-2 and IFN-α regimen may well enhance the antitumor response in patients with metastatic melanoma: the use of this combination produced a 54% response rate in a recent trial. IL-2 has been tested in the treatment of a variety of hematologic malignancies, with occasional responses documented. The combination of IL-2 and melatonin has been evaluated in several clinical trials involving patients with hepatocellular carcinoma, non-small cell lung cancer, and renal cell cancer. Objective responses have occurred in all disease types, and some responses were better than those seen with the use of IL-2 alone. The combination of IL-2 and melatonin was also associated with less toxicity.

Interleukin-4

IL-4 is a lymphocyte-derived cytokine. Originally termed B-cell stimulatory factor, this 20-kDa glycoprotein was identified as a potent activator of B and T cells, including CD4$^+$ and CD8$^+$ populations, as well as macrophages, mast cells, and hematopoietic progenitors. In several reports, IL-4 demonstrated stronger stimulatory effects than IL-2 on primed murine CTLs. IL-4 induces the proliferation and differentiation of lymphocytes and upregulates MHC class II and Ig expression by stimulated macrophages and B cells. IL-4 inhibits the expression of several inflammatory cytokines (IL-1, IFN-γ, TNF, and IL-6) and enhances the antiproliferative effects of TNF in many tumor cell lines. IL-4 has been presented to CTLs in peripheral blood lymphocytes and in tumor-infiltrating lymphocyte (TIL) populations that preferentially kill autologous tumors. IL-4 is currently being investigated in clinical protocols involving patients with renal cell carcinoma and melanoma. IL-4 appears less effective than IL-2 in inducing antitumor responses in solid tumors but may have more activity than IL-2 against hematologic malignancies, specifically B-cell lymphomas and myelomas. Combinations of IL-2 and IL-4 have also been evaluated, with no significant responses reported to date.

Tumor Necrosis Factor-α

TNF-α is a 17-kDa protein first described as a serum component responsible for inducing hemorrhagic necrosis of certain tumors in vivo. Several cell types, including T and B cells, macrophages, neutrophils, endothelial cells, and some tumors produce TNF-α. This cytokine upregulates the production of IL-1, IL-6, GM-CSF, and intercellular adhesion molecule-1 production, acts as a costimulus for T-cell proliferation, and increases the expression of MHC class I antigens.

TNF-α alters the growth of some tumor cell lines in vitro and in vivo, perhaps by acting on tumor microvasculature. However, high systemic levels of TNF-α induce a septic shock-like syndrome associated with tissue injury, organ failure, and cachexia. Clinical cancer trials of TNF-α have largely been disappointing; however, TNF alone or with IFN-α in hyperthermic isolated limb perfusion protocols for patients with melanoma and sarcoma has been associated with significant tumor responses that have obviated amputation in some patients. Unfortunately, regional toxic side effects have also been reported and have resulted in ischemic compartment syndromes in affected limbs.

Interferon γ

IFN γ is a 20-kDa glycoprotein that is produced by activated lymphocytes in response to various stimuli and induces the development of CTLs, NK cells, and macrophages. IFN γ exerts direct cytotoxic effects and upregulates the expression of MHC antigens and adhesion molecules. IFN γ has demonstrated divergent properties in different tumor models: in certain murine systems, IFN γ promotes tumorigenicity and metastatic potential, whereas in other models it has demonstrated antineoplastic activity. Clinically, the most encouraging data have come from studies involving patients with malignant mesothelioma, in whom intrapleural IFN γ therapy response rates were approximately 15%.

Interferon-α

IFN-α is a leukocyte-secreted cytokine that possesses tumoricidal effects and also increases the activity of cytotoxic effectors, including NK cells and macrophages. Systemic administration of IFN-α has been associated with upregulation of MHC class I antigen expression to a greater degree than that seen with administration of IFN-γ. IFN-α also increases expression of tumor antigens capable of eliciting MAb recognition. IFN-α has been evaluated in the treatment of several human malignancies, particularly renal cell carcinoma, melanoma, and hematologic malignancies.

IFN-α is currently recommended as an initial treatment for patients with hairy cell and chronic myelogenous leukemias. INF-α is capable of inducing hematologic and karyotypic remissions in patients with these diseases.

Recently, Kirkwood and associates from the Eastern Cooperative Oncology Group (1996) published the most compelling evidence to date regarding the efficacy of systemically administered IFN alfa-2b in patients with malignant melanoma. In a multicenter randomized trial comparing adjuvant high-dose IFN alfa-2b for 52 weeks with observation for the same period, a significant prolongation of relapse-free and overall survival was observed in the treatment group. The patients most likely to benefit from this therapy were those with regional lymph node metastases. The associated toxicity was significant, however, and a substantial proportion of patients could not tolerate fully planned doses or experienced significant or life-threatening side effects, including myelosuppression, hepatotoxicity, and neurologic symptoms.

Combinations of IFN-α and standard chemotherapy agents have been evaluated in the treatment of several solid tumor types. Though occasional responses have been observed, the addition of IFN-α to established chemotherapy regimens has not produced dramatic changes in response rates. The combination of INF-α and standard chemotherapy doses, however, appear to alter the pharmacokinetics and toxicity profiles of many therapies, in some cases adversely.

Interleukin-1

IL-1 is a 17-kDa cytokine initially recognized for its effect as an endogenous pyrogen. It was first shown to be produced by cells of the monocyte/macrophage lineage in response to perceived host stress or enhanced metabolic activity. Subsequently, IL-1 was found to be produced by NK cells, fibroblasts, T-cell lines, and some tumor cell lines. Properties attributed to IL-1 include participation in inflammatory responses, septic shock, T_H cell responses, and induction of other cytokines and adhesion molecules such as TNF, GM-CSF, IL-2, IL-2 receptor, IL-3, IL-4, IL-6, IL-7, and ICAM-1. Endotoxins, exotoxins, TNF-α, and GM-CSF stimulate IL-1 expression. IL-1 has been observed to induce cytotoxic effects in certain tumors, but its toxicity has limited its clinical utility. Antitumor effects of IL-1 administration have been disappointing, but phase II trials of combinations of IL-2 and IL-1 have suggested activity in patients with a variety of metastatic solid tumor malignancies. Furthermore, studies indicate that IL-1 may play a role in enhancing platelet recovery following chemotherapy.

Interleukin-6

IL-6 is a 25-kDa glycoprotein that functions as a growth factor and is capable of augmenting the in vitro cytotoxic capacity of T-cell subsets. Its release by various cell types—including T and B cells, platelets, macrophages, and fibroblasts—may be induced by TNF, IL-2, IL-3, GM-CSF, and IL-7. IL-6 has been shown to exert variable influences on the growth of tumor cells in vitro and when administered systemically. This cytokine demonstrated significant antineoplastic activity in tumor-bearing mice, the effect of which was abolished by sublethal irradiation of the animals. In a melanoma model, IL-6 differentially regulated the growth of metastatic and nonmetastatic cells. IL-6 has been clinically evaluated both as a platelet growth factor and as an antineoplastic agent. It appears to function more effectively in the former role than in the latter. Results of recent studies in a variety of tumor types have been mixed, although anecdotal reports of response by melanoma patients are encouraging. Side effects of IL-6 therapy include anemia, neurologic symptoms, cardiac arrhythmias, and constitutional symptoms.

Interleukin-7

IL-7 is a 25-kDa glycoprotein secreted by keratinocytes, DCs, and certain T-cell populations. IL-7 acts as a costimulator of lymphocyte growth and differentiation both independently and in concert with IL-2. IL-7 upregulates the expression of IL-6 and down-regulates the expression of the potent immunosuppressant TGF-β. In a direct comparison with IL-2, IL-7 was a more potent generator of antitumor CTLs in a murine model. In addition, intratumoral injection of high doses of IL-7 resulted in tumor rejection and decreased tumor growth in a proportion of animals treated. Mice that rejected tumors after IL-7 administration were found to be specifically immune to subsequent tumor challenge. Currently, there are no specific clinical protocols involving direct administration of IL-7. However, one phase I protocol is evaluating IL-7 in a gene therapy tumor vaccine model. This protocol will be discussed in the section on gene therapy.

Interleukin-12

IL-12 was purified and cloned after its identification as a stimulator of several cytotoxic lymphocyte populations, particularly NK cells. This cytokine is normally produced by B cells and cells of the monocyte/macrophage lineage. The molecule exists as a disulfide-linked heterodimer composed of 40- and 35-kDa subunits, both of which are required for biologic activity. Because of this unique structure, IL-12 has a longer half-life (measured in hours) than other cytokines. Its longer duration of action may allow less frequent dosing and may result in decreased toxicity. IL-12 has been observed to upregulate and induce IFN-γ in cultured T and NK cells, act synergistically with IL-2, and block the production of IL-4. IL-12 may also induce TNF, GM-CSF, and IL-3 in lymphocyte populations. Recently, IL-12 was shown to stimulate T_H1 helper cells, which characteristically secrete IL-2, IFN-γ, and TNF-γ. T_H2 cells are less affected by IL-12. Systemic and intratumoral administration of recombinant IL-12 to tumor-bearing animals caused growth inhibition of established primary and metastatic lesions that was at least partially dependent on CTLs. Mice were specifically immune to tumor rechallenge in certain systems. Clinical trials of IL-12 have recently been initiated, and signs of response have been seen in patients with metastatic renal cell cancer.

Colony-Stimulating Factors

Interleukin-3

IL-3 is a T-cell–derived pleuripotent hematopoietic growth factor with a molecular weight of approximately 28 kDa. In a comparison with several other cytokines, exogenous IL-3 administration significantly enhanced the immunogenicity of irradiated tumor cells, including a nonimmunogenic tumor. In the clinical setting, IL-3 has primarily been used for bone marrow rescue, with responses principally involving leukocytes and platelets. Studies of combinations of IL-3 and other colony-stimulating factors are also ongoing.

Granulocyte Colony-Stimulating Factor

Granulocyte colony-stimulating factor (G-CSF) is an approximately 20-kDa glycoprotein required for the growth and differentiation of hematopoietic precursors of the granulocyte lineage. Cells of the monocyte/macrophage lineage are the primary producers of G-CSF, which is not species-specific and therefore demonstrates biologic activity in both human and murine models. Clinical trials using this cytokine have demonstrated its efficacy in reducing the period of myelosuppression after chemotherapy for solid and hematologic malignancies, and after bone marrow transplantation.

Granulocyte-Macrophage Colony-Stimulating Factor

GM-CSF is a 22-kDa glycoprotein secreted by stimulated T cells. It is integral to the development of hematopoietic progenitor cells, as well as mature neutrophils, eosinophils, and macrophages, in bone marrow and peripheral circulation. This cytokine is involved in the generation of bone marrow–derived DCs participating in antigen presentation to unprimed T_H cells and CTLs. GM-CSF may also induce the expression of TNF and prostaglandin E2 in activated macrophages and may synergize with G-CSF in certain systems. GM-CSF–treated monocytes display enhanced Ab-directed cytotoxicity and phagocytosis in vitro. Clinical trials using this cytokine have reported increased peripheral granulocyte counts after myelosuppressive treatment in cytopenic patients. GM-CSF may also act to enhance cytokine levels in treated patients, thereby promoting antineoplastic inflammatory responses.

Vaccines

The essential task of vaccination is to activate the host's immune system. This should be achieved by offering the antigens that T cells can recognize in the most effective way, that is, ensuring that they are adequately presented and in the context of appropriate costimulatory signals. The goal of vaccination approaches in human cancer is to induce tumor-specific, long-lasting immune response that leads to tumor elimination. The induction of tumor immunity can be viewed as a three-step process: presentation of tumor-associated antigens (TAAs); selection and activation of TAA-specific T cells as well as nonantigen-specific effectors; and homing of TAA-specific T cells to the tumor site and recognition of restriction elements, leading to the elimination of tumor cells.

In the development of tumor vaccines, two different principles can be followed. One is to identify specific TAAs present on the target tumor and to treat the patient with these TAAs. The other approach is to vaccinate patients using whole tumor cells or cell lysates in which the specific TAAs are not known. Both approaches will be discussed in this section.

Vaccination with Molecularly Defined Antigens

Much effort has been expended to identify TAAs and their epitopes, in some instances, as in melanoma, a large but as yet incomplete number of TAAs have been identified. Some TAAs represent physiologically important proteins that are generally overexpressed in malignancies; these would be ideal targets for vaccines that could be used on a large scale. Vaccination with normal proteins has many advantages, chief among them the low cost and safe production. This approach may be effective even in the face of ongoing selective pressure if the antigens (proteins) used are essential determinants in carcinogenesis (e.g., RAS and p53). However, vaccination with normal proteins is also associated with risk of generating cross-reactivity against normal tissues and, hence, autoimmune disease. Furthermore, technical problems in terms of tumor escape by selection probably require further investigation of TAAs. Representative immunologic monitoring that correlates well with clinical effects is lacking at present. This interferes with pinpointing the exact reasons for the disappointing results so far. Progress in this field is desirable but will be difficult.

A good example of a TAA generally overexpressed in malignancies is wild-type p53, which is overexpressed in a great variety of tumors and is also expressed in normal tissues. Selective tumor eradication may be obtained through targeting of such proteins in malignancies. In contrast, targeting of mutant p53 and mutated RAS would require a vaccine with antigens that matched the mutation present in the individual tumor.

A more restricted specificity can be obtained by using antigens that represent proteins expressed only in certain tissues or groups of tissues. Examples of these are carcinoembryonic antigen (CEA) in colorectal and other epithelial tumors and Her-2/neu in breast and ovarian cancers. In these examples, tumor specificity depends on the overexpression rather than expression of a mutated protein.

As mentioned at the beginning of this section, TAAs have been identified that are restricted in their expression to certain malignancies. If a viral agent is involved in a crucial step of carcinogenesis, it may constitute a valuable source of target antigens of nonself origin. Thus, tumors such as hepatocellular carcinoma and cervical carcinoma could be controlled by vaccination with hepatitis B virus and human papilloma virus, respectively.

PEPTIDE-BASED VACCINES. The ideal vaccine should present no more antigens than necessary to obtain the desired immunologic reaction. The most pure antigen-containing vaccine would be multiple synthetic peptides containing only oligopeptide epitopes of TAAs that can be recognized by the patient's immune system in an HLA-restricted way. To cover a wide range of HLA types, the vaccine would be either HLA type-matched or contain a cocktail of epitopes for the various HLA alleles. The goal would be to load these peptides onto MHC molecules of APCs in vivo. Peptide vaccination is effective against viral antigens and in tumor challenge experiments in animals.

Peptide vaccination has been tested in recent and ongoing clinical trials, but no large-scale evaluation of its clinical use has been published as of this writing. Some of these phase I and II studies, carried out in stage IV melanoma, showed peptide-specific or clinical responses in a significant percentage of patients. Evaluation of studies in which clinical responses were weak or absent showed that loss of antigen expression by the tumor and MHC class I downregulation (selection) accounted for the failure of peptide vaccination. In a study in 23 patients with metastatic breast cancer, treatment with synthetic sialyl-Tn epitopes linked to keyhole limpet hemocyanin together with Detox-B adjuvant with or without cyclophosphamide pretreatment produced only a single partial response and a few cases of stable disease. Similar results were obtained in patients with metastatic cervical cancer with human papilloma virus-16 (HPV-16)–derived peptide bound to the T_H cell-activating peptide PADRE in incomplete Freund's adjuvant. In that trial, clinical responses appeared linked to recognition of PADRE and not to recognition of HPV peptide. In fact, in vitro responses to the HPV peptide could only be demonstrated in patients with no clinical response. Like the patients in the trials of peptide vaccines in melanoma, these patients were found to be immunocompromised.

RECOMBINANT VIRAL AND BACTERIAL VACCINES. Recombinant techniques make it possible to introduce antigens or just epitopes into viral vectors and will eventually make it possible to induce costimulatory molecules and cytokines as well. Viral infection and resulting tissue damage should attract professional APCs necessary for adequate antigen presentation. Direct infection of APCs could result in endogenous processing. Although cross-reaction in Abs recognizing the viral vector constitutes a major problem at the moment, particularly in adenovirus vectors, recombinant viral vaccines seem very promising.

Various virus vaccines have now been tested in the clinical setting. A vaccinia virus vaccine containing CEA has been extensively tested and has been reported to be effective in the induction of immune responses in humans. Vaccinia virus vaccines containing epitopes from HPV-16 and HPV-18, for application in cervical cancer, has reached that stage. Several canary chickenpox virus–based vaccines including single antigens (e.g., wild-type p53), developed by Pasteur-Merieux, are currently being investigated in phase I and phase II clinical trials.

NAKED DNA VACCINES. Naked DNA vaccines encoding tumor antigens result in some degree of systemic tumor protection in animal experiments, but unlike virus vaccines, naked DNA vaccines are unable to elicit amplification and generation of danger signals. Nevertheless, some degree of inflammation and attraction of APCs and presentation by such cells has been reported with naked DNA vaccines. Mechanisms involved in this type of immunization remain largely unclear.

IDIOTYPE ANTIBODY VACCINES. The idiotype is the variable binding part of an Ab and fits like a mold to the antigen. Vaccination with a TAA-specific Ab (so-called idiotype antibody vaccination) causes formation of autologous Abs against the vaccine. The variable part of these induced Abs fits to the mold and therefore strongly resembles the TAA. Thus, the TAA (mimic) is available for recognition by the immune system in a completely different environment. Idiotype antibody vaccination has two advantages. First, it allows vaccination without the need for significant quantities of the purified antigen. Second, and also of great practical importance, it allows the induction of a response against nonprotein antigens. This strategy has now reached the stage of clinical trials.

VACCINATION WITH UNDEFINED ANTIGENS. When the TAAs for a given tumor are not well defined, an alternative approach is to use autologous tumor cells to create a vaccine. Use of whole tumor cells increases the likelihood that a sufficient number of TAAs will be included in the vaccine. The use of such autologous vaccines in the form of whole tumor cells, lysates, apoptotic cells, or HSP extracts has one major advantage: the vaccine represents the whole spectrum of unique and shared antigens expressed by the individual tumor. Thus, the possibility of inducing an immune response with a variety of antigens also expressed on the target is increased, and the risk of tumor escape is theoretically reduced. However, this approach also has several disadvantages. The use of malignant tissue as the crude base from which a vaccine is produced can be expected to increase the risk of side effects. Synthetic preparation of such a vaccine is impossible and likely to remain so in the future. Cost of vaccination can be expected to grow along with the complexity of the vaccine.

DC-MEDIATED VACCINATION. Because of their unique ability to induce primary immune responses, DCs are attractive vectors for cancer immunotherapy. DCs present antigens to both T_H cells and CTLs, leading to activation of many clones with broad specificity. Activation of T_H cells permits recruitment of nonantigen-specific effectors including NK cells, eosinophils, and macrophages, resulting in diverse immune responses.

DCs are now believed to play a central role as APCs in tumor immunology. Several successful methods have been devised for loading the MHC molecules of DCs with appropriate epitopes. These methods, which often use the endogenous antigen processing pathway of these APCs, include pulsing with peptides, protein, or cell lysates; cross priming with apoptotic cells; fusion with whole tumor cells or RNA; and transfection with viral vectors. The distinct advantages of using peptides, implying a restricted number of antigens, have been discussed earlier (see the section on peptide-based vaccines). Using the whole antigenic repertoire of the tumor may lead to stimulation of different T-cell precursors, resulting in a larger repertoire of effector lymphocytes, both CTLs and T_H. Moreover, the application of a larger array of antigens theoretically reduces the chance of selection and tumor escape.

A number of ongoing and reported clinical trials have used TAA-loaded DCs as a vaccine in human cancer. Significant clinical responses have been observed in several preliminary trials and in three separate studies that were examined, respectively, including a pioneer study based on injection of blood-derived DCs loaded with lymphoma idiotype; administration of peptide-pulsed APCs generated by culturing monocytes with GM-CSF; vaccination with monocyte-derived DCs loaded with melanoma peptides; and injection of monocyte-derived DCs pulsed with prostate-specific membrane antigen peptide. Intranodal injection of immature monocyte-derived DCs pulsed with synthetic melanoma peptides or tumor induced delayed-type hypersensitivity reactivity toward vaccine antigens in 11 patients. Most recently, a reported study demonstrated that vaccination with melanoma peptide loaded mature monocyte-derived DCs led to substantial immune responses in blood. Nouri-Shirazi et al. (2000) demonstrated that vaccination of patients with stage IV melanoma with DCs derived from CD34$^+$ cells and pulsed with multiple antigens—including KLH protein, flu-matrix peptide, and melanoma peptides—led to significant primary and recall immune responses in blood. While trials reported to date prove the safety and tolerability of DC-mediated vaccination and have demonstrated limited clinical responses with this approach, several parameters need to be optimized in future trials to ensure optimal conditions for induction of therapeutic antitumor immunity. These parameters include the source and the preparation of TAAs and the DC loading strategy; the subset of DCs and the method of generation (ex vivo culture or in vivo mobilization); the DC activation/maturation status; DC dose, route, and frequency of injection; and the combination of DC-mediated vaccination with other therapies—for example, the combination of DC-mediated vaccination with biologic response modifiers such as IL-2.

DCs can be loaded with antigen in several ways, and the TAAs loaded can be either defined or undefined. Published data on vaccination with DCs consist of phase I and II studies including small series of patients. Nestle and colleagues reported on the efficacy of tumor lysate-pulsed and peptide-pulsed DCs in patients with metastatic melanoma, using biopsy material as the source of antigen. Injection of peptide- or protein-pulsed DC in prostate carcinoma patients has been reported to result in clinical response rates of 10% to 30%. No side effects in terms of autoimmunity have been found. DCs pulsed with K-ras–mutated peptides elicited immunologic but no clinical responses in patients with pancreatic cancer. An update of a multicenter trial with K-ras given with GM-CSF demonstrated specific immune responses in 50% of patients and prolonged survival. In contrast, a small pilot study using monocyte-derived macrophages instead of DCs as an APC vaccine in the treatment of colorectal cancer resulted in only one patient with stable disease of short duration.

Distributed as sentinels throughout the body, DCs are poised to capture antigens, migrate to draining lymphoid organs, and, after a process of maturation, select antigen-specific lymphocytes to which they present the processed antigen, thereby inducing immune responses. DCs present antigen to T_H cells, which in turn regulate multiple effectors, including CTLs, B cells, NK cells, macrophages, and eosinophils, all of which contribute to the protective immune responses. The DC system has several key features: (a) the existence of different DC subsets that have some biologic functions in common but also display unique functions, such as polarization of T-cell responses towards T_H1 or T_H2 cells or regulation of B-cell responses; (b) the functional specialization of DCs according to their differentiation/maturation stages; and (c) the plasticity of DCs, which is determined by the microenvironment (e.g., cytokines) and is seen in the ability of these cells to differentiate into either DCs (enhanced antigen presentation) or macrophages (enhanced antigen degradation); the ability of DCs to induce either immunity or tolerance; and the polarization of T-cell responses. Because of these unique properties, DCs represent both vectors and targets for immunologic intervention in numerous diseases and are optimal candidates for vaccination protocols in both cancer and infectious diseases.

TUMOR CELL–BASED VACCINATION. Whole tumor cells—live irradiated cells transduced with different genes, dead cells, and lysed cells—have been used in vaccines. Tumor cell–based vaccines may be limited in their effect by the very factors that kept the tumor itself from provoking an adequate immune response in the first place. Attempts to improve the efficacy of tumor cell–based vaccines by adding adjuvants, such as BCG, turned out to be effective, at least with immunogenic tumors. One reason may be that the irradiated tumor cells go into apoptosis and are subsequently presented by autologous DCs through cross-priming. BCG was shown to play an additional role by stimulating maturation of DCs. More sophisticated attempts to enhance immunogenicity came with genetic modification technologies that permitted the introduction of allogeneic MHC genes into tumor cells, even in vivo. The latest technique in this field is the introduction of cytokine genes or costimulatory molecules into the genome of the vaccine tumor cells. This should result in modification of the microenvironmental conditions in the area of the tumor cells so that anergy is overcome and tumor lysis takes place. One promising cytokine used for this purpose is GM-CSF, which is known to contribute to the maturation of DCs, and can therefore enhance antigen presentation by the tumor cells. Various preparations obtained from tumor tissue have now been evaluated in clinical vaccination studies, often in combination with a nonspecific immune stimulant as an adjuvant. The vaccines tested include both irradiated viable tumor cells and tumor cell lysates.

WHOLE-TUMOR-CELL VACCINES. Vaccination with tumor cells is one of the oldest ideas in tumor immunology. The past two decades have seen many publications on clinical applications of this approach. However, expression of immunogenic molecules in these vaccines was not documented and, with the exception of some Ab reactions, immune responses could not be adequately assessed.

Initial phase II studies in melanoma and renal cell carcinoma, in which autologous tumor cells along with a bacterial adjuvant were administered after a low dose of cyclophosphamide, elicited clinical responses in five of 64 and five of 26 cases, respectively. Both these studies were carried out in patients bearing a high burden of metastatic disease (no resections were carried out). The use of allogeneic cells instead of autologous tumor resulted in similar response rates in melanoma. More recently, a phase II study reported that the autologous tumor cell vaccine modified by the hapten dinitrophenyl as an adjuvant treatment to surgery in metastatic melanoma that resulted in survival rates markedly higher than those seen with surgery alone. In renal cell carcinoma, Robson stage 1 to 4, treatment of patients with stages II and III disease was reported to improve survival compared to survival in a historical control group. These results, however, need to be confirmed by prospective randomized studies.

Randomized controlled trials evaluating the effect of tumor cell vaccination plus BCG in colorectal cancer have been conducted. Though the latest reports mention the administration of viable cells, careful reading reveals that cells were irradiated with a dose that ensures that the vaccine cells will go into apoptosis within 24 hours. The authors reported an improved overall survival. Notably, apart from local effects of BCG, there was no toxicity. These studies demonstrated clearly significant improvements in overall survival in stage II disease. In stage III disease, however, the latest study failed to show statistically significant improvements. Whole tumor-cell vaccination plus BCG in a study by Hoover et al. (1993) did show a significant effect in patients with stage III colon cancer. Moreover, adjuvant autologous tumor cell vaccination in metastatic (stage IV) colorectal cancer also appeared effective. There is clearly enough evidence to warrant further evaluation of the use of autologous cellular vaccine on a larger scale in stage II colon cancer and, if a better characterization of antigen expression by the autologous vaccine can be carried out, to justify a trial in which patients with stage III colon cancer are randomly assigned to active specific immunotherapy or other treatment modalities.

Cytokine-modified cellular vaccines consisting of autologous or allogeneic tumor cells transduced with genes encoding IL-2, IL-4, IL-7 and IL-12 have been tested. The most important end points of these trials were induction or increase of CTLs, Ab-specific antitumor response, or both. Toxicity and any evidence of clinical activity were also considered. In one study, the gene for IFN-γ was introduced via a retroviral vector into autologous tumor cells cultured from patients with malignant melanoma, and the cells were then used as vaccine. Thirteen of the 20 entered patients completed this protocol, and eight patients showed a humoral IgG response against autologous and allogeneic melanoma cells. Two patients with significant increases in serum IgG had clinical tumor regression, specifically at superficial lymph node levels. Lotze et al. (1994) have initiated phase I and II clinical trials in which melanoma lesions are directly injected with IL-12-gene-engineered autologous fibroblasts. These authors have obtained a high expression of heterodimeric IL-12 from the transduced fibroblasts after selection. Eighteen patients, seven of whom presented with malignant melanoma, have been treated with weekly injections, and three patients with recurrent melanoma showed shrinkage of the injected lesions as well as distant lesions by more than 50% without significant side effects.

Two further phase I clinical studies with autologous tumor cells are worth mentioning. One involved vaccination of patients with metastatic melanoma with irradiated, autologous tumor cells transduced with the gene encoding GM-CSF. In this trial, 21 patients were given intradermal and subcutaneous injections of 10^7 cells 1, 2, or 4 weeks apart. Metastatic lesions resected after vaccination were densely infiltrated, and extensive tumor destruction was evident in 11 of 16 patients examined. Antimelanoma CTLs and Ab responses were associated with tumor destruction. A similar trial with autologous, irradiated, GM-CSF-gene–transduced vaccine was conducted by Simons and coworkers (1997) in patients with renal cancer. Patients were treated in a randomized, double-blind dose escalation study with equivalent doses of autologous cells with or without GM-CSF gene transfer. In the 16 evaluable patients, no dose-limiting side effects were found. An intense eosinophil infiltrate was detected at sites of DTH responses to GM-CSF vaccine but not in patients receiving nontransduced cells. An objective partial response (PR) was observed in a patient treated with GM-CSF-gene–transduced cells.

Studies with autologous tumor cells were also carried out in patients with metastatic melanoma using IL-2- or IFN-γ-gene-transduced vaccines. In both studies 12 patients were given up to 10^7 irradiated cells one to three times. With the IL-2-gene–transduced vaccine, antiautologous tumor CTLs were increased in four of seven patients tested, but no clinical responses were observed. No objective clinical responses were found in patients given IFN-γ vaccine.

Another study involved patients with metastatic melanoma treated with IL-7-gene-transduced autologous irradiated cells. Melanoma cells were transduced using a ballistic gene transfer technique and injected subcutaneously at weekly intervals for 3 weeks. No significant toxic effects but also no objective clinical responses were observed. In three of six cases, an increase in melanoma-specific cytolytic T cells was found. Limitations of the autologous vaccine approach—disease progression before sufficient cells have grown in culture or the inability to grow tumor cells in culture acquired from the tumor—result in vaccination of only 10% to 50% of eligible individuals.

One way to obviate culturing of tumor cells in vitro to carry out gene transfer is to establish allogeneic cell lines derived from the tumor type that is the target of therapy. These cell lines can be easily grown, transduced, and used as a single, standardized reagent. Two clinical trials have been conducted of vaccination with IL-2- or IL-4-gene–transduced allogeneic melanoma cells, using Melan-A/MART-1-, tyrosinase-, gp100-, and MAGE-3-positive cells in patients with advanced-stage HLA-A2+ melanoma. In the first protocol, patients were injected subcutaneously at 2-week intervals with IL-2-gene–transduced and irradiated melanoma cells at a dose of 5 or 15×10^7 cells. Evaluation of the specific CTL response with mixed lymphocyte-tumor cultures and with limiting dilution analysis showed that vaccination with cells bearing the appropriate antigens and releasing IL-2 locally could expand a T-cell response against melanoma-associated antigens of autologous, nontransduced tumors but only in a minority of patients. In the IL-2 study, a mixed clinical response was noted in two patients. The local and systemic side effects of treatment were mild. The amount of cytokine released by tumor cells appears to be an important parameter in conferring immunogenicity to the transduced cells. A variation on these themes is the clinical trial being conducted by Lotze et al. (1994) at the Pittsburgh Cancer Institute. Their strategy is to isolate patients' fibroblasts and then modify them with a retroviral vector containing the gene for IL-4. Once a sufficient number of IL-4–producing fibroblasts has been generated, they are mixed with a sample of autologous tumor obtained by a biopsy and re-administered back to the patient. The rationale for the use of the IL-4 gene is that this cytokine induces the switch from uncommitted T_H cells into

T$_H$2 cells, which are involved in Ab-mediated immunity. Nine patients have entered this study, and in two of these patients, an initial T-cell infiltrate into tumor has been observed.

LYSATE VACCINES. Few data exist to support the clinical efficacy of lysate vaccination. A large randomized study (250 patients) of treatment with vaccinia plus melanoma oncolysate compared to vaccinia alone showed no effect, except in a very small subgroup of young high-risk males. This result is difficult to interpret for methodologic reasons. In a phase II study in which 95 patients with stage I and II breast cancer were treated with lysate of tumor tissue, no clinical effect was evident.

HEAT SHOCK PROTEIN VACCINATION. HSPs such as hsp 70 and hsp 96 are naturally occurring intracellular substances that are supposed to chaperone a wide array of antigenic proteins present in the cell, channeling these proteins into both the MHC class I and MHC class II processing pathways. HSPs are also related to signals associated with tissue damage, signaling danger and thus triggering DC-mediated antigen presentation. Isolation of these immunologic adjuvants from the tumor thus obviates antigen identification in a particular patient or of composing a cocktail of epitopes from TAAs the individual tumor might be carrying without the need for a vaccine composed of viable cells. Evidence exists for receptor-mediated endocytosis of HSPs by macrophages and DCs. Vaccination with these HSPs in animal models can thus induce CTL-mediated systemic antitumor immunity. The practical importance of HSPs is supported by the observation that immunogenicity of tumor cells is related to the hsp 70 they release. Reviewing the existing evidence, one can even conclude that HSPs are the predominant source of antigen in the natural setting. Clinical trials to evaluate the efficacy of hsp 96 are underway in pancreatic, renal, gastric, and colorectal cancer and melanoma.

Adoptive Transfer

In adoptive transfer, selected effector cells are infused into the patient either systemically or locally into the tumor. Before infusion, the effector cells are expanded in vitro to evade mechanisms that inhibit expansion in vivo. The effector cells may be antigen specific (CTLs) or nonspecific (LAK cells). Several trials of adoptive transfer have been conducted.

The source of the effectors can be the tumor, as in TILs or peripheral blood mononuclear cells. Peripheral blood mononuclear cells are easier to obtain, but the frequency of tumor-specific lymphocyte precursors is expected to be much lower in the blood than at the tumor site. Generally, autologous lymphocytes have to be used because the host can rapidly reject allogeneic cells and allogeneic cells will attack normal tissues, inducing a graft-versus-host type of reaction. However, it has also been demonstrated that transplanted allogeneic immune cells can recognize malignant cells as being non-self and mount a therapeutic response known as graft-versus-disease effect. By depletion of subsets of cells, the graft-versus-disease effect remains intact, whereas no graft-versus-host effect occurs. This phenomenon of preferential tumor cell killing by certain subsets of allogeneic bone marrow cells is now being further evaluated for its use in solid tumors.

With the discovery of IL-2 and the ability to efficiently expand T cells in culture, the idea of adoptive transfer became a true possibility. As has previously been discussed, systemic IL-2 induces an anticancer response but with high levels of toxicity. These findings stimulated interest in adoptive immunotherapy—transfer of specific immune cells with antitumor activity to the tumor-bearing host—as a less toxic alternative. The vast majority of clinical trials of this approach have used IL-2–generated LAK cells and, more recently, TILs.

LAK Cell Therapy

LAK cells are a heterogeneous population of cells made up of T cells and NK cells harvested from the peripheral blood that develop antitumor activity after being incubated in high concentrations of IL-2. The mechanism of selective cellular killing by LAK cells is unknown; however, these cells maintain their antitumor activity in vivo with exogenous IL-2 administration. LAK cells were first described in 1980, and clinical studies to determine the safety of infusional therapies were initiated shortly thereafter at the National Cancer Institute (NCI). The first series, including 25 patients, was published in 1985 and demonstrated the effectiveness of the therapy: regression of metastatic cancer of several histologic subtypes was seen. The follow-up series of 178 consecutive patients treated with LAK cells at the NCI revealed a complete response (CR) rate of 14% and a partial response (PR) of 30%, with the best results seen in renal cell carcinoma (35% CR + PR), melanoma (21% CR + PR), and non-Hodgkin's lymphoma (57% CR + PR). Other institutions have reported various response rates with LAK cell therapy for melanoma (0%–56%; composite, 18%), renal cell (0%–50%; composite, 27%), lymphoma (0%–100%; composite, 50%), and colorectal (0%–100%; composite, 9%). The composite results are from pooled data from nine studies. The difference in results between institutions was most likely due to differences in the numbers of infused LAK cells, the length of time cells were incubated in IL-2, and the dose and method of systemic IL-2 administration. The duration of response was usually less than 6 months; however, long-term CRs have been reported. Significant toxic effects related to the systemically administered IL-2 were reported in most studies. In a prospective randomized study in which patients were assigned to IL-2 alone or IL-2 with LAK, the latter treatment resulted in an improved response rate but only a trend toward improved overall survival.

With the NCI report in 1988 describing the enhanced antitumor activity of TILs (see the next section), most clinical attention has shifted away from LAK cells. However, some recent reports have looked at development of LAK cells in IL-12 instead of IL-2 and at new ways to use LAK cells, such as in the treatment of myelodysplastic syndrome. The regional use of LAK cells, such as intraperitoneal or intrapleural therapy and even intralesional therapy in neurologic malignancies, has also been reported.

TIL Therapy

TILs are reported to be 50 to 100 times more potent on a cell-to-cell basis than LAK cells in terms of antitumor activity, as demonstrated in animal models. TILs are derived from an individual's surgically resected tumor by cell separation. These T cells have been shown to be cytotoxic for tumor cells, and this killing has been demonstrated to be limited to the individual's tumor, suggesting HLA restriction. In fact, it is now widely accepted that TILs recognize and lyse tumor cells by CD3/TCR interaction with HLA class I/peptide complexes on the tumor cell surface. Many of the involved TCRs, HLA class I molecules, and even peptides involved in this specific recognition are now known, and the peptides are being investigated in vaccine trials.

In 1988, the NCI reported the first clinical trial with TILs, which demonstrated complete and partial regression of melanoma in some patients. The follow-up series of 86 patients with melanoma revealed an overall response rate (CR + PR) of 34%. This response rate is almost twice the composite response rate for LAK cells in melanoma and has been confirmed at other institutions, with some variation in results. As with the LAK cell trials, variable results with TILs appear to be related to IL-2 dose and method of administration; TIL number; and, most important, TIL culture characteristics. Better results are seen with cultures grown over shorter periods, which are predominantly CD8+ and demonstrate in vitro antitumor activity.

In renal cell carcinoma, the response rate with TIL therapy does not appear to be significantly improved compared to the response rate with LAK cell therapy. Some response has been seen with TIL therapy in the treatment of both primary lung cancer and the often associated malignant effusions. Several groups have used TIL therapy in ovarian cancer with and without chemotherapy, with some success. Intraperitoneal TIL infusions and IL-2 resulted in some marginal clinical activity and the results with TIL in combination with chemotherapy were very promising. TIL therapy plus cyclophosphamide resulted in a CR of 14% and a PR rate of 57% and TIL therapy plus cisplatin resulted in a CR rate of 70% and a PR rate of 20%. Studies of TIL therapy in other malignancies are currently underway.

Limitations of TIL therapies include the need for surgically resected tumor and 4 to 6 weeks to grow TIL cultures. Some groups have overcome the necessity of surgery by isolating tumor- associated lymphocytes from malignant ascites or effusions. The culture expansion time can be decreased with nonspecific stimulation and cytokines but often at the expense of the tumor-specific cytotoxicity of the TILs. Because tumor-specific cytotoxicity is the best predictor of clinical response, the goal is efficient culture conditions with improved tumor reactivity. Current advances have included repeat in vitro stimulation with tumor cells and, most recently, with newly identified, HLA-presented, immunodominant peptides. In vitro peptide stimulation has resulted in TILs 50 to 100 times more potent than TILs grown conventionally. This enhanced efficiency may allow for clinically effective peripheral blood lymphocyte cultures, eliminating the need for surgically resected tumor. Other attempts to improve adoptive immunotherapy have included in vivo stimulation with tumor immunization and subsequent harvest of the draining lymph nodes as the source of TILs. In preliminary clinical trials, this method has not produced any apparent improvement in response. Some other groups have modified TILs with transduced cytokine genes to enhance their potency; others are experimenting with combinations of TILs with other immunomodulators or chemotherapies. Clinical studies investigating these methods are being performed.

Monoclonal Antibody Therapy

Whereas a number of investigations have focused on immunotherapy protocols designed to alter or enhance cell-mediated antitumor activity, manipulation of the humoral immune system represents a relatively underexplored area of inquiry. For decades, it has been known that tumors possess antigens that, although relatively weak immunogenically, may be recognized as foreign by the immunocompetent host. For certain tumors, Abs to these antigens have been identified that have been useful in clinical determinations of disease presence or recurrence as in the case of CEA for assessing colorectal cancer, AFP for testicular tumors and hepatocellular carcinoma, and prostate-specific antigen for prostate carcinoma.

Monoclonal Antibody Production

MAbs are generated by fusing B cells to a murine myeloma cell line, resulting in a hybridoma that produces large quantities of a single Ab with unique specificity. MAbs have been evaluated as therapeutic as well as diagnostic tools in cancer therapy with varying degrees of success. MAb therapy is limited by physical characteristics of tumors, including variations in tumor vascularity and cellular density that often inhibit the ability of MAbs to sufficiently penetrate bulky tumors. Construction of Abs that recognizes only tumor tissue and ignore nonneoplastic cells is also difficult. Furthermore, tumor-antigen heterogeneity impedes the ability of MAbs to generate clinically significant tumoricidal effects. Probably the most significant obstacle to the efficacy of MAbs is the reaction to the murine component of the Ab that is recognized as foreign by human hosts, resulting in the generation of human antimouse Ab reactions that destroy circulating MAbs and enhance their serum clearance. Attempts to reduce the immunogenicity of MAbs have included the use of Ab fragments that lack the Fc domain (the portion binding the effector cell). However, reduced binding affinity typically accompanies the loss of this portion of the Ab. Humanized MAbs have also been attempted.

Treatment Strategies

One strategy used to enhance the clinical efficacy of MAbs has been to combine Abs with known cellular toxins to create immunotoxins. Several clinical trials have evaluated various forms of ricin immunotoxins. Although transient antitumor responses have occurred in a minority of patients, these immunotoxins have been associated with consistent toxic effects, including fatigue/myalgias, capillary leak syndromes, elevation of hepatic transaminase levels, and bone marrow suppression. In two studies involving patients with breast carcinoma, substantial neurotoxicity was observed that was attributed to cross-reactivity to antigens contained within neural tissue.

Another strategy involves the construction of bispecific MAbs that target additional effectors of the immune system as well as tumor antigens. For example, some MAbs have dual specificity for tumor antigens and the CD3/TCR or CD16/FcRIII receptor on NK cells. This technology has been used in clinical trials directed toward B-cell neoplasms, but results so far have been disappointing.

Other MAb-therapy models have used drug immunoconjugates in which the Ab is fused to a chemotherapeutic drug such as doxorubicin. Radioimmunoconjugates have also been created in which radioactive sources such as I^{125} and I^{131} have been combined with MAbs to elicit antineoplastic responses. Limitations common to all these manipulations continue to be the generation of human antimouse antibody reactions and host side effects induced by cross-reactivity with rapidly dividing normal cells (e.g., bone marrow cells).

Clinical Results

Results of clinical trials of MAbs have been disappointing overall, but a few responses have been noted. JD118, a murine IgM MAb specific for neoplastic B cells, destroys human leukemia and lymphoma cells in the presence of human complement. HD37, an anti-CD19 MAb, induced cell cycle arrest in several Burkitt's lymphoma cell lines in vitro and in a xenograft model. Also, treatment with an antiganglioside MAb caused objective antitumor responses in patients with metastatic melanoma as well as neuroblastoma. Finally, a large randomized trial demonstrated that adjuvant therapy with 17-1A , a murine MAb recognizing a 37-kDa cell surface glycoprotein, induced improved remission durations and extended overall survival in patients with resected, locally metastatic colorectal carcinomas. Although MAb therapy remains a theoretically intriguing focus of attention, it has yet to overcome the problems of significant toxicity and host inactivation.

Gene Therapy

The concept of gene therapy is based on the theory that the host response to tumorigenesis is deficient and might be improved given the introduction of either novel genes or excess levels of existing genes. A variety of strategies have been conceived to exploit this basic concept. Most gene therapy models have focused on melanoma and renal cell carcinoma because these two tumor types are considered more immunogenic than most other solid-organ malignancies and have demonstrated spontaneous regressions. Furthermore, tumor antigens and cell-mediated immune responses to these neoplasms have been demonstrated in vitro and in vivo.

As discussed earlier in this chapter, biologic therapies for solid tumors originally concentrated on cytokines in an effort to augment host immune responses; likewise, early gene therapies have concentrated on cytokines. The large systemic doses of cytokines required to sustain biologically significant levels of these cytokines in tissues have been associated with substantial toxicity and only modest antitumor responses. Insertion of the gene encoding a cytokine within a biologic (typically viral) vector capable of infecting designated target cells offers an alternative delivery system in which relatively low, continuous concentrations of cytokines are delivered directly into tumor or effector cells.

The introduction of novel genetic information (DNA) into eukaryotic cells has been accomplished by chemical, physical, and biologic means. The gene transfer techniques of calcium phosphate transfection and electroporation have been useful in the laboratory but are limited in their clinical application. The most widely used biologic gene transfer vehicles are modified RNA and DNA viruses. Murine retroviral vectors have been the most extensively studied. Retroviral vectors can transduce dividing cells and allow stable integration of proviral sequences via a receptor-mediated process of endocytosis. This process has certain limitations, however. Despite the introduction of safety features in viral and packaging systems, recombination events and the generation of wild-type virus can occur. There is also the absolute requirement for target cell replication at the time of retroviral infection to permit integration. With retroviral vectors, viral titers of moderate magnitude have been achieved.

Adeno-associated viruses (AAVs) and adenoviruses represent two additional viral vectors that have been evaluated in gene transfer models. AAVs are single-stranded DNA (4.5 kb) parvoviruses that are not pathogenic in humans and may integrate into the host genome at specific regions in chromosome 19. Recombinant AAV vectors (RVVs) allow the insertion of relatively small DNA constructs of up to 4 kb. AAV vectors may not require target cell replication for integration, and multiple concatemeric copies may be integrated per cell. High AAV titers may also be achieved. Adenovirus-based vectors are currently being used for many gene transfer efforts because these vectors combine the characteristics of high achieved titers and infection of nondividing cells with a broad host range and a tropism for epithelial tissue. Consequently, adenovirus-based vectors transduce 80% to 90% of cells, in contrast to RVVs, which transduce between 5% and 20% of targets following multiple transduction attempts at high multiplicity of infection ratios. Adenoviruses are composed of double-stranded DNA of approximately 35 kb. Recombinant adenovirus vectors may accommodate up to 7.5 kb of inserted DNA. Limitations of adenoviral vectors include the fact that proviral DNA is not integrated but, rather, episomally inserted into target cells, resulting in transient gene expression. Furthermore, host immune reactions have been observed directed toward recognition of adenoviral proteins. These reactions have resulted in decreased gene expression and have necessitated repeated delivery of adenoviral vectors to the host.

Clearly, each vector system has advantages and disadvantages in different tumor models. A problem common to all vectors (although less so for adenoviral vectors) is that of low-level gene expression. Investigators have tried to optimize proviral gene expression using a variety of gene promoters and induction sequences. The cytomegalovirus promoter has been used in a variety of systems, and this approach has been successful in several tissue types. Regrettably, the cytomegalovirus promoter also induces gene expression in nontargeted cells and relatively low-level expression in certain in vivo systems. To direct gene expression more precisely, tissue-specific promoters have been developed, including the insulin promoter (for pancreatic islet cell transduction), the tyrosinase promoter (for melanoma), the albumin promoter (for tumors of the liver), the CEA promoter (for gastrointestinal tumors, breast tumors, and lung adenocarcinomas), and the TCR promoter (for targeting T lymphocytes). Though theoretically intriguing and logical, the use of these promoters in various viral constructs has not yet been demonstrated to be superior to the use of nonspecific high-level promoters such as cytomegalovirus in any models.

Target Cells for Gene Therapy

LYMPHOCYTES. Various cells have been evaluated as targets of gene therapy, including lymphocytes, fibroblasts, and tumor cells. Early interest in activated lymphocytes was motivated by trials of LAK cells and TILs, demonstrating antitumor activity in adoptive immunotherapy protocols. Initial studies of genetic modification of lymphocyte populations, including PBL, seemed promising and demonstrated successful transduction and selection of cells secreting proviral genetic elements. Rosenberg et al. at the NCI (1993) pioneered early efforts to transduce TIL, and initial reports suggested high-level gene expression, particularly of TNF. However, experience has demonstrated that lymphocytes are difficult to transduce with retroviral vectors because only a small percentage of cells are dividing during transduction and repeated transduction results in significant cell death. Similar difficulties exist with AAV vectors, and it is impossible to transduce lymphocytes with adenoviral constructs. Furthermore, evidence of transcriptional silencing of gene products has tempered enthusiasm for transduction of lymphocytes. Finally, the debate continues regarding whether TILs selectively locate within tumors in greater numbers than peripheral blood lymphocytes. Although the gene-marking studies used to generate these data advanced the field of gene therapy in terms of quantitation of gene copy number within large groups of untransduced cells, the clinical ramifications of this effort have been minimal except to move investigators away from transduction of mature lymphocytes. Transduction of stem cells and progenitor cells has proven to be more efficient than transduction of mature lymphocytes and has been successful in the treatment of patients with adenosine deaminase deficiency. The transduction of drug resistance genes in hematologic and solid tumors using retroviral vectors is currently being tested in clinical protocols.

FIBROBLASTS. Given the recent findings that the particular properties of transduced cells do not necessarily affect antitumor effects, investigators have sought to transduce cells that are hardier than lymphocytes and are easier to grow and maintain in vitro and in vivo. Several studies (principally involving IL-2 and IL-12) have evaluated the transduction of fibroblast cell lines, such as NIH/3T3 cells, which after transduction are reintroduced into a tumor-bearing host, either alone or in mixing experiments with tumor cells as vaccines. Transduction efficiencies have been high, and antineoplastic responses have been observed. It may well be more cost-effective and less labor-intensive to maintain fibroblasts in culture than to attempt to grow tumor explants for ex vivo protocols.

TUMOR CELLS. A variety of tumor cell lines are easily maintained in vitro and can maintain excellent growth kinetics despite multiple transduction attempts with cytokine and other types of genes. In addition, re-administration of nondividing, irradiated tumor cells to patients has the theoretical advantage of stimulating a specific immune response in the host, as in a vaccine model. Safety concerns about tumor growth following re-administration have necessitated irradiation that still allows for continued proviral gene expression, albeit for shorter periods and at somewhat lower levels than with nonirradiated cells. This model has been used with varying degrees of success by many investigators and is currently being evaluated in most of the tumor-directed gene therapy clinical protocols.

Cytokines in Gene Therapy

The introduction and expression of cytokine genes in tumor cells may modify their phenotype and alter the tumor-host relationship. With virtually all inflammatory cytokines, introduction of the cytokine into tumors has been found to decrease tumorigenicity in vivo. Reduced primary tumor growth is largely due to the infiltration and activation of host effector cells. The composition and activity of the cellular infiltrate depend on the cytokine used, the amount produced, the ability of the host to generate responses, and inherent properties of the tumor. It has been difficult to demonstrate regression of established lesions in certain systems, probably because murine tumors appear to grow faster than cytokine-transduced cells.

In both the immunocompetent and the immunodeficient host, the initial response to tumor inoculation involves nonspecific inflammatory immune mechanisms. A major question yet to be resolved is how this initial response relates to the development of the specific immunity that often follows primary tumor rejection. The mechanism of this "cross-talk" is unknown but presumably relates to the processing and presentation of antigens capable of generating target-specific tumor immunity. Gene therapy using cytokines as immunologic effectors has been attempted for virtually all known cytokines, with favorable in vivo and in vitro results in most systems. Rather than providing an exhaustive review of gene therapy with cytokines—a subject reviewed in detail in other texts—we will provide a brief analysis of selected cytokine gene therapy models.

INTERLEUKIN-2. Gene-modified, IL-2–secreting tumors have consistently demonstrated dose-dependent decreased tumorigenicity regardless of histologic features, immunogenicity, or metastatic potential without alterations in in vitro tumor growth or morphology. Nanogram levels (50–5,000 IU/10^6 cells daily) of human IL-2 were produced in several engineered tumor cell lines. IL-2-transduced cells did not demonstrate changes in MHC antigens or adhesion molecules. An important observation is that IL-2-producing cells mixed in vitro with autologous or allogeneic lymphocytes generate enhanced in vitro lymphocyte cytotoxicity at levels that could not be reproduced by the addition of recombinant IL-2 to cultures.

The growth of parental tumors is inhibited when tumor cells mixed with IL-2–producing cells are injected at the tumor site, an effect not observed when the modified and unmodified cells are injected at sites remote from the tumor. This local "bystander" effect has been observed by several investigators.

T cells are not required for decreased in vivo tumorigenicity. IL-2–modified human and murine melanomas and sarcomas have retarded or absent growth in congenitally athymic (nude) mice, with such tumors generating a mononuclear cell infiltrate. In immunologically competent animals, IL-2 induced CTL-mediated tumor rejection in a murine colon cancer model. Decreased tumorigenicity was shown to depend on NK cells in a nonimmunogenic murine fibrosarcoma and was associated with granulocyte activity in a murine breast carcinoma system. The development of specific systemic immunity was reported in syngeneic animals rejecting weakly immunogenic tumors of varying histologic subtypes. At least one group has reported that an IL-2–dose-dependent window exists in the optimal generation of protective immunity to parental tumor challenge.

The observation that tumor killing in the immunologically competent host occurred in the absence of $CD4^+$ cells led to a hypothesis that the T_H cell response may be insufficient (because of unfavorable antigen–MHC complex presentation) to drive cytotoxic T. cell generation against the tumor and that IL-2 could overcome this deficiency. Virtually all investigators have concluded that primary tumor rejection may be induced by nonspecific inflammatory responses (NK cells, neutrophils, or macrophages) but that T-cell–dependent systemic immunity develops in the same host.

IL-2 has been compared with several other inflammatory agents (IFN-gamma, IFN-alfa, IL-7, GM-CSF) in tumor-directed gene therapy investigations. IL-2 was equal or superior to most other cytokines in the mediation of antitumor effects, particularly in T-cell–deprived animals. This finding, and the considerable clinical experience with this cytokine, has led to the development and approval of several clinical protocols studying the effects of IL-2–producing vectors and tumors.

INTERLEUKIN-4. Despite the reported antiproliferative effects of IL-4, in vitro growth of IL-4–transduced tumors of several histologic subtypes producing 2,000 to 10,000 $IU/10^6$ cells every 48 hours was unaltered compared with the growth of parental cells. IL-4–secreting cells were rejected after injection in immunocompetent and immunodeficient mice. This effect was reversed by administration of anti-IL-4 MAb. Reduced tumorigenicity was also demonstrated for untransduced murine melanoma cells and plasmacytoma cells when mixed with IL-4 producers before injection. Significant tumor regression was also observed in established plasmacytomas after intralesional injection of exogenous IL-4 or autologous tumor cells producing this cytokine.

IL-4–producing tumors in syngeneic mice initially induced the infiltration of eosinophils and later induced the accumulation of macrophages in several tumor models. Tepper et al. (1989) demonstrated that tumor rejection was abolished in syngeneic immunocompetent animals when the hosts were depleted of mature granulocytes. Tumors were rejected in lymphocyte-depleted mice, but protective (T-cell-dependent) immunity against parental tumor rechallenge was not observed, suggesting that nonspecific effectors were involved in primary tumor rejection and confirming the requirement of T cells for the generation of immunologic memory.

In two reports, the induction of systemic immunity was observed in immunocompetent animals rejecting IL-4–producing tumors. Tumor-specific immunity was completely abolished by MAb depletion of CTLs and incompletely inhibited by depletion of T_H cells. The systemic immunity demonstrated in this model might have been due to enhanced tumor antigen presentation by the macrophage infiltrate induced by IL-4. Several clinical trials of IL-4–enhanced tumor-specific immunity are currently in progress.

TUMOR NECROSIS FACTOR-α. Several investigators have studied the properties of tumor cell lines engineered to produce TNF. TNF-transduced cells do not demonstrate altered cell growth or cell morphology in vitro. However, the efficiency of gene transduction of TNF-sensitive cells is low because of cell death, suggesting that TNF-resistant cells are selected in such cultures. Deleterious host effects were not observed after injection of tumor cells producing TNF at levels less than 100 ng/10^6 cells every 24 hours; however, tumors producing much higher levels of this cytokine did demonstrate significant host toxicity and death. Inoculation of TNF-secreting tumors into syngeneic mice resulted in dose-dependent decreased tumorigenicity that was reversed by MAbs to TNF. Parental murine sarcomas were rejected by gene-modified cells injected at the same anatomic site, but not when the two cell types were implanted at different sites. Antineoplastic effects, however, have not been consistently observed in all nude mice models.

Blankenstein et al. (1991) noted that the cellular infiltrate surrounding a TNF-producing murine plasmacytoma was predominantly composed of macrophages and that the antitumor effect in this model was abolished by anti-type 3 complement receptor MAb that inhibited the migration of inflammatory cells such as neutrophils, NK cells, and macrophages. These findings emphasize the role of non-T-cell effectors in TNF-mediated antineoplastic responses. However, Asher et al. (1991) noted that immunologically intact animals experiencing complete regression of murine sarcomas were found to be specifically immune to subsequent tumor challenge and to have a predominantly lymphocytic infiltrate. Selective depletion of CTLs or T_H cells completely abrogated the development of protective immunity in syngeneic mice. This finding documented the importance of T-cell–mediated immunity in this particular TNF tumor model.

Asher et al. (1991) attempted to resolve the disparity between their findings and observations regarding the role of macrophages in inducing TNF-mediated antitumor responses by suggesting that TNF secreted in a membrane-bound form might be incapable of recruiting other effectors. A therapeutic distinction between the membrane-bound and secretory forms of TNF was later described. Although both forms of TNF demonstrated biologic activity in vitro, only the secretory form reduced tumorigenicity in vivo. The mechanisms responsible for these divergent effects of the two TNF molecules remain unclear, but clinical protocols using secretory TNF gene-modified autologous tumors are in progress.

INTERLEUKIN-7. Tumor models using cells engineered to secrete IL-7 in the range of 1 to 80 ng/10^6 cells every 24 hours demonstrated significant antineoplastic effects. No alterations of in vitro growth or cell morphology were observed in IL-7–secreting cells. An IL-7–producing melanoma cell line expressed lower levels of TGF-β mRNA and protein than did untransduced or IL-2–transduced cells. Expression of the melanoma antigens MAGE-1 and MAGE-3 was not altered by cytokine gene transfer.

IL-7–transduced cell lines had decreased tumorigenicity in immunocompetent syngeneic mice. Animals rejecting these tumors were immunologically protected against tumor rechallenge. In nude mice, however, growth of gene-modified tumors was either unchanged or slightly decreased compared with that of parental tumor cells. Histologic analyses of the cellular infiltrates surrounding these tumors in immunocompetent animals showed a predominance of lymphocytes, although eosinophils and basophils were also present. Specifically, increased numbers (fivefold greater) of T_H and CTLs were recruited to IL-7–secreting tumor sites compared with parental tumors. Lymphocyte depletion analyses performed using MAbs to CD4$^+$ cells, CD8$^+$ cells, macrophages (anti-CR3$^+$), and NK cells were performed. Tumor rejection was inhibited by anti-CD4$^+$ MAbs in a plasmacytoma line, and dependence of the antitumor response on CD8$^+$ cells was demonstrated in a murine glioma model. Selective depletion of macrophages, but not NK cells, also inhibited tumor rejection, but to a lesser degree than treatment with MAbs for T cells.

Lymphocytes isolated from tumors transduced with IL-7 demonstrated significantly enhanced cytotoxicity toward parental tumor targets. Interestingly, allogeneic lymphocytes cocultured with IL-7–producing melanoma cell lines demonstrated increased cytotoxicity toward parental tumors compared with untransduced cells; this effect could not be duplicated by the addition to culture of recombinant IL-7. This stimulation of in vitro cytotoxicity was comparable to that produced by IL-2–transduced cells of the same tumor cell lines. It appears that IL-7 acts primarily through T-cell–mediated mechanisms in generating antineoplastic effects, although the ability of IL-7 to downregulate TGF-β production may be a distinct component of its biologic activity. The relative importance of T_H and CTLs in mediating tumor rejection may vary from tumor to tumor. Currently, Economou et al. are conducting a phase I clinical protocol involving vaccination of patients with melanomas with autologous-irradiated melanoma cells producing IL-7 contained within a retroviral construct. A few patients have been treated, but the results of therapy are as yet unreported.

INTERLEUKIN-12. Recent reports have described the transfection of IL-12 into NIH/3T3 cells. These IL-12–producing fibroblasts were mixed with murine melanoma cells in syngeneic mice and reduced tumorigenicity in most animals treated. IL-12–transduced murine colon carcinoma cells grew more slowly than unmanipulated tumors, resulting in delay in the formation of pulmonary and hepatic metastases. Antitumor activity was also recently demonstrated in a murine fibrosarcoma model using a vaccinia virus vector. The question of which T-cell subsets are most responsible for IL-12's antitumor effect is as yet unclear, as T_H and CTLs appear to act differently, depending on the specific model tested.

GRANULOCYTE-MACROPHAGE   COLONY-STIMULATING   FACTORS. Dranoff et al. (1993) compared the effects of gene therapy with GM-CSF and at least nine other cytokines in a murine model. The investigators used both live and irradiated genetically modified tumors producing high levels of GM-CSF (300 ng/10^6 cells every 24 hours) in syngeneic mice. This report was noteworthy in several respects. First, it demonstrated that vaccination of irradiated parental tumors alone resulted in some degree of antitumor immunity. Second, systemic murine toxicity was described, apparently induced by injection of tumor cells secreting high concentrations of GM-CSF. Third, in contrast to observations made by other investigators, systemic immunity was not conferred upon animals treated with live IL-2–producing tumors, although these cells were the only type to be rejected in this comparative analysis. However, irradiated tumors producing GM-CSF alone and live cells secreting a combination of IL-2 and GM-CSF did induce resistance to subsequent tumor challenge. Finally, MAb depletion of several effector cell subsets demonstrated dependence on both T_H and CTLs for the establishment of systemic immunity induced by GM-CSF–secreting murine melanoma cells.

A recent report from Johns Hopkins on renal cell carcinoma patients randomly assigned to treatment with either a GM-CSF gene-transduced autologous tumor cell vaccine or a nontransduced autologous tumor cell vaccine demonstrated only one objective partial responder out of 16 evaluable patients in the GM-CSF–transduced tumor cell group.

Tumor Suppressor Genes

Tumor suppressor genes are recessively functioning genes, both copies of which must be mutated to elicit phenotypic alterations supporting malignancy in the host. It has been hypothesized that delivering one copy of the wild-type (wt) gene could reverse a neoplastic process.

The tumor suppressor gene *p53* is mutated in a wide variety of tumors, including head and neck squamous cell cancer, non-small cell lung cancer, and colorectal carcinoma, and in premalignant conditions such as Barrett's esophagitis. *p53* is the tumor suppressor gene most widely studied in clinical gene therapy trials to date. The *p53* gene encodes a 393-amino acid phosphoprotein that forms complexes with a series of viral proteins. Other areas within the gene interact with other proteins, allowing *p53* oligomers to form and resulting in transactivation of gene expression. The wt form of *p53* appears to regulate the cell cycle and to control cell growth and proliferation, at least in part through the mechanism of apoptosis (programmed cell death). *p53* also has a role in controlling transcriptional regulation and DNA replication. Mutated *p53* allows unregulated cell growth to occur, while restoring wt *p53* restores cell cycle regulation and renders cells apoptotic or in G1 arrest of the cell cycle.

A variety of viral constructs have been evaluated that contain wt *p53* in several tumor systems. Roth et al. (1996) demonstrated that retroviral vectors containing wt *p53* can suppress in vivo and in vitro growth of human lung carcinoma cell lines that contain deleted or mutated *p53*. Conversely, tumor cell lines containing wt *p53* are not significantly altered by the retroviral construct. The so-called bystander effect phenomenon has also been observed in these studies, reduction in the growth of nontransduced cells co-culture with a transduced population.

Several models involving adenoviral vectors containing wt *p53* have also been evaluated. Apoptosis has been observed in tumor cells whose genome contained mutated or deleted *p53* following transduction with adenoviral wt *p53*. *p53* constructs have also been shown to act synergistically with cisplatin in inducing apoptosis in human lung tumors grown in nude mice. These results have led to several clinical gene therapy protocols involving wt *p53* introduced through a variety of delivery systems. Clinical responses have been modest to date, although the toxicity of therapy appears minimal. In addition, viral vectors containing related cell-cycle-control genes (*p21* and *p16*) are currently being evaluated and may soon be used in clinical protocols.

Suicide Gene Therapy

A gene therapy strategy that has been used with some degree of success in central nervous system tumor models is so-called suicide gene therapy. This technique involves the transduction of cells with a gene that renders the cells sensitive to killing by systemic administration of a compound toxic to all cells containing the gene. Most commonly, the gene for the herpes simplex virus driven by the thymidine kinase promoter has been introduced via both adenoviral and retroviral vectors. Following transduction, the host is treated with gancyclovir, which is toxic to all herpes simplex virus–containing cells. Additional cell killing has been observed in nontransduced cells in proximity to the transduced population, suggesting a bystander effect in this model. This strategy is currently employed in more than 20 approved clinical protocols worldwide, most of which are directed toward treatment of brain tumors.

Therapy with the B7 Costimulatory Molecules

B7 is the ligand for the CD28 receptor of lymphocytes. Antigen presentation to T cells and subsequent T-cell activation depend on binding to CD28, yet most tumors lack B7 molecules on their surface. Murine models of B7 tumor transfection have demonstrated antineoplastic responses and the generation of systemic immunity. Gene therapy studies involving the delivery of B7 in patients with melanoma are currently underway.

B7 is commonly confused with but is structurally and functionally different from the HLA-B7 molecule, a MHC class I haplotype also being studied in gene therapy models involving patients with melanoma and colorectal cancer. These models involve intratumoral injection of nonviral, liposomally delivered gene constructs. HLA therapy has demonstrated some antineoplastic responses in patients with melanoma but no documented responses in studies evaluating direct injection of liver metastases from colorectal carcinoma.

Antisense Gene Therapy

Antisense gene therapy strategies involve the creation of genetic sequences that are complementary to specific regions of RNA known to be critical for gene expression and transcription. Typically, regions of interest for antisense binding involve oncogene coding regions. Oncogenes act predominantly to promote neoplastic cell growth. Antisense constructs may be directed toward oncogenes and may be composed of oligonucleotides that bind to double-stranded DNA, thereby interfering with transcription. Other alternatives include antisense RNA, which may bind to single-stranded DNA or to mRNA and interfere with transcription, splicing, and translation.

Antisense oligonucleotides have been tested in phase II clinical studies, but efficacy has been limited by rapid host-induced degradation by nuclease in vivo. Antioncogenic oligonucleotides have been constructed to disrupt expression of *abl, fos, kit, myc, src,* and *ras* gene families, again with limited clinical consequence. Roth et al. (1997) described a model in which an antisense RNA construct was used to induce tumoricidal activity in a human lung cancer cell line expressing K-*ras*. The anti-K-*ras* retroviral constructs reduced tumorigenicity of a cell line with a homozygous K-*ras* mutation in nude mice. These observations have led to clinical trials involving direct intratumor injection of anti-K-*ras* retroviral particles in patients with unresectable pulmonary malignancies. Also, an adenoviral anti- K-*ras* construct has been reported recently to have potent antitumor activity in murine models involving human cancer cell lines.

Antiangiogenic Therapy

A crucial step for the continuous growth of tumors and the development of metastases is angiogenesis—the induction of vasculature. A tumor mass that is less than 0.5 mm in diameter can receive sufficient oxygen and nutrients by diffusion, but any increase in tumor mass beyond 0.5 mm requires the proliferation and morphogenesis of vascular endothelial cells. The process of angiogenesis consists of multiple, sequential, interdependent steps. It begins with local degradation of the basement membrane surrounding capillaries, which is followed by invasion of the surrounding stroma by the underlying endothelial cells in the direction of the angiogenic stimulus. Endothelial cell migration is accompanied by the proliferation of endothelial cells and their organization into three-dimensional structures that join with other similar structures to form a network of new blood vessels.

Classes of Antiangiogenic Agents

At this writing, 20 angiogenesis inhibitors produced by the biotechnology and pharmaceutical industry are being evaluated in phase I and II clinical trials in patients with advanced metastatic cancer, and seven are being evaluated in phase III trials. Antiangiogenic agents currently used in the clinic can be divided into several broad classes on the basis of the biologic activity of the compounds used.

The first class of compounds, metalloproteinase inhibitors, block degradation of the basement membrane. Most of the studies of metalloproteinase inhibitors reported to date have been phase I studies in which the major side effect associated with treatment was musculoskeletal and joint pain due to defects in collagen remodeling.

A second class of antiangiogenic agents includes those designed to inhibit endothelial cell function. These include TNP-470, thalidomide, squalamine, combretastatin A-4 prodrug, and endostatin. Less is known about the biologic effects of these drugs than about to the first class of angiogenesis inhibitors, and most of these drugs designed to inhibit endothelial cell function are currently in phase I or phase II trials. How these drugs exert their antiangiogenic activities in in vivo models is not fully understood at this time; perhaps well-designed clinical trials will shed some light on the mechanisms of action of these drugs.

A third class of antiangiogenic agents specifically targets an angiogenic factor or factors. These agents include tyrosine kinase inhibitors of the receptors of such factors as vascular endothelial growth factor (VEGF), basic fibroblast growth factor (bFGF), and platelet-derived growth factor (PDGF). In addition, Abs directed against these receptors or the factors themselves are either in clinical trials or in the process of being developed for clinical trials. In preclinical trials in animal models, most of these agents inhibited tumor growth, but very few caused tumor regression. This suggests that tumor regression, which is the typical end point for successful cytotoxic chemotherapy, may not be an appropriate end point for antiangiogenic therapies. Thus, it will be necessary to redefine the end points for biologic therapy.

Because endothelial cell survival has recently been recognized as an important characteristic of the development of a neovascular blood supply, drugs that target survival factors are beginning to be introduced into clinical trials. These drugs include antagonists to integrins that are present on the endothelial cell surface. In addition, as VEGF currently is thought of as both a survival factor for endothelial cells and an angiogenic factor, anti-VEGF therapy may affect the survival of tumor endothelial cells.

Antiangiogenic Activity of Interferon

In addition to their well-recognized activity as antiviral agents, IFNs regulate multiple biologic activities, such as cell growth, differentiation, oncogene expression, host immunity, and tumorigenicity. IFNs can also inhibit a number of steps in the angiogenic process. IFN exerts antiproliferative effects, especially on tumor cells and also on endothelial cells in vitro. IFN-α can inhibit bFGF-induced endothelial proliferation. IFN-γ also can inhibit endothelial proliferation. IFN-α and IFN-γ have been shown to be cytostatic to human dermal microvascular endothelial cells and human capillary endothelial cells.

Systemic therapy using recombinant IFNs produces antiangiogenic effects in vascular tumors, including life-threatening infantile hemangioma, Kaposi's sarcoma, giant cell tumor of the mandible, and bladder carcinoma. These tumors have been shown to produce the high levels of bFGF often detectable in the urine or serum of these patients. IFN-α and IFN-β, but not IFN-γ, down-regulate the expression of bFGF mRNA and protein in human carcinoma cells. Indeed, systemic administration of human IFN-α decreased the in vivo expression of bFGF, decreased blood vessel density, and inhibited tumor growth of a human bladder carcinoma implanted orthotopically in nude mice.

Antiangiogenic Therapy in Combination with Other Antineoplastic Approaches

The combination of an antiangiogenic drug (or drugs), such as TNP-470, with a conventional cytotoxic agent, such as cisplatin, paclitaxel, or cyclophosphamide, can significantly improve the antitumor efficacy of the cytotoxic drug. These effects of combination therapy, which have also been observed for the combination of radiation therapy and angiogenesis inhibitors, point to a potential new use of angiogenesis inhibitors.

A more rational, yet futuristic, approach to the treatment of patients with malignancies is to determine the molecular alterations that lead to the various processes involved in tumor growth. Angiogenesis is but one component of the process of tumor growth and metastasis, and overexpression of other genes involved in protection from apoptosis, cell proliferation, and cell invasion (i.e., an individual tumor's malignant fingerprint) must be examined. With the rapid development of gene chip technology, it may be possible in the future to determine the malignant fingerprint of individual tumors and to develop therapies that specifically target the molecular phenotype of an individual tumor. Antiangiogenic therapy may therefore be one component of diverse biologic therapy delivered in combination with anti-growth factor therapy or with agents that induce apoptosis in tumor cells and tumor vessel endothelial cells.

Molecular Profiling: Treatment Tailored to the Individual Patient

The concept of employing tumor characteristics, such as histologic features, to predict the best treatment for an individual patient has long been part of the practice of oncology. A significant refinement of this histology-based approach to selection of treatment has been the application of molecular markers, an approach best exemplified in the use of markers in the treatment of human leukemias. For solid tumors, the development of tumor markers for the prediction of therapeutic response has generally been much slower. However, the *HER2/neu* gene is an impressive positive example of a tumor marker useful in solid tumors. The *HER2/neu* gene encodes a 185-kD protein belonging to the transmembrane type I tyrosine kinase receptor family, which also includes the EGF receptor, HER3, and HER4. Clinical studies demonstrated that HER2 amplification or overexpression is a marker of poor prognosis for patients with lymph node–positive breast cancer. A major question, however, has been whether this poor prognosis is irrevocable or can be bypassed by some intervention. In 1994, the Cancer and Leukemia Group B (CALGB) demonstrated that the poor clinical outcome of patients with lymph node–positive breast cancer with HER2 overexpression can be overcome by adequate dose-intensive regimens of cyclophosphamide, doxorubicin, and 5-FU. The HER2-negative group, however, experienced no benefit from the dose escalation. These data raised the possibility that the adverse effects of HER2 overexpression can be specifically overcome by effective doses of doxorubicin. The most definitive test of the HER2-doxorubicin interaction was seen in two studies: the reanalysis of the National Surgical Adjuvant Breast and Bowel Project trial B-11, and the 10-year follow-up of the analysis of the complete cohort in CALGB trial 8541. Important in the analysis was that the HER2 determination was rigorously validated through concurrent analysis by immunohistochemistry, differential polymerase chain reaction, and fluorescent in situ hybridization. Patients with HER2-positive tumors responded with improved overall survival when treated with dose-intensive cyclophosphamide, doxorubicin, and 5-FU chemotherapy, whereas HER2-negative patients showed no benefit with dose escalation. Although the mechanism of this interaction and putative resistance is unclear, there is evidence that inhibition of HER2 signaling is associated with a decreased ability of the cell to repair DNA damage such as is seen after exposure to chemotherapy.

HER2 is an example of how the molecular profile of a cancer may allow prediction of its response to standard chemotherapeutic agents. In most cases, the mechanism for oncogene-associated relative resistance or sensitivity of a tumor to chemotherapy is uncertain. However, many markers may themselves be suitable targets for molecularly based therapeutics. Given the surface location of HER2 on cells and the overexpression that occurs mainly in cancerous states, the HER2 oncoprotein represented one such attractive target for Ab-directed therapies. One such Ab, 4D5, suppressed cancer cell growth both in vitro and in vivo animal studies. When coupled with standard chemotherapeutic agents, 4D5 showed additive and potentially synergistic antiproliferative effects. The humanized form of the murine 4D5 Ab (Herceptin) was developed for clinical applications. Based on a phase II clinical trial that showed improvement in response rates in patients receiving Herceptin, a phase III study was conducted in which individuals with metastatic breast cancer were randomly assigned to chemotherapy alone or chemotherapy plus weekly Herceptin. The results showed that patients treated with chemotherapy and Herceptin exhibited an improvement in all measures: response rate (49% vs. 32% with chemotherapy alone), median duration of response (9.3 vs. 5.9 months with chemotherapy alone), and time to progression at 7.6 months (vs. 4.6 months with chemotherapy alone). Thus, as predicted in the in vitro investigations, the combination of chemotherapy and Herceptin led to a more favorable outcome.

Because oncogenes are signaling molecules that rely on protein-protein interactions to conduct their signals, interruption of these interactions was predicted to disrupt critical pathways that maintain the cancerous state. Inhibition of the enzymatic activity of certain oncogenes, such as the genes encoding ras proteins and kinases, with small chemically derived molecules has been both an attractive and ultimately successful approach. Some of the most notable clinical successes have been in the treatment of leukemias. There is currently a rich developmental pipeline for these kinase inhibitors, with many potential agents being tested (or soon to be ready for testing) in the clinical setting. The targets include the ras proteins PDGF and EGF and the VEGF receptors. The number and diversity of targets make molecular profiling a necessary adjunct to therapeutic decision making. Thus, a comprehensive approach for target detection will no longer remain solely of academic interest but is predicted to become a clinical necessity.

Postgenome Challenge for Molecular Medicine

The recently completed sequencing of the entire human genome will have incalculable effects on science and society. The data on gene expression and putative gene functions inferred from sequence similarities and motif analysis will provide a powerful means of assessing the transcriptional activity of the genome in the cells and tissue before, during, and after the development of disease. However, completion of the human genome sequence is just the beginning. The current challenge is to generate a comprehensive understanding of the software and the hardware of the cell and the organism. Less than 2% of the noninfectious human disease burden is monogenic in nature. The rest (98%) is polygenic (caused by multiple genes at once) or epigenetic (caused by nongenetic or postgenetic alterations in cellular molecules). Consequently, fully elucidating the causal mechanisms driving carcinogenesis and cancer progression will require analysis tools ranging from direct DNA sequencing, to mRNA expression monitoring, to protein sequencing, and protein localization studies to metabolic or physiologic profiling.

A further essential phase will be a description of the normal range of human polymorphisms (base variations in the genome), which may provide a starting point for correlating genetic variance with disease states. The final physiologic state is further complicated because biologic diversity causally associated with disease may be due to posttranslational processes regulated by the cellular environment. These changes cannot be inferred from known DNA variance. Thus, a complete understanding of the molecular basis of cancer will depend on a multidisciplinary approach combining genetics, pathology, protein structure and function analysis, cell biology, and clinical medicine.

Finding all the expressed human genes is a different task from sequencing the genome itself. This is because the actual expressed genes and their regulatory elements make up only a small proportion of the genome. The number of expressed human genes may be 100,000. However, at any point in time, for any individual cell in any given tissue, the number of genes in use may be as few as 10,000. Of this 10,000, only a proportion may be susceptible to the influence of carcinogenic events. Thus, an important goal for molecular profiling of cancer is to identify a subset of expressed genes that is correlated with or causally related to the development and progression of cancer. Setting aside hereditary susceptibility, it is likely that the majority of cancers originate in tissue that starts with a completely normal genome and that carcinogenic events produce heritable genetic alterations that expand in microscopic premalignant states, such as hyperplasia and dysplasia, before frank malignant cancer ensues. Identification of the important genetic derangements and the causally important genes and proteins will depend on direct analysis of actual human cancer tissues, combined with insights gained using animal and cell culture methods. The massive profiling of genes associated with cancer progression is now possible using new technology for microdissection and array hybridization.

In response to this challenge, investigators in both the public and private sectors have been perfecting complementary DNA (cDNA) arrays (so-called gene chips) that can be used to survey patterns of gene expression. Changes in the pattern can then be correlated with histomorphology, clinical behavior, or response to treatment. Typically, the cDNA arrays take the form of rows and rows of oligonucleotide strands lined up in dots on a miniature silicon chip, glass slide, or sheet of nitrocellulose. The microarrays work as follows. First, the RNA is extracted from the tumor tissue, amplified, and labeled with a fluorescent or radioactive probe. This of course assumes that the highly labile RNA is preserved when the tissue is extracted. The labeled total RNA, containing the mRNA of the expressed genes, is applied to the surface of the chip or sheet. After appropriate hybridization, the relative intensity of the signal for each spot on the chip corresponds to the abundance of its matching mRNA species and hence reflects the expression level for its gene. With appropriate pattern recognition software, it is possible to assemble a global score for the gene study set represented on the substratum. Tremendous progress has been made in the use of cDNA arrays to analyze gene expression patterns in human cancer cell lines and human cancer tissue.

Once a putative marker (or set of markers) is identified by cDNA array analysis of cancer tissue samples, the next step is to validate these markers in a large population of human tumors. This exhaustive process has now been telescoped into a high-throughput miniaturized tissue array. The array consists of 1,000 cylindrical tissue biopsies, each from a different patient, all distributed on a single glass slide. Tumor arrays are ideal for comparing large numbers of solid tumor samples. Full automation of tumor array creation and screening is envisioned as a means to expeditiously correlate marker levels over large study sets of tumors.

Molecular analysis of pure cell populations in their native tissue environment will be an important component of the next generation of medical genetics. Accomplishing this goal is much more difficult than just grinding up a piece of tissue and applying the extracted molecules to a panel of assays. This is because tissues are complicated three-dimensional structures composed of large numbers of different types of interacting cell populations. The cell subpopulation of interest may constitute a tiny fraction of the total tissue volume—for example, one goal may be to analyze the genetic changes in the premalignant cells or malignant cells, but these subpopulations are frequently located in microscopic regions occupying less than 5% of the tissue volume. Culturing cell populations from fresh tissue is one means of reducing contamination. However, cultured cells may not accurately represent the molecular events taking place in the actual tissue they were derived from. Assuming the tissue cells of interest can be successfully isolated and grown in culture, the gene expression pattern of the cultured cells will be influenced by the culture environment and may be quite different from the gene expression pattern in the native tissue state. This is because the cultured cells are separated from the tissue elements that regulate gene expression, such as soluble factors, extracellular matrix molecules, and cell-cell communication. Thus, the problem of cellular heterogeneity has been a significant barrier to the molecular analysis of normal and diseased tissue. This problem can now be overcome by new developments in the field of tissue microdissection. Laser-capture microdissection (LCM) has been developed to provide scientists with a fast and dependable method of capturing and preserving specific cells from tissue, under direct microscopic visualization. With the ease of procuring a homogeneous population of cells from a complex tissue using LCM, the approaches to molecular analysis of pathologic processes are significantly enhanced. The mRNA from microdissected tumors has been used as the starting material to produce cDNA libraries, microarrays, differential display, and other techniques used to find new genes or mutations. The development of LCM allows investigators to determine specific gene expression patterns from tissues of individual patients. Pure populations of cells can be obtained, and RNA can be extracted, copied to cDNA, and hybridized to thousands of genes on a cDNA microarray. In this manner, an individualized molecular profile can be obtained for each histologically identified pathologic subtype. Using such multiplex analysis, investigators will be able to correlate the pattern of expressed genes with etiology, premalignant progression, and response to treatment. A patient's risk for disease and appropriate choice of treatment could, in the future, be personalized based on the profile. A growing clinical database of such results could be used to develop a minimal subset of key markers that will lead to a revolutionary approach for early detection and accurate diagnosis of disease.

Beyond Functional Genomics to Cancer Proteomics

While DNA is an information archive, proteins do all the work of the cell. The existence of a given DNA sequence does not guarantee the synthesis of a corresponding protein. The DNA sequence is also not sufficient to describe protein structure, function, and cellular location. This is because protein complexity and versatility stems from context-dependent posttranslational processes such as phosphorylation, sulfation, and glycosylation. Moreover, the DNA code does not provide information about how proteins link together into networks and functional machines in the cell. In fact, the activation of a protein signal pathway causing a cell to migrate, die, or initiate division can take place immediately, before any changes occur in DNA/RNA gene expression. Consequently, the technology to drive the molecular medicine revolution into the third phase is emerging from protein analytical methods. An important goal will be to apply this knowledge at the level of human tissue itself.

The term proteome denotes all the proteins expressed by a genome. Proteomics is proclaimed as the next step after genomics.

A goal of investigators in this exciting field is to assemble a complete library of all the human proteins. Only a small percentage of the proteome has been cataloged in 2002. Because PCR for proteins does not exist, sequencing the order of the up to 20 possible amino acids in a given protein remains relatively slow and labor-intensive work compared with nucleotide sequencing. Although a number of new technologies are being introduced for high-throughput protein characterization and discovery, the mainstay of protein identification continues to be two-dimensional gel electrophoresis. When a mixture of proteins is applied to the two-dimensional gel, individual proteins in the mixture are separated out into signature locations on the display, depending on their individual size and charge. Each signature is a spot on the gel that can constitute a unique single protein species. The protein spot can be procured from the gel, and a partial amino acid sequence can be read. In this manner, known proteins can be monitored for changes in abundance with treatment or new proteins can be identified. An experimental two-dimensional gel image can be captured and overlaid digitally with known archived two-dimensional gels. In this way, it is possible to immediately highlight proteins that are differentially abundant in one state versus another (e.g., tumor vs. normal or before and after hormone treatment). The use of LCM in combination with proteomics allows for studying protein expression of specific subpopulations of cells within a tumor. This approach allows for studying these cells in their normal microenvironment and avoids the problems of tissue heterogeneity and contamination.

Using a protein biochip that classified protein populations into molecular weight classes, Paweletz et al. showed distinct protein patterns of normal, premalignant, and malignant cancer cells microdissected from human tissue. Furthermore, they reported that different histologic types of cancer and normal tissue (ovarian, esophageal, prostate, breast, and hepatic) exhibited distinct protein profiles. Such a means to rapidly display a pattern of expressed proteins from microscopic tissue cellular populations will potentially be an important enabling technology for pharmacoproteomics, molecular pathology, and drug intervention. Proteomic array technologies of the future will be used to rapidly generate displays of signal pathway profiles. Investigators will be able to assess the status of defined pathways that control mitogenesis, apoptosis, survival, and a host of other physiologic states. The information flow through these circuits, separately or through cross talk, may dictate clinical behavior and susceptibility to therapy.

CONCLUSION

Biologic cancer therapies hold enormous promise; many different forms of biologic therapy, from cytokines to vaccines, have been shown to induce tumor regression in many human clinical trials. Although the response rates are not high, they are encouraging because the best results in trials in animals have been in small-volume disease and prevention, not in the treatment of established large cancers. Because most biologic therapies rely on the induction of host immune responses, patients with end-stage, bulky disease and poor nutritional status may not respond optimally. Therefore, most biologic modalities may not have been adequately tested clinically to date. Furthermore, more specific and possibly more potent therapies are just now entering clinical trials. Advances in biotechnology offer the promise of even more sophisticated therapeutics. The next generation of biologic therapies will most likely consist of multimodality biologic treatments targeting both humoral and cellular immunity against multiple tumor antigens.

RECOMMENDED READING

Cytokines

Anderson CM, Buzaid AC, Grimm EA. Interaction of chemotherapy and biological response modifiers in the treatment of melanoma. *Cancer Treat Res* 1996;87:357.

Bukowski RM, Olencki T, Wang Q, et al. Phase II trial of interleukin-2 and interferon-alpha in patients with renal cell carcinoma: clinical results and immunologic correlates of response. *J Immunother* 1997;20:301.

Brunda MJ, Luistro L, Rumennik L, et al. Antitumor activity of interleukin-12 in preclinical models. *Cancer Chemother Pharmacol* 1996;38[suppl]:S16.

de Vries MR, Rinkes IH, van de Velde CJ, et al. Isolated hepatic perfusion with tumor necrosis factor alpha and melphalan: experimental studies in pigs and phase I data from humans. *Recent Results Cancer Res* 1998;147:107.

Dutcher JP. Therapeutic strategies for cytokines. *Curr Opin Oncol* 1995;7:566.

Eggermont AMM. Treatment of melanoma in-transit metastases confined to the limb. *Cancer Surv* 1996;26:335.

Kirkwood JM, Strawderman MH, Ernstoff MS, et al. Interferon alpha-2b adjuvant therapy of high-risk resected cutaneous melanoma: the Eastern Cooperative Oncology Group trial EST 1684. *J Clin Oncol* 1996;14:7.

Kopp WC, Holmlund JT. Cytokines and immunological monitoring. *Cancer Chemother Biol Response Modif* 1996;16:189.

Nooijen PT, Eggermont AM, Schalkwijk L, et al. Complete response of melanoma-in-transit metastasis after isolated limb perfusion with tumor necrosis factor alpha and melphalan without massive tumor necrosis: a clinical and histopathological study of the delayed-type reaction pattern. *Cancer Res* 1998;58:4880.

Parkinson DR. Present status of biological response modifiers in cancer. *Am J Med* 1995;99(6A):54S.

Platanias LC. Interferons: laboratory to clinic investigations. *Curr Opin Oncol* 1995;7:560.

Ruegg C, Yilmaz A, Bieler G, et al. Evidence for the involvement of endothelial cell integrin aVb3 in the disruption of the tumor vasculation induced by TNF and IFN-gamma. *Nat Med* 1998;4:408.

Stouthard JM, Goey H, de Vries EG, et al. Recombinant human interleukin 6 in metastatic renal cell cancer: a phase II trial. *Br J Cancer* 1996;73:789.

Veltri S, Smith JW 2nd. Interleukin-1 trials in cancer patients: a review of the toxicity, antitumor and hematopoietic effects. *Stem Cells* 1996;14:164.

Monoclonal Antibodies

Greiner JW, Guadagni F, Roselli M, et al. Novel approaches to tumor detection and therapy using a combination of monoclonal antibody and cytokine. *Anticancer Res* 1996;16:2129.

Jurcic JG, Scheinberg DA, Houghton AN. Monoclonal antibody therapy of cancer. *Cancer Chemother Biol Response Modif* 1996; 16:168.

Koda K, Nakajima N, Saito N, et al. A human natural antibody to adenocarcinoma that inhibits tumour cell migration. *Br J Cancer* 1998;78:1313.

Cellular Therapy

Adema GJ, Hartgers F, Verstraten R, et al. A dendritic-cell-derived C-C chemokine that preferentially attracts naive T cells. *Nature* 1997;387:713.

Aoki Y, Takakuwa K, Kodama S, et al. Use of adoptive transfer of tumor-infiltrating lymphocytes alone or in combination with cisplatin-containing chemotherapy in patients with epithelial ovarian cancer. *Cancer Res* 1991;51:1934.

Banchereau J, Schuler-Thurner B, Palucka AK, et al. Dendritic cells as vectors for therapy. *Cell* 2001;106:271.

Banchereau J, Briere F, Caux C, et al. Immunobiology of dendritic cells. *Annu Rev Immunol* 2000;18:767.

Banchereau J, Steinman RM. Dendritic cells and the control of immunity. *Nature* 1998;392:245.

Chang AE, Yoshizawa H, Sakai K, et al. Clinical observations on adoptive immunotherapy with vaccine-primed T-lymphocytes secondarily sensitized to tumor *in vitro*. *Cancer Res* 1993;53:1043.

Cella M, Sallusto F, Lanzavecchia A. Origin, maturation and antigen presenting function of dendritic cells. *Curr Opin Immunol* 1997;9:10.

Colaco CA. Why are dendritic cells central to cancer immunotherapy? *Mol Med Today* 1999;5:14.

Goedegebuure PS, Douville LM, Li H, et al. Adoptive immunotherapy with tumor-infiltrating lymphocytes and interleukin-2 in patients with metastatic malignant melanoma and renal cell carcinoma: a pilot study. *J Clin Oncol* 1995;13:1939.

Gong J, Chen D, Kashiwaba M, et al. Induction of antitumor activity by immunization with fusions of dendritic and carcinoma cells. *Nat Med* 1997;3:58.

Nouri-Shirazi M, Banchereau J, Fay J, et al. Dendritic cell based tumor vaccines. *Immunol Lett* 2000;74:5.

Rivoltini L, Kawakami Y, Robbins P, et al. Efficient induction of tumor reactive CTL from peripheral blood and tumor-infiltrating lymphocytes of melanoma patients by *in vitro* stimulation with the human melanoma antigen MART-1 peptide. *J Exp Med* 1996;184: 647.

Rosenberg SA, Lotze MT, Aebersold PM, et al. Prospective randomized trial of high dose interleukin-2 alone or with lymphokine activated killer cells for the treatment of patients with advanced cancer. *J Natl Cancer Inst* 1993;85:622.

Rosenberg SA, Packard BS, Aebersold PM, et al. Use of tumor-infiltrating lymphocytes and interleukin-2 in the immunotherapy of patients with metastatic melanoma, special report. *N Engl J Med* 1988;319:1676.

Rosenberg SA, Spiess P, Lafreniere R. A new approach to the adoptive immunotherapy of cancer with tumor-infiltrating lymphocytes. *Science* 1986;223:1318.

Rosenberg SA, Yannelli JR, Yang JC, et al. Treatment of patients with metastatic melanoma with autologous tumor-infiltrating lymphocytes and interleukin-2. *J Natl Cancer Inst* 1994;86:1159.

Toes RE, van der Voort EI. Schoenberger SP, et al. Enhancement of tumor outgrowth through CTL tolerization after peptide vaccination is avoided by peptide presentation on dendritic cells. *J Immunol* 1998;160:4449.

Vaccines

Hellstrom I, Hellstrom KE. Tumor vaccines: a reality at last? *J Immunother* 1998;21:119.

Linehan DC, Goedegebuure PS, Eberlein TJ. Vaccine therapy for cancer. *Ann Surg Oncol* 1996;3:219.

Immunoadjuvants and Immunomodulators

Akporiaye ET, Hersh EM. Immune adjuvants. In: DeVita Jr VT, Hellman S, Rosenberg SA, eds. *Biologic therapy of cancer,* 2nd ed. Philadelphia: Lippincott, 1995.

Hsueh EC, Gupta RK, Qi K, et al. TA90 immune complex predicts survival following surgery and adjuvant vaccine immunotherapy for stage IV melanoma. *Cancer J Sci Am* 1997;3:364.

Schultz N, Oratz R, Chen D, et al. Effect of DETOX as an adjuvant for melanoma vaccine. *Vaccine* 1995;13:503.

Tumor Antigen Vaccines

Borysiewicz LK, Fiander A, Nimako M, et al. A recombinant vaccinia virus encoding human papillomavirus types 16 and 18, E6 and E7 proteins as immunotherapy for cervical cancer. *Lancet* 1996;347:1523.

Cormier JN, Salgaller ML, Prevette T, et al. Enhancement of cellular immunity in melanoma patients immunized with a peptide from MART-1:Melan A. *J Sci Am* 1997;3:37.

Finn OJ, Jerome KR, Henderson RA, et al. MUC-1 epithelial tumor mucin-based immunity and cancer vaccines. *Immunol Rev* 1995;145:61.

Goydos JS, Elder E, Whiteside TL, et al. A phase I trial of a synthetic mucin peptide vaccine. Induction of specific immune reactivity in patients with adenocarcinoma. *J Surg Res* 1996;63:298.

Jager E, Ringhoffer M, Altmannsberger M, et al. Immunoselection in vivo: independent loss of MHC class I and melanocyte differentiation antigen expression in metastatic melanoma. *Int J Cancer* 1997;71:142.

Marchand M, van Baren N, Weynants P, et al. Tumor regressions observed in patients with metastatic melanoma treated with an antigenic peptide encoded by gene MAGE-3 and presented by HLA-A1. *Int J Cancer* 1999;80:219.

McLaughlin JP, Schlom J, Kantor JA, et al. Improved immunotherapy of a recombinant carcinoembryonic antigen vaccinia vaccine when given in combination with interleukin-2. *Cancer Res* 1996;56:2361.

Miles DW, Towlson KE, Graham R, et al. A randomised phase II study of sialyl-Tn and DETOX-B adjuvant with or without cyclophosphamide pretreatment for the active specific immunotherapy of breast cancer. *Br J Cancer* 1996;74:1292.

Rosenberg SA, Yang JC, Schwartzentruber DJ, et al. Immunologic and therapeutic evaluation of a synthetic peptide vaccine for the treatment of patients with metastatic melanoma. *Nat Med* 1998;4:321.

Tumor Cell-Based Vaccines

Abdel-Wahab Z, Weltz C, Hester D, et al. A phase I clinical trial of immunotherapy with interferon-gamma gene-modified autologous melanoma cells. Monitoring the humoral immune response. *Cancer* 1997;80:401.

Arienti F, Sule-Suso J, Belli F, et al. Limited antitumor T cell response in melanoma patients vaccinated with interleukin-2 gene-transduced allogeneic melanoma cells. *Hum Gene Ther* 1996;7:1955.

Berd D, Maguire Jr HC, McCue P, et al. Treatment of metastatic melanoma with an autologous tumor-cell vaccine: clinical and immunologic results in 64 patients. *J Clin Oncol* 1990;8:1858.

Berd D, Maguire Jr HC, Schuchter LM, et al. Autologous hapten-modified melanoma vaccine as postsurgical adjuvant treatment after resection of nodal metastases. *J Clin Oncol* 1997;15:2359.

Belli F, Arienti F, Sule-Suso J, et al. Active immunization of metastatic melanoma patients with interleukin-2-transduced allogeneic melanoma cells: evaluation of efficacy and tolerability. *Cancer Immunol Immunother* 1997;44:197.

Bremers AJ, Parmiani G. Immunotherapy for colon cancer [letter]. *Lancet* 1999;353:1524.

Del Vecchio M, Parmiani G. Cancer vaccination: *Forum Trends Exp Clin Med* 1999;9:239.

Elliott GT, McLeod RA, Perez J, et al. Interim results of a phase II multicenter clinical trial evaluating the activity of a therapeutic allogeneic melanoma vaccine (theraccine) in the treatment of disseminated malignant melanoma. *Semin Surg Oncol* 1993;9:264.

Hoover HC Jr, Brandhorst JS, Peters LC, et al. Adjuvant active specific immunotherapy for human colorectal cancer: 6.5-year median follow-up of a phase III prospectively randomized trial. *J Clin Oncol* 1993;11:390.

Hu X, Chakraborty NG, Sporn JR, et al. Enhancement of cytolytic T lymphocyte precursor frequency in melanoma patients following immunization with the MAGE-1 peptide loaded antigen presenting cell-based vaccine. *Cancer Res* 1996;56:2479.

Lotze MT, Rubin JT, Carty S, et al. Clinical protocol: gene therapy of cancer: a pilot study of IL-4-gene-modified fibroblasts admixed with autologous tumor to elicit an immune response. *Hum Gene Ther* 1994;5:41.

Lytle GH, McGee JM, Yamanashi WS, et al. Five-year survival in breast cancer treated with adjuvant immunotherapy. *Am J Surg* 1994;168:19.

Moller P, Sun Y, Dorbic T, et al.. Vaccination with IL-7 gene-modified autologous melanoma cells can enhance the anti-melanoma lytic activity in peripheral blood of patients with a good clinical performance status: a clinical phase I study. *Br J Cancer* 1998;77:1907.

Nemunaitis J, Bohart C, Fong T, et al. Phase I trial of retroviral vector-mediated interferon (IFN)-gamma gene transfer into autologous tumor cells in patients with metastatic melanoma. *Cancer Gene Ther* 1998;5:292.

Palmer K, Moore J, Everard M, et al. Gene therapy with autologous, interleukin 2-secreting tumor cells in patients with malignant melanoma. *Hum Gene Ther* 1999;10:1261.

Repmann R, Wagner S, Richter A. Adjuvant therapy of renal cell carcinoma with active-specific-immunotherapy (ASI) using autologous tumor vaccine. *Anticancer Res* 1997;17:2879.

Simons JW, Jaffee EM, Weber CE, et al. Bioactivity of autologous irradiated renal cell carcinoma vaccines generated by *ex vivo* granulocyte-macrophage colony-stimulating factor gene transfer. *Cancer Res* 1997;57:1537.

Soiffer R, Lynch T, Mihm M, et al. Vaccination with irradiated autologous melanoma cells engineered to secrete human granulocyte-macrophage colony-stimulating factor generates potent antitumor immunity in patients with metastatic melanoma. *Proc Natl Acad Sci USA* 1998;95:13141.

Wallack MK, Sivanandham M, Balch CM, et al. A phase III randomized, double-blind multi-institutional trial of vaccinia melanoma oncolysate-active specific immunotherapy for patients with stage II melanoma. *Cancer* 1995;75:34.

Wallack MK, Sivanandham M, Balch CM, et al. Surgical adjuvant active specific immunotherapy for patients with stage III melanoma: the final analysis of data from a phase III, randomized, double-blind, multicenter vaccinia melanoma oncolysate trial. *J Am Coll Surg* 1998;187:69.

Wallack MK, Sivanandham M, Whooley B, et al. Favorable clinical responses in subsets of patients from a randomized, multi-institutional melanoma vaccine trial. *Ann Surg Oncol* 1996;3:110.

Dendritic Cell-Based Vaccines

Chakraborty NG, Sporn JR, Tortora AF, et al. Immunization with a tumor cell-lysate-loaded autologous antigen-presenting-cell-based vaccine in melanoma. *Cancer Immunol Immunother* 1998;47:58.

Gjertsen MK, Bakka A, Breivik J, et al. Vaccination with mutant ras peptides and induction of T-cell responsiveness in pancreatic carcinoma patients carrying the corresponding RAS mutation. *Lancet* 1995;346:1399.

Hennemann B, Beckmann G, Eichelmann A, et al. Phase I trial of adoptive immunotherapy of cancer patients using monocyte-derived macrophages activated with interferon gamma and lipopolysaccharide. *Immunol Immunother* 1998;45:250.

Salgaller ML, Tjoa BA, Lodge PA, et al. Dendritic cell-based immunotherapy of prostate cancer. *Crit Rev Immunol* 1998;18:109.

Viral Oncolysate Vaccines

Freedman RS, Edwards CL, Bowen JM, et al. Viral oncolysates in patients with advanced ovarian cancer. *Gynecol Oncol* 1988;29:337.

Hersey P. Active immunotherapy with viral lysates of micrometastases following surgical removal of high risk melanoma. *World J Surg* 1992;16:251.

Morton DL, Foshag LJ, Hoon DSB, et al. Prolongation of survival in metastatic malignant melanoma after active specific immunotherapy with a new polyvalent melanoma vaccine. *Ann Surg* 1992;216:463.

Sivanandham M, Scoggin S, Tanaka N, et al. Therapeutic effect of a vaccinia colon oncolysate prepared with interleukin-2 gene encoded vaccinia virus studied in syngeneic CC-36 murine colon hepatic metastasis model. *Cancer Immunol Immunother* 1994;38:259.

Gene Therapy

Asher AL, Mule JJ, Kasid A, et al. Murine tumor cells transduced with the gene for tumor necrosis factor-alpha. *J Immunol* 1991;146:3227.

Blankenstein TH, Qin Z, Uberla K, et al. Tumor suppression after cell-targeted tumor necrosis factor alpha gene transfer. *J Exp Med* 1991;173:1047.

Descamps V, Duffour M-T, Mathieu M-C, et al. Strategies for cancer gene therapy using adenoviral vectors. *J Mol Med* 1996;74: 183.

Dranoff G, Jaffee E, Lazenby A, et al. Vaccination with irradiated tumor cells engineered to secrete murine granulocyte-macrophage colony-stimulating factor stimulates potent, specific, and longlasting anti-tumor immunity. *Proc Natl Acad Sci USA* 1993;90: 3539.

Gunzburg WH, Salmons B. Development of retroviral vectors as safe, targeted gene delivery systems. *J Mol Med* 1996;74:171.

Mastrangelo MJ, Berd D, Nathan FE, et al. Gene therapy for human cancer: an assay for clinicians. *Semin Oncol* 1996;23:4.

Miller AR, McBride WH, Hunt K, et al. Cytokine-mediated gene therapy for cancer. *Ann Surg Oncol* 1994;1:436.

Rosenberg SA, Anderson WF, Blaese M, et al. The development of gene therapy for the treatment of cancer. *Ann Surg* 1993;218:455.

Roth JA, Cristiano RJ. Gene therapy for cancer: what have we done and where are we going? *J Natl Cancer Inst* 1997;89:21.

Roth JA, Nguyen D, Lawrence DD, et al. Retroviral-mediated wild type p53 gene transfer to tumors of patients with lung cancer. *Nat Med* 1996;2:985.

Simons JW, Jaffee EM, Weber CE, et al. Bioactivity of autologous irradiated renal cell carcinoma vaccines generated by *ex vivo* granulocyte-macrophage colony-stimulating factor gene transfer. *Cancer Res* 1997;57:1537.

Toloza EM, Hunt K, Miller AR, et al. Transduction of murine and human tumors using recombinant adenovirus vectors. *Ann Surg Oncol* 1997;4:70.

Zhang WW. Antisense oncogene and tumor suppressor gene therapy of cancer. *J Mol Med* 1996;74:191.

Zhang Y, Mukhopadhyay T, Donehower LA, et al. Retroviral vectormediated transduction of K-ras antisense RNA into human lung cancer cells inhibits expression of the malignant phenotype. *Hum Gene Ther* 1993;4:451.

Angiogenesis

Fidler IJ, Ellis LM. The implications of angiogenesis to the biology and therapy of cancer metastasis. *Cell* 1994;79:185.

Folkman J. Angiogenesis in cancer, vascular, rheumatoid and other disease. *Nat Med* 1995;1:27.

Liotta LA, Steeg PS, Settler-Stevenson WG. Cancer metastasis and angiogenesis: an imbalance of positive and negative regulation. *Cell* 1991;64:327.

General

Clark JI, Weiner LM. Biologic treatment of human cancer. *Curr Probl Cancer* 1995;19:185.

Clark JW. Biological response modifiers. *Cancer Chemother Biol Response Modif* 1996;16:239.

Coley W. Further observations upon the treatment of malignant tumors with the toxins of erysipelas and *Bacillus prodigiosus* with a report of 160 cases. *Bull Johns Hopkins Hosp* 1986;7:157.

Del Prete G, Maggi E, Romagnani S. Human Th1 and Th2 cells: functional properties, mechanisms of regulation and role in disease. *Lab Invest* 1994;70:299.

DeVita VT, Hellman S, Rosenberg SA, eds. *Biologic therapy of cancer,* 2nd ed. Philadelphia: Lippincott, 1995.

Rosenberg SA, Kawakami Y, Robbins PF, et al. Identification of the genes encoding cancer antigens: implications for cancer immunotherapy. *Adv Cancer Res* 1996;70:145.

Nutrition in Cancer Patients

Paula M. Termuhlen

Cancer patients face unique problems that can result in nutritional depletion during the perioperative period. For example, cancer cachexia is a well-described condition in which the abnormal metabolic priorities of the patient (host) and tumor alter the body's usual protein and energy requirements. Furthermore, tumors of the head and neck or gastrointestinal tract often compromise nutrition by interfering with ingestion, digestion, and absorption. Preoperative and postoperative chemotherapy and radiation therapy can adversely affect the integrity and function of the alimentary tract, contributing to the difficulty of maintaining adequate nutrition.

Nutrition plays an essential role in the recovery and rehabilitation of cancer patients. Adequate protein, calories, and essential micronutrients help maintain a reasonable quality of life for these patients. Surgeons caring for cancer patients must be knowledgeable about the general principles of nutritional assessment and the unique nutritional problems of cancer patients if optimal recovery from treatment is to be achieved.

CANCER CACHEXIA

Cachexia of malignancy, a nutritional problem unique to cancer patients, is a syndrome of progressive involuntary weight loss and intractable anorexia. Without effective intervention, cancer cachexia will result in death. The physical and biochemical features of this syndrome include tissue wasting, skeletal muscle atrophy, myopathy, anergy, anemia, and glucose intolerance. In addition, patients are unable to absorb and use nutrients adequately.

Not all tumors produce the same degree of cachexia, and much variation is observed among individual patients. Greater weight loss is associated with a tumor in a visceral organ (e.g., pancreas or stomach) than with a tumor in a nonvisceral organ (e.g., breast). Based on common indices of nutritional assessment, protein-calorie malnutrition exists preoperatively in up to 50% of patients with cancer. Cancer cachexia may also have prognostic significance. Patients who have no weight loss at the time of surgery demonstrate lower morbidity and higher survival rates than those who have had moderate to severe weight loss, regardless of tumor type.

Anorexia

The etiology of cancer cachexia is multifactorial, but the most obvious contributing factor is anorexia due to the presence of a malignancy or to its treatment. Many patients report altered taste perception that contributes to decreased food intake; however, this alteration appears to be an individual phenomenon unrelated to specific tumor types or sites. Adjuvant therapy, such as chemotherapy and radiation therapy, often causes nausea and vomiting and thus food aversion. In addition, radiation therapy can cause mucosal damage, malabsorption, and diarrhea, all of which contribute to reduced oral intake.

Substrate Utilization

Aside from anorexia, other causes of cancer cachexia are abnormal host carbohydrate, protein, and lipid metabolism. Studies have shown that even with adequate caloric intake, specific substrate utilization is abnormal and insufficient for adequate nutritional support.

Glucose

Glucose intolerance and insulin resistance are often found in cancer patients, and studies have documented abnormal glucose clearance in patients with many different tumors, including lung and colorectal cancers. A diabetes-like state develops in patients with cachexia that is a result of accentuated gluconeogenesis in the liver. Tumors can augment gluconeogenesis by the increased peripheral release of metabolic substrates such as lactate. In addition, unidentified mediators cause increased gluconeogenesis in the liver by the induction of associated enzymes. The increase in gluconeogenesis contributes to nutritional depletion by causing host energy to be used inefficiently in futile metabolic cycles.

Protein

Depletion of protein in cachectic patients manifests as skeletal muscle atrophy, visceral organ atrophy, and hypoalbuminemia. Protein wasting results from altered nitrogen metabolism. This effect is seen in cancer patients who are unable to adapt to decreased food intake and nonstressed patients suffering from simple starvation. Even when cancer patients are given supplemental nutrition, such as total parenteral nutrition, whole-body protein turnover rates remain elevated. Studies in animals suggest that tumors use nitrogen released from tissues at the expense of the malnourished host. There is evidence of decreased protein synthesis and increased protein breakdown in skeletal muscle, which contributes to tissue wasting. Hypoalbuminemia is consistently found in cancer patients and is most likely related to increased albumin turnover. Overall, hepatic production of proteins appears increased in cancer patients, but this is offset by increased turnover in the peripheral body cell mass.

Lipids

Lipid metabolism is also abnormal, resulting in depletion of lipid stores and hyperlipidemia. Increased turnover of lipid stores plays a role because glucose infusions in weight-losing patients fail to suppress lipolysis. Hyperlipidemia results from a decrease in the amount of lipoprotein lipase, which transports triglycerides from blood into adipose tissue. Abnormally high or even normal serum insulin levels appear to not promote fat storage in cancer patients and thus to contribute to hyperlipidemia.

Metabolic Rate

The abnormal carbohydrate, protein, and lipid metabolism of the host is accompanied by an inability to adjust the metabolic rate to food intake. Although some patients with weight loss have documented hypermetabolism, this finding is inconsistent in large studies, varying among individual patients and tumor types. Host and tumor-secreted factors have been the focus for identifying the mechanism of the metabolic changes in cancer cachexia. To date, no tumor-produced substance having a systemic effect has been isolated. However, factors secreted by the host as part of the immune response to a tumor appear to play a role in cancer cachexia.

The cytokine tumor necrosis factor (TNF) has not only local immune effects but also systemic effects that produce clinical results similar to those seen in cachexia. TNF, also known as cachectin, has a cytotoxic effect on tumors and inhibits lipoprotein lipase, resulting in hyperlipidemia. Receptors for TNF are found ubiquitously, but particularly in the liver, adipose tissue, and muscle cells, which are key sites for abnormal metabolism in cancer patients. In healthy volunteers, TNF has been shown to increase temperature and heart rate as well as peripheral protein turnover. One theory is that cytokines such as TNF released by the immune system in response to a tumor promote an acute-phase response that reroutes nutrients from the periphery to the liver. Ultimately, this response becomes unregulated, resulting in anorexia and abnormal carbohydrate, protein, and lipid metabolism.

PREOPERATIVE ASSESSMENT OF NUTRITIONAL STATUS

Malnutrition, as commonly manifested by weight loss, exists in more than 50% of cancer patients. Traditionally, malnourished patients without cancer who have undergone major operative procedures have had higher rates of morbidity (e.g., poor wound healing, increased wound infection rates, prolonged postoperative ileus) than their well-nourished counterparts. That finding is perhaps due to the fact that underlying the malnutrition is a depressed immune system, which is often found in cancer patients as well.

Cancer patients should undergo a thorough preoperative nutritional assessment, and high-risk patients should be identified. Many nutritional assessment techniques exist. Most are based on a complete history and physical examination as well as documentation of changes in weight over time. Other studies include anthropomorphic studies, measurements of serum albumin and transferrin, tests of immune function by assessment of delayed cutaneous hypersensitivity, and estimates of energy expenditure. However, for most patients nutritional status can be adequately assessed through a comprehensive history and physical examination.

Preoperatively, malnourished patients should have a full nutritional assessment, including an estimate of the patient's basal energy expenditure (BEE), which can be calculated indirectly by the Harris-Benedict equation:

Male: BEE = 66.5 + 13.7(wt) + 5(ht) − 6.7(age)

Female: BEE = 66.5 + 9.6(wt) + 1.8(ht) − 4.7(age)

where: wt is weight in kilograms, ht is height in centimeters, and age is in years.

The metabolic cart assessment, based on a patient's carbon dioxide production, is a clinical method of determining energy expenditure that gives a more personalized assessment but is cumbersome, time-consuming, and expensive.

PREOPERATIVE NUTRITIONAL SUPPLEMENTATION

It has been difficult to establish a clear benefit to short-term preoperative nutritional supplementation in terms of decreased morbidity and mortality. However, there is some evidence to suggest a benefit to severely malnourished patients if preoperative nutritional supplementation is given for at least 7 to 10 days. More thorough preoperative nutritional supplementation should be considered for the nutritionally high-risk patient who may be grossly underweight (80% of standard weight for height) or grossly overweight (120% of standard weight for height). A recent weight loss of 12% or more of usual body weight is particularly important because patients with acute-onset protein-calorie malnutrition and associated hypoalbuminemia have a higher mortality rate than those with a marasmic or adapted form of protein-calorie malnutrition that has occurred over a longer time. Alcoholic patients are also at high risk for being nutritionally depleted, as are patients with malabsorptive syndromes, short gut, gastrointestinal fistulas, renal failure requiring dialysis, abscesses, and large healing wounds. In addition, patients with systemic infections and associated fever have increased metabolic needs that place them at high risk for the complications associated with nutritional depletion. Stopping oral intake and providing only intravenous solutions perioperatively for hydration adds additional risk. Although preoperative nutritional support remains controversial except in severely malnourished patients, postoperative nutritional supplementation is a key therapeutic modality in helping patients recover.

POSTOPERATIVE NUTRITIONAL SUPPLEMENTATION

Acute Phase

Postoperative nutritional support can be divided into two phases: acute and chronic. Patients recovering from a major operative procedure will need nutritional supplementation until they demonstrate the ability to obtain full nourishment independently. Both enteral and parenteral means of support are available. It has been recognized that enteral feeding should be used whenever possible, and many patients have enteral feeding tubes placed at surgery so that feeding can begin early in the postoperative period. If enteral feeding cannot meet the patient's nutritional needs, then parenteral feeding should be instituted, alone or in conjunction with enteral feeding. In general, the goals for nutritional support are approximately 25 kcal and 1.5 g of protein per kilogram of body weight per day.

Chronic Phase

The chronic phase of postoperative nutritional support is related to the longer-term consequences of a particular operation and adjuvant therapy. Many operative procedures produce prolonged inability to obtain adequate nutrition orally. These include pancreaticoduodenectomy with prolonged gastric emptying, esophagectomy with gastric stasis and regurgitation, and gastrectomy with dumping syndrome. Patients undergoing operations in the head and neck region are also at particular risk for inadequate oral nutrition. For most of these patients, an enteral feeding tube can be placed into the jejunum during the operation and used for long periods. Patients are often discharged with feeding tubes in place. Thus, a patient's quality of life is enhanced by the ability to manage nutrition outside a hospital. Beyond supplying sufficient protein and calories, supplementation may include vitamins, iron, and pancreatic enzymes.

NUTRITIONAL COMPLICATIONS OF ADJUVANT THERAPY

Additional nutritional problems can arise with adjuvant therapy. Patients may receive chemotherapy or radiation therapy as part of their treatment plan before or after surgery, or both. These therapies have various adverse effects. Mucosal inflammation and pain are the initial post-radiation therapy complaints that prevent patients from obtaining adequate nutrition. Late effects such as loss of taste, fibrosis, stricture formation, obstruction, and fistulization also may occur. Each chemotherapeutic agent has its own systemic side effects, although many agents produce nausea and vomiting as well as fluid and electrolyte imbalances.

FUTURE CONSIDERATIONS

Studies are underway to address the unique nutritional needs and metabolic abnormalities of cancer patients. Specific amino acids such as glutamine and arginine seem to be easily used by the intestine and promote more efficient nitrogen retention during stress. Arginine also seems to enhance immune function and is a potentially fruitful target for research. A promising enteral product includes supplemental arginine, RNA, and omega-3 fatty acids as part of its formula. Each of these substances individually stimulates the immune system. In one clinical trial, fewer infections and wound complications, in addition to shorter hospital stays, were documented in cancer patients who underwent major operative procedures and received this product compared with those who received a common standard enteral product as part of their nutritional support.

Future nutritional research in cancer patients will continue to focus on providing optimal nutrition in a safe and efficacious fashion. In addition, therapeutic nutritional intervention with substrates that stimulate the immune system may provide yet another modality for improving the general health of cancer patients. Furthermore, advances in molecular biology may someday result in the development of highly sophisticated products that combine nutrient substrates and antineoplastic pharmacologic agents in synergistic formulations designed to control or eradicate tumor cells while maintaining adequate nutrition.

RECOMMENDED READING

Buzby GP, Mullen JL, Matthews DC, et al. Prognostic nutritional index in gastrointestinal surgery. *Am J Surg* 1980;139:160.

Daly JM, Lieberman MD, Goldfine J, et al. Enteral nutrition with supplemental arginine, RNA, and omega-3 fatty acids in patients after operation: immunologic, metabolic, and clinical outcome. *Surgery* 1992;112:56.

Daly JM, Redmond HP, Lieberman MD, et al. Nutritional support of patients with cancer of the gastrointestinal tract. *Surg Clin North Am* 1991;71:523.

Heys SD, Park KGM, Garlick PJ, et al. Nutrition and malignant disease: implications for surgical practice. *Br J Surg* 1992;79:614.

Kern KA, Norton JA. Cancer cachexia. *JPEN* 1988;12:286.

McClave SA, Mitoraj TE, Theilmeier KA, et al. Differentiating subtypes (hypoalbuminemic vs. marasmic) of protein calorie malnutrition: incidence and clinical significance in a university hospital setting. *JPEN* 1992;16:337.

Meguid MM, Debonis D, Meguid V, et al. Complications of abdominal operations for malignant disease. *Am J Surg* 1988;156:341.

Shike M, Brennan MF. Supportive care of the cancer patient. In: DeVita VT, Hellman S, Rosenberg SA, eds. *Cancer: principles and practice of oncology,* 3rd ed. Philadelphia: Lippincott, 1989.

Shikova SA, Blackburn GL. Nutritional consequences of major gastrointestinal surgery: patient outcome and starvation. *Surg Clin North Am* 1991;71:509.

Shils ME. Nutrition and diet in cancer. In: Shils ME, Young VR, eds. *Modern nutrition in health and disease,* 7th ed. Philadelphia: Lea & Febiger, 1987.

Tchekmedyian NS, Zahyna D, Halpert C, et al. Clinical aspects of nutrition in advanced cancer. *Oncology* 1992;49[suppl 2]:3.

Pharmacotherapy of Cancer

Judy L. Chase and Phillip B. Ley

A basic understanding of cancer pharmacotherapy and related toxicities is mandatory for the full integration of the surgical oncologist into a multidisciplinary cancer care program. To intelligently discuss surgical options with patients, knowledge of the available treatment regimens and their potential for toxicity is essential.

This chapter includes a discussion of basic principles of chemotherapy, an overview of the mechanisms of drug action and drug resistance, and a tabular listing of the drugs available and their common toxicities, and a tabular listing of approved biologic agents used in oncology. Finally, a summary of cancer pain management and the treatment of chemotherapy-induced emesis (CIE) is included.

The reader should be aware that a complete discussion of cancer chemotherapy is beyond the scope of this brief overview. The drug and dosage regimens listed are representative examples only and do not constitute a listing of all available protocols. For specific prescribing information, the practitioner is advised to consult individual manufacturer package inserts or one of the referenced texts.

BASIC PRINCIPLES OF CHEMOTHERAPY

Cancer chemotherapeutic agents are the result of drug design and, largely, empiricism. Their use has developed based on an understanding of tumor growth characteristics, the cell cycle, drug mechanisms of action, and drug resistance. It is hoped that new techniques and advances in molecular biology will allow improvements in drug design to extend the possibility of complete chemotherapeutic response and possibly the cure of patients currently deemed beyond salvage.

Tumor Growth and Kinetics

Kinetic aspects of tumor growth have been well described. Two concepts that underscore our knowledge of the kinetics of tumor growth are Skipper's laws and Gompertzian growth. Skipper's laws apply to cells in the proliferating compartment of a tumor. First, the doubling time of proliferating cells is constant, creating a straight line on a semilog plot. Second, cell kill by a particular drug at a given dose is constant, irrespective of body burden. In most solid tumors, however, only a portion of cells within the tumor—the growth fraction—is proliferating at any given time. This partially accounts for the refractory nature of many solid tumors to chemotherapy.

Human tumors follow a pattern of Gompertzian, rather than straight-line, growth. Gompertzian growth describes a cell population decreasing as a result of cell death and increasing because of proliferation. Also, cell subpopulations may have ceased to proliferate but have not died, further swaying the growth curve from a straight semilog plot. The normal Gompertzian growth curve is sigmoid in shape. Maximum tumor growth rate occurs at approximately 30% of maximum tumor volume, where nutrient and oxygen supply to the greatest number of tumor cells is optimized. This portion of the curve is also where drug efficacy against a particular tumor may best be estimated.

The cell cycle is an important fundamental concept to understand when designing chemotherapeutic agents and treatment regimens. The cell cycle is divided into five components. The resting or nonproliferating cell is in the G0 phase, entering the active portion of the cycle following stimulation. DNA synthesis occurs during the S phase and is followed by the postsynthetic G2 phase. Mitosis occurs during the M phase and precedes the postmitotic G1 phase.

The cell cycle becomes important in drug selection because the cells in the growth fraction are more susceptible to certain agents. In a broad sense, antineoplastic agents may be classified on the basis of their activity in relation to the cell cycle. Most antimetabolites, etoposide, hydroxyurea, vinca alkaloids, and bleomycin are cell cycle–specific agents that are most effective against tumors with a high growth fraction. In contrast, alkylating agents, antineoplastic antibiotics, fluorouracil, floxuridine, and procarbazine exert their effect independent of the cell cycle and generally show more activity against slow-growing tumors.

Drug Mechanisms and Therapeutics

Knowledge of the basic action mechanisms of chemotherapeutic agents is critical in selecting drugs for an effective chemotherapy combination regimen, minimizing toxicity and drug interactions, and preventing emergence of drug-resistant clones. Agents may damage the DNA template by alkylation, cross-linking, double-strand cleavage by topoisomerase II, intercalation, and blockage of RNA synthesis. Spindle poisons may arrest mitosis. Antimetabolites block enzymes necessary for DNA synthesis. Hormonal agents and their antagonists may influence cellular signal transduction, and biologic response modifiers may influence the host's immune response to the tumor alone or in the context of concomitantly administered drugs.

Combination chemotherapy frequently is used in an effort to forestall the development of drug resistance to antineoplastic agents and to achieve synergism with reduced toxicity. The Goldie-Coldman hypothesis assumes that at the time of diagnosis, most tumors possess resistant clones. Multiple mechanisms of drug resistance develop during cancer progression. The most well studied of these involves the *mdr* gene, which codes for membrane-bound P-glycoprotein. P-glycoprotein serves as a channel through which cellular toxins (i.e., chemotherapeutic agents) may be excreted from the cell. Additional mechanisms of drug resistance are decreased drug transport into cells, reduction of drug activation, drug metabolism enhancement, development of alternative metabolic pathways, drug inhibition of enzyme targets overcome by gene amplification, and impairment of drug binding to target. A single drug may be subject to one or more mechanisms.

Interestingly, normal human cells never develop drug resistance. As a result, several caveats of combination chemotherapy have emerged. Drugs shown active as single agents should be chosen, and drugs selected for combined use should have different mechanisms of action. Ideally, drugs with different dose-limiting toxicities should be administered together, although toxicity overlap may necessitate dose reduction, as with myelosuppression. Finally, drug combinations with similar patterns of resistance should be avoided.

Different patterns of chemotherapy administration are used in particular settings with specific goals. Induction chemotherapy is usually high dose and given in combination to induce complete remission. Consolidation is a repetition of an induction regimen in a complete responder to prolong remission or increase the cure rate. Chemotherapy given with an intent similar to that of consolidation but with higher doses than induction or with different agents at high doses is known as intensification. Maintenance regimens are low-dose, long-term protocols intended to delay tumor cell regrowth after complete remission. Induction, consolidation, intensification, and maintenance usually apply to hematologic malignancies but also may describe solid tumor regimens as well.

Neoadjuvant treatment in the preoperative or perioperative period is used more commonly with solid tumors, such as locally advanced breast carcinoma, soft-tissue sarcomas of the extremities, and, more recently, rectal carcinoma and squamous cell carcinoma of the head and neck. It is often given in combination with radiation therapy to improve survival, resectability, and organ preservation.

Palliative chemotherapy may be given to control symptoms or, if the toxicity profile is favorable, prolong life for incurable patients. Salvage chemotherapy involves the use of a potentially curative, high-dose protocol in patients failing or recurring after different standard treatment plans have been attempted.

Adjuvant chemotherapy is administered following curative surgery or radiation therapy as a short-course, high-dose regimen to destroy a low number of residual tumor cells. Several factors determine the effectiveness of adjuvant regimens, including tumor burden, drug dose and schedule, combination chemotherapy, and drug resistance. The drug(s) must be active locally against residual cells as well as distantly against clinically occult metastatic deposits. Extensive literature supports the use of adjuvant chemotherapy for breast, colon, rectal, and anal carcinomas and for ovarian germ cell tumors, osteosarcoma, and pediatric solid tumors. No definitive benefit has been reported yet for pancreatic, gastric, and testicular carcinomas or for cervical cancer and melanoma, although investigative adjuvant therapy protocols are ongoing and open for patient enrollment.

Most chemotherapeutic agents exhibit very steep dose-response profiles and have low therapeutic indices, making a high-dose, short-term administration desirable. This can be accomplished through regional dose intensification. One example is intraperitoneal chemotherapy of ovarian or gastric cancer with high risk of peritoneal recurrence, or low-volume intraperitoneal disease, pseudomyxoma peritonei, and peritoneal mesothelioma.

Another type of regional dose intensification is intraarterial therapy, which requires regional tumor confinement and a unique tumor blood supply and is most commonly used in hepatic artery infusion for primary or metastatic liver tumors that are surgically unresectable for cure. Intraarterial chemotherapy also has been used for brain gliomas and some head and neck tumors. Isolated perfusion of a specific anatomic site, usually the extremities, is one more type of regional dose intensification that allows for the delivery of very high doses to the involved site with little systemic toxicity; it is often combined with hyperthermia. The largest body of literature discusses its use in all stages of melanoma, although limb perfusion for extremity sarcoma has been reported.

CHEMOTHERAPEUTIC AGENTS

Fundamental knowledge of the drugs available for cancer treatment, their mechanisms of action, general dose ranges, dominant toxicities, and indications for use is important to the general surgeon caring for cancer patients. Table 24-1 lists the available agents and their mechanisms, doses, and toxicities. Table 24-2 lists the available biologic agents, their U.S. Food and Drug Administration (FDA) indications and dosages. Table 24-3 lists commonly used combination chemotherapeutic regimens.

MANAGEMENT OF CANCER PAIN

The vast majority of patients with advanced cancer and as many as 60% of patients with any stage of disease experience significant pain. However, cancer pain frequently is undertreated for a multitude of reasons and fears that are largely unfounded. Effective management of cancer pain is achieved best with a multidisciplinary approach, including pain specialists, oncologists, nurses, pharmacists, physiatrists, physical and occupational therapists, psychologists, psychiatrists, primary care physicians, social workers, clergy, and hospice caregivers. Open lines of communication are of paramount importance to the successful management of cancer pain.

Cancer pain may be due to direct tumor involvement of bone, nerves, viscera, blood vessels, or mucous membranes and can occur postoperatively, after radiation therapy, or after chemotherapy. Narcotic use should follow the basic principles of cancer pain management, beginning with an agent that has the potential to provide relief; individualization of the agent, route, dose, and schedule; titration to efficacy; and provision of relief for breakthrough pain. Side effects should be anticipated and treated. Change from one route of administration to another should be done with equianalgesic doses, and the oral route should be used whenever possible. In cancer patients receiving chemotherapy, combination analgesics employing an acetaminophen component may not be the best choice for treatment of chronic pain secondary to the risk of masking a neutropenic fever and the risk of acetaminophen toxicity if large doses are required. In addition, combination products using an aspirin component are discouraged secondary to the antiplatelet and antipyretic effects. The nonsteroidal antiinflammatory agents are a useful adjunct to the treatment of cancer pain but must be used with caution secondary to the antiplatelet effects. The practitioner should be aware of various adjuncts to pain management, including steroids, antidepressants, anxiolytics, and neuroleptics, as well as neuroablative, neurostimulatory, and anesthetic procedures.

Table 24-4 is a compilation of various nonnarcotic and narcotic analgesic agents for treating cancer pain and includes dose ranges and expected toxicities.

MANAGEMENT OF CHEMOTHERAPY-INDUCED EMESIS

Because many surgical patients receive neoadjuvant and adjuvant chemotherapy, the surgeon may be called on to treat CIE, which is often a dose-limiting toxicity that may lead patients to refuse further therapy. Three physiologic areas are included in the pathogenesis of CIE: (a) the emetic center in the lateral reticular formation of the medulla, (b) vagal and splanchnic afferents from the gastrointestinal tract to the central nervous system, and (c) the chemoreceptor trigger zone in the area postrema of the medulla. Chemotherapeutic agents and their metabolites may trigger the latter two directly.

Three patterns of emesis tend to occur in association with chemotherapy. Acute emesis occurs within 24 hours of chemotherapy. Delayed emesis occurs more than 24 hours after the cessation of chemotherapy administration and is predisposed by female gender, high-dose cisplatin, and prior episodes of acute emesis. Anticipatory emesis may occur before retreatment in patients whose prior episodes of emesis were poorly controlled, occurring in up to 25% of patients who received prior chemotherapy. Younger age and history of motion sickness also predispose to CIE.

Table 24-5 lists the emetogenic potential of many of the individual chemotherapeutic agents. As chemotherapeutic agents are combined, the combination will have a higher emetogenic potential than the individual agents and appropriate prevention of nausea and vomiting will be required. The emetogenic potential of many agents is dose-dependent. Therefore, additional antiemetic prophylaxis/treatment may be required with higher chemotherapy dosages.

The treatment of CIE underwent a veritable revolution with the introduction of the first selective serotonin antagonist, ondansetron. Currently there are three FDA-approved selective serotonin antagonists available for the treatment and prevention of CIE (ondansetron, dolasetron, and granisetron). These agents have also found great utility in the prevention of postoperative nausea and vomiting and radiation therapy–induced nausea and vomiting. Intravenous (IV) administration is not necessary in most cases of noncisplatin-induced emesis, because efficacy by oral administration is comparable. They also have the advantage of not causing sedation, and therefore can be safely administered in combination with other agents. High-dose IV metoclopramide has been found effective in treating CIE, although less so than ondansetron, but its extrapyramidal side effects are a major problem. These extrapyramidal side effects may occur with any of the antidopaminergic agents including metoclopramide, haloperidol, droperidol, and the phenothiazines. The extrapyramidal side effects can be treated/prevented by co-administration

Table 24-1.   Cancer chemotherapeutic agents: mechanisms, doses, and toxicities

Drug	Dose and Schedule	Toxicity
Alkylating agents		
Altretamine (hexamethylmelamine)	4–12 mg/kg/d or 260 mg/m² PO divided doses × 14–21 d	Nausea and vomiting, myelosuppression, paresthesias, CNS toxicity
Busulfan	2–8 mg PO daily	Myelosuppression, pulmonary fibrosis, aplastic anemia, skin hyperpigmentation
Carmustine	150–200 mg/m² IV every 6–8 wk	Delayed myelosuppression, nausea and vomiting, hepatotoxicity
Chlorambucil	0.1–0.2 mg/kg/d PO × 3–6 wk (average 4–10 mg/d)	Myelosuppression, pulmonary fibrosis, hyperuricemia
Carbolplatin	300–360 mg/m² IV every 4 wk	Myelosuppression, nausea and vomiting, peripheral neuropathy, ototoxicity
Cisplatin	40–120 mg/m² IV every 3 wk 20 mg/m²/d IV × 5 days every 3–4 wk	Nephrotoxicity, nausea and vomiting, peripheral neuropathy, myelosuppression, ototoxicity
Cyclophosphamide	40–50 mg/kg IV in divided doses over 2–5 days 1–5 mg/kg/d PO	Myelosuppression, hemorrhagic cystitis, immunosuppression, alopecia, stomatitis, SIADH
Dacarbazine	2.0–4.5 mg/kg/d IV × 10 d, or 250 mg/m²/d IV × 5 d (melanoma) 150 mg/m²/d IV × 5 d, or 375 mg/m² IV every 15 d (Hodgkin's disease)	Myelosuppression, nausea and vomiting, flulike syndrome, hepatoxicity, alopecia, flushing
Ifosfamide	1.2 g/m² IV daily × 5 d	Myelosuppression, hemorrhagic cystitis, somnolence, confusion
Lomustine	130 mg/m² PO every 6 wk	Delayed myelosuppression, nausea and vomiting, hepatotoxicity, neurotoxicity

Drug	Dose	Toxicity
Mechlorethamine	0.4 mg/kg IV single dose or in divided doses of 0.1–0.2 mg/kg/d	Myelosuppression, nausea and vomiting, phlebitis, gonadal dysfunction
Melphalan	2–6 mg PO daily × 14–21 d 10 mg PO daily × 7–10 d 16 mg/m^2 IV every 2 wk	Myelosuppression, anorexia, nausea and vomiting, gonadal dysfunction
Procarbazine	4–6 mg/kg/d PO daily 100 mg/m^2/d PO × 14 d	Myelosuppression, nausea and vomiting, lethargy, depression, paresthesias, headache, flulike syndrome
Streptozocin	500 mg/m^2/d IV × 5 d 1,000–1,500 mg/m^2 IV weekly	Renal toxicity, nausea and vomiting, diarrhea, altered glucose metabolism, liver dysfunction
Thiotepa	0.3–0.4 mg/kg IV every 1–4 wk	Myelosuppression, nausea and vomiting, mucositis, skin rashes
Antimetabolites		
Capecitabine	2,000–2,500 mg/m^2/d PO × 14 d	Diarrhea, stomatitis, nausea and vomiting, hand-foot syndrome, myelosuppression
Cladribine	4 mg/m^2/d IV continuous infusion × 7 d	Myelosuppression, fever, rash
Cytarabine	100–200 mg/m^2/d IV infusion × 5–7 d 3 g/m^2 IV every 12 hr × 4–12 doses	Myelosuppression, nausea and vomiting, diarrhea, stomatitis, hepatotoxicity, fever, conjunctivitis, CNS toxicity
Fludarabine	25 mg/m^2/d IV × 5 d	Myelosuppression, nausea and vomiting, fever, malaise, pulmonary infiltrates
Floxuridine	0.1–0.6 mg/kg/d × 5–14 d continuous arterial infusion	Hepatotoxicity, gastritis, mucositis
5-Fluorouracil	300–500 mg/m^2/d IV × 3–5 d 10–15 mg/kg IV weekly 200–300 mg/m^2/d IV continuous infusion	Stomatitis, myelosuppression, diarrhea, nausea and vomiting, cerebellar ataxia

continued

Table 24-1. *Continued*

Drug	Dose and Schedule	Toxicity
Gemcitibine	1,000 mg/m^2 IV weekly	Myelosuppression, fever, flulike syndrome, rash, mild nausea and vomiting
Hydrea (hydroxyurea)	80 mg/kg PO every 3 d 20–30 mg/kg PO daily	Myelosuppression, mild nausea and vomiting, rash
6-Mercaptopurine	1.5–2.5 mg/kg/d PO (average 100–200 mg/d)	Myelosuppression, nausea and vomiting, anorexia, diarrhea, cholestasis
Methotrexate	2.5–5.0 mg PO daily (low dose) 50 mg/m^2 IV every 2–3 wk (low dose) 1–12 g/m^2 IV every 1–3 wk (high dose) 5–10 mg/m^2 (max 15 mg) intrathecal every 3–7 d	Mucositis, myelosuppression, pulmonary fibrosis, hepatotoxicity, nephrotoxicity, diarrhea, skin erythema
Pentostatin	4 mg/m^2 IV every 7–14 d	Nephrotoxicity, CNS depression, myelosuppression, nausea and vomiting, conjunctivitis
6-Thioguanine	2 mg/kg PO daily	Myelosuppression, hepatotoxicity, stomatitis
Natural products		
Antitumor antibiotics		
Bleomycin	10–20 U/m^2 IV, IM, or SC once-twice weekly	Pneumonitis, pulmonary fibrosis, fever, anaphylaxis, hyperpigmentation, alopecia
Dactinomycin	0.5 mg/day IV × 5 d max 0.015 mg/kg/d IV × 5 d max (children)	Stomatitis, myelosuppression, anorexia, nausea and vomiting, diarrhea, alopecia
Daunorubicin	30–45 mg/m^2/d IV × 3 d 40 mg/m^2 IV every 2 wk (liposomal)	Myelosuppression, cardiotoxicity, stomatitis, alopecia, nausea and vomiting
Doxorubicin	60–90 mg/m^2 IV every 21 d 20–30 mg/m^2/d IV × 3 d, every 3–4 wk 20 mg/m^2 IV every 3 wk (liposomal)	Myelosuppression, cardiotoxicity, stomatitis, alopecia, nausea and vomiting

Epirubicin	100–120 mg/m² IV every 3–4 wk	Myelosuppression, nausea and vomiting, cardiotoxicity, alopecia
Idarubicin	12 mg/m²/d IV × 3 d every 3 wk	Myelosuppression, nausea and vomiting, stomatitis, alopecia, cardiotoxicity
Mitomycin C	20 mg/m² IV every 6–8 wk	Myelosuppression, nausea and vomiting, anorexia, alopecia, stomatitis
Mitoxantrone	12 mg/m²/d IV × 3 d	Myelosuppression, cardiotoxicity, alopecia, stomatitis, nausea and vomiting
Mitotic inhibitors		
Estramustine	10–16 mg/kg/d PO	Myelosuppression, ischemic heart disease, thrombophlebitis, hepatotoxicity, nausea and vomiting
Docetaxel	60–100 mg/m² IV every 21 d	Myelosuppression, fluid retention, hypersensitivity, paresthesias, rash alopecia
Paclitaxel	135–175 mg/m²/d IV infusion every 3 wk 80 mg/m²/d IV infusion weekly	Myelosuppression, peripheral neuropathy, alopecia, mucositis, anaphylaxis, dyspnea
Vinblastine	4–12 mg/m² IV every 1–2 wk	Myelosuppression, paralytic ileus, alopecia, nausea, stomatitis
Vincristine	0.4–1.4 mg/m² IV weekly (2.0 mg/wk max)	Peripheral neuropathy, paralytic ileus, SIADH
Vinorelbine	30 mg/m² IV weekly	Peripheral neuropathy, myelosuppression, nausea and vomiting, hepatic dysfunction
Topoisomerase inhibitors		
Etoposide	50–100 mg/m²/d IV × 3–5 d 100 mg/m²/d PO × 5 d	Myelosuppression, nausea and vomiting, diarrhea, fever, hypotension with infusion, alopecia
Irinotecan	125 mg/m² IV weekly 350 mg/m² IV every 3 wk	Myelosuppression, diarrhea, nausea and vomiting, anorexia

continued

Table 24-1. *Continued*

Drug	Dose and Schedule	Toxicity
Teniposide	80–90 mg/m^2/d IV × 5 d	Myelosuppression, nausea and vomiting, alopecia, hepatotoxicity, hypotension with infusion
Topotecan	1.5 mg/m^2/d IV × 5 d	Myelosuppression, fever, flulike syndrome, nausea and vomiting
Enzymes		
Asparaginase	6,000 IU/m^2 IM 3X/wk 1,000 IU/kg/d IV × 10 d	Allergic reactions, nausea and vomiting, liver dysfunction, CNS depression, hyperglycemia
Pegasparaginase	2,500 IU/m^2 IM or IV every 14 d	Hypersensitivity reactions, hepatotoxicity, fever, nausea and vomiting
Hormonal agents		
Adrenocorticoids		
Dexamethasone	0.5–4.0 mg PO, IV, IM daily	Fluid retention, hyperglycemia, hypertension, infection
Methylprednisolone	4–200 mg/day PO, IV daily	
Prednisone	5–100 mg/day PO	
Estrogens		
Diethylstilbestrol	1–15 mg/day PO	Fluid retention, feminization, uterine bleeding, nausea and vomiting, thrombophlebitis
Estradiol	0.15–3.0 mg/day PO	
Progestins		
Medroxyprogesterone	400–1,000 mg/week PO or IM	Weight gain, fluid retention, feminization, cardiovascular effects
Megestrol	160 mg/day PO	

Antiestrogens		
Taxoxifen	10 mg PO bid	Hot flashes, nausea and vomiting, altered menses
Toremifene	60 mg PO daily	
Aromatase inhibitors		
Aminoglutethimide	250 mg PO bid–qid	Rash, electrolytes disturbance, drowsiness, nausea, anorexia
Anastrozole	1 mg PO daily	
Androgens		
Testosterone	200–400 mg IM every 2–4 wk (long acting)	Masculinization, amenorrhea, gynecomastia, nausea, water retention, changes in libido, skin hypersensitivity, hepatotoxicity
Methyltestosterone	50–200 mg PO daily	
Fluoxymesterone	10–40 mg PO daily	
Antiandrogens		
Bicalutamide	50 mg PO daily	Hot flashes, decreased libido, impotence, diarrhea, nausea and vomiting, gynecomastia, hepatotoxicity
Flutamide	250 mg PO tid	
Nilutamide	150–300 mg PO daily	
LHRH Analogues		
Leuprolide	1 mg SC daily 7.5 mg IM monthly, 22.5 mg IM every 3 mo, or 30 mg IM every 4 mo	Hot flashes, menstrual irregularity, sexual dysfunction, edema
Goserelin	3.6–10.8 mg implant SC every 3 mo	

bid, twice daily; CNS, central nervous system; IM, intramuscularly; IV, intravenously; LHRH, luteinizing hormone-releasing hormone; PO, orally; qid, four times daily; SC, subcutaneously; SIADH, syndrome of inappropriate antidiuretic secretion; tid, three times daily.

Table 24-2. Biologic agents used in oncology

Cytokine	Indications	Dose and Schedule	Toxicity
Interferon-alfa (Roferon-A[R], Intron A[R])	Melanoma, chronic myelogenous leukemia, hairy-cell leukemia, Kaposi's sarcoma, chronic hepatits B and C	3–50 million IU/m^2/d or 3 × per wk	Flulike syndrome, anorexia, depression, fatigue
Interluekin-2 (Aldesleukin, Proleukin[R])	Renal cell carcinoma, metastatic melanoma	72,000 IU/kg every 8 hr × 5 d	Chills, fever, edema, hepatotoxicity, nephrotoxicity, hypotension, mental status changes, anemia, thrombocytopenia, diarrhea, nausea and vomiting
Interleukin-11 (Oprelvekin, Neumega[R])	Thrombocytopenia	50 μg/kg SC once daily	Fluid retention, peripheral edema, dyspnea, tachycardia, atrial arrythmias, dizziness, blurred vision
Filgrastim (G-CSF) (Neupogen[R])	Non-myeloid malignancy, neutropenia	5–10 μg/kg/day IV or SC	Hypersensitivity, bone pain, fever, malaise
Sargramostim (GM-CSF) (Leukine[R])	Acceleration of myeloid recovery. BMT failure or engraftment delay. Induction for acute myelogenous leukemia. Mobilization after autologous peripheral blood progenitor cells.	250 μg/m^2/day IV or SC	Rash, fluid retention, bone pain, cardiac arrythmia, dyspnea, hypersensitivity

Epoetin alfa (Erythropoietin; Epogen[R], Procrit[R])	Anemia associated with chronic renal failure, cancer chemotherapy or aids treatments. Reduction of blood transfusions in surgery patients.	Initial dose: 50–150 U/kg IV or SC 3 × per wk May increase to 300 U/kg 3 × per wk	Hypertension, hypersensitivity, fever, tachycardia, nausea, fatigue
Monoclonal antibody			
Rituximab (Rituxin[R])	Non-Hodgkin's lymphoma	375 mg/m² IV infusion weekly × 4 doses	Hypersensitivity, infusion-related fever and chills/rigors, hypotension
Trastuzumab (Herceptin[R])	Breast cancer	Initial dose: 4 mg/kg IV infusion Maintenance dose: 2 mg/kg IV infusion weekly	Infusion-related fever and chills; cardiac dysfunction, including dyspnea, cough, peripheral edema; nausea/vomiting; hypersensitivity; hypotension; diarrhea
Alemtuzumab (Campath[R])	B-cell chronic lymphocytic leukemia	Initial dose: 3 mg/d IV infusion, if tolerated increase to 10 mg/d IV, if tolerated increase to 30 mg/d IV 3 × per wk	Infusion-related fever, chills, rash, nausea, hypotension, shortness of breath, opportunistic infections, neutropenia, thrombocytopenia
Gemtuzumab ozogamicin (Mylotarg[R])	Acute myeloid leukemia	9 mg/m² IV infusion every 14 d × 2 doses	Chills, fever, nausea, vomiting, headache, hypotension
Immunotoxin			
Denileukin diftitox (Ontak[R])	Cutaneous T-cell lymphoma	9 or 18 μg/kg/day IV × 5 d, repeat every 21 d	Acute hypersensitivity, including hypotension, dyspnea, rash, chest pain, tachycardia; vascular leak syndrome; dizziness; nausea; vomiting; diarrhea

Table 24-3. Commonly used combination chemotherapeutic regimens

Acromym	Cancer Use	Agents
ABVD	Hodgkin's lymphoma	Doxorubicin, bleomycin, vinblastine, dacarbazine
AC	Breast, sarcoma, neuroblastoma	Doxorubicin, cyclophosphamide
ACE, CAE	Small cell lung	Cyclophosphamide, doxorubicin, etoposide
AP	Ovarian, endometrial	Doxorubicin, cisplatin
BEACOPP	Hodgkin's lymphoma	Bleomycin, etoposide, doxorubicin, cyclophosphamide, vincristine, procarbazine, prednisone, filgrastim
BEP	Testicular	Bleomycin, etoposide, cisplatin
CABO	Head and neck	Cisplatin, methotrexate, bleomycin, vincristine
CAF	Breast	Cyclophosphamide, doxorubisin, fluorouracil
CAMP	Non–small cell lung	Cyclophosphamide, doxorubicin, methotrexate, procarbazine
CAP	Non–small cell lung	Cyclophosphamide, doxorubicin, cisplatin
CAVE	Small cell lung	Cyclophosphamide, doxorubicin, vincristine, etoposide
CEF	Breast	Cyclophosphamide, epirubicin, fluorouracil
CF	Head and neck	Cisplatin, fluorouracil
CHOP	Non-Hodgkin's lymphoma	Cyclophosphamide, doxorubicin, vincristine, prednisone
CHOP-Bleo	Non-Hodgkin's lymphoma	Cyclophosphamide, doxorubicin, vincristine, prednisone, bleomycin
CMF	Breast	Methotrexate, fluorouracil, cyclophosphamide
COMLA	Non-Hodgkin's lymphoma	Cyclophosphamide, vincristine, methotrexate, leucovorin, cytarabine
COPE	Small cell lung	Cyclophosphamide, vincristine, cisplatin, etoposide
CVD + IL-21	Malignant melanoma	Cisplatin, vinblastine, dacarbazine, aldesleukin, interferon-α
CYVADIC	Sarcoma (bone or soft tissue)	Cyclophosphamide, vincristine, doxorubicin, dacarbazine
DI	Soft tissue sarcoma	Doxorubicin, ifosfamide
EAP	Gastric, small bowel	Etoposide, doxorubicin, cisplatin
EC	Lung	Etoposide, carboplatin
EFP	Gastric, small bowel	Etoposide, fluorouracil, cisplatin
ELF	Gastric	Etoposide, leucovorin, fluorouracil

Acronym	Cancer type	Drugs
EP	Testicular, lung	Etoposide, cisplatin
ESHAP	Non-Hodgkin's lymphoma	Methylprednisolone, etoposide, cytarabine, cisplatin
FAC	Breast	Fluorouracil, doxorubicin, cyclophosphamide
FAM	Gastric, pancreas	Fluorouracil, doxorubicin, mitomycin
FAMTX	Gastric	Methotrexate, fluorouracil, leucovorin, doxorubicin
FAP	Gastric	Fluorouracil, doxorubicin, cisplatin
FU/LV	Colorectal	Fluorouracil, leucovorin
MACOP-B	Non-Hodgkin's lymphoma	Methotrexate, leucovorin, doxorubicin, prednisone, cyclophosphamide, vincristine, bleomycin,
MAID	Soft tissue sarcoma	Mesna, doxorubicin, ifosfamide, dacarbazine
m-BACOD	Non-Hodgkin's lymphoma	Methotrexate, leucovorin, doxorubicin, cyclophosphamide, vincristine, bleomycin, dexamethasone
MICE (ICE)	Sarcoma, lung	Ifosfamide, carboplatin, etoposide, mesna
MBC	Head and neck	Methotrexate, bleomycin, cisplatin
MOPP	Hodgkin's lymphoma	Mechlorethamine, vincristine, procarbazine, prednisone
MP	Multiple myeloma	Melphalan, prednisone
MP	Prostate gland	Mitoxantrone, prednisone
M-VAC	Bladder	Methotrexate, vinblastine, doxorubicin, cisplatin
PAC	Ovarian, endometrial	Cisplatin, doxorubicin, cyclophosphamide
PVB	Testicular, adenocarcinoma	Cisplatin, vinblastine, bleomycin
SMF	Pancreas	Streptozocin, mitomycin, fluorouracil
TCF	Esophageal	Paclitaxel, cisplatin, fluorouracil
TIP	Head and neck, esophageal	Paclitaxel, ifosfamide, mesna, cisplatin
VAC	Sarcoma	Vincristine, dactinomycin, cyclophosphamide
VAD	Multiple myeloma, acute lymphocytic leukemia	Vincristine, doxorubicin, dexamethasone
VC	Non-small cell lung	Vinorelbine, cisplatin
VIP	Testicular, genitourinary, lung	Etoposide, cisplatin, ifosfamide, mesna
5 + 2	Acute myelocytic leukemia	Cytarabine, daunorubicin or mitoxantrone
7 + 3	Acute myelocytic leukemia	Cytarabine, daunorubicin or mitoxantrone

Table 24-4.   Non-narcotic and narcotic analgesic agents use for treating cancer pain

Drug	How Supplied	Dose and Schedule	Toxicity
Non-Narcotics			
Acetaminophen	Various tablets, liquid, and suppository strengths	650–1,000 mg PO every 6 hr	Hepatic and renal impairment
Celecoxib (Celebrex)	Capsules: 100 mg and 200 mg	200 mg PO once daily	Dyspepsia, heartburn, nausea, epigastric pain, antiplatelet effects, bleeding, renal dysfunction
Ibuprofen	Tablets: 100 mg, 200 mg, 400 mg, 600 mg, and 800 mg Suspension: 100 and 200 mg/5 mL	400–800 mg PO every 6–8 hr	
Ketorolac (Toradol)	Injection: 15 and 30 mg/mL Tablets: 10 mg	15–30 mg IV/IM every 6 hr 10 mg PO every 6 hr (limit therapy to 5 d)	
Nabumetone (Relafen)	Tablets: 500 and 750 mg	500–750 mg PO twice daily	
Naproxen	Tablets: 200, 250, 375, and 500 mg Suspension: 125 mg/5 mL	250–500 mg PO twice daily	
Rofecoxib (Vioxx)	Tablets: 12.5 mg, 25 mg, and 50 mg Suspension: 12.5 and 25 mg/5 mL	25–50 mg PO once daily	
Tramadol (Ultram)	Tablets: 50 mg	50–100 mg PO every 4–6 hr	Dizziness, nausea, constipation, headache
Narcotics			
Codeine	Tablets: 15, 30, and 60 mg Oral solution: 15 mg/5 mL Tablets: 15, 30, and 60 mg with acetaminophen Injection: 30 and 60 mg	15–60 mg PO, IM, IV, or SC every 4–6 hr	Sedation, constipation, nausea, respiratory depression, occurs with all narcotic analgesics

Drug	Formulation	Dose	Comments
Fentanyl	Lozenges: 100, 200, 300, 400, 600, 800, 1,200, and 1,600 mcg	100–400 mcg PO every 2–3 hr	
	Transdermal patch: 25, 50, 75, and 100 μg/hr	Apply one patch every 72 hr	
Levorphanol	Tablets: 2 mg	2–4 mg PO/IV/IM every 6 hr	
	Injection: 2 mg/mL		
Hydrocodone	Tablets: 5, 7.5, and 10 mg with acetaminophen	5–10 mg PO every 4–6 hr	
Hydromorphone	Tablets: 1, 2, 3, 4, and 8 mg tablets	2–4 mg PO every 3–4 hr	
	Injection: 1, 2, 4, and 10 mg/mL	0.5–2 mg IV/IM every 3–4 hr	
	Oral liquid: 5 mg/5 mL		
	Suppository: 3 mg		
Methadone	Tablets: 5, 10, and 40 mg	10–20 mg PO every 4–6 hr	As above Delayed toxicity, accumulation
	Oral Solution: 1, 2, and 10 mg/mL		
	Injection: 10 mg/mL		
Meperidine	Tablets: 50 and 100 mg	5–15 mg IV/IM every 4–6 hr	As above: Seizures from normeperidine metabolite accumulation
	Oral syrup: 50 mg/5 mL	50–100 mg PO every 3–4 hr	
	Injection: 10, 25, 50, 75, and 100 mg	25–100 mg IV/IM every 3–4 hr	As above
Morphine	Tablets: 10, 15, and 30 mg	10–30 mg PO every 3–4 hr	
	Oral solution: 10, 20, and 100 mg/5 mL	30–200 mg PO every 8–12 hr	
	Extended release tablets/capsules: 15, 20, 30, 60, 100, and 200 mg		
	Injection: 1, 2, 4, 5, 8, 10, 15, 25, and 50 mg	2–10 mg IV/IM every 3–4 hr	
	Suppositories: 5, 10, 20, and 30 mg		
Oxycodone	Tablet/capsule: 5 mg	5–10 mg PO every 4–6 hr	As above
	Oral solution: 1 and 20 mg/mL		
	Tablets: 5, 7.5, and 10 mg with acetaminophen		
	Controlled release tablets: 10, 20, 40, 80, and 160 mg	20–160 mg PO every 8–12 hr	
Propoxyphene	Tablets: 65 mg tablets (as HCl)	65 mg PO every 4 hr	As above
	Tablets: 50, 65, and 100 mg with acetaminophen	50–100 mg PO every 4 hr	

Table 24-5. Emetogenic potential of individual chemotherapeutic agents

Frequency of Emesis[a]	Agents	
>90% Very highly emetogenic	Carmustine > 250 mg/m^2 Cisplatin > 50 mg/m^2 Cyclophosphamide > 1,500 mg/m^2 Dacarbazine	Ifosfamide > 1,500 mg/m^2 Mechlorethamine Streptozocin

60%–90%
Highly emetogenic
	Carboplatin
	Carmustine < 250 mg/m^2
	Cisplatin < 50 mg/m^2
	Cyclophosphamide
	  750–1,500 mg/m^2
	Cytarabine > 1 g/m^2
	Dactinomycin > 1.5 g/m^2
	Daunorubicin > 50 mg/m^2
		Doxorubicin > 60 mg/m^2
		Irinotecan
		Melphalan (IV)
		Methotrexate
		  > 1,000 mg/m^2
		Mitoxantrone > 15 mg/m^2
		Procarbazine

30%–60% Moderately emetogenic	Aldesleukin Altretamine (oral) Capecitabine (oral) Cyclophosphamide < 750 mg/m^2 Cyclophosphamide (oral) Dactinomycin < 1.5 g/m^2 Daunorubicin < 50 mg/m^2	Doxorubicin 20–60 mg/m^2 Epirubicin > 90 mg/m^2 Idarubicin Ifosfamide < 1,500 mg/m^2 Methotrexate 250–1,000 mg/m^2 Mitoxantrone < 15 mg/m^2 Temozolomide

10%–30%
Mildly emetogenic
	Asparaginase
	
	Cytarabine < cytarabine
	  > 1 g/m^2
	Daunorubicin (liposomal)
	Docetaxel
	Etoposide
	5-Fluorouracil
	  < 1,000 mg/m^2
	Gemcitabine
		Methotrexate
		  50–250 mg/m^2
		Mitomycin
		
		Paclitaxel
		Pegaspariginase
		Tenoposide
		Thiotepa
		
		Topotecan

<10% Not emetogenic	Bleomycin Busulfan (non-BMT) Chlorambucil (oral) Cladribine Doxorubicin (liposomal) Estramustine Floxuridine Fludarabine Hydroxyurea	Interferon-α Melphalan (oral) Mercaptopurine (oral) Methotrexate < 50 mg/m^2 Pentostatin 6-Thioguanine (oral) Vinblastine Vincristine Vinorelbine

[a]Proportion of patients who experience emesis in the absence of effective antiemetic prophylaxis.

Table 24-6. Anti-emetic agents for chemotherapy-induced emesis

Drug	Class/Mechanism	Dose and Schedule	Toxicity
Ondansetron	Selective serotonin receptor antagonist	8–32 mg IV daily	Headache, constipation, diarrhea, dizziness, ECG changes
Granisetron	Selective serotonin receptor antagonist	4–8 mg PO every 8 hr	
Dolasetron	Selective serotonin receptor antagonist	1–2 mg IV daily 2 mg PO daily 100 mg IV or PO	
Metoclopramide	Other—dopamine antagonist	0.5–2 mg/kg IV every 3–4 hr for highly emetogenic agents. 20–40 mg PO every 4–6 hr for less emetogenic agents.	Diarrhea, headache, dystonia, akathisia, extrapyramidal effects, sedation, ECG changes
Haloperidol	Other—dopamine antagonist	1–3 mg IV or PO every 3–6 hr	Dystonia, akathisia, hypotension, sedation, extrapyramidal effects
Droperidol	Other—dopamine antagonist	0.5–2.0 mg IV every 4 hr	Dystonia, extrapyramidal effects, sedation, anticholinergic effects (dry mouth, dizziness, blurred vision, etc.)
Prochlorperazine	Phenothiazine—dopamine antagonist	10 mg PO or IV every 4–6 hr 25 mg PR every 6 hr	
Chlorpromazine	Phenothiazine—dopamine antagonist	25–50 mg PO every 4–6 hr	Hyperglycemia, euphoria, insomnia, psychosis, GI upset
Dexamethasone	Other—corticosteroid	10–20 mg IV daily	
Methylprednisolone	Other—corticosteroid	4 mg PO every 6–12 hours 250–500 mg IV daily	
Lorazepam	Other—benzodiazepine	1–2 mg IV/PO/SL every 4–8 hr	Sedation, amnesia, confusion
Diphenhydramine	Antihistamine/anticholinergic	25–50 mg IV or PO every 6 hr	Sedation, anticholinergic effects (dry mouth, dizziness, blurred vision, etc.)
Dronabinol	Other—cannabinoid	5–10 mg/m² PO every 4–6 hr	Drowsiness, dizziness, euphoria, dysphoria, hypotension, hallucinations

ECG, electrocardiogram; GI, gastrointestinal; IV, intravenously; PO, orally; PR, as needed; SL, sublingually.

or pretreatment with an anticholinergic such as benztropine or diphenhydramine. Standard phenothiazines are less effective but serve as useful adjuncts in the treatment of CIE. Corticosteroids, especially dexamethasone and methylprednisolone, act via a mechanism that is still unclear. In combination with other agents, corticosteroids dramatically improve antiemetic efficacy and may reduce the incidence of unwanted side effects by permitting dosage reduction. Corticosteroids are especially useful in treating/preventing-delayed emesis. Lorazepam, a benzodiazepine, is useful in the prevention of anticipatory emesis and may reduce the incidence of dystonic reactions to metoclopramide. Most important, combinations of these agents, specifically ondansetron, dexamethasone, lorazepam, and metoclopramide, increase antiemetic efficacy and reduce troublesome side effects through presumed synergistic activity.

Table 24-6 lists available and commonly used antiemetic agents with their dose ranges and the known major side effects.

RECOMMENDED READING

Abramowicz M, ed. Drugs of choice for cancer chemotherapy. *Med Lett Drugs Ther* 1993;35:43.

Burnham T, ed. *Drug facts and comparisons,* 55th ed. St. Louis, MO: Facts and Comparisons, Wolters Kluwer, 2001.

DeVita V, Hellman S, Rosenberg S, eds. *Cancer: principles and practice of oncology,* 6th ed. Philadelphia: Lippincott, 2001.

Krakoff I. Cancer chemotherapeutic and biologic agents. *CA Cancer J Clin* 1991;41:264.

McEvoy G, ed. *AHFS drug information.* Easton, MD: American Society of Hospital Pharmacists, 2001.

Pazdur R, ed. *Cancer management: a multidisciplinary approach,* 3rd ed. Melville, NY: PRR Inc., 1999.

Perry M, ed. *The chemotherapy source book,* 2nd ed. Baltimore: Williams & Wilkins, 1996.

Portenoy R. Cancer pain management. *Semin Oncol* 1993;20[suppl 1]:19.

Subject Index